Exploring Medical Language

A Student-Directed Approach, 7th Edition

Exploring Medical Language

A Student-Directed Approach, 7th Edition

understand.

be understood.

Myrna LaFleur Brooks, RN, BEd
Founding President
National Association of Health Unit Coordinators
Faculty Emeritus
Maricopa County Community College District
Phoenix, Arizona

Contributing Author
Danielle LaFleur Brooks, MEd, MATLA
Faculty
Goddard College
Plainfield, Vermont

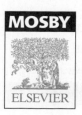

MOSBY
ELSEVIER

11830 Westline Industrial Drive
St. Louis, Missouri 63146

Vice President and Publisher: Andrew Allen
Publisher: Jeanne Wilke
Senior Developmental Editor: Linda Woodard
Publishing Services Manager: Julie Eddy
Project Manager: Andrea Campbell
Medical Illustrator: Jeanne Robertson

Printed in Canada

Last digit is the print number: 9 8 7 6 5 4 3 2

To Siena Grace, who has given me the cherished privilege
of being called "Grandma"

REVIEWERS

Gail Bicknell, HRT
Instructor (Retired)
School of Health and Public Safety
SAIT Polytechnic
Calgary, Alberta, Canada

Joyce K. Bohnert, RN
Stone Center
St. Joseph's Hospital
Phoenix, Arizona

William W. Bohnert, MD, FASC
Urology Associates, Ltd.
Scottsdale, Arizona

Richard K. Brooks, MD, FACP, FACG
Phoenix, Arizona

Chris Costa, HUC
Rise Services, Inc.
Phoenix, Arizona

Anne P. Curtis, RN, BSN
Red Cross Instructor
Health Sciences & Technology Instructor
Southwest Technology College
Cedar City, Utah

Laura E. Davis, MMd, BS, NCCPA
Otolaryngology, Head and Neck Surgery
Mayo Clinic
Scottsdale, Arizona

Patricia Faur, MAed, BA
Phoenix, Arizona

Pamela Fleming, RW, MPA, CMA, CPC
Professor
Quinsigamond Community College
Worcester, Massachusetts

Robert Lloyd Fortune, MD, FACS, FRCS(C)
Scottsdale, Arizona

Sharyn D. Gibson, EdD, RT(R)
Department Head and Professor
Radiologic Sciences
Armstrong Atlantic State University
Savannah, Georgia

Rose K. Goedenm, RHIA
Instructor
HIM Program
Dakota State University
Madison, South Dakota

Sheryl E. Goss, MS, RT(R), RDMS, RDCS, RVT
Program Director/Assistant Professor
Sonography
College Misericordia
Dallas, Pennsylvania

Karen R. Hardney, RT(T), MSEd
Assistant Professor
Chicago State University
Chicago, Illinois

Katherine Hawkins, BS
Program Chair
Medical Assisting Program
Ivy Tech Community College
Columbus, Indiana

Meg Holloway, MS, RN, ARNP
Breast Center
Shawnee Mission Medical Center
Shawnee Mission, Kansas

John Lampignano, MEd, RT(R)
Center for Teaching and Learning
GateWay Community College
Phoenix, Arizona

Deborah Lowry, CNM, MS
Planned Parenthood
Santa Barbara, California

Judy B. Merrick, NBCT 2001, Med
Instructor
West Florence High School
Florence, South Carolina

M. Caroline Owen, BA, MS
Professor
Our Lady of the Lake College
Baton Rouge, LA

Maria M. Pappas, PT
Associate Professor, Academic Coordinator of Clinical
   Education
MassBay Community College: Health Human Services
   and Education Institute
Framingham, Massachusetts

Janine Plavac, RN, BSN
Co-Director
Institute of Health Professions
Gainesville High School
Gainesville, Florida

Leslie A. Reed, MA, NCC
Director of Allied Health Certificate Programs
Mercyhurst College
North East, Pennsylvania

Helen Reid, RN, MSN, EdD
Dean of Health Occupations
Trinity Valley Community College
Kaufman, Texas

Toni Rodriguez, EdD, RRT
Respiratory Care Program
GateWay Community College
Phoenix, Arizona

Susan K. Shear, MHA, CPC
Assistant Professor
Bluegrass Community and Technical College
Danville, Kentucky

Stanley Shorb, MD
Affiliated Eye Specialists
Phoenix, Arizona

John D. Smith, PhD, HFI
Assistant Professor
Southern Illinois University–Edwardsville
Edwardsville, Illinois

CONTRIBUTORS

Carolyn Ehrlich, MSN Psy, NP
Private Practice, Psychiatry
Phoenix, Arizona
Appendix F–Behavioral Health Terms (Evolve website)

Kelly Eiden, MS, LD, CDS
Interim Dean, Division of Allied Health
Chair of Dietetics
Barnes Jewish College
St. Louis, Missouri
Appendix J–Nutritional Terms (Evolve website)

Erinn Kao, PharmD
GE Medical
St. Louis, Missouri
Appendix E–Pharmacology Terms

Catherine J. Cerulli, MEd
Director
Interwoven Healing Arts
Montpelier, Vermont
*Appendix G–Complementary and Alternative Medicine
    Therapies (Evolve website) and CAM boxes*

Sharon Tomkins Luzcu, RN, MA, MBA
Director
Health Services Management Program
GateWay Community College
Phoenix, Arizona
*Appendix F–Health Care Delivery/Managed Care Terms
    (Evolve website)*

Linda A. Mottle, MSN-HAS, RN
Program Director
Clinical Research Program
GateWay Community College
Phoenix, Arizona
Appendix I–Clinical Research Terms (Evolve website)

Welcome to the seventh edition of *Exploring Medical Language*. Medical terminology, like any living language, is not static. It has become the common currency of not only those in medical professions but also insurers, lawyers, equipment suppliers, pharmaceutical representatives, and others who interact with health care providers and consumers, all of whom need to both understand medical language and be understood. To keep apace of medical science and to communicate medical knowledge effectively, medical language must expand and change. The goal of this seventh edition is to reflect those changes with a presentation that is up to date, sound in its approach to language instruction, and visually supports the learning process.

NEW TO THIS EDITION

Along with the bold new look of the seventh edition, some outstanding features have been added to allow you to learn the language of medicine in an interactive and rewarding way. Many new medical documents have been inserted to bring medical terms from the classroom to the clinical setting. The student CD has been integrated with the text to enhance the learning system that has proven so valuable in past editions. Besides adding new material and deleting terms no longer in common use, many new illustrations, tables, images, and icons have been added to augment learning.

New to the Edition Are:

Two-page chapter openers use the Outline and Objectives to invite you into the chapter by informing you of the journey ahead.

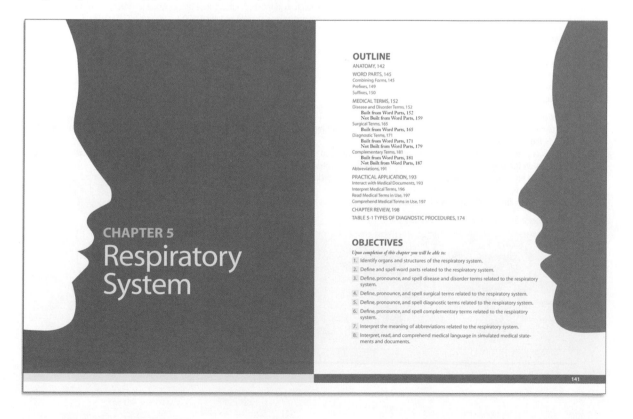

New illustrations give visual meaning to anatomic structure, disease processes, and procedures.

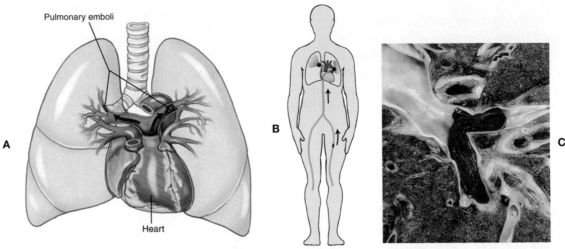

Figure 5-7

A, Bilateral pulmonary emboli. **B,** Pulmonary emboli usually originate in the deep veins of the lower extremities. **C,** Necropsy specimen of the lung showing a large embolus.

New tables collect collaborative information scattered throughout a chapter into one document to help you recognize the relationships of terms to one another.

TABLE 7-1

Prostate Cancer

Prostate cancer is the most commonly diagnosed cancer in men and the second most common cause of cancer death among men in the United States. Approximately 95% of all cancers of the prostate are adenocarcinomas arising from epithelial cells.

Diagnostic Procedures
1. Digital rectal examination (DRE)
2. Prostate-specific antigen (PSA)
3. Transrectal ultrasound
4. Transrectal ultrasonically guided biopsy
5. Magnetic resonance imaging with endorectal surface coil

Treatment
Treatment depends on the stage of the prostate cancer, the age of the patient, and choices of treatment by the patient and his physician. Options include the following:
1. **Radical prostatectomy (RP),** which may be performed by retropubic or perineal routes, laparoscopically, or with the use of robotic-assisted devices
2. **Radiation therapy,** which may be performed with an external beam or with radioactive seeds (brachytherapy)
3. **Bilateral orchidectomy** or **hormonal therapy** to reduce the production of testosterone, which fuels the growth of prostate cancer
4. **Chemotherapy,** treating cancer with drugs
5. **Watchful waiting,** with the intent to pursue active therapy on disease progression

Progression of Prostate Cancer

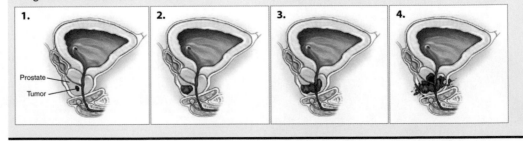

An **immunology section** added to Chapter 10 presents up-to-date immunology terms and information.

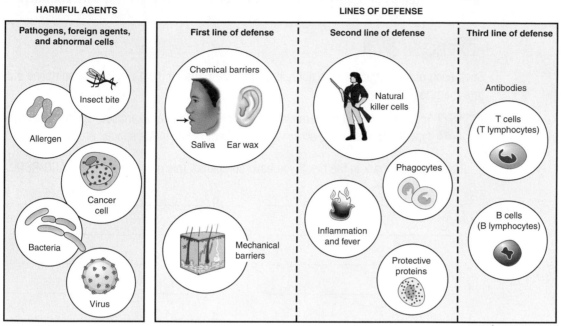

Figure 10-6
Three lines of defense provided by the immune system to protect the body against pathogens, foreign agents, and cancer.

Pronunciation exercises on the CD will assist you with one of the most difficult aspects of learning a new language—how to pronounce terms correctly. Easy directions guide you from the textbook to the CD, where you will hear each term pronounced. Terms can be heard as often as necessary to enable you to become proficient in speaking medical language.

EXERCISE 10

Practice saying aloud each of the disease and disorder terms built from word parts on p. 98.

 To hear the terms select Chapter 4, Chapter Exercises, Pronunciation.

☐ Place a check mark in the box when you have completed this exercise.

Spelling exercises on the CD will assist you in spelling medical terms with confidence. Easy directions guide you from the textbook to the CD, where you can listen to the terms from each word list to be spelled. You can listen to and spell the terms as often as necessary to become proficient in writing them with confidence.

EXERCISE 26

Spell each of the surgical terms not built from word parts on p. 113 by having someone dictate them to you.

 To hear and spell the terms select Chapter 4, Chapter Exercises, Spelling. You may type the terms on the screen or write them below in the spaces provided.

☐ Place a check mark in the box if you have compelted this exercise using your CD-ROM.

1. _____   6. _____

2. _____   7. _____

3. _____   8. _____

4. _____   9. _____

5. _____   10. _____

New icons and boxes help you understand and navigate the material in each chapter.

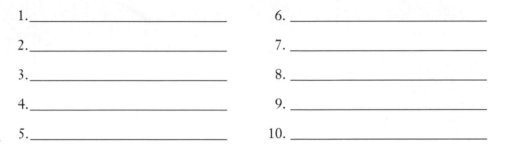

INCIDENTALOMA
refers to a mass lesion involving an organ that is discovered unexpectedly by the use of ultrasound, computed tomography scan, or magnetic resonance imaging and has nothing to do with the patient's symptoms or primary diagnosis.

PROGNOSIS
was used by Hippocrates to mean the same then as now: **to foretell the course of a disease.**

WEB LINK
For additional information on cancer visit the National Cancer Institute at www.nic.nih.gov

A **Practical Application** section featuring more than 60 medical documents (medical records, case studies, health care reports) designed to assist you with interacting, interpreting, reading, and comprehending medical language as it is used in health care settings.

PRACTICAL APPLICATION

EXERCISE 37   *Interact with Medical Documents*

B. Read the pathology report and answer the questions following it.

49785 LIGHT, Darla B.   _ □ ×

File Patient Navigate Custom Fields Help

| Patient Chart | Lab | Rad | Notes | Documents | Rx | Scheduling | Images | Billing |

Name: **LIGHT, Darla B.**   MR#: **49785**   Sex: **F**
                             DOB: **6/15/19XX**

PATHOLOGY REPORT

DATE/TIME COLL: Jun 12 20XX 12:00 AM
DATE RECEIVED: Jun 12 20XX 8:00 PM
DATE REPORTED: Jun 22 20XX
REPORT STATUS: FINAL REPORT

HISTORY: Previous incidence of melanoma and basal cell carcinoma, no metastases

PRE-OP: Melanoma vs. compound nevi

PROCEDURE: Tissue biopsy

SPECIMEN: Skin biopsy, anterior, proximal right arm

GROSS DESCRIPTION: One container is received. Specimen in formalin labeled with the patient's name is a shave biopsy of gray-white hair bearing skin measuring 0.4 x 0.3 cm in surface dimension and averaging 0.1 cm in thickness. The epidermal surface contains a symmetric, smooth bordered, pigmented lesion measuring 0.3 cm in greatest diameter. The specimen is bisected and totally submitted.

MICROSCOPIC EXAMINATION: A microscopic examination has been performed.

DIAGNOSIS: Lesion, anterior, proximal right arm: benign compound nevus.

Electronically signed by: J. Alvarez, MD, Pathologist, 6/22/20XX 10:48 AM

| Start | Log On/Off | Print | Edit |

---

1. Identify singular and plural forms of medical terms used in the pathology report. Write "p" for plural and "s" for singular next to the terms. Refer to Table 2-2 for plural endings.
   a. melanoma _____
   b. melanomata _____
   c. nevi _____
   d. nevus _____
   e. metastasis _____
   f. metastases _____
   g. biopsy _____
   h. biopsies _____

2. The skin biopsy was obtained from:
   a. near the shoulder on the back of the right arm
   b. near the shoulder on the front of the right arm
   c. near the wrist on the back of the right arm
   d. near the wrist on the front of the right arm

3. Use your medical dictionary to find the meanings of the following terms used in the pathology report:
   a. compound _____
   b. pigmented _____
   c. bisected _____
   d. microscopic _____

The **Read Medical Terms in Use** exercise featured on the CD as well as in the text allows you to hear the terms pronounced while reading a medical document.

EXERCISE **39**   *Read Medical Terms in Use*

Practice pronunciation of terms by reading aloud the following medical document. Use the pronunciation key following the medical term to assist you in saying the word.

 To hear these terms select Chapter 4, Chapter Exercises, Read Medical Terms in Use.

Emily visited the **dermatology** (*der*-ma-TOL-o-jē) clinic because of **pruritus** (prū-RĪ-tus) secondary to **dermatitis** (*der*-ma-TĪ-tis) involving her scalp, arms, and legs. A diagnosis of **psoriasis** (so-RĪ-a-sis) was made. **Eczema** (EK-ze-ma), **scabies** (SKĀ-bēz), and **tinea** (TIN-ē-a) were considered in the differential diagnosis. An **emollient** (e-MOL-yent) cream was prescribed. In addition the patient showed the **dermatologist** (der-ma-TOL-o-jist) the tender, discolored, thickened nail of her right great toe. Emily learned she had **onychomycosis** (*on*-i-kō-mī-KŌ-sis), for which she was given an additional prescription for an oral antifungal drug.

Chapter Review on CD-ROM clearly summarizes how to use the CD to play and practice, and to assess what you have learned upon completion of each chapter.

CHAPTER REVIEW

CHAPTER REVIEW ON CD-ROM

Use the CD-ROM that accompanies this textbook to play and practice what you have learned in this chapter. The Chapter Exercises, Practice Activities, Animations, and Games allow you to hear, see, and interact with the chapter content.

Chapter Exercises

Exercises in this section of your CD-ROM correlate to exercises in your textbook. You may have completed them as you worked through the chapter.
- ☐ Pronunciation
- ☐ Spelling
- ☐ Read Medical Terms in Use

Practice Activities

Practice in study mode, then test your learning in assessment mode. Keep track of your scores from assessment mode if you wish.

SCORE
- ☐ Picture It   _____
- ☐ Define Word Parts   _____
- ☐ Build Medical Terms _____
- ☐ Word Shop   _____
- ☐ Define Medical Terms _____
- ☐ Use It   _____
- ☐ Hear It and Type It: _____
  Clinical Vignettes

Animations
- ☐ Atelectasis
- ☐ Asthma
- ☐ Pneumothorax

Games
- ☐ Name that Word Part
- ☐ Term Storm
- ☐ Term Explorer
- ☐ Termbusters
- ☐ Medical Millionaire

Answers appear at the end of each chapter for quick confirmation upon completion of exercises.

ANSWERS

Exercise Figures

Exercise Figure
A. 1. sinus: sinus/o
    2. nose: nas/o, rhin/o
    3. tonsils: tonsill/o
    4. epiglottis: epiglott/o
    5. larynx: laryng/o
    6. trachea: trache/o
    7. pleura: pleur/o
    8. lobe: lob/o
    9. diaphragm: diaphragmat/o, phren/o
   10. adenoids: adenoid/o
   11. pharynx: pharyng/o
   12. lung: pneum/o, pneumat/o, pneumon/o, pulmon/o
   13. bronchus: bronch/o, bronchi/o
   14. alveolus: alveol/o

Exercise Figure
B. bronchi/ectasis

Exercise Figure
C. A. pneum/o/thorax,
    B. hem/o/thorax

Exercise Figure
D. adenoid/ectomy, aden/o/tome

Exercise Figure
E. thorac/o/centesis

Exercise Figure
F. bronch/o/scopy

Exercise Figure
G. endo/trache/al, laryng/o/scope

Exercise 1
1. h
2. a
3. g
4. c
5. f
6. d
7. e
8. b

Exercise 2
1. nasal septum
2. epiglottis
3. bronchioles
4. nose
5. diaphragm
6. mediastinum
7. tonsils

Exercise 3
1. larynx
2. bronchus
3. pleura
4. air, lung
5. tonsil
6. lung
7. diaphragm
8. trachea
9. alveolus
10. air, lung
11. thorax (chest)
12. adenoids
13. pharynx
14. nose
15. sinus
16. lobe
17. epiglottis
18. lung, air
19. nose
20. septum
21. diaphragm

Exercise 4
1. a. nas/o
   b. rhin/o
2. laryng/o
3. a. pneum/o
   b. pneumat/o
   c. pneumon/o
4. pulmon/o
5. tonsill/o
6. trache/o
7. adenoid/o
8. pleur/o
9. a. diaphragmat/o
   b. phren/o
10. sinus/o
11. thorac/o
12. alveol/o
13. pharyng/o
14. a. bronchi/o
    b. bronch/i
15. lob/o
16. epiglott/o
17. sept/o

Exercise 5
1. oxygen
2. breathe, breathing
3. mucus
4. imperfect, incomplete
5. straight
6. pus
7. blood
8. sleep

9. carbon dioxide
10. sound, voice

Exercise 6
1. spir/o
2. a. ox/o
   b. ox/i
3. atel/o
4. orth/o
5. py/o
6. muc/o
7. a. hem/o
   b. hemat/o
8. somn/o
9. phon/o
10. capn/o

Exercise 7
1. within
2. without, absence of
3. all, total
4. normal, good
5. many, much
6. fast, rapid

Exercise 8
1. endo-
2. eu-
3. a. a-
   b. an-
4. pan-
5. poly-
6. tachy-

Exercise 9
1. k
2. f
3. g
4. c
5. b
6. j
7. a
8. h
9. d
10. e

Exercise 10
1. c
2. e
3. a
4. h
5. b
6. i
7. f
8. d
9. g
10. j

BUILDING YOUR MEDICAL VOCABULARY

Exploring Medical Language prepares you to understand and be understood in ensuring your mastery of the language of medicine. This is accomplished by categorizing related terms into easily learned units and by introducing you to the structure of medical language. In this way, you will be equipped to understand the terms included in this text, as well as the new and unfamiliar terms you may encounter in a clinical setting.

Many medical terms are constructed from language elements known as *word parts*. The word parts, each with its own definition, combine to form specific medical terms. Retaining a proven aid to learning, this edition of *Exploring Medical Language* distinguishes medical terms that can be translated literally (or built) from word parts and provides a variety of exercises to help you learn the word parts and their meanings. Because the language of medicine is incomplete without them, terms not built from word parts are included in separate sections with their own exercises. These sections, if not part of your course of study, can be omitted easily.

Organization

Introductory Chapters

Chapters 1 through 3 provide a foundation for building medical vocabulary. Chapter 1 introduces the word part method of learning medical terminology and explains how prefixes, word roots, combining vowels, and suffixes are used to form terms. Chapter 2 establishes a base for the body system chapters that follow by providing information about body structure and by helping you build the terms related to color and oncology that apply to all body systems. Chapter 3 covers directional terms, anatomic planes, and regions and quadrants. All chapters are enhanced with many four-color illustrations, providing clarification of terms and procedures. Chapters 2 and 3 end with a practical application section, offering you additional opportunities to both evaluate your knowledge and apply what you have learned.

Body System Chapters

Chapters 4 through 16 present medical terms organized by body system. Each of these chapters opens by introducing the relevant anatomy. This section may either acquaint you with body structure and function or, if you have studied anatomy in a separate course, can serve as a review.

Body system word parts precede the medical terms. The medical term section is divided into four categories: **disease and disorder terms, surgical terms, diagnostic terms,** and **complementary terms.** Each category of terms is further divided into terms **built from word parts** and those **not built from word parts.** Considerable attention has been given in this edition to updating these terms, ensuring that they reflect current usage, including the newest techniques and procedures. Abbreviations and plurals are included. Boxed information throughout the chapters amplifies definitions, describes the derivation of specific terms, and gives historical information and references to websites. Exercises follow each group of terms, giving you the opportunity to review and rehearse new vocabulary immediately after it is presented. Each chapter ends with a practical application section, offering you an additional opportunity to evaluate your knowledge and apply what you have learned.

Spelling and pronunciation exercises on the Student CD are threaded throughout the chapter. In addition, practice activities, animations, and games on the Student CD are listed in the Chapter Review at the end of each chapter to help you become even more comfortable with reading, writing, and speaking medical terms.

Appendixes

Helpful appendixes supplement the information provided in the chapters. Appendixes A and B list, in alphabetical order, all the combining forms, prefixes, and suffixes from the entire book by word part and definition. Appendix C lists less commonly used word parts not presented in the chapters. Appendix D provides abbreviations to medical terms. Appendix E lists common pharmacology terms. The terms are listed by chapter and can be accessed easily as an extension to the terms included in each chapter.

Appendixes F through J present medical terms that are not related to a particular body system but are used frequently in the day-to-day health care environment. These terms that have a more general application fall into the categories of health care delivery/managed care, complementary and alternative medicine, behavioral health, clinical research, and nutrition. Appendixes F through J can be accessed on the Evolve website at *http://evolve.elsevier.com/LaFleur*.

Learning Aids

The seventh edition of *Exploring Medical Language* comes with a variety of learning aids intended to make your study of medical terminology as efficient and enjoyable as possible.

STUDENT CD

Your copy of *Exploring Medical Language* includes a complementary student CD, which features interactive exercises, activities, animations, and games designed to augment your learning and deepen your understanding of chapter content. With the CD, you can practice while you play. It also provides an "assessment-mode" for some of the activities so you can test yourself, assessing your learning and readiness for chapter exams. There are four parts to the CD:

1. Chapter Exercises

This portion of the CD correlates directly with exercises in your textbook chapters. As you work through the content of each chapter in the text, you will be invited to access "Pronunciation," "Spelling," and "Read Medical Terms in Use" exercises. The following CD chapter exercises were designed to give you an option to hear and see medical terms as you are learning them in the textbook:

- **Pronunciation**—Click and hear medical terms pronounced. Every medical term appears by term list as it is presented in the chapter.
- **Spelling**—Click, hear, and spell medical terms. Terms may be typed as you use the CD and/or you may write them in the spaces provided within the textbook chapter. The Spelling Chapter Exercises on the CD give you the opportunity to practice spelling of all terms presented in the textbook and gives you immediate feedback, alerting you to what you may still need help with.
- **Read Medical Terms in Use**—Click, hear pronunciation, and read the definitions of medical terms used in context. The Read Medical Terms in Use exercise on the CD will help you prepare for completing the activity in class.

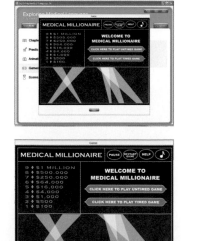

2. Practice Activities

Reinforce your learning of word parts and medical terms presented by engaging with additional activities beyond those in the textbook chapter. The Practice Activities portion of the CD features dual modes, allowing you to study and then assess your learning. In Study Mode, hints and access to the glossary are available, as are multiple tries for the correct answer and immediate feedback about the correctness of your answers. Assessment Mode provides an examlike setting, with scores reflecting the percentage of correct answers. Scores may be printed for your records. The Practice Activities on the CD are:

- **Picture It**—Label diagrams with combining forms related to anatomy
- **Define Word Parts**—Match word parts and combining forms with their definitions
- **Analyze Medical Terms**—Identify and label word parts and combining forms in medical terms built from word parts (Chapters 1-3 only)
- **Build Medical Terms**—Complete medical terms by typing missing word parts
- **Word Shop**—Build new medical terms using word parts and combining forms you have learned
- **Define Medical Terms**—Match medical terms not built from word parts with their definitions
- **Use It**—Complete a sentence by typing in the correct medical term
- **Hear It & Type It: Clinical Vignettes**—Click, hear pronunciation, and type the correct medical term used in context

3. Animations

View animations associated with the body system feature in the chapter. Animations detail anatomy, disease processes, and procedures.

4. Games

Play while you practice what you have learned in the textbook chapter. The following games have been designed to enhance your learning of word parts, terms built from word parts, terms not built from word parts, abbreviations, and the clinical use of the terms:

- **Name That Word Part**—See how many word parts and combining forms you can identify in 90 seconds. You may see your score increase with practice!
- **Term Storm**—It's raining word parts and combining forms. How many terms can you build in a round of this game? Click and drag to build whole terms.
- **Term Explorer**—Retrieve lost medallions of terminology from an ancient and mysterious cave. Solve word riddles by guessing letters and discovering the correct medical term not built from word parts.
- **Termbusters**—Identify the correct medical term from a look- and soundalike list to claim a hexagon on the game board. Win a round by creating an uninterrupted string of five hexagons. Can you win all three timed rounds?
- **Medical Millionaire**—Show that you are rich in medical terminology knowledge by answering questions of increasing difficulty.

FLASH CARDS

More than 480 flash cards come with *Exploring Medical Language*. Each flash card has a word part, combining form, suffix, or prefix on one side and the definition of the word part and chapter where it can be found on the opposite side.

MOSBY'S MEDICAL TERMINOLOGY ONLINE

Mosby's Medical Terminology Online to accompany *Exploring Medical Language* is a great resource to supplement your textbook. This web-delivered course supplement provides a range of visual, auditory, and interactive elements to reinforce your learning and synthesize concepts presented in the text. Objective-based quizzes at the end of each section and an end-of-module exam provide you with self-testing tools. In addition, related Internet resources may be accessed by links provided throughout the program. This online course supplement may be accessed if you have purchased the PIN code packaged with your book. If you did not purchase the PIN code, ask your instructor for information or visit *http://evolve.elsevier.com/LaFleur* to purchase it.

AUDIO CDS WITH PRONUNCIATIONS AND DEFINITIONS

The audio CDs that accompany *Exploring Medical Language* include pronunciations and definitions. Because the CDs include definitions, they are an additional tool for learning and reviewing terms. The CDs are especially helpful when using your book is impractical, such as when you are driving in a car, walking, or doing daily chores. You may purchase the audio CDs separately or packaged with the book for a small additional cost. This audio product is available for the Apple iPod® and is called *iTerms for Exploring Medical Language, ed 7*.

EVOLVE STUDENT RESOURCES

Visit the LaFleur companion website (*http://evolve.elsevier.com/LaFleur*) to access additional learning activities, including crosswords, electronic flashcards, a 5,000-term English/Spanish glossary, and more.

TO THE INSTRUCTOR

TEACH

Available in print, on CD, or on Evolve, TEACH Instructor Resources for *Exploring Medical Language* links all parts of the educational package by providing you with customizable lesson plans and lecture outlines based on learning objectives.

Each lesson plan features:
- A 3-column format that correlates chapter objective with content and teaching resources
- Lesson preparation checklists that make planning your class quick and easy
- Critical thinking questions to focus and motivate students
- Teaching resources that cross reference all of TEACH and Elsevier's curriculum solution
- Pretests and handouts that can be used in class or as homework

Each lecture online features:
- PowerPoint slides that present a compelling visual summary of the chapter's main points
- Practical, concise talking points that complement the slides
- Clicker questions to stimulate classroom discussions
- Unique ideas for moving beyond traditional lectures and getting students involved

For more information on the benefits of TEACH, visit online at *http://TEACH.elsevier.com* or call Faculty Support at 1-800-222-9570.

Mosby's Medical Terminology Online

Designed to work with *Exploring Medical Language*, this multidimensional online course supplement enhances students' understanding of the subject through an exciting range of visual, auditory, and interactive elements that amplify text content, synthesize concepts, and demonstrate the practical applications of health care terminology. Interactive tools reinforce learning by providing a variety of student and instructor communications options, interactive exercises, illustrations, animations and slide shows with audio narration, and instructor administrative tools. Students log on, complete lessons, and take quizzes and exams; the program records their results. You can tailor the program's content to the specific needs of your course, resulting in greater learning opportunities and flexibility. Included in this edition are:
- More word-building and pronunciation exercises
- Listen In activities in the threaded case studies
- English/Spanish glossary with more than 5,000 audio pronunciations and definitions
- Case studies and medical reports
- Quizzes and exams mapped to objectives

Contact your sales rep or visit *http://evolve.elsevier.com/LaFleur* for more information.

Evolve for Instructors

Evolve is an interactive learning environment that works in coordination with the textbook, providing Internet-based course management tools and content that reinforces and expands on the concepts you deliver in class. Evolve provides you with:
- Areas to post course syllabi outlines and lecture notes
- TEACH Instructor Resources for *Exploring Medical Language*
- ExamView test bank
- Image collection from the textbook
- PowerPoint lecture slides
- Discussion boards
- Calendar
- Electronic flash cards
- Spanish/English glossary
- Body Spectrum—an interactive coloring book
- Additional games and activities for students
- Web Links

Visit *http://evolve.elsevier.com/LaFleur* for more information.

To the newcomer, the language of medicine is like a vast, uncharted frontier. *Exploring Medical Language* guides you systematically along a path of vocabulary development that is interesting and enjoyable and that thoroughly prepares you to understand and be understood as a medical professional. While using this text, you will become familiar with the structure of medical language and the most effective strategies for learning medical terms. A variety of learning activities will allow you the practice to grow confident in your use of the terminology. Follow the guidelines below to get the most from this textbook as you embark on your journey of acquiring a new language.

Understand the Content of Chapter 1 Before Moving on to Chapter 2.

Chapter 1 is the most important chapter in the text. Here you are introduced to word parts—word roots, prefixes, suffixes, and combining vowels—and the rules for combining them to build medical terms. You will use this information in each of the subsequent chapters to analyze, construct, define, and spell terms built from word parts.

Use Each Chapter Section Fully to Help You Master the Medical Terms Presented

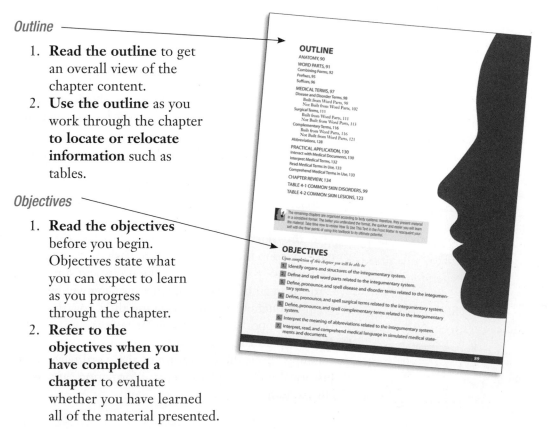

Outline

1. **Read the outline** to get an overall view of the chapter content.
2. **Use the outline** as you work through the chapter **to locate or relocate information** such as tables.

Objectives

1. **Read the objectives** before you begin. Objectives state what you can expect to learn as you progress through the chapter.
2. **Refer to the objectives when you have completed a chapter** to evaluate whether you have learned all of the material presented.

Anatomy

1. **Read the content,** using the illustrations to clarify the structure, location, and relationship of parts of the anatomy.
2. **Complete the exercises.**
3. **Check your answers** with the answer section, located at the end of each chapter. If you have studied anatomy previously, you can omit this section or use it as a review.

Word Parts

1. **Read each word part and its definition.**
2. **Complete the exercises.** Each list of words is followed by exercises that help you recall the definition of the word part and retrieve the word part when the definition is provided.
3. **Label the anatomic diagram** with the correct combining forms.
4. **Compare your answers** on both the diagram and the exercises with the answer section, located at the end of each chapter.
5. **Use the flash cards to help memorize the word parts.** Group the combining form flash cards separately for each body system. Gather the prefix and suffix flash cards from all of the chapters because you will be using them throughout the text; keeping them together provides the opportunity for frequent review.
6. **Read the information boxes** to enrich your understanding about the derivation of the word parts, their historical and complementary information, and website locations.

Medical Terms

1. **Become familiar with the presentation of terms.** The medical terms are presented in word lists and divided into four categories: *disease and disorder* terms, which are used to diagnose conditions; *surgical* terms, which are used to describe surgical procedures; *diagnostic* terms, which are used to describe diagnostic procedures and equipment; and *complementary* terms, which complete the vocabulary presented in a chapter by describing signs, symptoms, medical specialties, specialists, and related words. Understanding that the terms are categorized will assist you in the overall comprehension of medical language and how it is used. For example, you will soon learn that the suffix indicates whether a term is surgical, diagnostic, or procedural.

2. **Become familiar with the organization of terms** into those **built from word parts** and those **not built from word parts**. All of the medical terms in the text are arranged into one of these two categories that determine the learning strategy you will use. Terms built from word parts are constructed from specific language elements through application of certain rules. Learning the rules for analyzing and combining word parts will help you to master this set of terms. Terms not built from word parts may contain some of the word parts you know, but you cannot translate the term literally to arrive at its meaning; memorization is used to learn these terms.

3. **Read each of the terms and its definition.** If more information is necessary for comprehension of the term, it is included in parentheses after the definition.

4. **Pronounce each of the terms.** Use the pronunciation guide and listen to the terms pronounced on the Student CD to practice pronouncing the medical terms yourself.

5. **Complete all the exercises for each word list.** The exercises may seem repetitive, but they are provided to allow the practice needed to master the terms. Check your answers with the answers located at the end of each chapter.

6. **Spell each of the terms.** Hear the terms spoken and type them on the Student CD, or write the terms in the space provided in the text. Check your spelling by comparing the terms with those recorded in the word lists.

7. **Read the information boxes;** they contain information on the origin of terms, the distinguishing features and amplification of the words, complementary and alternative medicine terms, and references to websites.

8. **Use the appendixes** to assist you in building and defining terms built from word parts. Use Appendix A for a quick-reference, alphabetical listing of the meanings of word parts; use Appendix B to find the word part to match a definition.

9. **Label the diagrams** placed throughout this section by filling in the blanks with the correct word part. Check your answers against the Answers located at the end of each chapter.

10. **Read the abbreviation list** and complete the exercises.

Practical Application

1. **Complete the practical application exercises.** Use this as an opportunity to evaluate your comprehension of the content of the chapter and apply what you have learned by interacting with medical documents and clinical situations. Some questions will require you to recall terms from previous chapters.

2. **Compare your answers** with the answers located at the end of the chapter.

Chapter Review

1. **Use the CD for more practice if desired.** Complete Practice Activities in either study or assessment mode, watch animations, or play any of the five games included on the CD.

2. **Review the lists of word parts and medical terms** presented in the chapter. Highlight terms that need more practice.

3. **Use the Pronounce It activity on the CD** with the review list to evaluate and practice your pronunciation.

Appendixes

Use the appendixes to quickly locate alphabetically listed word parts, definitions, abbreviations, and pharmacology terms.

From the Author

After you've worked through a chapter, completing all of the exercises and correcting errors, you will have met the chapter objectives and will feel confident and eager to move on to the next chapter. I wish you the best as you begin your discovery of the language of medicine.

I welcome your comments. You may contact me at mbrooks6@cox.net.

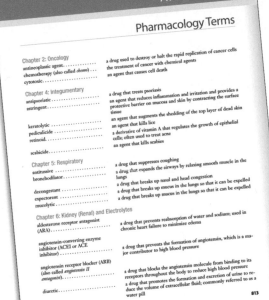

ACKNOWLEDGMENTS

I am grateful to many who assisted in the preparation of the seventh edition of *Exploring Medical Language*. They shared their knowledge, their imagination, and their precious time. With their help, I believe it is the most comprehensive edition yet.

I want to recognize three people who contributed so much to this work:

Danielle LaFleur Brooks, MEd, MATLA, my daughter, who came on board as contributing author, for breathing new life into the textbook and student CD, for revising several chapters and reviewing and advising on all others, for her extensive work on developing new games and clinical vignettes for the student CD, and for integrating the CD with the textbook.

Richard K. Brooks, MD, FACP, FACG, my husband, for reviewing and advising on all the chapters and medical documents, and for advising on the most recent developments in the medical field.

Chris Costa, for creating content and source documents for the Student CD, as well as dedicating time, energy, and expertise in reviewing all materials for consistency and correctness. It was a pleasure to collaborate and create with you, and I cherish the memories of the time we shared in bringing this edition to fruition.

I would also like to express my appreciation to **John Lampignano,** MEd, RT(R), for advising on the diagnostic imaging information in Chapters 2-16; **Toni Rodriguez,** EdD, RRT, for advising on *Chapter 5, Respiratory System;* **William W. Bohnert,** MD, FASC, and **Joyce K. Bohnert,** RN, for advising on *Chapter 6, Urinary System, and Chapter 7, Male Reproductive System;* **Meg Holloway,** MS, ARNP, for advising on *Chapter 8, Female Reproductive System;* **Deborah Lowry,** CNM, MS, for advising on *Chapter 9, Obstetrics and Neonatology;* **Robert Lloyd Fortune,** MD, FACS, FRCS(C), for advising on *Chapter 10, Cardiovascular, Lymphatic and Immune Systems and Blood;* **Stanley Shorb,** MD, for advising on *Chapter 12, Eye;* and **Laura E. Davis,** MMd, BS, NCCPA, for advising on *Chapter 13, Ear.* The information you shared helped us capture the current medical climate in the written and spoken word.

Thanks to **Linda A. Mottle,** MSN-HAS, RN, for updating *Appendix I, Clinical Research Terms;* **Catherine J. Cerulli,** MEd, for revising *Appendix G, Complementary and Alternative Medicine Therapies,* and for writing the chapter CAM term boxes; **Kelly Eiden,** MS, LD, CSD, for updating *Appendix J, Nutritional Terms;* **Carolyn Ehrlich,** MSN, Psy, NP, for updating *Appendix F, Behavioral Health Terms;* **Sharon Tomkins Luczu,** RN, MA, MBA, for updating *Appendix F, Health Care Delivery/Managed Care Terms;* and **Erinn Kao,** PharmD, for updating *Appendix E, Pharmacology Terms.* With your expert contributions, I feel confident that these specialty areas are accurate and complete.

I am indebted to **Gail Bicknell, Pat Faur, Meg Holloway,** and **Chris Costa** for their many hours spent reviewing the words and images, assuring accuracy on the printed pages. I'm grateful to Carolyn Kruse, who worked on updating pronunciation, both in print and audio.

Thanks to the Elsevier/Mosby staff: Jeanne Wilke for her continued ability to determine the needs of the user and thus providing us with the necessary resources to meet those needs; Linda Woodard, Senior Developmental Editor, who was always there for us and worked tirelessly to meet the demands of manuscript and ancillary preparation; Julie Eddy, Publishing Services Manager; and Andrea Campbell, Project Manager, for the time and effort in bringing our vision so clearly to the pages. I feel privileged to be associated with these dedicated, talented professionals.

It has been 25 years since I first put pen to paper to begin writing the script for a medial terminology textbook not yet titled. My coauthor was Winifred K. Starr (1921–1993). I would like to recognize her contribution in creating a sound system for learning medical language that has remained popular to this day. Her contributions to the earlier editions of the text continue to enrich the seventh edition.

Finally, I would like to acknowledge and thank the faculty who have adopted the text to use in their classrooms and online and to those who took their time to give us feedback I am forever grateful. And perhaps closest to my heart, I want to recognize the students, who over the years have worn thin the pages of previous editions to acquire their own language of medicine.

CONTENTS

PART I   **Introduction to Word Parts and Human Body Structure**

    1   Introduction to Word Parts, *2*
    2   Body Structure, Color, and Oncology, *18*
    3   Directional Terms, Anatomic Planes, Regions, and Quadrants, *62*

PART II   **Body Systems**

    4   Integumentary System, *88*
    5   Respiratory System, *140*
    6   Urinary System, *206*
    7   Male Reproductive System, *258*
    8   Female Reproductive System, *296*
    9   Obstetrics and Neonatology, *350*
  10   Cardiovascular, Immune, and Lymphatic Systems and Blood, *392*
  11   Digestive System, *470*
  12   Eye, *538*
  13   Ear, *578*
  14   Musculoskeletal System, *606*
  15   Nervous System and Behavioral Health, *676*
  16   Endocrine System, *734*

TABLES

  1-1   Guidelines for Using Combining Vowels, *9*
  1-2   Word Parts and Combining Form, *10*
  1-3   Techniques to Learn Medical Terms Built From Word Parts, *14*
  2-1   Pronunciation Guide, *34*
  2-2   Common Plural Endings, *49*
  3-1   Anatomic Planes and Diagnostic Images, *73*
  4-1   Common Skin Disorders, *99*
  4-2   Common Skin Lesions, *123*
  5-1   Types of Diagnostic Procedures, *174*
  7-1   Prostate Cancer, *270*
  8-1   Types of Hysterectomies, *315*
  8-2   Types of Surgeries Performed to Treat Malignant Breast Tumors, *315*
  8-3   Endoscopic Surgery, *328*
10-1   Types of Angiography, *432*
10-2   Understanding a Lipid Profile, *440*
11-1   Bariatric Surgery, *503*
14-1   Types of Arthroplasty, *644*
14-2   Procedures for Treatment of Compression Fractures Caused by Osteoporosis, *646*
14-3   Diagnostic Imaging Procedures Used for the Musculoskeletal System, *652*

APPENDIXES

A Combining Forms, Prefixes, and Suffixes Alphabetized According to Word Part, *772*

B Combining Forms, Prefixes, and Suffixes Alphabetized According to Definition, *785*

C Additional Combining Forms, Prefixes, and Suffixes, *798*

D Abbreviations, *800*

E Pharmacology Terms, *813*

Visit the Evolve website *(http://evolve.elsevier.com/LaFleur)* to access the following appendixes:

F Health Care Delivery/Managed Care Terms

G Complementary and Alternative Medicine Therapies

H Behavioral Health Terms

I Clinical Research Terms

J Nutritional Terms

Exploring Medical Language
A Student-Directed Approach, 7th Edition

Introduction to Word Parts

OUTLINE

ORIGINS OF MEDICAL LANGUAGE, 4

FOUR WORD PARTS, 5
Word Root, 5
Suffix, 6
Prefix, 6
Combining Vowel, 7
    Four Guidelines for Using Combining Vowels, 7
        Guideline One, 7
        Guideline Two, 7
        Guideline Three, 8
        Guideline Four, 8

COMBINING FORM, 9

TECHNIQUES FOR LEARNING MEDICAL TERMS BUILT FROM WORD PARTS, 10
Analyzing Medical Terms, 10
Defining Medical Terms, 11
Word Part List, 11
Building Medical Terms, 12

CHAPTER REVIEW, 15

TABLE 1-1 GUIDELINES FOR USING COMBINING VOWELS, 9

TABLE 1-2 WORD PARTS AND COMBINING FORM, 10

TABLE 1-3 TECHNIQUES TO LEARN MEDICAL TERMS BUILT FROM WORD PARTS, 14

OBJECTIVES

Upon completion of this chapter you will be able to:

1. Describe four origins of medical language.

2. Identify and define the four word parts and the combining form.

3. Analyze and define medical terms.

4. Build medical terms for given definitions.

ORIGINS OF MEDICAL LANGUAGE

Medicine has a language of its own, and its vocabulary includes terms built from **Greek and Latin word parts, eponyms, acronyms,** and **modern language** (Figure 1-1). Like a language of a people, medical language is dynamic and develops over time. As clinical settings, current practice, technology, and medical knowledge evolve with scientific advancement, medical language changes. Some words are discarded, the meanings of others are altered, and new words are added.

The majority of medical terms in use today are composed of **Greek and Latin word parts,** some of which were used by Hippocrates and Aristotle more than 2400 years ago. In *Exploring Medical Language*, these terms are taught through a step-by-step word-building process that includes learning the meanings of word parts and how they fit together to form medical terms. Acquiring this skill will enable you to learn scores of medical terms quickly, and it will give you the tools you need to understand new terms you encounter in school or on the job.

Medical terms that are **eponyms** or **acronyms,** or **based on modern language** need to be learned by memorization. Medical terms that cannot be literally translated through the meanings of their word parts will also be learned by memorization. Illustrations, notes on current use, historical information, and learning tips will be presented with these terms to help you become familiar with their meanings as easily as possible. Although it takes effort, memorization is a fundamental step that allows you to create a foundation of knowledge. You will find that *Exploring Medical Language* creates multiple opportunities for you to practice, and practice itself will help you internalize the meanings and use of medical terms.

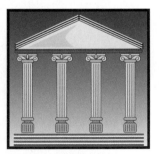

Greek and Latin
Terms built from Greek and Latin word parts such as *arthritis*

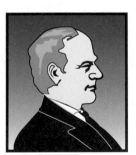

Eponyms
Terms derived from the name of a person, often a physician or scientist who was the first to identify a condition or technique such as *Parkinson disease*

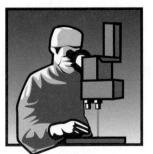

Acronyms
Terms formed from the first letters of the words in a phrase such as *laser* (light amplification by stimulated emission of radiation)

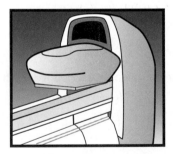

Modern language
Terms derived from the English language such as *nuclear medicine scanner*

FIGURE 1-1
Origins of medical language.

EXERCISE 1

Place the letter from the first column to identify the origin of the term in the second column. You may use an answer more than once. *To check your answers go to p. 16, Answers to Chapter 1 Exercises.*

a. components of Greek and Latin word parts

b. eponym

c. acronym

d. modern language

_B_ 1. Parkinson disease

_A_ 2. hepatitis

_C_ 3. SARS (severe acute respiratory syndrome)

_D_ 4. posttraumatic stress disorder

_A_ 5. arthritis

_D_ 6. nuclear medicine scanner

_C_ 7. AIDS (acquired immunodeficiency syndrome)

_B_ 8. Alzheimer disease

FOUR WORD PARTS

Most medical terms built from word parts consist of some or all of the following components:

1. Word root
2. Suffix
3. Prefix
4. Combining vowel

Word Root

The word root is the word part that is the core of the word. The word root contains the fundamental meaning of the word.

Examples:	
In the word	play/er, *play* is the word root.
In the medical term	arthr/itis, *arthr* (which means *joint*) is the word root.
In the medical term	hepat/itis, *hepat* (which means *liver*) is the word root.

> The word root is the core of the word; therefore, each medical term contains one or more word roots.

Complete the following: A word root is _the word part that_ _is the core of the word_

Answer: the word part that is the core of the word

SUFFIXES
frequently indicate:
- *procedures,* such as **-scopy,** meaning visual examination, or **-tomy,** meaning incision
- *conditions,* such as **-itis,** meaning inflammation
- *diseases,* such as **-oma,** meaning tumor.

Suffix

The suffix is a word part attached to the end of the word root to modify its meaning.

Examples:	
In the word	play/er, *-er* is the suffix.
In the medical term.	hepat/ic, *-ic* (which means *pertaining to*) is the suffix. *Hepat* is the word root for *liver;* therefore, *hepatic* means *pertaining to the liver.*
In the medical term.	hepat/itis, *-itis* (which means *inflammation*) is the suffix. The medical term *hepatitis* means *inflammation of the liver.*

 The suffix is used to modify the meaning of a word. Most medical terms have a suffix.

Complete the following: The suffix is <u>the word part attached to the end of the word root to modify its meaning</u>

Answer: the word part attached to the end of the word root to modify its meaning

PREFIXES
often indicate:
- *number* such as **bi-,** meaning two
- *position,* such as **sub-,** meaning under
- *direction,* such as **intra-,** meaning within
- *time,* such as **brady-,** meaning slow
- *negation,* such as **a-,** meaning without

Prefix

The prefix is a word part attached to the beginning of a word root to modify its meaning.

Examples:	
In the word	re/play, *re-* is the prefix.
In the medical term.	sub/hepat/ic, *sub-* (which means *under*) is the prefix. *Hepat* is the word root for *liver,* and *-ic* is the suffix for *pertaining to.* The medical term *subhepatic* means *pertaining to under the liver.*
In the medical term.	intra/ven/ous, *intra-* (which means *within*) is the prefix, *ven* (which means *vein*) is the word root, and *-ous* (which means *pertaining to*) is the suffix. The medical term *intravenous* means *pertaining to within the vein.*

 A prefix can be used to modify the meaning of a word. Many medical terms do not have a prefix.

Complete the following: The prefix is <u>the word part attached to the beginning of a word root to modify its</u>

Answer: the word part attached to the beginning of a word root to modify its meaning

Combining Vowel

The combining vowel is a word part, usually an *o*, used to ease pronunciation (Table 1-1).

The combining vowel is:

- Placed to connect two word roots
- Placed to connect a word root and a suffix
- **Not** placed to connect a prefix and a word root

Examples:

In the medical term..........	oste/o/arthr/itis
	o is the combining vowel used between two word roots *oste* (which means bone) and *arthr* (which means joint).
In the medical term..........	arthr/o/pathy,
	o is the combining vowel used between the word root *arthr* and the suffix *-pathy* (which means *disease*).
In the medical term..........	sub/hepat/ic,
	the combining vowel is **not** used between the prefix *sub-* and the word root *hepat*.

Four Guidelines for Using Combining Vowels

Guideline One

When connecting a word root and a suffix, a combining vowel is used if the suffix does not begin with a vowel (Table 1-1).

Example:

In the medical term..........	arthr/o/pathy,
	the suffix *-pathy* does not begin with a vowel; therefore, a combining vowel is used.

Guideline Two

When connecting a word root and a suffix, a combining vowel is usually not used if the suffix begins with a vowel.

Example:

In the medical term..........	hepat/ic,
	the suffix *-ic* begins with the vowel *i*; therefore, a combining vowel is not used.

VOWELS
are speech sounds represented by the letters *a, e, i, o, u,* and sometimes *y.*

Guideline Three

When connecting two word roots, a combining vowel is usually used even if vowels are present at the junction.

Example:	
In the medical term	oste/o/arthr/itis, *o* is the combining vowel used, even though the word root *oste* ends with the vowel *e*, and the word root *arthr* begins with the vowel *a*.

Guideline Four

When connecting a prefix and a word root, a combining vowel is **not** used.

Example:	
In the medical term	sub/hepat/ic, the combining vowel is **not** used between the prefix *sub-* and the word root *hepat*.

 The combining vowel is used to ease pronunciation; therefore *not all medical terms have combining vowels.* Medical terms introduced throughout the text that have combining vowels other than *o* are highlighted at their introduction.

Complete the following:

1. A combining vowel is ̲a̲ ̲w̲o̲r̲d̲ ̲p̲a̲r̲t̲,̲ ̲u̲s̲u̲a̲l̲l̲y̲ ̲a̲n̲ ̲O̲,̲ ̲u̲s̲e̲d̲ ̲t̲o̲
   ̲e̲a̲s̲e̲ ̲p̲r̲o̲n̲u̲n̲c̲i̲a̲t̲i̲o̲n̲

   Answer: a word part, usually an o, used to ease pronunciation

2. When connecting a word root and a suffix, a combining vowel is
   ̲u̲s̲e̲d̲ if the suffix does not begin with a vowel.

   Answer: used

3. When connecting a word root and a suffix, a combining vowel is usually not used if the suffix begins with a ̲v̲o̲w̲e̲l̲ .

   Answer: vowel

4. When connecting two ̲w̲o̲r̲d̲ ̲r̲o̲o̲t̲s̲ , a combining vowel is usually used, even if vowels are present at the junction.

   Answer: word roots

5. When connecting a prefix and a word root, a combining vowel is ̲n̲o̲t̲ used.

   Answer: not

TABLE 1-1

Guidelines for Using Combining Vowels

Combining Vowel Guideline	Example
1. When connecting a word root and a suffix, a **combining vowel** *Is Used* if the suffix *Does Not Begin* with a vowel.	arthr/**o**/pathy
2. When connecting a word root and a suffix, a **combining vowel** *Is Usually Not Used* if the suffix *Begins* with a vowel.	hepat/ic
3. When connecting two word roots a **combining vowel** *Is Usually Used* even if vowels are present at the junctions.	oste/**o**/arthr/itis
4. When connecting a **prefix** and a word root a combining vowel is *Not Used*.	sub/hepat/ic

COMBINING FORM

A combining form is a word root with the combining vowel attached, separated by a vertical slash (Table 1-2).

Examples: arthr/o

oste/o

ven/o

The combining form is not a word part per se; rather it is the word root and the combining vowel. *For learning purposes, word roots are presented together with their combining vowels as combining forms throughout the text.*

Complete the following: A combining form is <u>a word root with the</u> <u>combining vowel attached, separated by a verticle slash</u>

Answer: a word root with the combining vowel attached, separated by a vertical slash

 Word roots are presented as combining forms throughout the text.

EXERCISE   2

Match the phrases in the first column with the correct terms in the second column. *To check your answers, go to p. 16, Answers to Chapter 1 Exercises.*

_B_ 1. attached at the beginning

_A_ 2. usually an *o*

_D_ 3. all medical terms contain at least one

_E_ 4. attached at the end of a word root

_C_ 5. word root with combining vowel attached

a. combining vowel

b. prefix

c. combining form

d. word root

e. suffix

EXERCISE 3

Answer *T* for true and *F* for false.

_F_ 1. There are always prefixes at the beginning of medical terms.

_F_ 2. A combining vowel is always used when connecting a word root and a suffix that begins with the letter *o*.

_T_ 3. A prefix modifies the meaning of the word.

_T_ 4. A combining vowel is used to ease pronunciation.

_F_ 5. *I* is the most commonly used combining vowel.

_T_ 6. The word root is the core of a medical term.

_F_ 7. A combining vowel is used between a prefix and a word root.

_F_ 8. A combining form is a word part.

_T_ 9. A combining vowel is used when connecting a word root and a suffix if the suffix begins with the letter *g*.

TABLE 1-2

Word Parts and Combining Form

Word Parts	Definition	Example
1. Word root	The core of the word	hepat/itis
2. Suffix	Attached at the end of a word root to modify its meaning	hepat/itis
3. Prefix	Attached at the beginning of a word root to modify its meaning	sub/hepatic
4. Combining vowel	Usually an "o" used to ease pronunciation	hepat/o/megaly
Combining form	Word root with a combining vowel attached separated by a slash	hepat/o

---

TECHNIQUES FOR LEARNING MEDICAL TERMS BUILT FROM WORD PARTS

Analyzing Medical Terms

To analyze medical terms, divide them into word parts and label each word part and each combining form (Table 1-3 on p. 14). Follow the procedure below:

1. **Divide the term** into word parts with vertical slashes.

   Example: oste / o / arthr / o / pathy

2. **Label each word part** by using the following abbreviations.

   WR   Word Root

   P   Prefix

   S   Suffix

   CV   Combining Vowel

   WR   CV   WR   CV   S
   Example: oste / o / arthr / o / pathy

3. **Label the combining forms.**

Example:
$$\underbrace{\overset{WR}{oste} / \overset{CV}{o}}_{CF} / \underbrace{\overset{WR}{arthr} / \overset{CV}{o}}_{CF} / \overset{S}{pathy}$$

Analyze the following medical term:

o s t e o p a t h y

Answer:
$$\underbrace{\overset{WR}{oste} / \overset{CV}{o}}_{CF} / \overset{S}{pathy}$$

Complete the following: To analyze medical terms, <u>divide them into word parts and label each word part and each combining form.</u>

Answer: divide them into word parts and label each word part and each combining form

Defining Medical Terms

To define medical terms, apply the meaning of each word part contained in the term.

1. Begin by defining the suffix.
2. Then move to the beginning of the term to complete the definition.

Define the medical term: oste/o/arthr/o/pathy

Use the Word Part List below to find the meaning of the word parts.

Begin by defining the suffix *-pathy*. Then move to the beginning of the term and define the word roots *oste* and *arthr*:

oste/o/arthr/o/pathy means <u>disease of the bone and joint</u>

Answer: disease of the bone and joint

 Most medical terms built from word parts can be defined by beginning with the meaning of the suffix; however, this does not always apply.

Word Part List

Word Roots	Definition	Suffixes	Definition
arthr	joint	-itis	inflammation
hepat	liver	-ic	pertaining to
ven	vein	-ous	pertaining to
oste	bone	-pathy	disease
		-megaly	enlargement

Prefixes		Combining Vowel	
intra-	within	o	
sub-	under		

Complete the following: To define medical terms, *apply the meaning of each word part contained in the term* [handwritten]

Answer: apply the meaning of each word part contained in the term

EXERCISE 4

Using the Word Part List on p. 11 to identify the word parts and their meanings, analyze and define the following terms.

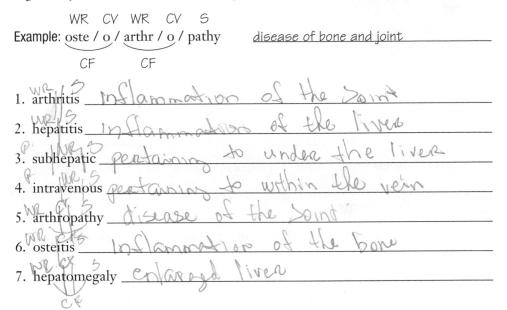

Example: oste / o / arthr / o / pathy   <u>disease of bone and joint</u>

1. arthritis   <u>Inflammation of the joint</u> [handwritten]
2. hepatitis   <u>Inflammation of the liver</u> [handwritten]
3. subhepatic   <u>pertaining to under the liver</u> [handwritten]
4. intravenous   <u>pertaining to within the vein</u> [handwritten]
5. arthropathy   <u>disease of the joint</u> [handwritten]
6. osteitis   <u>Inflammation of the bone</u> [handwritten]
7. hepatomegaly   <u>enlarged liver</u> [handwritten]

Building Medical Terms

To build medical terms, place word parts together to form words.

Using the Word Part List on p. 11 as a reference, build the medical term for the following:

disease of a joint

1. Find the word part for *disease*. Write the word part in the correct space below.
2. Find the word part for *joint*. Write the word part in the correct space below.
3. The suffix does not begin with a vowel, so a combining vowel is needed. Insert the combining vowel *o* in the correct space below.

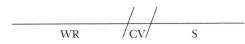

    WR   CV   S

Answer: arthr/o/pathy

Complete the following: To build medical terms means *to place word parts together to form words* [handwritten]

Answer: to place word parts together to form words

 Keep in mind that the beginning of the definition usually indicates the suffix.

EXERCISE 5

Using the Word Part List on p. 11 as a reference, build medical terms for the following definitions. *To check your answers, go to p. 16, Answers to Chapter 1 Exercises.*

Example: disease of a joint

<u>arthr</u> / <u>o</u> / <u>pathy</u>
WR /CV/   S

1. inflammation of a joint

    <u>arthr</u>   / <u>itis</u>
       WR   /   S

2. pertaining to the liver

    <u>hepa</u>   / <u>tic</u>
       WR   /   S

3. pertaining to under the liver

    <u>sub</u> / <u>hepa</u>   / <u>tic</u>
      P /   WR   /   S

4. pertaining to within the vein

    <u>Intra</u> / <u>ven</u>   / <u>ous</u>
      P   /   WR   /   S

5. inflammation of the bone

    <u>oste</u>   / <u>itis</u>
       WR   /   S

6. inflammation of the liver

    <u>hepa</u>   / <u>titis</u>
       WR   /   S

7. disease of the bone and joint

    <u>oste</u> /<u>o</u>/ <u>arthr</u>   /<u>o</u>/ <u>pathy</u>
      WR /CV/   WR   /CV/ S

8. enlargement of the liver

    <u>hepat</u>   /<u>o</u>/ <u>megaly</u>
       WR   /CV/   S

EXERCISE FIGURE A

Fill in the blanks to complete labeling of the diagram.
To check your answer, go to p. 16, Answers to Chapter 1 Exercises.

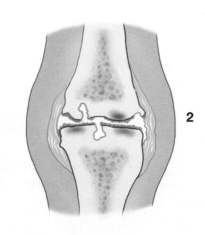

1. Normal knee joint   **2.** Knee joint showing

<u>oste</u> /<u>o</u>/ <u>arthr</u> / <u>itis</u>   .
bone / cv / joint / inflammation

TABLE 1-3
Techniques to Learn Medical Terms Built from Word Parts

• Analyzing	Divide medical terms into word parts	oste/o/arthr/o/pathy
	Label each word part	WR CV WR CV S oste/o/arthr/o/pathy
	Label each combining form	WR CV WR CV S oste/o/arthr/o/pathy CF CF
• Defining	Apply the meaning of each word part contained in the term *(begin by defining the suffix, then move to the beginning of the term)*	
	oste/o/arthr/o/pathy *disease of the bone and joint* WR WR S	
• Building	Place word parts together to form terms *(the beginning of the definition usually indicates the suffix)*	
	disease of the bone and joint	oste / / arthr / /pathy WR WR S
	Add combining vowels as needed	oste /o /arthr / o /pathy WR CV WR CV S

 At this time do not be concerned about which word root goes first when building a term that contains two word roots. The order is usually dictated by common practice; for surgical or diagnostic terms, word roots are sometimes arranged by the order of function or by the order in which an instrument may encounter a structure. As you practice and learn you will become accustomed to the accepted order.

SUMMARY

Word Parts and Combining Form

Word root—core of a word; example, **hepat**

Suffix—attached at the end of a word root to modify its meaning; example, **-ic**

Prefix—attached at the beginning of a word to modify its meaning; example, **sub-**

Combining vowel—usually an **o** used between two word roots or a word root and suffix to ease pronunciation; example, hepat **o** pathy

Combining form—word root plus combining vowel separated by a vertical slash; example, **hepat/o**

Techniques for Learning Medical Terms Built from Word Parts

Analyzing—dividing medical terms into word parts, then labeling each word part and combining form

Defining—applying the meaning of each word part contained in the medical term to derive its meaning

Building—placing word parts together to form words

arthr/o/pathy
combining form

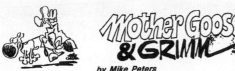

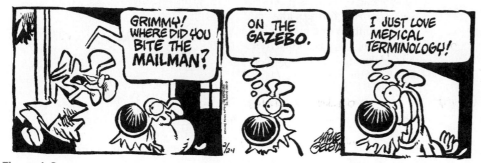

Figure 1-2

Reprinted by permission of Tribune Media Services.

CHAPTER REVIEW

To complete this chapter successfully, you do not need to know what the word parts, such as *arthr*, mean. You will learn these in subsequent chapters. **It is important that you have met these objectives:**

1. Can you describe four origins of medical language? *Greek & Latin, Eponyms, Acronyms modern languages*   yes ☒   no ☐ *combining*
2. Can you identify and define the four word parts and combining form? *Word root, Suffix* yes ☒ *Prefix* no ☐ *combining vowel*
3. Can you use word parts to analyze and define medical terms?   yes ☒   no ☐
4. Can you use word parts to build medical terms for a given definition?   yes ☐   no ☐

If you answered yes to these questions you need no further practice because you will be using these concepts repeatedly as you work your way through this text. Refer to this chapter to refresh your memory as needed. Move on to Chapter 2 and begin to build your medical vocabulary so that you will be better prepared than Grimm in Figure 1-2 to understand and use the language of medicine.

CHAPTER REVIEW ON CD-ROM

Use the CD-ROM that accompanies this textbook to play and practice what you have learned in this chapter. The Chapter Exercises, Practice Activities, Animations, and Games allow you to hear, see, and interact with the chapter content.

Chapter Exercises	**Practice Activities**	**Animations**	**Games**
Exercises in this section of your CD-ROM correlate to exercises in your textbook. You may have completed them as you worked through the chapter.	Practice in study mode, and then test your learning in assessment mode. Keep track of your scores from assessment mode if you wish.	☐ None for this chapter	☐ Medical Millionaire
☐ None for this chapter	SCORE ☐ Define Word Parts _21_ ☐ Analyze Medical Terms _6_ ☐ Build Medical Terms _____ ☐ Define Medical Terms _____		

ANSWERS

Exercise Figure
Exercise Figure
A. oste/o/arthr/itis

Exercise 1

1. b	5. a
2. a	6. d
3. c	7. c
4. d	8. b

Exercise 2

1. b   2. a   3. d   4. e   5. c

Exercise 3
1. *F*, a medical term may begin with the word root and have no prefix.
2. *F*, if the suffix begins with a vowel, the combining vowel is usually not used.
3. *T*
4. *T*
5. *F*, *o* is the combining vowel most often used.

6. *T*
7. *F*, a combining vowel is used between two word roots or between a word root and a suffix to ease pronunciation.
8. *F*, a combining form is a word root with a combining vowel attached and is not one of the four word parts.
9. *T*

Exercise 4
1.   WR   S
     arthr/itis
     inflammation of the joint
2.   WR   S
     hepat/itis
     inflammation of the liver
3.   P   WR   S
     sub/hepat/ic
     pertaining to under the liver
4.   P   WR S
     intra/ven/ous
     pertaining to within the vein

5.   WR CV S
     arthr/o/pathy
          CF
     disease of the joint
6.   WR   S
     oste/itis
     inflammation of the bone
7.   WR CV   S
     hepat/o/megaly
          CF
     enlargement of the liver

Exercise 5
1. arthr/itis
2. hepat/ic
3. sub/hepat/ic
4. intra/ven/ous
5. oste/itis
6. hepat/itis
7. oste/o/arthr/o/pathy
8. hepat/o/megaly

NOTES

CHAPTER 2

Body Structure, Color, and Oncology

OUTLINE

ANATOMY, 20

WORD PARTS, 23
Combining Forms, 23
Prefixes, 28
Suffixes, 29

MEDICAL TERMS, 31
Oncology, 31
Disease and Disorder Oncology Terms, 31
    Built from Word Parts, 31
Body Structure Terms, 37
    Built from Word Parts, 37
Complementary Terms, 41
    Built from Word Parts, 41
    Not Built from Word Parts, 46
Plural Endings for Medical Terms, 49
Abbreviations, 51

PRACTICAL APPLICATION, 52
Interact with Medical Documents, 52
Interpret Medical Terms, 54
Read Medical Terms in Use, 55
Comprehend Medical Terms in Use, 55

CHAPTER REVIEW, 56

TABLE 2-1 PRONUNCIATION GUIDE, 34

TABLE 2-2 COMMON PLURAL ENDINGS, 49

OBJECTIVES

Upon completion of this chapter you will be able to:

1. Identify anatomic structures of the human body.

2. Define and spell word parts related to body structure, color, and oncology.

3. Define, pronounce, and spell disease and disorder oncology terms.

4. Define, pronounce, and spell body structure terms.

5. Define, pronounce, and spell complementary terms related to body structure, color, and oncology.

6. Identify and use singular and plural endings.

7. Interpret the meaning of abbreviations related to body structure, and oncology.

8. Interpret, read, and comprehend medical language in simulated medical statements and documents.

ANATOMY

Organization of the Body

The structure of the human body falls into the following four categories: cells, tissues, organs, and systems. Each structure is a highly organized unit of smaller structures (Exercise Figure A).

CELL
was named about 300 years ago by Robert Hooke. On seeing cells through a microscope, he named them **cells** because they reminded him of miniature prison cells.

MEDICAL GENOMICS
A **genome** is the complete set of genes in a chromosome of each cell of a specific organism. **Genomics** is the study of the genome and its products and interactions. **Medical genomics** is the study of the genome and how it can be used in the cause, treatment, and prevention of disease. It is thought that it will alter twenty-first century medicine. **Gene therapy** is any therapeutic procedure in which genes are intentionally introduced into human body cells to achieve gene repair, gene suppression, or gene addition. Gene therapy is still in its infancy. The first human gene transfer was performed on a patient with malignant melanoma in 1989. Since then more than 30,000 patients have received gene therapy.

Go to Evolve at http://evolve.elsevier.com/ for an appendix of clinical research terms.

Term	Definition
cell	basic unit of all living things (Figure 2-1). The human body is composed of trillions of cells, which vary in size and shape according to function.
cell membrane	forms the boundary of the cell
cytoplasm	gel-like fluid inside the cell
nucleus	largest structure within the cell, usually spherical and centrally located. It contains chromosomes for cellular reproduction and is the control center of the cell.
chromosomes	located in the nucleus of the cell. There are 46 chromosomes in all normal human cells, with the exception of mature sex cells, which have 23.
genes	regions within the chromosome. Each chromosome has several thousand genes that determine hereditary characteristics.
DNA (deoxyribonucleic acid)	comprises each gene; is a chemical that regulates the activities of the cell
tissue	group of similar cells that performs a specific task (Exercise Figure B)
muscle tissue	composed of cells that have a special ability to contract, usually producing movement

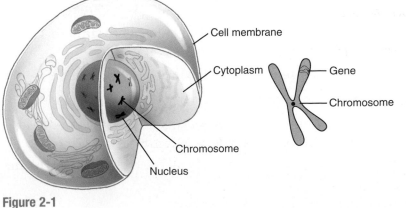

Figure 2-1
Body cell.

Term	Definition
nervous tissue	found in the nerves, spinal cord, and brain. It is responsible for coordinating and controlling body activities.
connective tissue	connects, supports, penetrates, and encases various body structures. Adipose (fat), osseous (bone) tissues, and blood are types of connective tissue.
epithelial tissue	the major covering of the external surface of the body; forms membranes that line body cavities and organs and is the major tissue in glands
organ	two or more kinds of tissues that together perform special body functions. For example, the skin is an organ composed of epithelial, connective, muscle, and nerve tissue.
system	group of organs that work together to perform complex body functions. For example, the cardiovascular system consists of the heart, blood vessels, and blood. Its function is to transport nutrients and oxygen to the cells and remove carbon dioxide and other waste products.

Body Cavities

The body is not a solid structure as it appears on the outside, but has five cavities (Figure 2-2), each containing an orderly arrangement of the internal organs.

Term	Definition
cranial cavity	space inside the skull (cranium) containing the brain
spinal cavity	space inside the spinal column containing the spinal cord
thoracic, or chest, cavity	space containing the heart, aorta, lungs, esophagus, trachea, and bronchi
abdominal cavity	space containing the stomach, intestines, kidneys, liver, gallbladder, pancreas, spleen, and ureters
pelvic cavity	space containing the urinary bladder, certain reproductive organs, parts of the large intestine, and the rectum
abdominopelvic cavity	both the pelvic and abdominal cavities

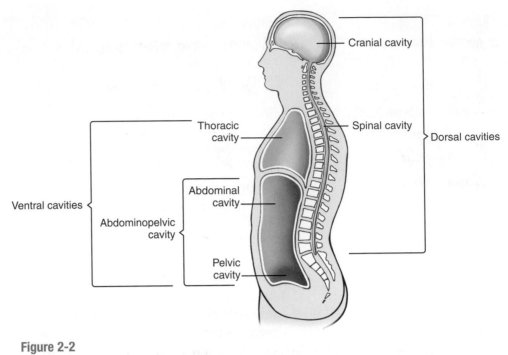

Figure 2-2
Body cavities.

EXERCISE 1

Match the anatomic terms in the first column with the correct definitions in the second column. *To check your answers, go to p. 58, Answers to Chapter 2 Exercises.*

h	1. chromosomes	a. type of connective tissue
E	2. nucleus	b. regions within the chromosome
D	3. cytoplasm	c. covers external body surface, lines body cavities and organs
K	4. cell	d. gel-like fluid inside the cell
G	5. muscle tissue	e. contains chromosomes
F	6. nerve tissue	f. coordinates body activities
C	7. epithelial tissue	g. usually produces movement
A	8. bone	h. contain genes
B	9. genes	i. chest cavity
J	10. DNA	j. a chemical that regulates the activities of the cell
		k. basic unit of all living things

EXERCISE 2

Match the anatomic terms in the first column with the correct definitions in the second column.

H 1. spinal cavity
B 2. thoracic cavity
C 3. organ
E 4. cranial cavity
G 5. pelvic cavity
A 6. system
F 7. abdominal cavity

a. group of organs functioning together
b. chest cavity
c. composed of two or more tissues
d. found in the skin
e. space inside the skull
f. contains the stomach
g. contains the urinary bladder
h. contains the spinal cord

WORD PARTS

Begin building your medical vocabulary by learning the word parts listed next. The list may appear long to you; however, the many exercises that follow are designed to help you understand and remember the word parts.

Combining Forms of Body Structure

Reminder: the word root is the core of the word. The combining form is the word root with the combining vowel attached, separated by a vertical slash.

Combining Form	Definition
aden/o	gland
cyt/o	cell
epitheli/o	epithelium
fibr/o	fiber
hist/o	tissue
kary/o	nucleus
lip/o	fat
my/o	muscle
neur/o	nerve
organ/o	organ
sarc/o	flesh, connective tissue
system/o	system
viscer/o	internal organs

EPITHELIUM
originally meant **surface over the nipple.** Epi means **upon,** and **thela** means **nipple** (or projecting surfaces of many kinds).

Fill in the blanks with combining forms in this diagram of the organization of the body.

To check your answers, go to p. 58, Answers to Chapter 2 Exercises.

2. Tissue
CF: _hist/o_

1. Cell
CF: _cyt/o_

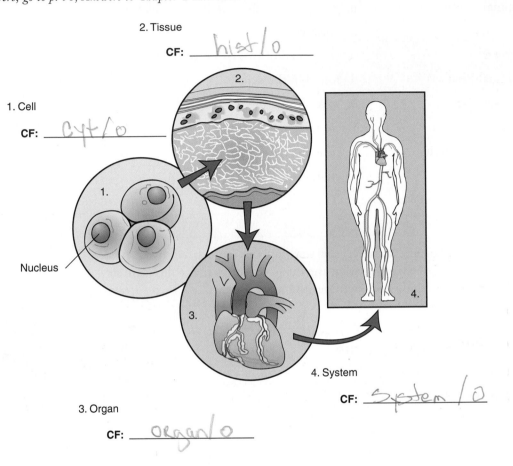

Nucleus

4. System
CF: _system/o_

3. Organ
CF: _organ/o_

EXERCISE   3

Write the definitions of the following combining forms.

1. sarc/o _flesh, connective tissue_   8. neur/o _nerve_

2. lip/o _fat_   9. organ/o _organ_

3. kary/o _nucleus_   10. system/o _system_

4. viscer/o _internal organs_   11. epitheli/o _epithelium_

5. cyt/o _cell_   12. fibr/o _fiber_

6. hist/o _tissue_   13. aden/o _gland_

7. my/o _muscle_

Fill in the blanks with combining forms in this diagram of types of tissues.

To check your answers, go to p. 58, Answers to Chapter 2 Exercises.

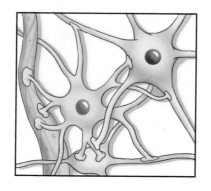

2. Epithelium

CF: _____epitheli / o_____

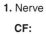

1. Nerve

CF: _____neur / o_____

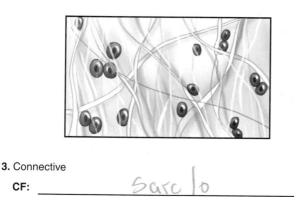

3. Connective

CF: _____sarc / o_____

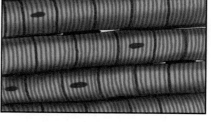

4. Muscle

CF: _____my / o_____

EXERCISE **4**

Write the combining form for each of the following.

1. internal organs _____viscer / o_____

2. epithelium _____epitheli / o_____

3. organ _____organ / o_____

4. nucleus _____kary / o_____

5. cell _____cyt / o_____

6. tissue _____hist / o_____

7. nerve _____neur / o_____

8. muscle _____my / o_____

9. fat _____lip / o_____

10. system _____system / o_____

11. connective tissue, flesh _____sarc / o_____

12. fiber _____fibr / o_____

13. gland _____aden / o_____

CANCER

Carcin and *cancer* are derived from Latin and Greek words meaning *crab*. They originated before the nature of malignant growth was understood. One explanation was that the swollen veins around the diseased area looked like the claws of a crab.

Combining Forms Commonly Used with Body Structure Terms

Combining Form	Definition
cancer/o, carcin/o	cancer (a disease characterized by the unregulated, abnormal growth of new cells)
eti/o	cause (of disease)
gno/o	knowledge
iatr/o	physician, medicine (also means treatment)
lei/o	smooth
onc/o	tumor, mass
path/o	disease
rhabd/o	rod-shaped, striated
somat/o	body

EXERCISE 5

Write the definitions of the following combining forms.

1. onc/o _tumor, mass_

2. carcin/o _cancer_

3. eti/o _cause_

4. path/o _disease_

5. somat/o _body_

6. cancer/o _cancer_

7. rhabd/o _Rod shaped, striated_

8. lei/o _smooth_

9. gno/o _knowledge_

10. iatr/o _physician, medicine_

EXERCISE 6

Write the combining form for each of the following.

1. disease _path/o_

2. tumor, mass _onc/o_

3. cause (of disease) _eti/o_

4. cancer a. _cancer/o_
         b. _carcin/o_

5. body _somat/o_

6. smooth _lei/o_

7. rod-shaped, striated _rhabd/o_

8. knowledge _gno/o_

9. physician, medicine _iatr/o_

Combining Forms that Describe Color

Combining Form	Definition
chlor/o	green
chrom/o	color
cyan/o	blue
erythr/o	red
leuk/o	white
melan/o	black
xanth/o	yellow

ERYTHRO
Aristotle noted "two colors of blood" and applied the term **erythro** to the dark red blood.

EXERCISE 7

Write the definitions of the following combining forms.

1. cyan/o _____blue_____

2. erythr/o _____red_____

3. leuk/o _____white_____

4. xanth/o _____yellow_____

5. chrom/o _____color_____

6. melan/o _____black_____

7. chlor/o _____green_____

EXERCISE 8

Write the combining form for each of the following.

1. blue _____cyan/o_____

2. red _____erythr/o_____

3. white _____leuk/o_____

4. black _____melan/o_____

5. yellow _____xanth/o_____

6. color _____chrom/o_____

7. green _____chlor/o_____

Prefixes

Reminder: prefixes are placed at the beginning of word roots to modify their meanings.

Prefix	Definition
dia-	through, complete
dys-	painful, abnormal, difficult, labored
hyper-	above, excessive
hypo-	below, incomplete, deficient
meta-	after, beyond, change
neo-	new
pro-	before

EXERCISE 9

Write the definitions of the following prefixes.

1. neo- _____ *new* _____
2. hyper- _____ *above, excessive* _____
3. meta- _____ *after, beyond, change* _____
4. hypo- _____ *below* _____
5. dys- _____ *painful, abnormal* _____
6. dia- _____ *through, complete* _____
7. pro- _____ *before* _____

EXERCISE 10

Write the prefix for each of the following.

1. new _____ *neo* _____
2. above, excessive _____ *hyper* _____
3. below, incomplete, deficient _____ *hypo* _____
4. beyond, after, change _____ *meta* _____
5. abnormal, painful, labored, difficult _____ *dys* _____
6. through, complete _____ *dia* _____
7. before _____ *pro* _____

Suffixes

 Reminder: suffixes are placed at the end of word roots to modify their meanings.

Suffix	Definition
-al, -ic, -ous...............	pertaining to
-cyte	cell
(NOTE: the combining form for cell is *cyt/o*; the suffix for cell is *-cyte*, ending with an *e*.)	
-gen.....................	substance or agent that produces or causes
-genesis..................	origin, cause
-genic	producing, originating, causing
-logist	one who studies and treats (specialist, physician)
-logy	study of
-oid	resembling
-oma	tumor, swelling
-osis.....................	abnormal condition (means *increase* when used with blood cell word roots)
-pathy	disease
-plasia	condition of formation, development, growth
-plasm...................	growth, substance, formation
-sarcoma.................	malignant tumor
-sis......................	state of
-stasis	control, stop, standing

 Some suffixes are made of a word root plus a suffix; they are presented as suffixes for ease of learning. For example, **-pathy** is made up of the word root **path** and the suffix **-y.** When analyzing a medical term, divide the suffixes as learned. For example, **somatopathy** should be divided somat/o/pathy and **not** somat/o/path/y.

Refer to Appendix A and Appendix B for alphabetized lists of word parts and their meanings.

INCIDENTALOMA
refers to a mass lesion involving an organ that is discovered unexpectedly by the use of ultrasound, computed tomography scan, or magnetic resonance imaging and has nothing to do with the patient's symptoms or primary diagnosis.

EXERCISE 11

Match the suffixes in the first column with their correct definitions in the second column.

_I_	1. -logy	a. producing, originating, causing
_L_	2. -osis	b. cell
_D_	3. -pathy	c. specialist, physician
_F_	4. -plasm	d. new
_G_	5. -al, -ic, -ous	e. disease
_J_	6. -stasis	f. growth, substance, formation
_H_	7. -oid	g. pertaining to
_B_	8. -cyte	h. resembling
_P_	9. -genesis	i. study of
_C_	10. -logist	j. control, stop, standing
_N_	11. -oma	k. substance that produces
_K_	12. -gen	l. abnormal condition
_Q_	13. -sarcoma	m. condition of formation, development, growth
_M_	14. -plasia	n. tumor, swelling
_A_	15. -genic	o. state of
_O_	16. -sis	p. origin, cause
		q. malignant tumor

SARCOMA has been used since the time of ancient Greece to describe any fleshy tumor. Since the introduction of cellular pathology, the meaning was restricted to mean a **malignant connective tissue tumor.**

EXERCISE 12

Write the definitions of the following suffixes.

1. -logist _Specialist, physican_
2. -pathy _New_
3. -logy _Study of_
4. -ic _Pertaining to_
5. -stasis _Control, stop, standing_
6. -cyte _Cell_
7. -osis _abnormal condition_
8. -ous _pertaining to_
9. -plasm _growth, substance, formation_
10. -al _Pertaining to_
11. -plasia _condition of formation_
12. -oid _Resembling_
13. -gen _Substance that produces_

14. -genic _producing, originating, causing_

15. -oma _tumor, swelling_

16. -genesis _origin, cause_

17. -sarcoma _malignant tumor_

18. -sis _state of_

> Practice two things in your dealings with disease: either help or do not harm the patient.
> **Hippocrates** 460–375 BC

MEDICAL TERMS

Oncology

Oncology is the study of tumors. Tumors develop from excessive growth of cells from a body part. Tumors, or masses, are benign (noncancerous) or malignant (cancerous). The names of tumors are often made of the word root for the body part and the suffix **-oma,** as in the term *my/oma*.

Oncology terms are introduced in this chapter because of their relation to cells and cell abnormalities. This is an introductory list only. More oncology terms appear in subsequent chapters and are presented with the introduction of the related body systems.

Disease and Disorder Oncology Terms

> Medical terms built from word parts can be translated literally to find their meanings. The terms are learned by completing all of the analyzing, defining, and word-building exercises.

Built from Word Parts

The following terms are built from word parts you have already learned and can be translated literally to find their meanings. Further explanation of terms beyond the definition of their word parts, if needed, is included in parentheses. At first the list of terms may seem long to you; however, many of the word parts are repeated in many of the words. You will soon find that knowing parts of the terms makes learning the words easy. Analyzing, defining, and word-building exercises are used to learn these terms and their meanings.

Term	Definition
adenocarcinoma . . . . (*ad*-e-nō-*kar*-si-NŌ-ma)	cancerous tumor of glandular tissue
adenoma . . . . (ad-e-NŌ-ma)	tumor composed of glandular tissue (benign)
carcinoma (Ca) . . . . (*kar*-si-NŌ-ma)	cancerous tumor (malignant) (Exercise Figure C)
chloroma . . . . (klo-RŌ-ma)	tumor of green color (malignant, arising from myeloid tissue)
epithelioma . . . . (ep-i-*thē*-lē-Ō-ma)	tumor composed of epithelium (may be benign or malignant)
fibroma . . . . (fi-BRŌ-ma)	tumor composed of fiber (fibrous tissue) (benign)

> **TNM STAGING SYSTEM OF CANCER**
>
> AJCC (American Joint Commission on Cancer) has devised a classification widely used to stage certain types of cancer properly.
>
> **T** refers to size and the extent of the primary tumor (ranked 0-4).
>
> **N** denotes the involvement of the lymph nodes (ranked 0-4).
>
> **M** defines whether there is metastasis (0 = none; 1 = present).
>
> **For example, $T_2 N_1 M_0$**
>
> **T_2** refers to the primary tumor of 2 cm.
>
> **N_1** means spread of tumor to ipsilateral (same side) lymph nodes.
>
> **M_0** means no distant metastasis.
>
> This system helps communicate the extent of cancer and is frequently cited by oncologists, surgeons, and radiation oncologists.

Disease and Disorder Oncology Terms—*cont'd*
Built from Word Parts

> **MESOTHELIOMA**
> Is a rare form of cancer most common in the lungs and most often caused by inhalation exposure to asbestos.

Term	Definition
fibrosarcoma (fī-brō-sar-KŌ-ma)	malignant tumor composed of fiber (fibrous tissue)
leiomyoma (lī-ō-mī-Ō-ma)	tumor composed of smooth muscle (benign)
leiomyosarcoma (*lī*-ō-*mī*-ō-sar-KŌ-ma)	malignant tumor of smooth muscle
lipoma (li-PŌ-ma)	tumor composed of fat (benign tumor)
liposarcoma (lip-ō-sar-KŌ-ma)	malignant tumor of fat
melanocarcinoma (*mel*-a-nō-*kar*-si-NŌ-ma)	cancerous black tumor (malignant)
melanoma (mel-a-NŌ-ma)	black tumor (primarily of the skin) (Exercise Figure C)
myoma (mī-Ō-ma)	tumor composed of muscle (benign)
neoplasm (NĒ-ō-plazm)	new growth (of abnormal tissue or tumor)
neuroma (nū-RŌ-ma)	tumor composed of nerve (benign)
rhabdomyoma (*rab*-dō-mī-Ō-ma)	tumor composed of striated muscle (benign)
rhabdomyosarcoma (*rab*-dō-*mī*-ō-sar-KŌ-ma)	malignant tumor of striated muscle (Exercise Figure C)
sarcoma (sar-KŌ-ma) (NOTE: sarc/o also is presented in this chapter as a word root.)	tumor of connective tissue (such as bone or cartilage) (highly malignant) (Exercise Figure C)

EXERCISE 13

Practice saying aloud each of the disease and disorder oncology terms built from word parts on pp. 31-32. Use Table 2-1, p. 34, for explanation of the pronunciation key.

 To hear the terms select Chapter 2, Chapter Exercises, Pronunciation.

☐ Place a check mark in the box when you have completed this exercise.

EXERCISE FIGURE C

Fill in the blanks to complete labeling of these diagrams of types of cancers.

To check your answers, go to p. 58, Answers to Chapter 2 Exercises.

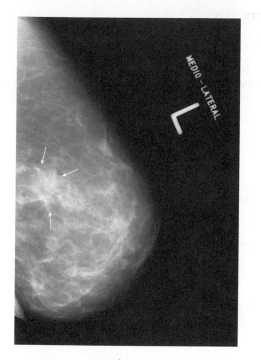

<u>carcin / oma</u>   of the breast
1.   cancer / tumor

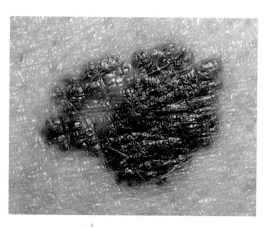

<u>melan / oma</u>
2.   black / tumor

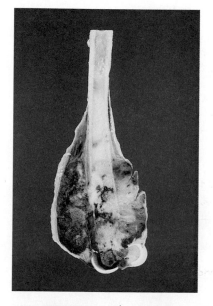

<u>Sarc / oma</u>   of the femur
3.   connective / tumor
      tissue

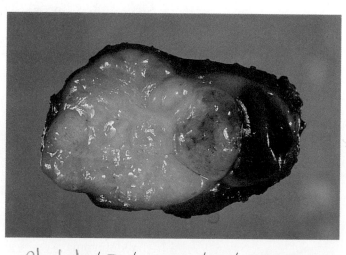

<u>Rhabd / o / my / o / sarcoma</u>
4.   striated / cv / muscle / cv / malignant tumor

TABLE 2-1

Pronunciation Guide

The following is a simple guide to use for practicing pronunciation of the medical terms. The pronunciations are only approximate; however, they are adequate to meet the needs of the beginning student.

In respelling for pronunciation, words are minimally distorted to indicate phonetic sound.

Example: doctor (dok-tor)
gastric (gas-trik)

A special mark called the macron (‾) is used to indicate the long vowel sounds.

Example: donate (dō -nāt)
hepatoma (hep-a-tō -ma)
ā as in *ate, say*
ē as in *eat, beet, see*
ī as in *I, mine, sky*
ō as in *oats, so*
ū as in *unit, mute*

Vowels with no markings have the short sound.

Example: discuss (dis-kus)
medical (med-i-kal)
a as in *at, lad*
e as in *edge, bet*
i as in *itch, wish*
o as in *ox, top*
u as in *sun, come*

An accent mark indicates the stress on a certain syllable. The primary accent is indicated by capital letters, and the secondary accent (which is stressed, but not as strongly as the primary accent) is indicated by italics.

Example: altogether (*all*-tū -GETH-er)
pancreatitis (*pan*-krē -a-TĪ -tis)

EXERCISE 14

Analyze and define the following disease and disorder oncology terms. Refer to Chapter 1, pp. 10-11, to review analyzing and defining techniques. **This is an important exercise; do not skip any portion of it.**

Example: lei / o / my / o / sarcoma   malignant tumor of smooth muscle

1. sarcoma ___ Sarc / oma - tumor of connective tissue
2. melanoma ___ melan / oma   black tumor
3. epithelioma ___ epitheli / oma   tumor composed of epith
4. lipoma ___ lip / oma   tumor composed of fat
5. neoplasm ___ neo / plasm   new growth
6. myoma ___ my / oma   tumor composed of muscle
7. neuroma ___ neur / oma   tumor composed of nerve
8. carcinoma ___ carcin / oma   cancerous tumor
9. melanocarcinoma ___ melano / carcin / oma   cancerous black
10. rhabdomyosarcoma ___ malignant tumor of striated muscle
11. leiomyoma ___ lei / o / my / oma   tumor composed of smooth
12. rhabdomyoma ___ tumor composed of striated muscle
13. fibroma ___ fibr / oma   tumor composed of fiber
14. liposarcoma ___ lipo / sarcoma - malignant tumor of fat

15. fibrosarcoma _fibro / sarcoma_
16. adenoma _aden / oma_
17. adenocarcinoma _aden / o / carcin / oma_
18. chloroma _chlor / oma_

EXERCISE 15

Build medical disease and disorder oncology terms for the following definitions by using the word parts you have learned. If you need help, refer to p. 12 to review word-building techniques. **Once again, this is an integral part of the learning process; do not skip any part of this exercise.**

Example: a tumor composed of fat   _lip / oma_
                                         WR / S

1. black tumor   _melan_ / _oma_
                          WR   /   S

2. cancerous tumor   _carcin_ / _oma_
                          WR   /   S

3. new growth   _neo_ / _plasm_
                          P   /   S(WR)

> When analyzing medical terms that have a suffix containing a word root, it may appear, as in the word **neoplasm,** that the term is composed of only a prefix and a suffix. Keep in mind that the word root is embedded in the suffix and is indicated in the *Building Medical Terms* exercises by S (WR).

4. tumor composed of epithelium   _epitheli_ / _oma_
                                    WR   /   S

5. tumor of connective tissue   _sarc_ / _oma_
                                    WR   /   S

6. cancerous black tumor   _melan_ / o / _carcin_ / _oma_
                                    WR   /CV/ WR   /   S

7. tumor composed of nerve   _neur_ / _oma_
                                    WR   /   S

8. tumor composed of muscle   _my_ / _oma_
                                    WR /   S

9. malignant tumor of striated muscle   _rhabd_ / o / _my_ / o / _sarcoma_
                                          WR   /CV/ WR /CV/   S

10. tumor composed of smooth muscle   _lei_ / o / _my_ / _oma_
                                          WR /CV/ WR /   S

11. tumor composed of striated muscle   _rhabd_ / o / _my_ / _oma_
                                          WR   /CV/ WR /   S

12. malignant tumor of smooth muscle

lei /o/ my /o/ ma
<u>WR</u> /<u>CV</u>/ <u>WR</u> /<u>CV</u>/ <u>S</u>

13. malignant tumor of fat

lip /o/ sarcoma
<u>WR</u> /<u>CV</u>/ <u>S</u>

14. tumor composed of fiber (fibrous tissue)

fibr / oma
<u>WR</u> / <u>S</u>

15. malignant tumor of fiber (fibrous tissue)

fibr /o/ sarcoma
<u>WR</u> /<u>CV</u>/ <u>S</u>

16. tumor composed of glandular tissue

aden / oma
<u>WR</u> / <u>S</u>

17. cancerous tumor of glandular tissue

aden /o/ carcin/ oma
<u>WR</u> /<u>CV</u>/ <u>WR</u> / <u>S</u>

18. tumor of green color

chlor / oma
<u>WR</u> / <u>S</u>

EXERCISE 16

Spell each of the disease and disorder oncology terms built from word parts on pp. 31-32 by having someone dictate them to you.

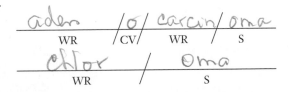 To hear and spell the terms select Chapter 2, Chapter Exercises, Spelling.

You may type the terms on the screen or write them below in the spaces provided.

1. _____   11. _____

2. _____   12. _____

3. _____   13. _____

4. _____   14. _____

5. _____   15. _____

6. _____   16. _____

7. _____   17. _____

8. _____   18. _____

9. _____   19. _____

10. _____

Body Structure Terms

Built from Word Parts

The following terms are built from word parts you have already learned and can be translated literally to find their meanings. Further explanation of terms beyond the definition of their word parts, if needed, is included in parentheses. By analyzing, defining, and building the terms in the exercises that follow, you will come to know the terms.

Term	Definition
cytogenic .... (sī-tō-JEN-ik)	producing cells
cytoid .... (SĪ-toid)	resembling a cell
cytology .... (sī-TOL-o-jē)	study of cells
cytoplasm .... (SĪ-tō-plazm)	cell substance
dysplasia .... (dis-PLĀ-zha)	abnormal development (see Figure 2-6)
epithelial .... (ep-i-THĒ-lē-al)	pertaining to epithelium
erythrocyte (RBC)........... (e-RITH-rō-sīt)	red (blood) cell (Exercise Figure D)
erythrocytosis .... (e-rith-rō-sī-TŌ-sis)	increase in the number of red (blood) cells
histology .... (his-TOL-o-jē)	study of tissue
hyperplasia .... (hī-per-PLĀ-zha)	excessive development (number of cells) (Exercise Figure E) (see Figure 2-6)
hypoplasia .... (hī-pō-PLĀ-zha)	incomplete development (of an organ or tissues)
karyocyte .... (KĀR-ē-ō-sīt)	cell with a nucleus
karyoplasm .... (KĀR-ē-ō-plazm)	substance of a nucleus
leukocyte (WBC) .... (LŪ-kō-sīt)	white (blood) cell (Exercise Figure D)
leukocytosis............... (lū-kō-sī-TŌ-sis)	increase in the number of white (blood) cells
lipoid .... (LIP-oid)	resembling fat

> 🧠 **Ellipsis** is the practice of omitting an essential part of a word by common consent. Note this practice in the terms **leukocyte** (white **blood** cell) and erythrocyte (red **blood** cell). The word root for blood is omitted.

EXERCISE FIGURE D

Fill in the blanks to label this diagram of blood cells.

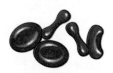

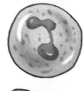

1. erthr/o/ cyte
    red /cv/ cell(s)

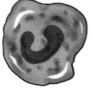

2. leuk/o/ cyte
    white /cv/ cell(s)

To check your answers, go to p. 58, Answers to Chapter 2 Exercises.

EXERCISE FIGURE E

Fill in the blanks to label the diagram.

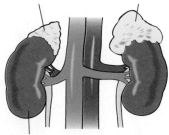

Normal adrenal gland

Excessive development (abnormal adrenal gland)

Kidney

hyper / plasia
excessive / development

To check your answers, go to p. 58, Answers to Chapter 2 Exercises.

COMPLEMENTARY AND ALTERNATIVE MEDICINE (CAM)

According to the National Institutes of Health, **CAM** is defined as "a group of diverse medical and health care systems, practices, and products that are not presently considered to be a part of conventional medicine."

Complementary medicine is used in conjunction with conventional medicine.

Alternative medicine is used in place of conventional medicine.

Integrative medicine is the combination of mainstream medical therapies and evidence-based CAM therapies.

Use of CAM has increased dramatically in recent years as health care consumers search for a multitude of ways to treat illness and promote wellness.

CAM terms

Look for the CAM terms appearing throughout the text.

Go to Evolve at: *http://www. evolve.elsevier.com/LaFleur* for a complete list of CAM definitions.

Body Structure Terms—*cont'd*

Built from Word Parts

Term	Definition
myopathy . . . . (mī-OP-a-thē)	disease of the muscle
neuroid . . . . (NŪ-rōyd)	resembling a nerve
somatic . . . . (sō-MAT-ik)	pertaining to the body
somatogenic . . . . (sō-ma-tō-JEN-ik)	originating in the body (organic as opposed to psychologic)
somatopathy . . . . (sō-ma-TOP-a-thē)	disease of the body
somatoplasm . . . . (sō-MAT-ō-plazm)	body substance
systemic . . . . (sis-TEM-ik)	pertaining to a (body) system (or the body as a whole)
visceral . . . . (VIS-er-al)	pertaining to the internal organs

EXERCISE 17

Practice saying aloud each of the body structure terms built from word parts on pp. 37-38.

To hear the terms select Chapter 2, Chapter Exercises, Pronunciation.

☐ Place a check mark in the box when you have completed this exercise.

EXERCISE 18

Analyze and define the following body structure terms.

Example: <u>WR CV S</u> cyt / o / genic _producing cells_____

1. cytology _cyt / o / logy - study of cells_____
2. histology _hist / o / logy - study of tissue_____
3. visceral _VIS / eral - pertaining to the internal organs_
4. karyocyte _kary / o / cyte - cells w/ nucleus_____
5. karyoplasm _kary / o / plasm - substance of a nucleus_
6. systemic _syste / mic - pertaining to a (body) system_
7. cytoplasm _cyto / plasm cell substance_____

8. somatic _so/matic - pertaining to the body_

9. somatogenic _somat/o/genic - originating in the body_

10. somatoplasm _somat/o/plasm - body substance_

11. somatopathy _somat/o/pathy - disease of the body_

12. neuroid _neur/oid - Resembling a nerve_

13. myopathy _my/o/pathy - disease of the muscle_

14. erythrocyte _erythr/ocyte - Red blood cell_

15. leukocyte _leuk/ocyte - white blood cell_

16. epithelial _epith/elial - pertaining to epithelium_

17. lipoid _li/poid - Resembling fat_

18. hyperplasia _hyper/plasia - excessive development_

19. erythrocytosis _erythr/o/cyt/o/sis - increase of number of Red cells_

20. leukocytosis _leuk/o/cyt/osis - increase number of white blood cells_

21. hypoplasia _hyp/o/plasia - incomplete development of organ or tissue_

22. cytoid _cyt/oid - Resembling a cell_

23. dysplasia _dys/plasia - abnormal development_

EXERCISE 19

Build medical terms for the following body structure definitions by using the word parts you have learned.

Example: producing cells   cyt / o / genic
                     WR /CV/ S

1. cell substance   Cyt /o/ plasm
                        WR /CV/ S

2. substance of a nucleus   Kary /o/ plasm
                        WR /CV/ S

3. pertaining to the body   Somat / ic
                        WR / S

4. disease of the muscle   my /o/ pathy
                        WR /CV/ S

5. body substance   Somat /o/ plasm
                        WR /CV/ S

6. pertaining to the internal organs   Vis / ceral
                        WR / S

7. originating in the body

     somat / o / genic
     WR   /CV/   S

8. disease of the body

     somat / o / pathy
     WR   /CV/   S

9. red (blood) cell

     erythr / o / cyte
     WR   /CV/   S

10. resembling a nerve

     neur / oid
     WR   S

11. pertaining to a (body) system

     system / ic
     WR   S

12. white (blood) cell

     leuk / o / cyte
     WR   /CV/   S

13. cell with a nucleus

     kary / o / cyte
     WR   /CV/   S

14. resembling fat

     lip / oid
     WR   S

15. study of cells

     cyt / o / logy
     WR   /CV/   S

16. excessive development (of cells)

     hyper / plasia
     P   S(WR)

17. resembling a cell

     cyt / oid
     WR   S

18. pertaining to epithelium

     epitheli / al
     WR   S

19. study of tissue

     hist / o / logy
     WR   /CV/   S

20. increase in the number of red (blood) cells

     erythr / o / cyt / osis
     WR   /CV/   WR   S

21. incomplete development (of an organ or tissue)

     hypo / plasia
     P   S(WR)

22. increase in the number of white (blood) cells

     leuk / o / cyt / osis
     WR   /CV/   WR   S

23. abnormal development

     dys / plasia
     P   S(WR)

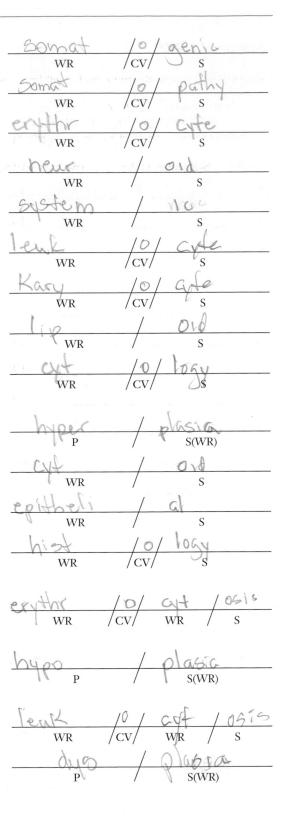

EXERCISE 20

Spell each of the body structure terms built from word parts on pp. 37-38 by having someone dictate them to you.

To hear and spell the terms select Chapter 2, Chapter Exercises, Spelling. You may type the terms on the screen or write them below in the spaces provided.

☐ Place a check mark in the box if you have completed this exercise using your CD-ROM.

1. _____
2. _____
3. _____
4. _____
5. _____
6. _____
7. _____
8. _____
9. _____
10. _____
11. _____
12. _____

13. _____
14. _____
15. _____
16. _____
17. _____
18. _____
19. _____
20. _____
21. _____
22. _____
23. _____
24. _____

Complementary Terms

Complementary terms complete the vocabulary presented in the chapter by describing signs, symptoms, medical specialties, specialists, and related words.

Built from Word Parts

The following terms are built from word parts you have already learned and can be translated literally to find their meanings. Further explanation of terms beyond the definition of their word parts, if needed, is included in parentheses.

Term	Definition
cancerous . . . . (KAN-ser-us)	pertaining to cancer
carcinogen . . . . (kar-SIN-o-jen)	substance that causes cancer
carcinogenic . . . . (*kar*-sin-ō-JEN-ik)	producing cancer
cyanosis . . . . (sī-a-NŌ-sis)	abnormal condition of blue (bluish discoloration of the skin caused by inadequate supply of oxygen in the blood) (Figure 2-3)

Complementary Terms—*cont'd*
Built from Word Parts

Term	Definition
diagnosis (Dx) . . . . (dī-ag-NŌ-sis)	state of complete knowledge (identifying a disease)
etiology . . . . (ē-tē-OL-o-jē)	study of causes (of diseases)
iatrogenic. . . . . (ī-*at*-rō-JEN-ik)	produced by a physician (the unexpected results from a treatment prescribed by a physician)
iatrology. . . . . (ī-a-TROL-o-jē)	study of medicine
metastasis (mets) . . . . (*pl.* metastases) (me-TAS-ta-sis) (me-TAS-ta-sēz)	beyond control (transfer of disease from one organ to another, as in the transfer of malignant tumors) (Figure 2-4)
neopathy . . . . (nē-OP-a-thē)	new disease
oncogenic . . . . (*ong*-kō-JEN-ik)	causing tumors
oncologist . . . . (ong-KOL-o-jist)	a physician who studies and treats tumors
oncology . . . . (ong-KOL-o-jē)	study of tumors (a branch of medicine concerned with the study of malignant tumors)
pathogenic. . . . . (path-ō-JEN-ik)	producing disease
pathologist. . . . . (pa-THOL-o-jist)	a physician who studies diseases (examines biopsies and performs autopsies to determine the cause of disease or death)
pathology. . . . . (pa-THOL-o-jē)	study of disease (a branch of medicine dealing with the study of the causes of disease and death)
prognosis (Px) . . . . (prog-NŌ-sis)	state of before knowledge (prediction of the outcome of disease)
xanthochromic. . . . . (*zan*-thō-KRŌ-mik)	pertaining to yellow color
xanthosis . . . . (zan-THŌ-sis)	abnormal condition of yellow (discoloration)

ONCOLOGY AND ONCOLOGIC
are used to name the medical specialty and health care nursing units devoted to the treatment and care of cancer patients.

PROGNOSIS
was used by Hippocrates to mean the same then as now: **to foretell the course of a disease.**

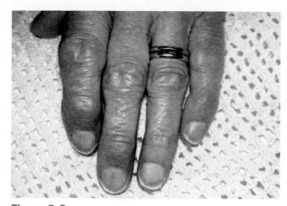

Figure 2-3

Cyanosis in an elderly patient.

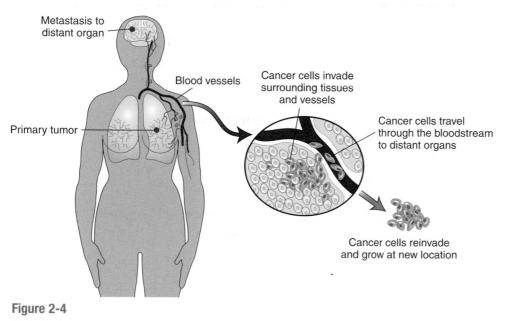

Figure 2-4

Metastasis.

EXERCISE 21

Practice saying aloud each of the complementary terms built from word parts on pp. 41-42.

 To hear the terms select Chapter 2, Chapter Exercises, Pronunciation.

☐ Place a check mark in the box when you have completed this exercise.

EXERCISE 22

Analyze and define the following complementary terms.

         WR CV S

Example: path / o / genic   *producing disease*

            CF

1. pathology   *path/o/logy - study of disease*

2. pathologist   *path/o/logist - physician who studies disease*

3. metastasis _Meta/stasis ~ beyond control_

4. oncogenic _Onc/o/genic ~ causing tumors_

5. oncology _Onc/o/logy - Study of tumors_

6. neopathy _neo/pathy ~ new disease_

7. cancerous _Cancer/ous - pertaining t cancer_

8. carcinogenic _Carci/o/genic - producing cancer_

9. cyanosis _Cyan/osis - abnormal condition of blue_

10. etiology _eti/o/logy - study of the cause of disease_

11. xanthosis _Xanth/osis - abnormal condition of yellow_

12. xanthochromic _Xanth/o/chrom/ic - pertaining to yellow_

13. carcinogen _carcin/o/gen - substance that causes cancer_

14. oncologist _oncol/o/gist - physician who studies and treats tumors_

15. prognosis _progn/o/sis - state of before knowledge_

16. diagnosis _diagn/o/sis - state of complete knowledge_

17. iatrogenic _iatr/o/genic produced by a physician_

18. iatrology _iatr/o/logy - study of medicine_

EXERCISE 23

Build medical terms for the following definitions of complementary terms by using the word parts you have learned.

Example: producing disease path / o / genic
                                   WR / CV / S

1. pertaining to yellow color   Xanth / o / chrom / ic
                                  WR / CV / WR / S

2. beyond control   meta / stasis
                                    P / S(WR)

3. new disease   neo / pathy
                                   P / S(WR)

4. study of the cause (of disease) eti / o / logy
                                    WR / CV / S

5. study of tumors   onc / o / logy
                                 WR / CV / S

6. study of diseases   path / o / logy
                                 WR / CV / S

7. a physician who studies diseases path / o / logist
                                     WR / CV / S

8. abnormal condition of yellow   Xanth / osis
                                   WR / S

9. causing tumors   onc / o / genic
   _____   WR /CV/ S

10. pertaining to cancer   cancer / ous
    _____   WR   /   S

11. abnormal condition of blue   cyan / osis
    _____   WR / S

12. producing cancer   carcin / o / genic
    _____   WR   /CV/ S

13. substance that causes cancer   carcin / o / gen
    _____   WR   /CV/ S

14. physician who studies and treats tumors   oncol / o / gist
    _____   WR   /CV/ S

15. study of medicine   iatr / o / logy
    _____   WR /CV/ S

16. state of complete knowledge   diagn / o / sis
    _____   P   / WR / S

17. produced by a physician   iatr / o / genic
    _____   WR /CV/ S

18. state of before knowledge   progn / o / sis
    _____   P   / WR / S

EXERCISE 24

Spell each of the complementary terms built from word parts on pp. 41-42 by having someone dictate them to you.

To hear and spell the terms select Chapter 2, Chapter Exercises, Spelling. You may
type the terms on the screen or write them below in the spaces provided.

☐ Place a check mark in the box if you have completed this exercise using your CD-ROM.

1. _____   10. _____

2. _____   11. _____

3. _____   12. _____

4. _____   13. _____

5. _____   14. _____

6. _____   15. _____

7. _____   16. _____

8. _____   17. _____

9. _____   18. _____

Neoadjuvant therapy is a cancer treatment that precedes other treatment, such as administering chemotherapy or radiation therapy to a patient before surgery. **Adjuvant chemotherapy** is the use of chemotherapy after or in combination with another form of cancer treatment such as administering chemotherapy after surgery or with radiation therapy. **Brachytherapy** is the use of radiotherapy in which the source of radiation is placed within or close to the area being treated, such as implantation of radiation sources into the breast to treat cancer.

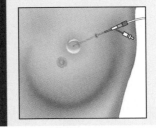

IDIOPATHIC is derived from the Greek word **idios** meaning **one's own** and **path** or **disease.** The term probably originated from the idea that disease of unknown origin comes from within oneself and is not acquired from without.

INFLAMMATORY AND INFLAMMATION are spelled with two *m*'s. *Inflame* and *inflamed* have one *m*.

MALIGNANT is derived from the Latin word root **mal** meaning **bad,** as used in **malicious, malaise, malady,** and **malign.**

Complementary Terms

Not Built from Word Parts

 Medical terms not built from word parts cannot be translated literally to find their meanings. *The terms are learned by memorizing the whole word by using recall and spelling exercises.*

The terms in this list are not built from word parts. The terms are commonly used in the medical world and you will need to know them. *In some of the words, you may recognize a word part; however, these terms cannot be literally translated to find the meaning.* New knowledge may have changed the meanings of the terms since they were coined; some terms are eponyms, some are acronyms, and some have no apparent explanation for their names. Memorization is used in the following exercises to learn the terms.

Term	Definition
benign (be-NĪN)	not malignant, nonrecurrent, favorable for recovery (Figure 2-5)
carcinoma in situ (kar-si-NŌ-ma) (in-SĪ-too)	cancer in the early stage before invading surrounding tissue (Figure 2-6)
chemotherapy (chemo) (kē-mō-THER-a-pē)	treatment of cancer with drugs
encapsulated (en-KAP-sū-lā-ted)	enclosed in a capsule, as with benign tumors (Figure 2-7)
exacerbation (eg-*zas*-er-BĀ-shun)	increase in the severity of a disease or its symptoms
idiopathic (id-ē-ō-PATH-ik)	pertaining to disease of unknown origin
inflammation (in-fla-MĀ-shun)	response to injury or destruction of tissue characterized by redness, swelling, heat, and pain
in vitro (in VĒ-trō)	within a glass, observable within a test tube
in vivo (in VĒ-vō)	within the living body
malignant (ma-LIG-nant)	tending to become progressively worse and to cause death, as in cancer (Figure 2-5)
radiation therapy (XRT) (rā-dē-A-shun) (THER-a-pē)	treatment of cancer with a radioactive substance, x-ray, or radiation (also called **radiation oncology** and **radiotherapy**) (Figure 2-8)
remission (rē-MISH-un)	improvement or absence of signs of disease

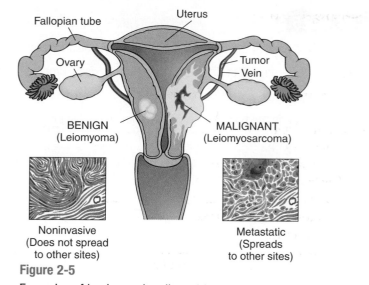

Fallopian tube

Uterus

Ovary

Tumor
Vein

BENIGN
(Leiomyoma)

MALIGNANT
(Leiomyosarcoma)

Noninvasive
(Does not spread
to other sites)

Metastatic
(Spreads
to other sites)

Figure 2-5

Examples of benign and malignant tumors.

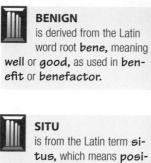

BENIGN
is derived from the Latin word root **bene**, meaning **well** or **good**, as used in **benefit** or **benefactor**.

SITU
is from the Latin term **situs**, which means **position** or **place**. Think of **in situ** as meaning "in place" or "not wandering around."

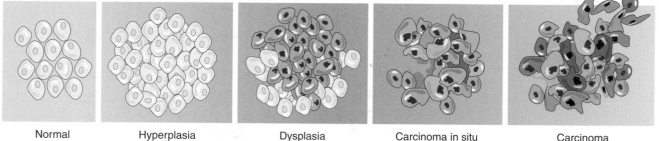

Normal

Hyperplasia

Dysplasia

Carcinoma in situ
(severe dysplasia)

Carcinoma
(invasive)

Figure 2-6

Progression of cell growth.

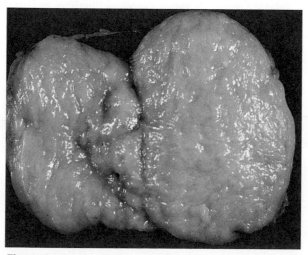

Figure 2-7

An encapsulated benign tumor.

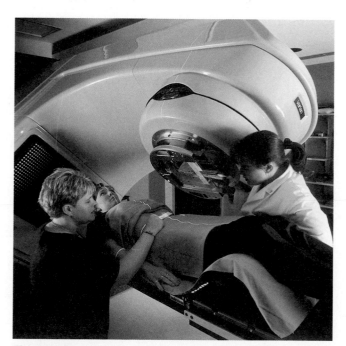

Figure 2-8

Radiation therapist preparing the patient for cancer therapy.

EXERCISE 25

Practice saying aloud each of the complementary terms not built from word parts on p. 46.

 To hear the terms select Chapter 2, Chapter Exercises, Pronunciation.

☐ Place a check mark in the box when you have completed this exercise.

EXERCISE 26

Write the definitions for the following terms.

1. benign _not malignant, nonrecurrent_
2. malignant _tending to become progressively worse_
3. remission _improvement or absence of signs of disease_
4. idiopathic _pertaining to disease of unknown origin_
5. inflammation _Response to injury or destruction of tissue_
6. chemotherapy _treatment of cancer with drugs_
7. radiation therapy _treatment of cancer with Radioactive substance_
8. encapsulated _enclosed with a capsule, benign tumors_
9. in vitro _within a glass_
10. in vivo _within the living body_
11. carcinoma in situ _Cancer in the early stages_
12. exacerbation _Increase in the severity disease or its symptom_

EXERCISE 27

Spell each of the complementary terms not built from word parts on p. 46 by having someone dictate them to you.

 To hear and spell the terms select Chapter 2, Chapter Exercises, Spelling. You may type the terms on the screen or write them below in the spaces provided.

☐ Place a check mark in the box if you have completed this exercise using your CD-ROM.

1. _____
2. _____
3. _____
4. _____
5. _____
6. _____

7. _____
8. _____
9. _____
10. _____
11. _____
12. _____

Refer to Appendix E for pharmacology terms related to oncology.

Plural Endings for Medical Terms

Most medical terms originate from Greek and Latin; therefore, plural endings differ from those used in English. Table 2-2, Common Plural Endings, lists the most common singular and plural endings used in medical terminology. When appropriate, both singular and plural endings are included in the word lists throughout the text, such as metastasis/metastases on p. 42.

TABLE 2-2
Common Plural Endings

Singular Endings	Plural Formation	Singular Form		Plural Form	
-a	-ae	verteb**ra**		vertebr**ae**	
-ax	-aces	thor**ax**		thor**aces**	
-is	-es	test**is**		test**es**	
-ix	-ices	append**ix**		append**ices**	
-ma	-mata	carcino**ma**		carcino**mata**	
-on	-a	gangli**on**		gangli**a**	
-sis	-ses	metasta**sis**		metasta**ses**	
-um	-a	ov**um**		ov**a**	
-us	-i	fung**us**		fung**i**	
-nx	-nges	lary**nx**		lary**nges**	
-y	-ies	biops**y**		biops**ies**	

Complete the following exercises to become familiar with how plurals are formed. Do not be concerned about the meaning of these terms; concentrate only on the plural endings.

EXERCISE 28

Convert each of the following terms from singular to plural. Refer to Table 2-2, Plural Endings, on p. 49 for guidance.

1. etiology _etiologies_
2. *Staphylococcus* _Staphylococci_
3. cyanosis _cyanoses_
4. bacterium _bacteria_
5. nucleus _nuclei_
6. pharynx _pharynges_
7. sarcoma _sarcomata_
8. carcinoma _carcinomata_
9. anastomosis _anastomoses_
10. pubis _pubes_
11. prognosis _prognoses_
12. spermatozoon _spermatozoa_
13. fimbria _fimbriae_
14. thorax _thoraces_
15. appendix _appendices_

EXERCISE 29

Circle the correct singular or plural form in each sentence.

1. During a colonoscopy the gastroenterologist noted that the patient had several (**diverticula, diverticulum**) in his transverse colon.

2. Bronchogenic carcinoma was diagnosed in the patient's left (**bronchus, bronchi**).

3. Bilateral (two sides) orchiditis is inflammation of the (**testes, testis**).

4. The light brown mole with notched borders turned out to be a (**melanomata, melanoma**).

5. Multiple (**embolus, emboli**) were observed on the lung scan.

6. Many (**diagnosis,** **diagnoses**) of benign tumors are picked up during whole-body scanning.

7. Diagnostic studies have shown (**metastasis,** **metastases**) of the patient's carcinoma of the breast to both her lungs and brain.

Abbreviations

Abbreviations are frequently used verbally and in writing to communicate in the medical and health care setting. Abbreviations of the terms included in the chapter are listed below.

Ca	carcinoma
chemo	chemotherapy
Dx	diagnosis
mets.	metastasis
Px.	prognosis
RBC	red blood cell
XRT	radiation therapy
WBC.	white blood cell

Refer to Appendix D for a complete list of abbreviations and for the ISMP's list of error-prone abbreviations, which include The Joint Commission's "do not use" list.

EXERCISE 30

Write the term for each of the abbreviations in the following paragraph.

A 55-year-old white woman was admitted to the oncology unit with a **Dx** _diagnosis_ of **Ca** _carcinoma_ of the breast, **mets** _metastasis_ to the lung. Her **Px** _prognosis_ was tentative. Laboratory tests, including **RBC** _Red Blood Cell_ _____ _____ and **WBC** _White_ _Blood_ _cell_ counts, were ordered. She will receive both **chemo** _Chemotherapy_ and **XRT** _Radiation therapy_.

PRACTICAL APPLICATION

EXERCISE 31   *Interact with Medical Documents*

A. Below is a physician's progress note. Complete the record by writing the medical terms in the blanks that correspond to the numbered definitions.

University Hospital and Medical Center
4700 North Main Street • Wellness, Arizona 54321 • (987) 555-3210

PATIENT NAME: Morris Greeley   **CASE NUMBER:** 830293-ONC
DATE OF BIRTH: 08/03/19XX   **DATE:** 02/12/20XX

PROGRESS NOTE

SUBJECTIVE: Mr. Greeley arrives today for a 1. *Chemotherapy* treatment for 2. *adeno carcinoma* of the sigmoid colon.

He had an anterior sigmoid resection in October. 3. *pathology* study revealed 4. *Malignant* tumor cells in two of six lymph nodes.

The 5FU/Leucovorin protocol is being administered weekly for 6 weeks. Today is his sixth infusion. We plan to start 5. *Radiation Therapy* after a 2-week hiatus from the chemotherapy.

The patient continues to do well and is receiving significant support from his family. He has had no hair loss, oral ulcerations, abdominal pain, nausea, or diarrhea.

OBJECTIVE: Vital signs show a temperature of 98. Pulse is 60. Respirations 20. Blood pressure is 152/65. His current weight is 183 pounds. HEENT: Tongue and pharynx are normal. PULMONARY: Clear to auscultation. HEART: Regular rate and rhythm without a murmur, rub, or gallop. ABDOMEN: Soft and nontender. No masses or organomegaly. EXTREMITIES: No edema or 6. *cyanosis*.

ASSESSMENT:
1. Adenocarcinoma of the sigmoid colon with 7. *metastasis* to regional lymph nodes.

PLAN:
1. 5FU/Leucovorin protocol as outlined above, treatment six of six today, followed by radiation therapy after 2-week period of rest.

Brian Smith, MD

BS/mcm

---

1. treatment of cancer by using drugs
2. cancerous tumor of glandular tissue
3. study of disease
4. tending to become progressively worse

5. treatment of cancer by using radioactive substance, x-rays, or radiation
6. abnormal condition of blue
7. beyond control

EXERCISE **31**   *Interact with Medical Documents—cont'd*

B. Read the office visit report and answer the following questions.

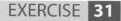

| 49920 THATCH, MARTIN R. | ＿□✕ |

File Patient Navigate Custom Fields Help

| Patient Chart | Lab | Rad | Notes | Documents | Rx | Scheduling | Images | Billing |

Name: **THATCH, MARTIN R.**   MR#: **49920**   Sex: **M**
DOB: **5/12/19XX**

POSTOPERATIVE OFFICE VISIT

ENCOUNTER DATE: 10/21/20XX

The patient is a 45-year-old white male who underwent removal of a 2.5-cm firm mass of the lateral portion of the proximal right thigh one week ago. Inspection of operative site shows a normal healing wound. Preoperative lab work showed a normal erythrocyte and leukocyte count. Histology of the surgical specimen revealed an encapsulated lipoma. The etiology of the lipoma is unknown, but it is definitely a benign lesion. His prognosis is excellent.

Electronically signed by: Ronald Bryan, MD 10/21/20XX 11:15 AM

| Start | Log On/Off | Print | Edit |

---

1. The firm mass was confirmed as a lipoma from the surgical specimen in which area of study?
   a. cell
   b. tissue
   c. blood
   d. plasma

2. The lipoma was
   a. spreading.
   b. enclosed in a capsule.
   c. inflamed.
   d. blue in color.

3. *Erythr* and *leuk* refer to the _____ of cells.
   a. size
   b. shape
   c. amount
   d. color

4. Write the plural form of
   a. prognosis _prognoses_
   b. lipoma _lipomata_
   c. histology _histologies_

EXERCISE **32**   *Interpret Medical Terms*

To test your understanding of the terms introduced in this chapter, circle the words that correctly complete each sentence. The italicized words refer to the correct answer.

1. Mr. Roberts was diagnosed as having a cancerous *tumor of connective tissue*, or (**sarcoma**, **melanoma**, **lipoma**). The doctor said the tumor was *becoming progressively worse*; that is, it was (**benign**, **malignant**, **pathogenic**).

2. The blood test showed an *increased amount of red blood cells*, or (**erythrocytosis**, **leukocytosis**, **cyanosis**).

3. (**Organic**, **Visceral**, **Systemic**) means *pertaining to internal organs*.

4. A *tumor composed of fat*, or (**neuroma**, **carcinoma**, **lipoma**), is benign, or (**recurrent**, **nonrecurrent**, **cancerous**).

5. Many substances are thought to be *cancer producing*, or (**carcinogenic**, **carcinogen**, **cancerous**).

6. *Etiology* is the study of (**the causes of disease**, **tissue disease**, **the causes of tumors**).

7. A *tumor* may be called a (**cytoplasm**, **neoplasm**, **karyoplasm**).

8. The pain *originated in the body*, or was (**somatogenic**, **oncogenic**, **pathogenic**).

9. Any *disease of a muscle* is called (**myoma**, **myopathy**, **somatopathy**).

10. The term for *abnormal development* is (**hypoplasia**, **dysplasia**, **hyperplasia**).

11. The term that means *produced by a physician* is (**diagnosis**, **iatrogenic**, **prognosis**).

12. The incidence of malignant *black tumor* (**fibrosarcoma**, **fibroma**, **melanoma**) is increasing in the white population. One *study of disease* (**pathology**, **pathogenic**, **liposarcoma**) finding influencing *state of before knowledge* (**cancer in situ**, **in vitro**, **prognosis**) may be tumor thickness.

13. The term that means *within the living organism* is (**in vitro**, **in vivo**, **encapsulated**).

14. A (**liposarcoma**, **fibroma**, **myoma**) is a *malignant tumor*.

15. (**DNA**, **RBC**, **WBC**) regulates the *activities of a cell*.

EXERCISE **33**   *Read Medical Terms in Use*

Practice pronunciation of terms by reading aloud the following medical document.

Use the pronunciation key after each medical term to assist you in saying the words. The script contains medical terms not yet presented. Treat them as information only; you will learn more about them as you continue to study. Or, if desired, look for their meanings in your medical dictionary.

 To hear these terms select Chapter 2, Chapter Exercises, Read Medical Terms in Use.

cytology - study of cells

A 54-year-old woman presented to the office with a 3-week history of bloody diarrhea. She had been diagnosed with ulcerative colitis at age 25 years. She was referred for a colonoscopy. The examination revealed a suspicious lesion in the transverse colon. A biopsy was performed and a **cytology** (sī-TOL-o-jē) specimen was obtained. The **pathologist** (pa-THOL-o-jist) made a **diagnosis** (dī-ag-NŌ-sis) of **carcinoma** (kar-si-NŌ-ma) of the colon. Advanced **dysplasia** (dis-PLĀ-zha) and **inflammation** (in-fla-MĀ-shun) existed in the specimen. The patient underwent surgery and was found to have no evidence of **metastasis** (me-TAS-ta-sis). Her entire colon was removed because of a high risk for developing a **malignant** (ma-LIG-nant) lesion in the remaining colon. She made an uneventful recovery and was referred to an **oncologist** (ong-KOL-o-jist) for consideration of **chemotherapy** (kē-mō-THER-a-pē). Her **prognosis** (prog-NŌ-sis) is generally positive. **Radiation therapy** (rā-dē-Ā-shun) (THER-a-pē) is not indicated in this case.

EXERCISE **34**   *Comprehend Medical Terms in Use*

Test your comprehension of terms in the previous medical document by answering *T* for true and *F* for false.

F   1. The cancer has spread from the colon to other surrounding organs.

T   2. The specimen is described as having abnormal development.

F   3. The patient's prognosis is carcinoma of the colon.

T   4. The patient's colon was removed to avoid development of a malignant lesion in the remaining colon.

F   5. The patient was referred to a pathologist for consideration of treatment for the cancer with drugs.

 WEB LINK
For additional information on cancer visit the National Cancer Institute at www.nic.nih.gov.

CHAPTER REVIEW

CHAPTER REVIEW ON CD-ROM

Use the CD-ROM that accompanies this textbook to play and practice what you have learned in this chapter. The Chapter Exercises, Practice Activities, Animations, and Games allow you to hear, see, and interact with the chapter content.

Chapter Exercises

Exercises in this section of your CD-ROM correlate to exercises in your textbook. You may have completed them as you worked through the chapter.

☐ Pronunciation
☐ Spelling
☐ Read Medical Terms in Use

Practice Activities

Practice in study mode, then test your learning in assessment mode. Keep track of your scores from assessment mode if you wish.

SCORE

☐ Define Word Parts   _____
☐ Plural Endings   _____
☐ Analyze Medical Terms   _____
☐ Build Medical Terms   _____
☐ Define Medical Terms   _____
☐ Use It   _____
☐ Hear It and Type It: _____
   Clinical Vignettes

Animations

☐ Breast Cancer Metastasis

Games

☐ Name that Word Part
☐ Term Storm
☐ Termbusters
☐ Medical Millionaire

REVIEW OF WORD PARTS

Can you define and spell the following word parts?

Combining Forms

aden/o	erythr/o	leuk/o	rhabd/o
cancer/o	eti/o	lip/o	sarc/o
carcin/o	fibr/o	melan/o	somat/o
chlor/o	gno/o	my/o	system/o
chrom/o	hist/o	neur/o	viscer/o
cyan/o	iatr/o	onc/o	xanth/o
cyt/o	kary/o	organ/o	
epitheli/o	lei/o	path/o	

Prefixes

dia-
dys-
hyper-
hypo-
meta-
neo-
pro-

Suffixes

-al	-logist	-pathy
-cyte	-logy	-plasia
-gen	-oid	-plasm
-genesis	-oma	-sarcoma
-genic	-osis	-sis
-ic	-ous	-stasis

REVIEW OF TERMS

Can you build, analyze, define, spell, and pronounce the following terms *built from word parts?*

Oncology	**Body Structure**	**Complementary**
adenocarcinoma	cytogenic	cancerous
adenoma	cytoid	carcinogen
carcinoma (Ca)	cytology	carcinogenic
chloroma	cytoplasm	cyanosis
epithelioma	dysplasia	diagnosis (Dx)
fibroma	epithelial	etiology
fibrosarcoma	erythrocyte (RBC)	iatrogenic
leiomyoma	erythrocytosis	iatrology
leiomyosarcoma	histology	metastasis (mets)
lipoma	hyperplasia	neopathy
liposarcoma	hypoplasia	oncogenic
melanocarcinoma	karyocyte	oncologist
melanoma	karyoplasm	oncology
myoma	leukocyte (WBC)	pathogenic
neoplasm	leukocytosis	pathologist
neuroma	lipoid	pathology
rhabdomyoma	myopathy	prognosis (Px)
rhabdomyosarcoma	neuroid	xanthochromic
sarcoma	somatic	xanthosis
	somatogenic	
	somatopathy	
	somatoplasm	
	systemic	
	visceral	

Can you define, pronounce, and spell the following terms *not built from word parts?*

Complementary

benign
carcinoma in situ
chemotherapy (chemo)
encapsulated
exacerbation
idiopathic
inflammation
in vitro
in vivo
malignant
radiation therapy (XRT)
remission

ANSWERS

Exercise Figures

Exercise Figure

A. 1. cell: cyt/o
   2. tissue: hist/o
   3. organ: organ/o
   4. system: system/o

Exercise Figure

B. 1. neur/o
   2. epitheli/o
   3. sarc/o
   4. my/o

Exercise Figure

C. 1. carcin/oma
   2. melan/oma
   3. sarc/oma
   4. rhabd/o/my/o/sarcoma

Exercise Figure

D. 1. erythr/o/cyte
   2. leuk/o/cyte

Exercise Figure

E. hyper/plasia

Exercise 1

1. h   6. f
2. e   7. c
3. d   8. a
4. k   9. b
5. g   10. j

Exercise 2

1. h   5. g
2. b   6. a
3. c   7. f
4. e

Exercise 3

1. flesh, connective   7. muscle
   tissue   8. nerve
2. fat   9. organ
3. nucleus   10. system
4. internal organs   11. epithelium
5. cell   12. fiber
6. tissue   13. gland

Exercise 4

1. viscer/o   8. my/o
2. epitheli/o   9. lip/o
3. organ/o   10. system/o
4. kary/o   11. sarc/o
5. cyt/o   12. fibr/o
6. hist/o   13. aden/o
7. neur/o

Exercise 5

1. tumor, mass
2. cancer
3. cause (of disease)
4. disease
5. body
6. cancer
7. rod-shaped, striated
8. smooth
9. knowledge
10. physician, medicine

Exercise 6

1. path/o   5. somat/o
2. onc/o   6. lei/o
3. eti/o   7. rhabd/o
4. a. cancer/o   8. gno/o
   b. carcin/o   9. iatr/o

Exercise 7

1. blue   5. color
2. red   6. black
3. white   7. green
4. yellow

Exercise 8

1. cyan/o   5. xanth/o
2. erythr/o   6. chrom/o
3. leuk/o   7. chlor/o
4. melan/o

Exercise 9

1. new
2. above, excessive
3. after, beyond, change
4. below, incomplete, deficient
5. painful, abnormal, difficult, labored
6. through, complete
7. before

Exercise 10

1. neo-   5. dys-
2. hyper-   6. dia-
3. hypo-   7. pro-
4. meta-

Exercise 11

1. i   9. p
2. l   10. c
3. e   11. n
4. f   12. k
5. g   13. q
6. j   14. m
7. h   15. a
8. b   16. o

Exercise 12

1. one who studies and treats (specialist, physician)
2. disease
3. study of
4. pertaining to
5. control, stop, standing
6. cell
7. abnormal condition
8. pertaining to
9. growth, substance, formation
10. pertaining to
11. condition of formation, development, growth
12. resembling
13. substance or agent that produces or causes
14. producing, originating, causing
15. tumor, swelling
16. origin, cause
17. malignant tumor
18. state of

Exercise 13

Pronunciation Exercise

Exercise 14

1. WR   S
   sarc/oma
   tumor composed of connective tissue
2. WR   S
   melan/oma
   black tumor
3. WR   S
   epitheli/oma
   tumor composed of epithelium
4. WR   S
   lip/oma
   tumor composed of fat
5. P   S(WR)
   neo/plasm
   new growth
6. WR   S
   my/oma
   tumor composed of muscle
7. WR   S
   neur/oma
   tumor composed of nerve
8. WR   S
   carcin/oma
   cancerous tumor
9. WR CV WR   S
   melan/o/carcin/oma
       CF
   cancerous black tumor

10. WR CVWR CV   S
    rhabd/o/my/o/sarcoma
         CF   CF
    malignant tumor of striated muscle
11. WRCVWR S
    lei/o/my/oma
       CF
    tumor composed of smooth muscle
12. WR   CVWR S
    rhabd/o/my/oma
         CF
    tumor composed of striated muscle
13. WR S
    fibr/oma
    tumor composed of fiber (fibrous
        tissue)
14. WR CV   S
    lip/o/sarcoma
       CF
    malignant tumor of fat
15. WR CV   S
    fibr/o/sarcoma
        CF
    malignant tumor of fiber
        (fibrous tissue)
16. WR   S
    aden/oma
    tumor composed of glandular tissue
17. WR CV WR   S
    aden/o/carcin/oma
        CF
    cancerous tumor composed of
        glandular tissue
18. WR   S
    chlor/oma
    tumor of green color

Exercise 15
1. melan/oma
2. carcin/oma
3. neo/plasm
4. epitheli/oma
5. sarc/oma
6. melan/o/carcin/oma
7. neur/oma
8. my/oma
9. rhabd/o/my/o/sarcoma
10. lei/o/my/oma
11. rhabd/o/my/oma
12. lei/o/my/o/sarcoma
13. lip/o/sarcoma
14. fibr/oma
15. fibr/o/sarcoma
16. aden/oma
17. aden/o/carcin/oma
18. chlor/oma

Exercise 16
Spelling Exercise; see text p. 36.

Exercise 17
Pronunciation Exercise

Exercise 18
1. WR CV S
   cyt/o/logy
       CF
   study of cells
2. WR CV S
   hist/o/logy
       CF
   study of tissue
3. WR S
   viscer/al
   pertaining to internal organs
4. WR CV S
   kary/o/cyte
        CF
   cell with a nucleus
5. WR CV S
   kary/o/plasm
        CF
   substance of a nucleus
6. WR   S
   system/ic
   pertaining to a (body) system
7. WR CV S
   cyt/o/plasm
       CF
   cell substance
8. WR   S
   somat/ic
   pertaining to the body
9. WR CV S
   somat/o/genic
         CF
   originating in the body
10. WR CV S
    somat/o/plasm
          CF
    body substance
11. WR CV S
    somat/o/pathy
          CF
    disease of the body
12. WR   S
    neur/oid
    resembling a nerve
13. WR CV S
    my/o/pathy
        CF
    disease of the muscle

14. WR CV S
    erythr/o/cyte
          CF
    red (blood) cell
15. WR CV S
    leuk/o/cyte
         CF
    white (blood) cell
16. WR   S
    epitheli/al
    pertaining to epithelium
17. WR S
    lip/oid
    resembling fat
18. P   S(WR)
    hyper/plasia
    excessive development (of cells)
19. WR CV WR S
    erythr/o/cyt/osis
          CF
    increase in the number of red (blood)
        cells
20. WR CV WR S
    leuk/o/cyt/osis
        CF
    increase in the number of white
        (blood) cells
21. P   S(WR)
    hypo/plasia
    incomplete development
        (of an organ or tissue)
22. WR S
    cyt/oid
    resembling a cell
23. P   S(WR)
    dys/plasia
    abnormal development

Exercise 19
1. cyt/o/plasm
2. kary/o/plasm
3. somat/ic
4. my/o/pathy
5. somat/o/plasm
6. viscer/al
7. somat/o/genic
8. somat/o/pathy
9. erythr/o/cyte
10. neur/oid
11. system/ic
12. leuk/o/cyte
13. kary/o/cyte
14. lip/oid
15. cyt/o/logy
16. hyper/plasia
17. cyt/oid
18. epitheli/al
19. hist/o/logy
20. erythr/o/cyt/osis

21. hypo/plasia
22. leuk/o/cyt/osis
23. dys/plasia

Exercise 20
Spelling Exercise; see text p. 41.

Exercise 21
Pronunciation Exercise

Exercise 22
1. WR CV S
   path/o/logy
     CF
   study of disease
2. WR CV S
   path/o/logist
     CF
   a physician who studies diseases
3. P   S(WR)
   meta/stasis
   beyond control (transfer of disease)
4. WR CV S
   onc/o/genic
     CF
   causing tumors
5. WR CV S
   onc/o/logy
     CF
   study of tumors
6. P   S(WR)
   neo/pathy
   new disease
7. WR   S
   cancer/ous
   pertaining to cancer
8. WR CV S
   carcin/o/genic
        CF
   producing cancer
9. WR   S
   cyan/osis
   abnormal condition of blue (bluish
     discoloration of the skin)
10. WR CV S
    eti/o/logy
       CF
    study of causes (of disease)
11. WR   S
    xanth/osis
    abnormal condition of yellow
12. WR CV WR S
    xanth/o/chrom/ic
         CF
    pertaining to yellow color

13. WR CV S
    carcin/o/gen
        CF
    substance that causes cancer
14. WR CV S
    onc/o/logist
       CF
    physician who studies and treats tumors
15. P WR S
    pro/gno/sis
    state of before knowledge
16. P WR S
    dia/gno/sis
    state of complete knowledge
17. WR CV S
    iatr/o/genic
        CF
    produced by a physician
18. WR CV S
    iatr/o/logy
        CF
    study of medicine

Exercise 23
1. xanth/o/chrom/ic
2. meta/stasis
3. neo/pathy
4. eti/o/logy
5. onc/o/logy
6. path/o/logy
7. path/o/logist
8. xanth/osis
9. onc/o/genic
10. cancer/ous
11. cyan/osis
12. carcin/o/genic
13. carcin/o/gen
14. onc/o/logist
15. iatr/o/logy
16. dia/gno/sis
17. iatr/o/genic
18. pro/gno/sis

Exercise 24
Spelling Exercise; see text p. 45.

Exercise 25
Pronunciation Exercise

Exercise 26
1. not malignant, nonrecurrent, favor-
   able for recovery
2. tending to become progressively
   worse and to cause death, as in cancer
3. improvement or absence of signs of
   disease
4. pertaining to disease of unknown
   origin

5. response to injury or destruction of
   tissue; signs are redness, swelling,
   heat, and pain
6. treatment of cancer with drugs
7. treatment of cancer with radioactive
   substance, such as x-ray or radiation
8. enclosed in a capsule, as in benign
   tumors
9. within a glass, observable within a
   test tube
10. within the living body
11. cancer in the early stage before in-
    vading the surrounding tissue
12. increase in the severity of a disease or
    its symptoms

Exercise 27
Spelling Exercise; see text p. 48.

Exercise 28
1. etiologies
2. staphylococci
3. cyanoses
4. bacteria
5. nuclei
6. pharynges
7. sarcomata
8. carcinomata
9. anastomoses
10. pubes
11. prognoses
12. spermatozoa
13. fimbriae
14. thoraces
15. appendices

Exercise 29
1. diverticula
2. bronchus
3. testes
4. melanoma
5. emboli
6. diagnoses
7. metastases

Exercise 30
diagnosis; carcinoma; metastasis; prognosis; red blood cell; white blood cell; chemotherapy; radiation therapy

Exercise 31
A. 1. chemotherapy
2. adenocarcinoma
3. pathology
4. malignant
5. radiation therapy
6. cyanosis
7. metastasis

Exercise 31

B. 1. b
2. b
3. d
4. a. prognoses
   b. lipomata
   c. histologies

Exercise 32

1. sarcoma, malignant
2. erythrocytosis
3. visceral
4. lipoma, nonrecurrent
5. carcinogenic

6. causes of disease
7. neoplasm
8. somatogenic
9. myopathy
10. dysplasia
11. iatrogenic
12. melanoma, pathology, prognosis
13. in vivo
14. liposarcoma
15. DNA

Exercise 33

Reading Exercise

Exercise 34

1. *F*, "no evidence of metastasis" (transfer of disease from one organ to another) means the cancer has not spread to surrounding organs.
2. *T*
3. *F*, prognosis means "prediction of the outcome of disease"; diagnosis means "identifying a disease."
4. *T*
5. *F*, an oncologist treats patients with cancer; a pathologist studies body changes caused by disease usually from a specimen in a laboratory setting.

CHAPTER 3
Directional Terms, Anatomic Planes, Regions, and Quadrants

OUTLINE

ANATOMIC POSITION, 64

WORD PARTS, 64
Combining Forms, 64
Prefixes, 66
Suffixes, 66

DIRECTIONAL TERMS, 67

ANATOMIC PLANES, 72

ABDOMINOPELVIC REGIONS, 75

ABDOMINOPELVIC QUADRANTS, 78
Abbreviations, 80

PRACTICAL APPLICATION, 81
Interact with Medical Documents, 81
Interpret Medical Terms, 82
Read Medical Terms in Use, 83
Comprehend Medical Terms in Use, 83

CHAPTER REVIEW, 84

TABLE 3-1 ANATOMIC PLANES AND DIAGNOSTIC IMAGES, 73

OBJECTIVES

Upon completion of this chapter you will be able to:

1. Define and spell word parts related to directional terms.

2. Define, pronounce, and spell terms used to describe directions with respect to the body.

3. Define, pronounce, and spell terms used to describe the anatomic planes.

4. Define, pronounce, and spell terms used to describe the abdominopelvic regions.

5. Identify and spell the four abdominopelvic quadrants.

6. Interpret the meaning of abbreviations presented in this chapter.

7. Interpret, read, and comprehend medical language in simulated medical statements and documents.

ANATOMIC POSITION

In the description and use of body directions and planes, the body is assumed to be in the standard, neutral position of reference called the *anatomic position*. In this position, the body is viewed as standing erect, arms at the side, palms of the hands facing forward, and feet placed side by side (Figure 3-1).

WORD PARTS

Combining Forms of Directional Terms

Word parts you need to learn to complete this chapter are listed on the following pages. The exercises at the end of each list will help you learn their definitions and spelling.

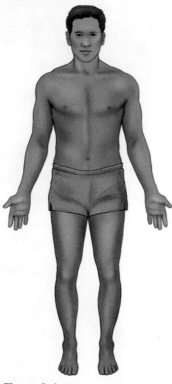

Figure 3-1
Anatomic position.

Combining Form	Definition
anter/o	front
caud/o	tail (downward)
cephal/o	head (upward)
dist/o	away (from the point of attachment of a body part)
dors/o	back
infer/o	below
later/o	side
medi/o	middle
poster/o	back, behind
proxim/o	near (the point of attachment of a body part)
super/o	above
ventr/o	belly (front)

EXERCISE FIGURE A

Fill in the blanks with directional combining forms. *To check your answers, go to p. 86, Answers to Chapter 3 Exercises.*

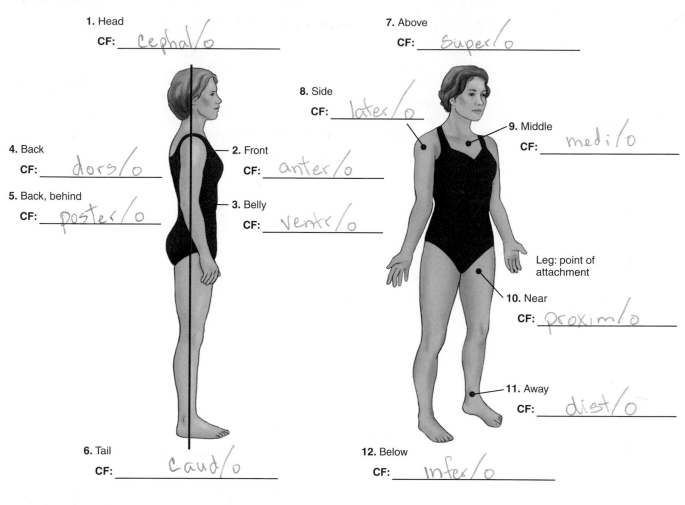

1. Head   CF: _cephal/o_

7. Above   CF: _super/o_

8. Side   CF: _later/o_

9. Middle   CF: _medi/o_

4. Back   CF: _dors/o_

2. Front   CF: _anter/o_

5. Back, behind   CF: _poster/o_

3. Belly   CF: _ventr/o_

Leg: point of attachment

10. Near   CF: _proxim/o_

11. Away   CF: _dist/o_

6. Tail   CF: _caud/o_

12. Below   CF: _infer/o_

EXERCISE 1

Write the definitions for the following combining forms.

1. ventr/o _belly (front)_
2. cephal/o _head (upward)_
3. later/o _side_
4. medi/o _middle_
5. infer/o _below_
6. proxim/o _near_
7. super/o _above_
8. dist/o _away_
9. dors/o _back_
10. caud/o _tail (downward)_
11. anter/o _front_
12. poster/o _back, behind_

EXERCISE 2

Write the combining form for each of the following.

1. side — *later/o*
2. above — *super/o*
3. head — *cephal/o*
4. away (from the point of attachment of a body part) — *dist/o*
5. front — *anter/o*
6. middle — *medi/o*

7. back — *dors/o*
8. belly — *ventr/o*
9. tail — *caud/o*
10. below — *infer/o*
11. back, behind — *dors/o*
12. near (the point of attachment of a body part) — *proxim/o*

Prefixes

Prefix	Definition
bi-	two
uni-	one

Suffixes

Suffix	Definition
-ad	toward
-ior	pertaining to

Refer to Appendix A and Appendix B for alphabetized lists of word parts and their meanings.

 Many suffixes mean **pertaining to.** You have already learned three of them in Chapter 2: **-al, -ic,** and **-ous.** You will learn more in subsequent chapters. With practice, you will learn which suffix is most commonly used with a particular word root or combining form.

EXERCISE 3

Match the prefixes and suffixes in the first column with their correct definitions in the second column.

_C_ 1. -ad   a. one

_B_ 2. -ior   b. pertaining to

_D_ 3. bi-   c. toward

_A_ 4. uni-   d. two

Write the definitions of the following prefixes and suffixes.

1. -ior   *pertaining to*
2. -ad   *toward*
3. bi-   *two*
4. uni-   *one*

DIRECTIONAL TERMS

The following terms are built from word parts you have already learned and can be translated literally to find their meanings. Further explanation of terms beyond the definition of their word parts, if needed, is included in parentheses.

Term	Definition
caudad (KAW-dad)	toward the tail (downward) (Figure 3-2)
cephalad (SEF-a-lad)	toward the head (upward) (Figure 3-2)
lateral (lat) (LAT-e-ral)	pertaining to a side (Figure 3-3)
medial (med) (MĒ-dē-al)	pertaining to the middle (Figure 3-3)
unilateral (ū-ni-LAT-er-al)	pertaining to one side (only)
bilateral (bī-LAT-er-al)	pertaining to two sides
mediolateral (*mē-dē-ō-LAT-er-al*)	pertaining to the middle and to the side
distal (DIS-tal)	pertaining to away (from the point of attachment of a body part) (Figure 3-4)
proximal (PROK-si-mal)	pertaining to near (to the point of attachment of a body part) (Figure 3-4)
inferior (inf) (in-FĒR-ē-or)	pertaining to below (Figure 3-5)
superior (sup) (sū-PĒR-ē-or)	pertaining to above (Figure 3-5)
caudal (KAW-dal)	pertaining to the tail (similar to **inferior** in most instances related to human anatomy) (Figure 3-5)
cephalic (se-FAL-ik)	pertaining to the head (Figure 3-5)
anterior (ant) (an-TĒR-ē-or)	pertaining to the front (Figure 3-5)

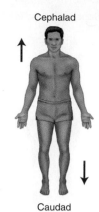

Cephalad

Caudad

Figure 3-2
Caudad and cephalad.

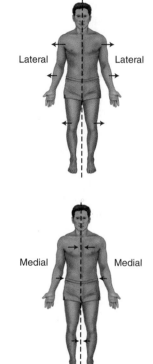

Lateral   Lateral

Medial   Medial

Figure 3-3
Lateral and medial.

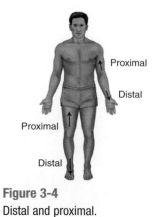

Proximal

Distal

Proximal

Distal

Figure 3-4
Distal and proximal.

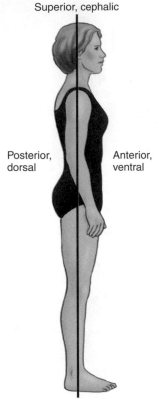

Superior, cephalic

Posterior, dorsal

Anterior, ventral

Inferior, caudal

Figure 3-5
Superior and inferior, cephalic and caudal, posterior and anterior, dorsal and ventral.

DIRECTIONAL TERMS—*cont'd*

Term	Definition
posterior . . . . (pos-TĒR-ē-or)	pertaining to the back (Figure 3-5)
dorsal. . . . . (DOR-sal)	pertaining to the back (Figure 3-5)
ventral . . . . (VEN-tral)	pertaining to the belly (front) (Figure 3-5)
anteroposterior (AP) . . . . (*an*-ter-ō-pos-TĒR-ē-or)	pertaining to the front and to the back (Exercise Figure C)
posteroanterior (PA). . . . . (*pos*-ter-ō-an-TĒR-ē-or)	pertaining to the back and to the front (Exercise Figure C)

EXERCISE 5

Practice saying aloud each of the directional terms on pp. 67-68.

To hear the terms select Chapter 3, Chapter Exercises, Pronunciation.

☐ Place a check mark in the box when you have completed this exercise.

EXERCISE 6

Analyze and define the following directional terms.

1. cephalad _Cephal/ad – toward head_
2. cephalic _Cephal/ic – pertaining to the head_
3. caudad _Caud/ad – toward the tail_
4. caudal _Caud/al – pertaining to the tail_
5. anterior _anteri/or – pertaining to the front_
6. posterior _posteri/or – pertaining to the back_
7. dorsal _dors/al – pertaining to the back_
8. superior _superi/or – pertaining to above_
9. inferior _inferi/or – pertaining to below_
10. proximal _proxim/al – pertaining to near body_
11. distal _dist/al – pertaining to away body_
12. lateral _later/al – pertaining to a side_
13. medial _medi/al – pertaining to the middle_
14. ventral _Ventr/al – pertaining to the belly_

15. posteroanterior *poster/o/anterior - pertaining to back and front*
16. unilateral *uni/later/al - pertaining to one side*
17. mediolateral *medi/o/later/al - pertaining to middle & one side*
18. anteroposterior *anter/o/posterior - pertaining to front & back*
19. bilateral *bi/later/al - pertaining to two side*

EXERCISE FIGURE B

Fill in the blanks to label the diagram.

1. ___*Superior*___
   above / pertaining to

2. ___*Cephal / ic*___
   head / pertaining to

3. ___*Cephal / ad*___
   head / toward

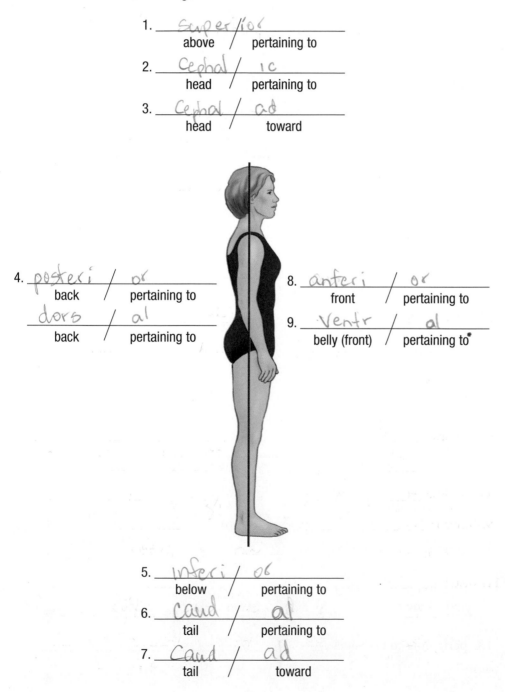

4. ___*posteri / or*___
   back / pertaining to
   ___*dors / al*___
   back / pertaining to

8. ___*anteri / or*___
   front / pertaining to

9. ___*Ventr / al*___
   belly (front) / pertaining to

5. ___*inferi / or*___
   below / pertaining to

6. ___*Caud / al*___
   tail / pertaining to

7. ___*Caud / ad*___
   tail / toward

EXERCISE **7**

Build directional terms for the following definitions by using the word parts you have learned.

1. toward the head (upward)   <u>Cephal</u> / <u>ad</u>
                    WR   S

2. pertaining to the head   <u>cephal</u> / <u>ic</u>
                WR   S

3. pertaining to the tail   <u>caud</u> / <u>ad</u>
              WR   S

4. pertaining to the front   <u>anteri</u> / <u>or</u>
               WR   S

5. pertaining to the back   <u>posterR</u> / <u>ior</u>
               WR   S

                            <u>dors</u> / <u>al</u>
                            WR   S

6. pertaining to above   <u>super</u> / <u>ior</u>
            WR   S

7. pertaining to below   <u>infer</u> / <u>ior</u>
            WR   S

8. pertaining to near   <u>proxim</u> / <u>al</u>
          WR   S

9. pertaining to away   <u>dist</u> / <u>al</u>
           WR   S

10. pertaining to a side   <u>later</u> / <u>al</u>
            WR   S

11. pertaining to the middle   <u>medi</u> / <u>al</u>
               WR   S

12. toward the tail (downward)   <u>caud</u> / <u>al</u>
                 WR   S

13. pertaining to the belly   <u>ventr</u> / <u>al</u>
             WR   S

14. pertaining to the back
    and to the front   <u>poster</u> /o/ <u>anteri</u> / <u>or</u>
                   WR   CV   WR   S

15. pertaining to the middle
    and to the side   <u>medi</u> /o/ <u>later</u> / <u>al</u>
              WR   CV   WR   S

16. pertaining to one side (only)   <u>uni</u> / <u>later</u> / <u>al</u>
                       P   WR   S

17. pertaining to the front
    and to the back   <u>anteri</u> /o/ <u>poster</u> / <u>or</u>
              WR   CV   WR   S

18. pertaining to two sides   <u>bi</u> / <u>later</u> / <u>al</u>
               P   WR   S

EXERCISE FIGURE C

Fill in the blanks to label the diagram.

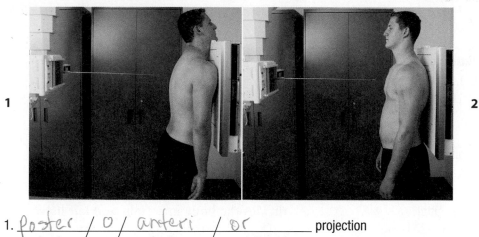

1. ___Poster___ / _O_ / ___anteri___ / ___or___ _____ projection
      back   / cv /   front   / pertaining to

2. ___anter___ / _O_ / ___posteri___ / ___or___ _____ projection
      front   / cv /   back   / pertaining to

EXERCISE 8

Spell each of the directional terms on pp. 67-68 by having someone dictate them to you.

To hear and spell the terms select Chapter 3, Chapter Exercises, Spelling. You may type the terms on the screen or write them below in the spaces provided.

☐ Place a check mark in the box if you have completed this exercise using your CD-ROM.

1. _____   11. _____

2. _____   12. _____

3. _____   13. _____

4. _____   14. _____

5. _____   15. _____

6. _____   16. _____

7. _____   17. _____

8. _____   18. _____

9. _____   19. _____

10. _____

ANATOMIC PLANES

Planes are imaginary flat fields used as points of reference to identify the position of parts of the body (Table 3-1). *In some of the following terms, you may recognize word parts you have already learned; however, the full meaning of the terms cannot be discerned by the definition of their word parts.*

Term	Definition
frontal or coronal............ (FRON-tal) (ko-RŌN-al)	vertical field passing through the body from side to side, dividing the body into anterior and posterior portions (Figure 3-6)
sagittal................... (SAJ-i-tal)	vertical field running through the body from front to back, dividing the body into right and left sides
midsagittal................ (mid-SAJ-i-tal)	divides the body into right and left halves (Figure 3-6)
transverse .... (trans-VERS)	horizontal field dividing the body into upper and lower portions (Figure 3-6)

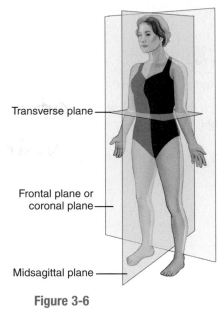

Transverse plane —

Frontal plane or
coronal plane —

Midsagittal plane —

Figure 3-6
Anatomic planes.

EXERCISE 9

Practice saying aloud each of the anatomic planes above.

 To hear the anatomic plane terms select Chapter 3, Chapter Exercises, Pronunciation.

☐ Place a check mark in the box when you have completed this exercise.

TABLE 3-1
Anatomic Planes and Diagnostic Images

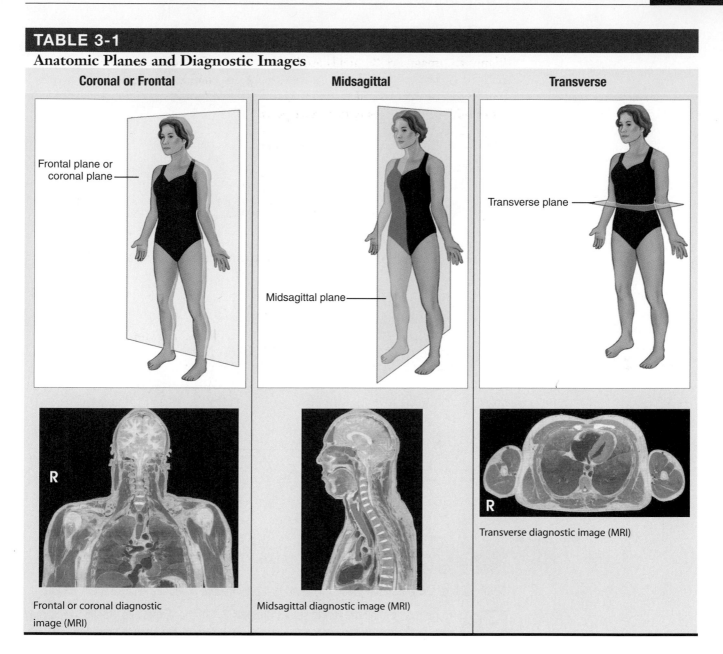

Coronal or Frontal	Midsagittal	Transverse

Frontal plane or coronal plane

Midsagittal plane

Transverse plane

Frontal or coronal diagnostic image (MRI)

Midsagittal diagnostic image (MRI)

Transverse diagnostic image (MRI)

EXERCISE 10

Fill in the blanks with the correct terms.

1. The plane that divides the body into upper and lower portions is the
   transverse plane.

2. The plane that divides the body into right and left halves is the
   midsagittal plane.

3. The plane that divides the body into anterior and posterior portions is the
   frontal or _coronal_ plane.

4. The plane that divides the body into right and left sides is the
   sagittal plane.

EXERCISE FIGURE D

Fill in the blanks with anatomic planes.

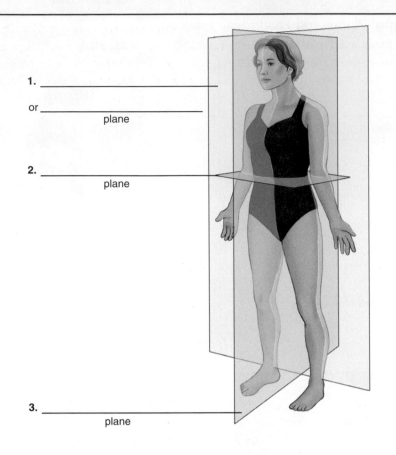

1. _____

or _____
          plane

2. _____
          plane

3. _____
          plane

EXERCISE 11

Spell each of the anatomic plane terms on p. 72 by having someone dictate them to you.

 To hear and spell the terms select Chapter 3, Chapter Exercises, Spelling. You may type the terms on the screen or write them below in the spaces provided.

☐ Place a check mark in the box if you have completed this exercise using your CD-ROM.

1. _____   4. _____

2. _____   5. _____

3. _____

ABDOMINOPELVIC REGIONS

To assist in locating medical problems with greater accuracy and for identification purposes, the abdomen and pelvis are divided into nine regions (Figure 3-7). *Although these terms are made up of word parts, most of the word parts are presented in later chapters;* therefore, memorization is the learning method used in the exercises that follow. The number in parentheses indicates the number of regions.

Term	Definition
umbilical region (1) . . . . (um-BIL-i-kal)	around the navel (umbilicus)
epigastric region (1) . . . . (*ep*-i-GAS-trik)	directly above the umbilical region
hypogastric region (1) . . . . (*hī*-pō-GAS-trik)	directly below the umbilical region
hypochondriac regions (2). . . . . (*hī*-pō-KON-drē-ak)	to the right and left of the epigastric region
lumbar regions (2). . . . . (LUM-bar)	to the right and left of the umbilical region
iliac regions (2) . . . . (IL-ē-ak)	to the right and left of the hypogastric region

UMBILICUS
is a term derived from the Latin **umbo,** which denoted the boss, or protuberant part, of a shield. Around the first century the term was used to designate either a raised or a depressed spot in the middle of anything.

HYPOCHONDRIAC
is derived from the Greek **hypo,** meaning **under,** and **chondros,** meaning **cartilage.** This ancient term was used by Hippocrates to refer to the region just below the cartilages of the ribs. In 1765 the term was first used to refer to people who experienced discomfort or painful sensations in this area but had no organic findings. Now, a person who falsely believes he or she has an illness is referred to as a **hypochondriac.**

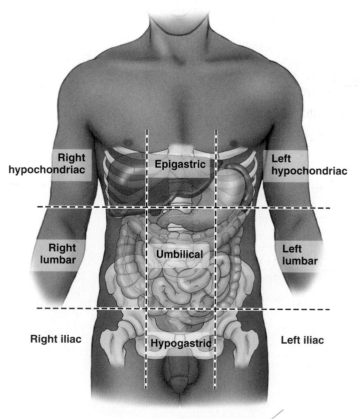

Figure 3-7
Abdominopelvic regions.

EXERCISE **12**

Practice saying aloud each of the abdominopelvic region terms on p. 75.

To hear the terms select Chapter 3, Chapter Exercises, Pronunciation.

☐ Place a check mark in the box when you have completed this exercise.

EXERCISE FIGURE **E**

Fill in the blanks with abdominopelvic regions.

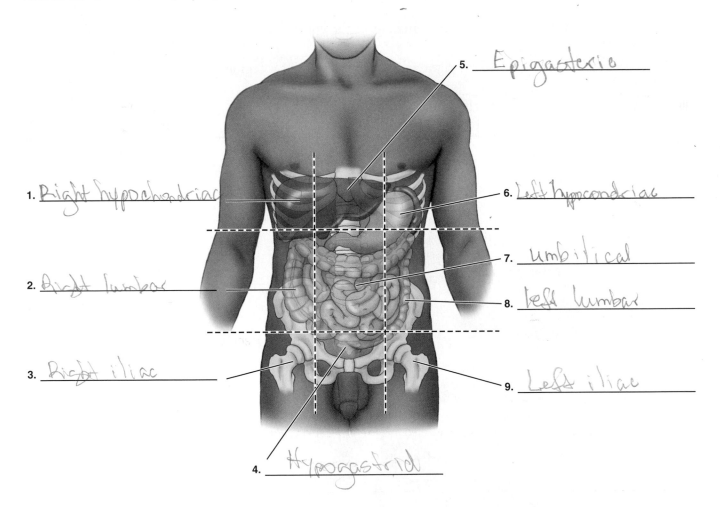

5. _Epigasteria_

1. _Right hypochondriac_

6. _Left hypocondriac_

7. _umbilical_

2. _Right lumbar_

8. _left lumbar_

3. _Right iliac_

9. _Left iliac_

4. _Hypogastrid_

EXERCISE 13

Fill in the blanks with the correct terms.

1. The regions to the right and left of the hypogastric region are the ___iliac___ regions.

2. The ___Epigastric___ region is directly above the umbilical region.

3. Inferior to the umbilical region is the ___hypogastrid___ region.

4. The ___hypocondriac___ are the regions to the right and left of the epigastric region.

5. Superior to the hypogastric region is the ___umbilical___ region.

6. To the right and the left of the umbilical region are the ___lumbar___ regions.

EXERCISE 14

Match the terms in the first column with the correct definitions in the second column.

__B__ 1. epigastric   a. inferior to the umbilical region

__D__ 2. hypochondriac   b. superior to the umbilical region

__A__ 3. hypogastric   c. right and left of the umbilical region

__E__ 4. iliac   d. right and left of the epigastric region

__C__ 5. lumbar   e. right and left of the hypogastric region

__G__ 6. umbilical   f. below the hypogastric region

                             g. inferior to the epigastric region

EXERCISE 15

Spell each of the abdominopelvic region terms on p. 75 by having someone dictate them to you.

 To hear and spell the terms select Chapter 3, Chapter Exercises, Spelling. You may type the terms on the screen or write them below in the spaces provided.

☐ Place a check mark in the box if you have completed this exercise using your CD-ROM.

1. _____   4. _____

2. _____   5. _____

3. _____   6. _____

ABDOMINOPELVIC QUADRANTS

The abdominopelvic area can also be divided into four quadrants by using imaginary vertical and horizontal lines that intersect at the umbilicus. These divisions are used by health professionals to locate an anatomic position to describe pain, incisions, markings, lesions, and so forth (Figure 3-8).

Term	Definition
right upper quadrant (RUQ).... (KWOD-rant)	refers to the area encompassing the right lobe of the liver, the gallbladder, part of the pancreas, portions of the small and large intestines, and the right kidney
left upper quadrant (LUQ)..... (KWOD-rant)	refers to the area encompassing the left lobe of the liver, the stomach, the spleen, part of the pancreas, portions of the small and large intestines, and the left kidney
right lower quadrant (RLQ).... (KWOD-rant)	refers to the area encompassing portions of the small and large intestines, the appendix, the right ureter, and the right ovary and uterine tube in women or the right spermatic duct in men
left lower quadrant (LLQ)...... (KWOD-rant)	refers to the area encompassing portions of the small and large intestines, the left ureter, and the left ovary and uterine tube in women or the left spermatic duct in men

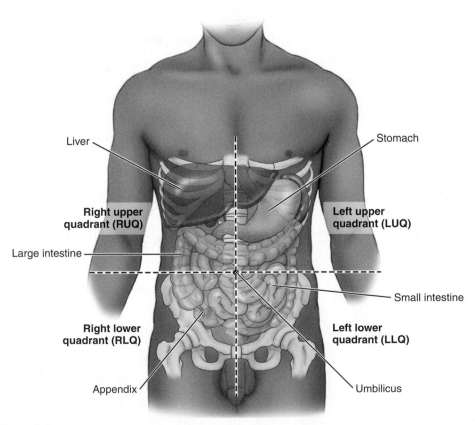

Figure 3-8
Abdominopelvic quadrants.

EXERCISE 16

Write the abbreviation for the abdominopelvic quadrant associated with the following organs.

RLQ 1. appendix
RUQ 2. right lobe of the liver
LLQ 3. left spermatic duct in men
LUQ 4. the stomach and the spleen
RLQ 5. right ovary and uterine tube in women
RUQ 6. gallbladder
RLQ 7. right ureter
LUQ 8. left kidney

EXERCISE FIGURE F

Fill in the blanks with abdominopelvic quadrants and the abbreviations for each.

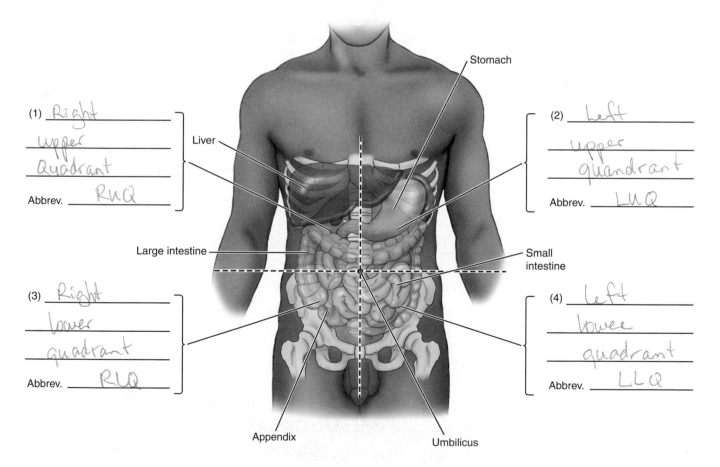

(1) _Right upper Quadrant_
Abbrev. _RuQ_

Liver

Stomach

(2) _Left upper quandrant_
Abbrev. _LuQ_

Large intestine

Small intestine

(3) _Right lower quadrant_
Abbrev. _RLQ_

(4) _left lower quadrant_
Abbrev. _LLQ_

Appendix

Umbilicus

EXERCISE 17

Spell each of the abdominopelvic quadrant terms on p. 78 by having someone dictate them to you.

 To hear and spell the terms select Chapter 3, Chapter Exercises, Spelling. You may type the terms on the screen or write them below in the spaces provided.

☐ Place a check mark in the box if you have completed this exercise using your CD-ROM.

1. _____   3. _____

2. _____   4. _____

Abbreviations

ant	anterior
AP	anteroposterior
inf	inferior
lat.	lateral
LLQ.	left lower quadrant
LUQ	left upper quadrant
med	medial
PA	posteroanterior
RLQ	right lower quadrant
RUQ	right upper quadrant
sup.	superior

Refer to Appendix D for a complete list of abbreviations.

EXERCISE 18

Write the meaning of each abbreviation in the space provided.

1. sup _____ Superior _____

2. ant _____ anterior _____

3. inf _____ Inferior _____

4. PA _____ Posteroanterior _____

5. AP _____ anteroposterior _____

6. med _____ medial _____

7. lat _____ lateral _____

PRACTICAL APPLICATION

EXERCISE **19**   *Interact with Medical Documents*

A. Complete the physician's progress note by writing the medical terms in the blanks. Use the list of definitions with corresponding numbers following the document.

University Hospital and Medical Center

4700 North Main Street • Wellness, Arizona 54321 • (987) 555-3210

PATIENT NAME: Zoe Parker   **CASE NUMBER:** 817254-DPQ
DATE OF BIRTH: 03/27/19XX   **DATE:** 11/24/20XX

PROGRESS NOTE

Mrs. Parker is here today for follow-up for degenerative joint disease of both knees. She arrived ambulatory with the assistance of a cane, walking slowly with a fairly steady gait.

On examination of the knees, there is marked crepitus that is palpable with pressure applied to the kneecaps with the knees flexed and extended, right greater than left. She has a range of motion from 11 degrees to 106 degrees in the right knee. Pain is evident at the end of extension at 11 degrees. The right knee is stable when stressed in an 1. _anteroposterior_, valgus, and varus manner.

On examination of the right ankle, there is some mild tenderness on palpation above the right ankle. The right ankle moves from 0 degrees of dorsiflexion to 25 degrees of plantar flexion. From the 2. _lateral_ joint line at the knee to the malleolus at the ankle, the right tib/fib is 1.5 cm shorter than the left. There is pigment change mainly on the 3. _posterior_ and 4. _medial_ aspect of the right lower leg. There is a slight bony deformity over the 5. _anterior_ aspect of the mid-tibial area.

IMPRESSION:
1. Degenerative joint disease of both knees, stable.

PLAN:
1. Patient is to continue on current medications unchanged.

Robert Means, MD

RM/mcm

---

1. pertaining to the front and to the back
2. pertaining to the side
3. pertaining to the back
4. pertaining to the middle
5. pertaining to the front

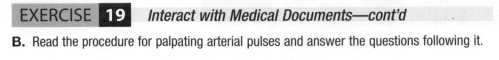

EXERCISE 19   *Interact with Medical Documents—cont'd*

B. Read the procedure for palpating arterial pulses and answer the questions following it.

PROCEDURE FOR PALPATING ARTERIAL PULSES

Palpate arteries with the distal pads of the first two fingers. The fingertips are used because they are the most sensitive parts of the hand. Unless contraindicated, simultaneous palpation is preferred.

Temporal: Palpate over the temporal bone on each side of the head lateral to each eyebrow.

Carotid: Palpate the anterior edge of the sternocleidomastoid muscle, just medial and inferior to the angle of the jaw. To avoid reduction of blood flow, do not palpate right and left carotid pulses simultaneously.

Apical: Palpate over the apex of the heart at the fourth or fifth intercostal space, left midclavicular line.

Brachial: Palpate in the groove between the biceps and triceps, just medial to the biceps tendon.

Radial: Palpate lateral and anterior side of wrist, proximal to the first metacarpal phalangeal joint.

Femoral: This pulse is inferior and medial to the inguinal ligament; if the patient is obese, the pulse is found midway between anterior superior iliac spine and pubic tubercle.

Dorsalis pedis: Lightly palpate the dorsal surface of the foot, with the foot slightly dorsiflexed.

Posterior tibial: This pulse is found posterior and slightly inferior to the medial malleolus of the ankle.

---

1. The temporal pulse is palpated
   a. just above the eyebrow.
   b. to the side of the eyebrow.
   c. below the eyebrow.
   d. to the middle of the eyebrow.

2. The radial pulse is palpated on the
   a. lateral and front of the wrist.
   b. lateral and back of the wrist.
   c. medial and back of the wrist.
   d. medial and front of the wrist.

3. The femoral pulse is located
   a. below and medial to the inguinal ligament.
   b. above and medial to the inguinal ligament.
   c. to the front and medial to the inguinal ligament.
   d. to the back and medial to the inguinal ligament.

4. When used with the foot, the directional term *dorsal* has a slightly different meaning. With the use of your medical dictionary, describe the dorsal surface of the foot. Hint: try *dorsum* and *dorsal pedis* as search terms.
   The dorsal surface of the foot is _the upper surface of the foot._

EXERCISE 20   *Interpret Medical Terms*

To test your understanding of the terms introduced in this chapter, complete the sentence by filling in the blank with the term that corresponds to the definition provided.

1. A polyp was found in the colon ___distal___ to the splenic flexure.
   (pertaining to away from the point of attachment of a body part)

2. The drainage catheter is placed over the right ___anterior___ pelvis.
   (pertaining to the front)

3. The incision was made at the _____Superior_____ pole of the lesion. **(pertaining to above)**

4. A(n) _____anteroposterior_____ chest radiograph is taken in the _____frontal_____ plane. **(pertaining to the front and to the back) (dividing the body into anterior and posterior portions)**

5. The patient complained of _____epigastric_____ pain. **(directly above the umbilical region)**

6. A _____unilateral_____ chest radiograph displays the anatomy in the _____midsagittal_____ plane. **(pertaining to a side) (divides the body into right and left sides)**

7. The patient was scheduled for an ultrasound-guided _____bilateral_____ thoracentesis. **(pertaining to two [both] sides)**

Practice pronunciation of terms by reading aloud the following medical document. Use the pronunciation key following the medical term to assist you in saying the word. The script contains medical terms not yet presented. Treat them as information only; you will learn more about them as you continue to study. Or, if desired, look for their meanings in your medical dictionary.

 To hear these terms select Chapter 3, Chapter Exercises, Read Medical Terms in Use.

The patient presented to her physician with pain in the right **lumbar** (LUM-bar) **region** and right **unilateral** (ū-ni-LAT-er-al) leg pain. The pain was felt in the **posterior** (pos-TĒR-ē-or) portion of the leg and radiated to the **distal** (DIS-tal) **lateral** (LAT-e-ral) portion of the extremity. There was some **proximal** (PROK-si-mal) muscle weakness reported of the affected leg. A lumbar spine radiograph was normal. If the pain does not respond to antiinflammatory medication, she will be referred to an orthopedist.

Test your comprehension of terms in the previous medical document by answering *T* for true and *F* for false.

___F___ 1. The patient had pain on both sides of her leg and to the right of the hypogastric region.

___T___ 2. The pain was felt at the back of the leg and radiated away from this point to the side of the extremity.

___T___ 3. The muscle weakness was felt near the point of attachment.

CHAPTER REVIEW

CHAPTER REVIEW ON CD-ROM

Use the CD-ROM that accompanies this textbook to play and practice what you have learned in this chapter. The Chapter Exercises, Practice Activities, Animations, and Games allow you to hear, see, and interact with the chapter content.

Chapter Exercises

Exercises in this section of your CD-ROM correlate to exercises in your textbook. You may have completed them as you worked through the chapter.

☐ Pronunciation
☐ Spelling
☐ Read Medical Terms in Use

Practice Activities

Practice in study mode, then test your learning in assessment mode. Keep track of your scores from assessment mode if you wish.

                    SCORE

☐ Picture It   _____
☐ Define Word Parts   _____
☐ Analyze Medical Terms _____
☐ Build Medical Terms   _____
☐ Define Medical Terms _____
☐ Use It   _____
☐ Hear It and Type It: _____
    Clinical Vignettes

Animations

☐ Directions of the Body

Games

☐ Name that Word Part
☐ Medical Millionaire

REVIEW OF WORD PARTS

Can you define and spell the following word parts?

Combining Forms		Prefixes	Suffixes
anter/o	medi/o	bi-	-ad
caud/o	poster/o	uni-	-ior
cephal/o	proxim/o		
dist/o	super/o		
dors/o	ventr/o		
infer/o			
later/o			

REVIEW OF TERMS

Can you define, pronounce, and spell the following terms?

Body Directional Terms	**Anatomic Planes**	**Abdominopelvic Regions**	**Abdominopelvic Quadrants**
anterior (ant)	frontal or coronal	epigastric region	left lower quadrant (LLQ)
anteroposterior (AP)	midsagittal	hypochondriac regions	left upper quadrant (LUQ)
bilateral	sagittal	hypogastric region	right lower quadrant (RLQ)
caudad	transverse	iliac regions	right upper quadrant (RUQ)
caudal		lumbar regions	
cephalad		umbilical region	
cephalic			
distal			
dorsal			
inferior (inf)			
lateral (lat)			
medial (med)			
mediolateral			
posterior			
posteroanterior (PA)			
proximal			
superior (sup)			
unilateral			
ventral			

ANSWERS

Exercise Figures

Exercise Figure

A. 1. head: cephal/o
   2. front: anter/o
   3. belly: ventr/o
   4. back: dors/o
   5. back, behind: poster/o
   6. tail: caud/o
   7. above: super/o
   8. side: later/o
   9. middle: medi/o
   10. near: proxim/o
   11. away: dist/o
   12. below: infer/o

Exercise Figure

B. 1. super/ior
   2. cephal/ic
   3. cephal/ad
   4. poster/ior, dors/al
   5. infer/ior
   6. caud/al
   7. caud/ad
   8. anter/ior
   9. ventr/al

Exercise Figure

C. 1. poster/o/anter/ior
   2. anter/o/poster/ior

Exercise Figure

D. 1. coronal or frontal plane
   2. transverse plane
   3. midsagittal plane

Exercise Figure

E. 1. hypochondriac
   2. lumbar
   3. iliac
   4. hypogastric
   5. epigastric
   6. hypochondriac
   7. umbilical
   8. lumbar
   9. iliac

Exercise Figure

F. 1. right upper quadrant (RUQ)
   2. left upper quadrant (LUQ)
   3. right lower quadrant (RLQ)
   4. left lower quadrant (LLQ)

Exercise 1
1. belly (front)
2. head (upward)
3. side
4. middle
5. below
6. near (point of attachment of a body part)
7. above
8. away (from the point of attachment of a body part)
9. back
10. tail (downward)
11. front
12. back, behind

Exercise 2
1. later/o
2. super/o
3. cephal/o
4. dist/o
5. anter/o
6. medi/o
7. dors/o
8. ventr/o
9. caud/o
10. infer/o
11. poster/o
12. proxim/o

Exercise 3
1. c
2. b
3. d
4. a

Exercise 4
1. pertaining to
2. toward
3. two
4. one

Exercise 5
Pronunciation Exercise

Exercise 6
1. WR   S
   cephal/ad
   toward the head
2. WR   S
   cephal/ic
   pertaining to the head
3. WR   S
   caud/ad
   toward the tail
4. WR   S
   caud/al
   pertaining to the tail
5. WR   S
   anter/ior
   pertaining to the front
6. WR   S
   poster/ior
   pertaining to the back
7. WR   S
   dors/al
   pertaining to the back
8. WR   S
   super/ior
   pertaining to above
9. WR   S
   infer/ior
   pertaining to below
10. WR   S
   proxim/al
   pertaining to near
11. WR   S
   dist/al
   pertaining to away
12. WR   S
   later/al
   pertaining to a side
13. WR   S
   medi/al
   pertaining to the middle
14. WR   S
   ventr/al
   pertaining to the belly (front)
15. WR CV WR S
   poster/o/anter/ior
        CF
   pertaining to the back and to the front
16. P   WR   S
   uni/later/al
   pertaining to one side
17. WR CV WR S
   medi/o/later/al
        CF
   pertaining to the middle and to the side
18. WR CV WR S
   anter/o/poster/ior
        CF
   pertaining to the front and to the back
19. P   WR   S
   bi/later/al
   pertaining to two sides

Exercise 7
1. cephal/ad
2. cephal/ic
3. caud/al
4. anter/ior
5. poster/ior, dors/al
6. super/ior
7. infer/ior
8. proxim/al
9. dist/al
10. later/al
11. medi/al
12. caud/ad
13. ventr/al
14. poster/o/anter/ior
15. medi/o/later/al
16. uni/later/al
17. anter/o/poster/ior
18. bi/later/al

Exercise 8
Spelling Exercise; see text p. 71.

Exercise 9
Pronunciation Exercise

Exercise 10
1. transverse
2. midsagittal
3. coronal or frontal
4. sagittal

Exercise 11
Spelling Exercise; see text p. 74.

Exercise 12
Pronunciation Exercise

Exercise 13
1. iliac
2. epigastric
3. hypogastric
4. hypochondriac
5. umbilical
6. lumbar

Exercise 14
1. b
2. d
3. a
4. e
5. c
6. g

Exercise 15
Spelling Exercise; see text p. 77.

Exercise 16
1. RLQ
2. RUQ
3. LLQ
4. LUQ
5. RLQ
6. RUQ
7. RLQ
8. LUQ

Exercise 17
Spelling Exercise; see text p. 80.

Exercise 18
1. superior
2. anterior
3. inferior
4. posteroanterior

5. anteroposterior
6. medial
7. lateral

Exercise 19
A. 1. anteroposterior
   2. lateral
   3. posterior or dorsal
   4. medial
   5. anterior
B. 1. b
   2. a
   3. a
   4. answers may vary: the upper surface of the foot; the surface opposite the sole

Exercise 20
1. distal
2. anterior
3. superior
4. anteroposterior; frontal (or coronal)
5. epigastric
6. lateral; sagittal
7. bilateral

Exercise 21
Reading Exercise

Exercise 22
1. *F*, "unilateral" means one side; "bilateral" means two sides. The right lumbar region is to the right of the umbilical region.
2. *T*
3. *T*

CHAPTER 4
Integumentary System

OUTLINE

ANATOMY, 90

WORD PARTS, 91
Combining Forms, 92
Prefixes, 95
Suffixes, 96

MEDICAL TERMS, 97
Disease and Disorder Terms, 98
    Built from Word Parts, 98
    Not Built from Word Parts, 102
Surgical Terms, 111
    Built from Word Parts, 111
    Not Built from Word Parts, 113
Complementary Terms, 116
    Built from Word Parts, 116
    Not Built from Word Parts, 121
Abbreviations, 128

PRACTICAL APPLICATION, 130
Interact with Medical Documents, 130
Interpret Medical Terms, 132
Read Medical Terms in Use, 133
Comprehend Medical Terms in Use, 133

CHAPTER REVIEW, 134

TABLE 4-1 COMMON SKIN DISORDERS, 99

TABLE 4-2 COMMON SKIN LESIONS, 123

The remaining chapters are organized according to body systems; therefore, they present material in a consistent format. The better you understand the format, the quicker and easier you will learn the material. Take time now to review How To Use This Text in the Front Matter to reacquaint yourself with the finer points of using this textbook to its ultimate potential.

OBJECTIVES

Upon completion of this chapter you will be able to:

1. Identify organs and structures of the integumentary system.

2. Define and spell word parts related to the integumentary system.

3. Define, pronounce, and spell disease and disorder terms related to the integumentary system.

4. Define, pronounce, and spell surgical terms related to the integumentary system.

5. Define, pronounce, and spell complementary terms related to the integumentary system.

6. Interpret the meaning of abbreviations related to the integumentary system.

7. Interpret, read, and comprehend medical language in simulated medical statements and documents.

ANATOMY

Function

The integumentary system is composed of the skin, nails, and glands. The skin forms a protective covering for the body that, when unbroken, prevents entry of bacteria and other invading organisms. The skin also protects the body from water loss and the damaging effects of ultraviolet light. Other functions include regulation of body temperature and synthesis of vitamin D (Figure 4-1).

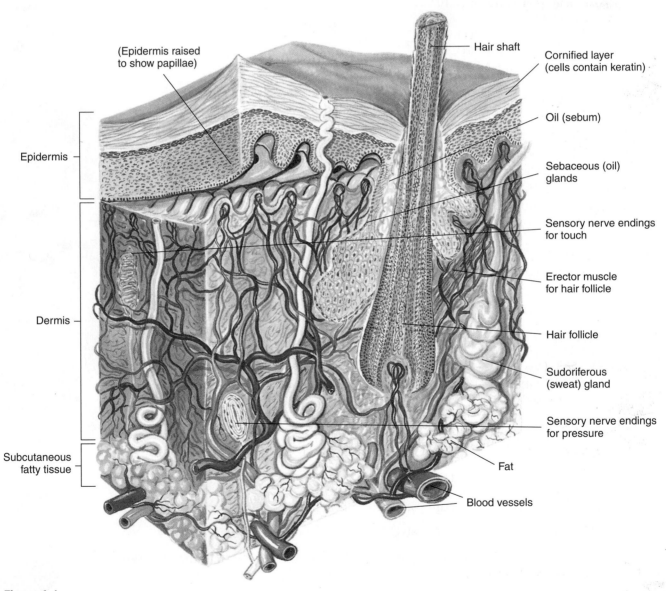

Figure 4-1
Structure of the skin.

The Skin

Term	Definition
epidermis	outer layer of skin
keratin	horny, or cornified, layer composed of protein. It is contained in the hair, skin, and nails.
melanin	color, or pigmentation, of the skin
dermis	inner layer of skin (also called the **true skin**)
sudoriferous (sweat) glands	tiny, coiled, tubular structures that emerge through pores on the skin's surface and secrete sweat
sebaceous glands	secrete sebum (oil) into the hair follicles where the hair shafts pass through the dermis

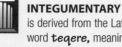

INTEGUMENTARY is derived from the Latin word **teqere,** meaning *to cover.*

Accessory Structures of the Skin

Term	Definition
hair	compressed, keratinized cells that arise from hair follicles, the sacs that enclose the hair fibers
nails	originate in the epidermis. Nails are found on the upper surface of the ends of the fingers and toes. The white area at the base of the nail is called the **lunula,** or **moon.**

EXERCISE 1

Match the terms in the first column with the correct definitions in the second column.

_C_   1. dermis

_D_   2. epidermis

_G_   3. hair

_B_   4. melanin

_F_   5. nail

_H_   6. sebaceous glands

_A_   7. sudoriferous glands

a. secrete sweat

b. responsible for skin color

c. true skin

d. outermost layer of the skin

e. white area at the nail's base

f. originates in the epidermis

g. composed of compressed, keratinized cells

h. secrete sebum

WORD PARTS

Word parts you need to learn to complete this chapter are listed on the following pages. The exercises at the end of each list will help you learn their definitions and spelling.

Combining Forms of the Integumentary System

Combining Form	Definition
cutane/o, derm/o, dermat/o....	skin
hidr/o.....................	sweat
kerat/o.................... (NOTE: *kerat/o* is also used to refer to the cornea of the eye; see Chapter 12.)	horny tissue, hard
onych/o, ungu/o.............	nail
seb/o.....................	sebum (oil)
trich/o	hair

Do not be concerned about which combining form to use for skin or nail. As you continue to study and use medical terms, you will become familiar with common usage of each word part.

EXERCISE FIGURE A

Fill in the blanks with combining forms in this diagram of a cross section of the skin.

1. Horny tissue   **CF:** _Kerat/o_

Melanin

Epidermis

Dermis

2. Hair   **CF:** _trich/o_

3. Skin
   CF: _cutane/o_
   CF: _derm/o_
   CF: _dermat/o_

Sebaceous gland

4. Sebum   **CF:** _seb/o_

Hair follicle

Sudoriferous gland

5. Sweat   **CF:** _hidr/o_

EXERCISE FIGURE B

Fill in the blanks with combining forms in this cross section of the finger with nail.

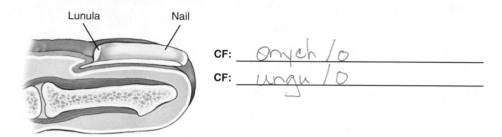

CF: ___onych /o___

CF: ___ungu /o___

EXERCISE 2

Write the definitions of the following combining forms.

1. hidr/o ___sweat___
2. derm/o ___skin___
3. onych/o ___nail___
4. trich/o ___hair___
5. kerat/o ___horny tissue___

6. dermat/o ___skin___
7. seb/o ___sebum (oil)___
8. ungu/o ___nail___
9. cutane/o ___skin___

EXERCISE 3

Write the combining form for each of the following.

1. hair ___trich/o___
2. sweat ___hidr/o___
3. nail   a. ___onych/o___
         b. ___ungu/o___
4. sebum ___seb/o___

5. skin   a. ___cutane/o___
          b. ___derm/o___
          c. ___dermat/o___
6. hard, horny tissue ___kerat/o___

Combining Forms Commonly Used with Integumentary System Terms

Combining Form	Definition
aut/o	self
bi/o	life
coni/o . . . . ,	dust
crypt/o	hidden
heter/o	other
myc/o	fungus
necr/o	death (cells, body)
pachy/o	thick
rhytid/o	wrinkles
staphyl/o	grapelike clusters
strept/o	twisted chains
xer/o	dry

The prefix **bi-,** which means **two,** was presented in Chapter 3. The word root **bi** means **life.**

EXERCISE 4

Write the definitions of the following combining forms.

1. necr/o _death (cells, body)_
2. staphyl/o _grapelike clusters_
3. crypt/o _hidden_
4. pachy/o _thick_
5. coni/o _dust_
6. myc/o _fungus_
7. bi/o _life_
8. heter/o _other_
9. strept/o _twisted chains_
10. xer/o _dry_
11. aut/o _self_
12. rhytid/o _wrinkles_

EXERCISE 5

Write the combining form for each of the following.

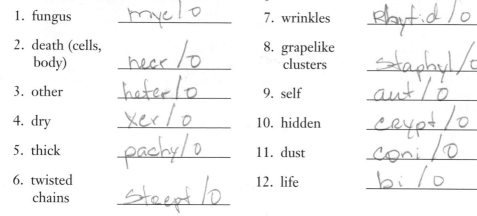

1. fungus   myel/o
2. death (cells, body)   necr/o
3. other   heter/o
4. dry   xer/o
5. thick   pachy/o
6. twisted chains   strept/o

7. wrinkles   Rhytid/o
8. grapelike clusters   staphyl/o
9. self   aut/o
10. hidden   crypt/o
11. dust   coni/o
12. life   bi/o

Prefixes

Prefix	Definition
epi-	on, upon, over
intra-	within
para-	beside, beyond, around, abnormal
per-	through
sub-	under, below
trans-	through, across, beyond

EXERCISE 6

Write the definitions of the following prefixes.

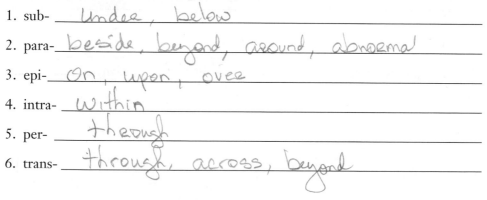

1. sub- Under, below
2. para- beside, beyond, around, abnormal
3. epi- On, upon, over
4. intra- Within
5. per- through
6. trans- through, across, beyond

EXERCISE 7

Write the prefix for each of the following.

1. within _____ *intra* _____

2. under, below _____ *sub* _____

3. on, upon, over _____ *epi* _____

4. beside, beyond, around, abnormal _____ *para* _____

5. through _____ *per* _____

6. through, across, beyond _____ *trans* _____

Suffixes

Suffix	Definition
-a	noun suffix, no meaning
-coccus (*pl.* -cocci)	berry-shaped (form of bacterium)
-ectomy	excision or surgical removal
-ia	diseased or abnormal state, condition of
-itis	inflammation
-malacia	softening
-opsy	view of, viewing
-phagia	eating or swallowing
-plasty	surgical repair
-rrhea	flow, discharge
-tome	instrument used to cut

Refer to Appendix A and Appendix B for alphabetical lists of word parts and their meanings.

EXERCISE 8

Match the suffixes in the first column with the correct definitions in the second column.

_C_	1. -coccus	a. inflammation
_E_	2. -ectomy	b. surgical repair
_A_	3. -itis	c. berry-shaped
_J_	4. -malacia	d. eating or swallowing
_I_	5. -opsy	e. excision or surgical removal
_H_	6. -rrhea	f. instrument used to cut
_D_	7. -phagia	g. thick
_B_	8. -plasty	h. flow, discharge
_F_	9. -tome	i. view of, viewing
_K_	10. -ia	j. softening
_L_	11. -a	k. diseased or abnormal state, condition of
		l. noun suffix, no meaning

EXERCISE 9

Write the definitions of the following suffixes.

1. -plasty _Surgical Repair_
2. -ectomy _excision or surgical Removal_
3. -malacia _softening_
4. -itis _inflammation_
5. -tome _instrument used to cut_
6. -phagia _eating or swallowing_
7. -rrhea _flow, discharge_
8. -coccus _berry-shaped_
9. -opsy _view of, viewing_
10. -ia _diseased or abnormal state_
11. -a _noun suffix, no meaning_

MEDICAL TERMS

The terms you need to learn to complete this chapter are listed on the following pages. The exercises at the end of each list will help you learn each word well enough to add it to your vocabulary.

Disease and Disorder Terms

Built from Word Parts

The following terms are built from word parts you have already learned and can be translated literally to find their meanings. Further explanation of terms beyond the definition of their word parts, if needed, is included in parentheses.

Term	Definition
dermatitis . . . . (*der*-ma-TĪ-tis)	inflammation of the skin (Table 4-1)
dermatoconiosis . . . . (*der*-ma-tō-kō-nē-Ō-sis)	abnormal condition of the skin caused by dust
dermatofibroma. . . . . (*der*-ma-tō-fī-BRŌ-ma)	fibrous tumor of the skin
hidradenitis . . . . (*hī*-drad-e-NĪ-tis)	inflammation of a sweat gland
leiodermia . . . . (lī-ō-DER-mē-a)	condition of smooth skin
onychocryptosis . . . . (*on*-i-kō-krip-TŌ-sis)	abnormal condition of a hidden nail (also called **ingrown nail**)
onychomalacia. . . . . (*on*-i-kō-ma-LĀ-sha)	softening of the nails
onychomycosis . . . . (*on*-i-kō-mī-KŌ-sis)	abnormal condition of a fungus in the nails (Exercise Figure C)
onychophagia . . . . (*on*-i-kō-FĀ-ja)	eating the nails (nail biting)
pachyderma. . . . . (pak-i-DER-ma)	thickening of the skin
paronychia. . . . . (par-ō-NIK-ē-a) (NOTE: the *a* from para- has been dropped. The fi- nal vowel in a prefix may be dropped when the word to which it is added begins with a vowel.)	diseased state around the nail (Exercise Figure C)
seborrhea . . . . (seb-o-RĒ-a)	discharge of sebum (excessive)
trichomycosis . . . . (*trik*-ō-mī-KŌ-sis)	abnormal condition of a fungus in the hair
xeroderma. . . . . (zē-rō-DER-ma)	dry skin

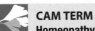

CAM TERM
Homeopathy is a system of medical treatment based on the theory that "like cures like." Homeopathic remedies, small doses of substances that would produce similar symptoms in a healthy person, stimulate the body's healing mechanisms to prevent or treat illness. Homeopathic treatments have reduced itchiness and improved skin conditions in patients with atopic dermatitis.

TABLE 4-1
Common Skin Disorders

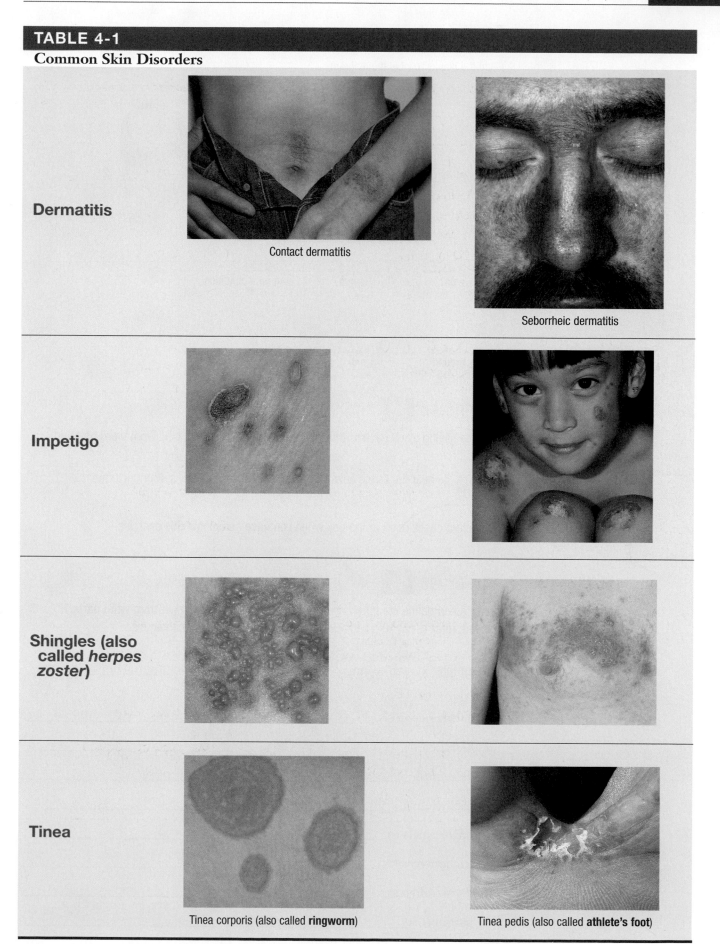

Dermatitis

Contact dermatitis

Seborrheic dermatitis

Impetigo

Shingles (also called *herpes zoster*)

Tinea

Tinea corporis (also called **ringworm**)

Tinea pedis (also called **athlete's foot**)

EXERCISE FIGURE C

Fill in the blanks to label the diagrams.

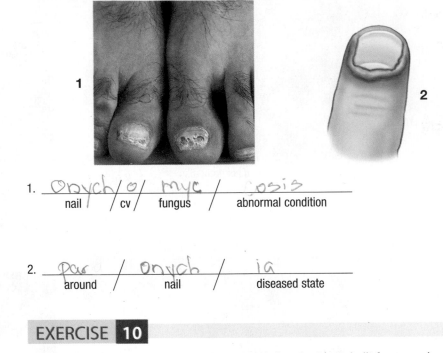

1. __Onych / o / myc / osis__
    nail / cv / fungus / abnormal condition

2. __Par / Onych / ia__
    around / nail / diseased state

EXERCISE 10

Practice saying aloud each of the disease and disorder terms built from word parts on
p. 98.

To hear the terms select Chapter 4, Chapter Exercises, Pronunciation.

☐ Place a check mark in the box when you have completed this exercise.

EXERCISE 11

Analyze and define the following disease and disorder terms built from word parts. If
needed, refer to pp. 10-11 to review analyzing and defining techniques.

              WR CV WR S
Example: onych/o/myc/osis   _abnormal condition of a fungus in the nails_

1. dermatoconiosis _abnormal condition of the skin caused by dust_
2. hidradenitis _inflammation of a sweat gland_
3. dermatitis _inflammation of the skin_
4. pachyderma _thickening of the skin_
5. onychomalacia _softening of the nail_
6. trichomycosis _abnormal condition of fungus in hair_
7. dermatofibroma _fibrous tumor of skin_
8. paronychia _diseased state around the nail_

9. onychocryptosis _abnormal condition of a hidden nail_
10. seborrhea _discharge of sebum_
11. onychophagia _eating the nails_
12. xeroderma _dry skin_
13. leiodermia _condition of smooth skin_

EXERCISE 12

Build disease and disorder terms for the following definitions by using the word parts you have learned. If you need help, refer to p. 12 to review word-building techniques.

Example: abnormal condition of a fungus in the hair   trich/o/myc/osis
                                                          WR /CV/ WR/ S

1. thickening of the skin   pachy / derm / a
                                   WR / WR / S

2. abnormal condition of a
   fungus in the nails   onych/o/ myc / osis
                                  WR /CV/ WR / S

3. discharge of sebum (excessive)   seb / o/ rrhea
                                    WR /CV/ S

4. inflammation of the skin   dermat / itis
                                   WR / S

5. fibrous tumor of the skin   dermat/o/ fibr / oma
                                   WR /CV/ WR / S

6. softening of the nails   onych / o/ malacia
                                   WR /CV/ S

7. inflammation of a sweat gland   hidr / aden / itis
                                   WR / WR / S

8. abnormal condition
   of a hidden nail   onych / o/ crypt / osis
                                   WR /CV/ WR / S

9. abnormal condition of the
   skin caused by dust   dermat/ o/ coni / osis
                                   WR /CV/ WR / S

10. eating the nails   onych / o/ phagia
                                   WR /CV/ S

11. diseased state around the nail par / onych / ia
                                    P / WR / S

12. dry skin   xer / o/ derm / a
                                   WR /CV/ WR / S

13. condition of smooth skin   lei / o/ derm / ia
                                   WR /CV/ WR / S

EXERCISE 13

Spell each of the disease and disorder terms built from word parts on p. 98 by having someone dictate them to you.

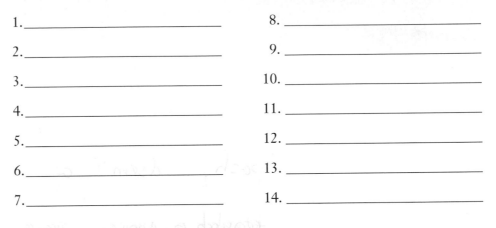 To hear and spell the terms select Chapter 4, Chapter Exercises, Spelling. You may type the terms on the screen or write them below in the spaces provided.

☐ Place a check mark in the box if you have completed this exercise using your CD-ROM.

1. _____   8. _____

2. _____   9. _____

3. _____   10. _____

4. _____   11. _____

5. _____   12. _____

6. _____   13. _____

7. _____   14. _____

Disease and Disorder Terms

Not Built from Word Parts

In some of the following terms, you may recognize word parts you have already learned; however, the full meaning of the terms cannot be discerned by the definition of their word parts.

ABSCESS
is derived from the Latin **ab,** meaning **from,** and *cedo,* meaning **to go.** The tissue dies and goes away, with the pus replacing it.

Term	Definition
abrasion................. (a-BRĀ-zhun)	scraping away of the skin by mechanical process or injury
abscess................. (AB-ses)	localized collection of pus
acne..................... (AK-nē)	inflammatory disease of the skin involving the sebaceous glands and hair follicles
actinic keratosis .... (ack-TIN-ik) (ker-a-TŌ-sis)	a precancerous skin condition of horny tissue formation that results from excessive exposure to sunlight (Figure 4-2, *A*). It may evolve into a squamous cell carcinoma.
albinism................. (AL-bi-niz-um)	congenital hereditary condition characterized by partial or total lack of pigment in the skin, hair, and eyes (Figure 4-3)
basal cell carcinoma (BCC) .... (BĀ-sal) (sel) (kar-si-NŌ-ma)	epithelial tumor arising from the epidermis. It seldom metastasizes but invades local tissue (Figure 4-2, *C*). Common in individuals who have had excessive sun exposure.

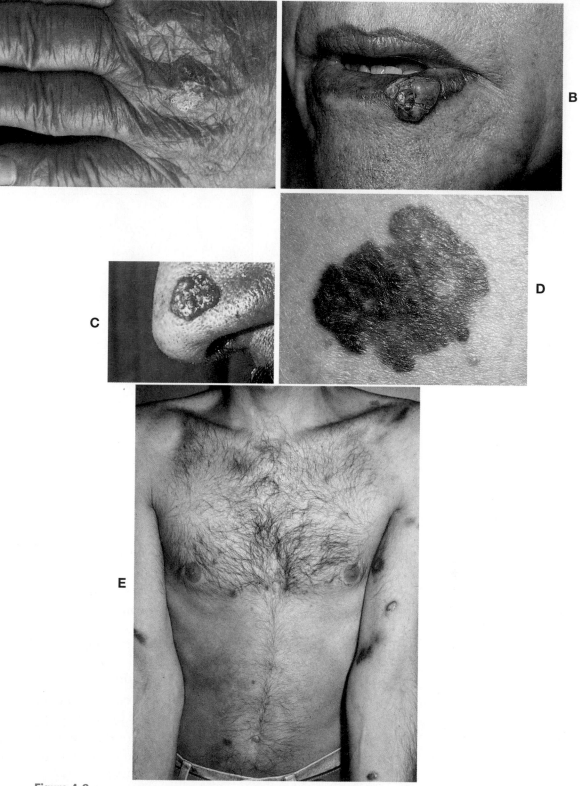

Figure 4-2

Percutaneous lesion and cancers of the skin. **A,** Actinic keratosis; **B,** squamous cell carcinoma; **C,** basal cell carcinoma; **D,** melanoma (covered in Chapter 2); **E,** Kaposi sarcoma.

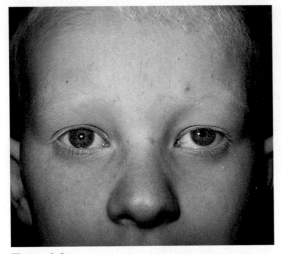

Figure 4-3
White hair and pale skin of a person with albinism. *Alb* is the Latin word root meaning *white*. *Leuk* is the Greek word root meaning *white*.

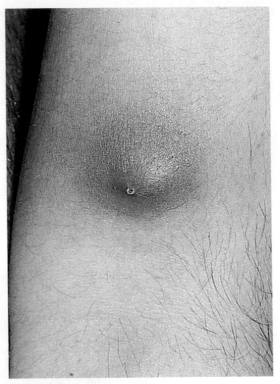

Figure 4-4
Furuncle resulting from a *Staphylococcus aureus* infection.

Disease and Disorder Terms—*cont'd*

Not Built from Word Parts

CANDIDA comes from the Latin **candidus,** meaning **gleaming white;** albicans is from the Latin verb **albicare,** meaning **to make white.** The growth of the fungus is white, and the infection produces a white discharge.

Term	Definition
candidiasis (kan-di-DĪ-a-sis)	an infection of the skin, mouth (also called **thrush**), or vagina caused by the yeast-type fungus *Candida albicans. Candida* is normally present in the mucous membranes; overgrowth causes an infection. Esophageal candidiasis is often seen in patients with AIDS (acquired immunodeficiency syndrome).
carbuncle (KAR-bung-kl)	skin infection composed of a cluster of boils caused by staphylococcal bacteria
cellulitis (sel-ū-LĪ-tis)	inflammation of the skin and subcutaneous tissue caused by infection, leading to redness, swelling, and fever
contusion (kon-TŪ-zhun)	injury with no break in the skin, characterized by pain, swelling, and discoloration (also called a **bruise**)
eczema (EK-ze-ma)	noninfectious, inflammatory skin disease characterized by redness, blisters, scabs, and itching

Term	Definition
fissure (FISH-ur)	slit or cracklike sore in the skin
furuncle (FER-ung-kl)	painful skin node caused by staphylococcal bacteria in a hair follicle (also called a **boil**) (Figure 4-4)
gangrene (GANG-grēn)	death of tissue caused by loss of blood supply followed by bacterial invasion (a form of necrosis)
herpes (HER-pēz)	inflammatory skin disease caused by herpes virus characterized by small blisters in clusters. Many types of herpes exist. *Herpes simplex*, for example, causes fever blisters; *herpes zoster*, also called **shingles,** is characterized by painful skin eruptions that follow nerves inflamed by the virus (Table 4-1).
impetigo. (im-pe-TĪ-gō)	superficial skin infection characterized by pustules and caused by either staphylococci or streptococci (Table 4-1)
Kaposi sarcoma (KAP-ō-sē) (sar-KŌ-ma)	a cancerous condition starting as purple or brown papules on the lower extremities that spreads through the skin to the lymph nodes and internal organs. Frequently seen with AIDS (Figure 4-2, *E*).
laceration. (*las*-er-Ā-shun)	torn, ragged-edged wound
lesion (LĒ-zhun)	any visible change in tissue resulting from injury or disease. It is a broad term that includes sores, wounds, ulcers, and tumors.
pediculosis (pe-*dik*-ū-LŌ-sis)	invasion into the skin and hair by lice
psoriasis (so-RĪ-a-sis)	chronic skin condition producing red lesions covered with silvery scales
rosacea (ro-ZĀ-shē-a)	chronic disorder of the skin that produces erythema, papules, pustules, and broken blood vessels, usually occurring on the central area of the face in people older than 30 years (Figure 4-5) (also called **acne rosacea**)

HERPES
is derived from the Greek *herpo,* meaning to *creep along.* It is descriptive of the course and type of skin lesion.

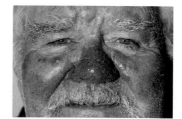

Figure 4-5
Rosacea.

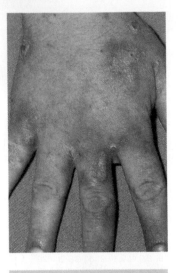

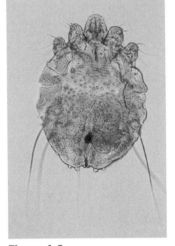

Figure 4-6
A, Scabies; **B,** scabies mite.

Disease and Disorder Terms—*cont'd*
Not Built from Word Parts

Term	Definition
scabies . . . . (SKĀ-bēz)	skin infection cased by the itch mite, characterized by papule eruptions that are caused by the female burrowing in the outer layer of the skin and laying eggs. This condition is accompanied by severe itching (Figure 4-6).
scleroderma. . . . . (skle-rō-DER-ma)	a disease characterized by chronic hardening (induration) of the connective tissue of the skin and other body organs
shingles . . . . (SHING-glz)	development of painful, inflamed blisters that follow the nerve routes; caused by the same virus that causes chickenpox (Table 4-1) (also called **herpes zoster**)
squamous cell carcinoma (SqCCA) . . . . (SQWĀ-mus) (sel) (kar-si-NŌ-ma)	a malignant growth that develops from scale-like epithelial tissue. Unlike basal cell carcinoma, there is a significant potential for metastasis. The most frequent cause is chronic exposure to sunlight (Figure 4-2, *B*).
systemic lupus erythematosus (SLE) . . . . (sis-TEM-ik) (LŪ-pus) (e-ri-thē-*ma*-TŌ-sus)	a chronic inflammatory disease involving the skin, joints, kidneys, and nervous system. This autoimmune disease is characterized by periods of remission and exacerbations. It also may affect other organs.
tinea. . . . . (TIN-ē-a)	fungal infection of the skin. The fungi may infect keratin of the skin, hair, and nails. Infections are classified by body regions such as *tinea capitis* (scalp), *tinea corporis* (body), and *tinea pedis* (foot). Tinea in general is also called **ringworm,** and tinea pedis specifically is also called **athlete's foot** (Table 4-1).
urticaria. . . . . (ur-ti-KAR-ē-a)	an itching skin eruption composed of wheals of varying size and shape. It is usually related to an allergy (also called **hives**). (See Table 4-2)

EXERCISE 14

Practice saying aloud each of the disease and disorder terms not built from word parts on pp. 102-106.

 To hear the terms select Chapter 4, Chapter Exercises, Pronunciation.

☐ Place a check mark in the box when you have completed this exercise.

EXERCISE 15

Fill in the blanks with the correct disease and disorder terms.

1. A chronic inflammatory disease affecting the skin, joints, and other organs is _Systemic_ _lupus_ _erythematosus_

2. A(n) _abscess_ is a localized collection of pus.

3. A cracklike sore in the skin is called a(n) _fissure_ .

4. The scraping away of the skin by mechanical process or injury is called a(n) _abrasion_ .

5. _psoriasis_ is a chronic skin condition characterized by red lesions covered with silvery scales.

6. An inflammatory skin disease caused by a virus and characterized by small blisters in clusters is called _herpes_ .

7. _pediculosis_ is the name given to the invasion of the skin and hair by lice.

8. A fungal infection of the skin, also known as *ringworm*, is called _tinea_ .

9. An injury with no break in the skin and characterized by pain, swelling, and discoloration is called a(n) _contusion_ .

10. _gangrene_ is the name given to tissue death caused by a loss of blood supply followed by bacterial invasion.

11. Any visible change in tissue resulting from injury or disease is called a _lesion_ .

12. _Kaposi_ _sarcoma_ is a cancerous condition starting as purple or brown papules on the lower extremities.

13. A horny tissue formation that results from excessive exposure to sunlight and is precancerous is called _actinic_ _keratosis_ .

14. A cluster of boils caused by staphylococcal bacteria is a _Carbuncle_ .

15. An inflammatory skin disease that involves the oil glands and hair follicles is called _acne_ .

16. _laceration_ is the name given to a torn, ragged-edged wound.

17. A painful skin node caused by staphylococcal bacteria in a hair follicle is called a(n) _furuncle_.

18. A malignant growth that develops from scalelike epithelial tissue is known as _squamous_ _cell_ carcinoma.

19. Inflammation of the skin and subcutaneous tissue caused by infection and creating redness, swelling, and fever is called _____.

20. _____ is the name given to a superficial skin infection characterized by pustules and caused by either staphylococci or streptococci.

21. _____ is a noninfectious inflammatory skin disease characterized by redness, blisters, scabs, and itching.

22. A skin inflammation caused by the itch mite is called _____.

23. _____ is an itching skin eruption composed of wheals.

24. An epithelial tumor commonly found on the face of individuals who have had excessive sun exposure is _____ _____ carcinoma.

25. _____ is a disease characterized by induration of the connective tissue.

26. _Candidiasis_ is an infection of the mouth, skin, or vagina caused by _Candida albicans._

27. A condition of painful, inflamed blisters that follow nerve routes is called _shingles_.

28. _rosacea_ is a chronic disorder of the skin that produces erythema, papules, pustules, and broken blood vessels.

29. A congenital hereditary condition characterized by partial or total lack of pigment in the skin, hair, and eyes is _albinism_.

EXERCISE 16

Match the words in the first column with their correct definitions in the second column.

_____ 1. abrasion

_____ 2. abscess

_____ 3. acne

_____ 4. actinic keratosis

_____ 5. basal cell carcinoma

_____ 6. carbuncle

_____ 7. cellulitis

_____ 8. contusion

_____ 9. eczema

_____ 10. fissure

_____ 11. furuncle

_____ 12. gangrene

_____ 13. scleroderma

_____ 14. rosacea

a. death of tissue caused by loss of blood supply and entry of bacteria

b. cracklike sore in the skin

c. cluster of boils

d. induration of connective tissue

e. noninfectious inflammatory skin disease having redness, blisters, scabs, and itching

f. scraped-away skin

g. involves sebaceous glands and hair follicles

h. painful skin node caused by staphylococci in a hair follicle

i. inflammation of skin and subcutaneous tissue with redness, swelling, and fever

j. localized collection of pus

k. injury characterized by pain, swelling, and discoloration

l. precancerous skin condition caused by excessive exposure to sunlight

m. usually occurring in the central area of the face in people older than 30 years

n. epithelial tumor commonly found in individuals who have had excessive sun exposure

o. red lesions with silvery scales

EXERCISE 17

Match the words in the first column with the correct definitions in the second column.

_____ 1. herpes

_____ 2. impetigo

_____ 3. Kaposi sarcoma

_____ 4. laceration

_____ 5. lesion

_____ 6. pediculosis

_____ 7. psoriasis

_____ 8. scabies

_____ 9. squamous cell carcinoma

_____ 10. systemic lupus erythematosus

_____ 11. tinea

_____ 12. urticaria

_____ 13. candidiasis

_____ 14. shingles

_____ 15. albinism

a. skin inflammation caused by the itch mite

b. fungal infection of the skin, hair, and nails

c. red lesions covered by silvery scales

d. inflammatory skin disease having clusters of blisters and caused by a virus

e. chronic inflammatory disease involving the skin, joints, kidney, and nervous system

f. a cancerous condition that starts as brown or purple papules on the lower extremities

g. composed of wheals

h. torn, ragged-edged wound

i. superficial skin condition having pustules and caused by staphylococci or streptococci

j. characterized by lack of pigment in the skin, hair, and eyes

k. infection of the skin, mouth, or vagina caused by a yeast-type fungus

l. invasion of the hair and skin by lice

m. visible change in tissue resulting from injury or disease

n. a malignant growth that develops from scalelike epithelial tissue

o. lesions caused by herpes zoster virus

p. cracklike sore in the skin

EXERCISE 18

Spell each of the disease and disorder terms not built from word parts on pp. 102-106 by having someone dictate them to you.

 To hear and spell the terms select Chapter 4, Chapter Exercises, Spelling. You may type the terms on the screen or write them below in the spaces provided.

☐ Place a check mark in the box if you have completed this exercise using your CD-ROM.

1. _____

2. _____

3. _____

4. _____

5. _____

6. _____

7. _____

8. _____

9. _____   20. _____

10. _____   21. _____

11. _____   22. _____

12. _____   23. _____

13. _____   24. _____

14. _____   25. _____

15. _____   26. _____

16. _____   27. _____

17. _____   28. _____

18. _____   29. _____

19. _____

Surgical Terms

Built from Word Parts

The following terms are built from word parts you have already learned and can be translated literally to find their meanings. Further explanation of terms beyond the definition of their word parts, if needed, is included in parentheses.

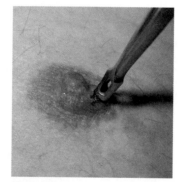

Figure 4-7
Punch biopsy.

Term	Definition
biopsy (bx) . . . . (BĪ-op-sē)	view of life (the removal of living tissue from the body to be viewed under the microscope) (Figure 4-7)
dermatoautoplasty . . . . (*der*-ma-tō-AW-tō-*plas*-tē)	surgical repair using one's own skin (skin graft) (also called **autograft**)
dermatoheteroplasty . . . . (*der*-ma-tō-HET-er-ō-*plas*-tē)	surgical repair using skin from others (skin graft) (also called **allograft**)
dermatome . . . . (DER-ma-tōm) NOTE: when two consonants of the same letter come together, one is sometimes dropped.	instrument used to cut skin (in thin slices for skin grafts)
dermatoplasty . . . . (DER-ma-tō-*plas*-tē)	surgical repair of the skin
onychectomy . . . . (on-i-KEK-to-mē)	excision of a nail
rhytidectomy . . . . (rit-i-DEK-to-mē)	excision of wrinkles (also called **facelift**)
rhytidoplasty . . . . (RIT-i-dō-*plas*-tē)	surgical repair of wrinkles

BIOPSY OF THE SKIN
may be performed by the dermatologist during an office visit. Common techniques include:
- **excisional biopsy** removes the entire lesion along with a margin of surrounding tissue
- **punch biopsy** removes a cylindrical portion of tissue with a specifically designed round knife (see Figure 4-7)
- **shave biopsy** removes a sample of tissue with a cut parallel to the surrounding skin

DERMATOME
also refers to the **dermatomic area,** the area of skin supplied by a specific sensory nerve root.

EXERCISE 19

Practice saying aloud each of the surgical terms built from word parts on p. 111.

To hear the terms select Chapter 4, Chapter Exercises, Pronunciation.

☐ Place a check mark in the box when you have completed this exercise.

EXERCISE 20

Analyze and define the following surgical terms.

Example: dermat/o/plasty   _surgical repair of the skin_

1. rhytidectomy _____

2. biopsy _____

3. dermatoautoplasty _____

4. onychectomy _____

5. rhytidoplasty _____

6. dermatoheteroplasty _____

7. dermatome _____

EXERCISE 21

Build surgical terms for the following definitions by using the word parts you have learned.

Example: surgical repair using one's own skin   dermat/o/aut/o/plasty
     WR /CV/ WR/CV/ S

1. excision of wrinkles
   _____/_____
   WR   S

2. view of life (removal of living tissue from the body)
   _____/_____
   WR   S

3. surgical repair using skin from others
   ____/__/____/__/____
   WR /CV/ WR /CV/ S

4. excision of a nail
   _____/_____
   WR   S

5. surgical repair of wrinkles
   _____/__/_____
   WR /CV/ S

6. surgical repair of the skin
   _____/__/_____
   WR /CV/ S

7. instrument used to cut skin
   _____/_____
   WR   S

EXERCISE 22

Spell each of the surgical terms built from word parts on p. 111 by having someone dictate them to you.

 To hear and spell the terms select Chapter 4, Chapter Exercises, Spelling. You may type the terms on the screen or write them below in the spaces provided.

☐ Place a check mark in the box if you have completed this exercise using your CD-ROM.

1. _____   5. _____

2. _____   6. _____

3. _____   7. _____

4. _____   8. _____

Surgical Terms

Not Built from Word Parts

In some of the following terms, you may recognize word parts you have already learned; however, the full meaning of the terms cannot be discerned by the definition of their word parts.

Term	Definition
cauterization .... (*kaw*-tur-ī-ZĀ-shun)	destruction of tissue with a hot or cold instrument, electric current, or caustic substance (also called **cautery**)
cryosurgery .... (*krī*-ō-SER-jer-ē)	destruction of tissue by using extreme cold, often by using liquid nitrogen (Figure 4-8)
débridement .... (dā-brēd-MA)	removal of contaminated or dead tissue and foreign matter from an open wound
dermabrasion .... (*derm*-a-BRĀ-zhun)	procedure to remove skin scars with abrasive material, such as sandpaper
excision .... (ek-SIZH-en)	removal by cutting
incision .... (in-SIZH-en)	surgical cut or wound produced by a sharp instrument
incision and drainage (I&D)... (in-SIZH-en) and (DRĀ-nij)	surgical cut made to allow the free flow or withdrawal of fluids from a lesion, wound, or cavity
laser surgery .... (LĀ-zer) (SER-jer-ē)	procedure using an instrument that emits a high-powered beam of light used to cut, burn, vaporize, or destroy tissue
Mohs surgery.............. (mōz) (SER-jer-ē)	technique of microscopically controlled serial excisions of skin cancers
suturing .... (SOO-cher-ing)	to stitch edges of a wound surgically (Figure 4-9)

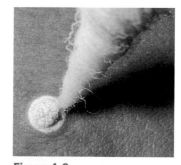

Figure 4-8
Cryosurgery performed with a nitrogen-soaked, cotton-tipped applicator.

MOHS SURGERY
allows for complete tumor removal while sparing surrounding normal tissue. It includes removing layers of tissue and examining them for tumor cells. If found, more tissue is removed until the margins are cancer free. It is used to treat recurrent skin cancers, especially lesions on the nose and ears, or areas that need tissue sparing. It is named after **Dr. Frederic E. Mohs,** Wisconsin, who first used the concept in 1936. The technique has evolved since that time.

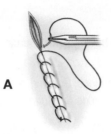

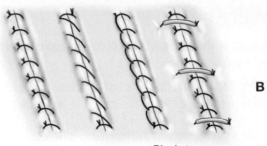

Intermittent   Continuous   Blanket   Retention
continuous

Figure 4-9
A, Suturing; **B,** types of sutures.

EXERCISE 23

Practice saying aloud each of the surgical terms not built from word parts on p. 113.

 To hear the terms select Chapter 4, Chapter Exercises, Pronunciation.

☐ Place a check mark in the box when you have completed this exercise.

EXERCISE 24

Fill in the blank with the correct surgical term.

1. _____ _____ is a technique of microscopically controlled serial excisions used for treatment of skin cancers.

2. A surgical cut or wound produced by a sharp instrument is called a(n) _____.

3. Destruction of tissue with a hot or cold instrument, electric current, or caustic substance is called _____.

4. _____ is to stitch the edges of a wound surgically.

5. A surgical cut made to allow the free flow or withdrawal of fluids from a lesion, wound, or cavity is called _____ _____ _____.

6. _____ is the removal of contaminated or dead tissue and foreign matter from an open wound.

7. Removal by cutting is known as _____.

8. _____ _____ is a procedure using an instrument that emits a high-powered beam of light used to cut, burn, vaporize, or destroy tissue.

9. The destruction of tissue by using extreme cold, often by using liquid nitrogen, is called _____.

10. _____ is a procedure to remove skin scars with abrasive material.

EXERCISE 25

Match the terms in the first column with their correct definitions in the second column.

_____ 1. suturing

_____ 2. dermabrasion

_____ 3. laser surgery

_____ 4. incision
       and drainage

_____ 5. cauterization

_____ 6. excision

_____ 7. Mohs surgery

_____ 8. débridement

_____ 9. cryosurgery

_____ 10. incision

a. destruction of tissue with a hot or cold instrument, electric current, or caustic substance

b. technique of microscopically controlled serial excisions of skin cancers

c. surgical cut or wound produced by a sharp instrument

d. surgical cut made to allow the free flow or withdrawal of fluids from a lesion, wound, or cavity

e. removal by cutting

f. removal of contaminated or dead tissue and foreign matter from an open wound

g. procedure using an instrument that emits a high-powered beam of light used to cut, burn, vaporize, or destroy tissue

h. procedure to remove skin scars with abrasive material, such as sandpaper

i. to stitch edges of a wound surgically

j. destruction of tissue by using extreme cold, often by using liquid nitrogen

EXERCISE 26

Spell each of the surgical terms not built from word parts on p. 113 by having someone dictate them to you.

 To hear and spell the terms select Chapter 4, Chapter Exercises, Spelling. You may type the terms on the screen or write them below in the spaces provided.

☐ Place a check mark in the box if you have compelted this exercise using your CD-ROM.

1. _____

2. _____

3. _____

4. _____

5. _____

6. _____

7. _____

8. _____

9. _____

10. _____

Complementary Terms

Built from Word Parts

The following terms are built from word parts you have already learned and can be translated literally to find their meanings. Further explanation of terms beyond the definition of their word parts, if needed, is included in parentheses.

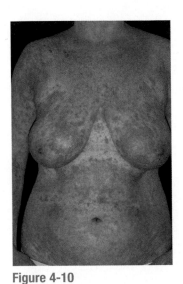

Figure 4-10
Exfoliative erythroderma. Erythroderma (red skin) may be caused by drugs, malignancy, psoriasis, and other conditions.

MRSA
or methicillin-resistant *Staphylococcus aureus,* is a strain of common bacteria that has developed resistance to penicillin and other antibiotics. It can produce skin and soft tissue infections and sometimes bloodstream infections and pneumonia, which can be fatal if not treated. MRSA is quite common in hospitals and long-term care facilities but is increasingly emerging as an important infection in the general population.

TRANSDERMAL
usually means entering through the skin and refers to the administration of a drug applied to the skin in ointment or patch form.
Percutaneous usually means performed through the skin, as in the insertion of a needle, catheter, or probe. See **percutaneous endoscopic gastronomy** highlighted in Chapter 11.

Term	Definition
dermatologist (*der*-ma-TOL-o-jist)	a physician who studies and treats skin (diseases)
dermatology (derm) (der-ma-TOL-o-jē)	study of the skin (a branch of medicine that deals with the diagnosis and treatment of skin diseases)
epidermal (*ep*-i-DER-mal)	pertaining to upon the skin
erythroderma (e-rith-rō-DER-ma)	red skin (abnormal redness of the skin) (Figure 4-10)
hypodermic (*hī*-pō-DER-mik)	pertaining to under the skin (Exercise Figure D)
intradermal (ID) (*in*-tra-DER-mal)	pertaining to within the skin (Exercise Figure D)
keratogenic (ker-a-tō-JEN-ik)	originating in horny tissue
leukoderma (lū-kō-DER-ma)	white skin (less color than normal)
necrosis (ne-KRŌ-sis)	abnormal condition of death (cells and tissue die because of disease)
percutaneous (per-kū-TĀ-nē-us)	pertaining to through the skin
staphylococcus (*pl.* staphylococci) (staph) (*staf*-il-ō-KOK-us) (*staf*-il-ō-KOK-sī)	berry-shaped (bacteria) in grapelike clusters (these bacteria cause many skin diseases) (Exercise Figure E)
streptococcus (*pl.* streptococci) (strep) (strep-tō-KOK-us) (strep-tō-KOK-sī)	berry-shaped (bacteria) in twisted chains (Exercise Figure E)
subcutaneous (subcut) (sub-kū-TĀ-nē-us)	pertaining to under the skin (Exercise Figure D)
transdermal (TD) (trans-DER-mel)	pertaining to through the skin (Exercise Figure D)
ungual (UNG-gwal)	pertaining to the nail
xanthoderma (zan-thō-DER-ma)	yellow skin (also called **jaundice**)

EXERCISE FIGURE **D**

Fill in the blanks to complete labeling the routes of administration diagrams.

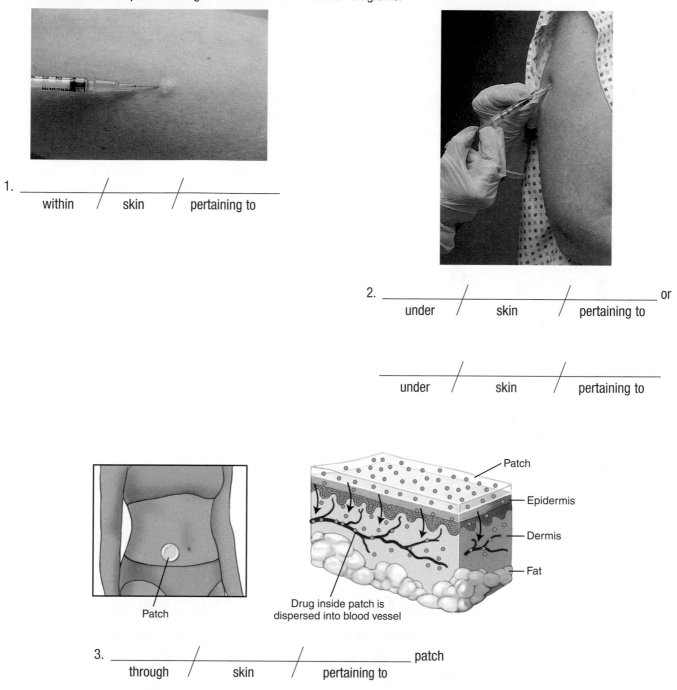

1. _____ / _____ / _____
   within / skin / pertaining to

2. _____ / _____ / _____ or
   under / skin / pertaining to

   _____ / _____ / _____
   under / skin / pertaining to

Patch

Epidermis

Dermis

Fat

Drug inside patch is
dispersed into blood vessel

Patch

3. _____ / _____ / _____ patch
   through / skin / pertaining to

EXERCISE FIGURE E

Fill in the blanks to label the diagrams.

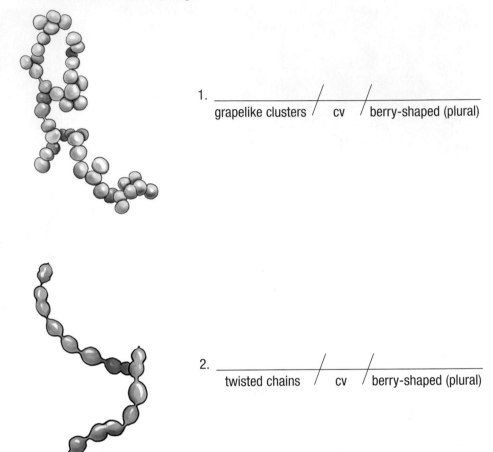

1. _____ / _____ / _____
   grapelike clusters / cv / berry-shaped (plural)

2. _____ / _____ / _____
   twisted chains / cv / berry-shaped (plural)

EXERCISE 27

Practice saying aloud each of the complementary terms built from word parts on p. 116.

To hear the terms select Chapter 4, Chapter Exercises, Pronunciation.

☐ Place a check mark in the box when you have completed this exercise.

EXERCISE 28

Analyze and define the following complementary terms.

Example: intra/derm/al   <u>pertaining to within the skin</u>
P   WR   S

1. ungual _____

2. transdermal _____

3. streptococcus _____

4. hypodermic _____

5. dermatology _____

6. subcutaneous _____

7. staphylococcus _____

8. keratogenic _____

9. dermatologist _____

10. necrosis _____

11. epidermal _____

12. xanthoderma _____

13. erythroderma _____

14. leukoderma _____

15. percutaneous _____

EXERCISE 29

Build complementary terms for the integumentary system by using the word parts you have learned.

Example: pertaining to under the skin   <u>hypo / derm / ic</u>
P / WR / S

1. study of the skin   _____ / / /
WR   CV   S

2. abnormal condition of death
   (of cells and tissue)

   _____/_____
   WR   /   S

3. pertaining to the nail

   _____/_____
   WR   /   S

4. berry-shaped bacteria in
   grapelike clusters (singular)

   _____//_____
   WR   /CV/   S

5. a physician who studies and
   treats skin (diseases)

   _____//_____
   WR   /CV/   S

6. pertaining to within the skin

   _____/_____/_____
   P   /   WR   /   S

7. pertaining to upon the skin

   _____/_____/_____
   P   /   WR   /   S

8. pertaining to under the skin

   _____/_____/_____
   P   /   WR   /   S

9. berry-shaped bacteria in
   twisted chains (singular)

   _____//_____
   WR   /CV/   S

10. originating in the horny
    tissue

    _Keter___/a/genic____
    WR   /CV/   S

11. white skin

    _____//_____/_____
    WR   /CV/ WR /   S

12. red skin

    _____//_____/_____
    WR   /CV/ WR /   S

13. yellow skin

    _____//_____/_____
    WR   /CV/ WR /   S

14. pertaining to through the skin

    _____/_____/_____
    P   /   WR   /   S

    _____/_____/_____
    P   /   WR   /   S

EXERCISE 30

Spell each of the complementary terms built from word parts on p. 116 by having someone dictate them to you.

To hear and spell the terms select Chapter 4, Chapter Exercises, Spelling. You may type the terms on the screen or write them on the following page in the spaces provided.

☐ Place a check mark in the box if you have completed this exercise using your CD-ROM.

1. _____   9. _____

2. _____   10. _____

3. _____   11. _____

4. _____   12. _____

5. _____   13. _____

6. _____   14. _____

7. _____   15. _____

8. _____   16. _____

Complementary Terms

Not Built from Word Parts

In some of the following terms, you may recognize word parts you have already learned; however, the full meaning of the terms cannot be discerned by the definition of their word parts.

Term	Definition
adipose (AD-i-pōs)	fat, fatty
allergy (AL-er-jē)	hypersensitivity to a substance
alopecia (al-ō-PĒ-sha)	loss of hair (Figure 4-11)
bacteria (*s.* bacterium) (bak-TĒR-ē-a) (bak-TĒR-ē-um)	single-celled microorganisms that reproduce by cell division and may cause infection by invading body tissue
cicatrix (SIK-a-triks)	scar
cyst (sist)	a closed sac containing fluid or semisolid material (Table 4-2)
cytomegalovirus (CMV) (*sī*-to-MEG-a-lō-*vī*-rus)	a herpes-type virus that usually causes disease when the immune system is compromised
diaphoresis (*dī*-a-fo-RĒ-sis)	profuse sweating
ecchymosis (ek-i-MŌ-sis)	escape of blood into the tissues, causing superficial discoloration; a "black and blue" mark (also called a **bruise**)
edema (e-DĒ-ma)	puffy swelling of tissue from the accumulation of fluid

ADIPOSE
contains the Latin word root **adip**, meaning **fat.** Adipose tissue is composed of fat cells arranged in lobules. **Lip** is the Greek word root for **fat.**

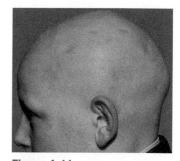

Figure 4-11
Alopecia totalis (loss of hair from the scalp) with absence of eyelashes.

ALOPECIA
is derived from the Greek **alopex**, meaning **fox.** One was thought to bald like a mangy fox.

DIAPHORESIS
is derived from Greek **dia**, meaning **through,** and **phoreo**, meaning **I carry.** Translated, it means the carrying through of perspiration.

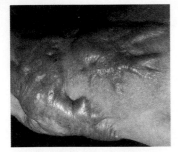

Figure 4-12
Burn keloid.

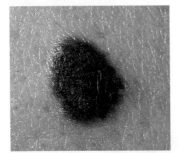

Figure 4-13
Nevus (also called **mole**).

 MACULE
is probably derived from the ancient Sanskrit word **mala,** meaning **dirt.**

 PETECHIA
is originally from the Italian **petechio,** meaning **flea bite.** The small hemorrhagic spot resembles the mark made by a flea.

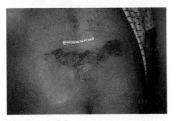

Figure 4-14
Stage 2 pressure ulcer (also called **decubitus ulcer** or **bed sore**).

Complementary Terms—*cont'd*
Not Built from Word Parts

Term	Definition
emollient (e-MOL-yent)	agent that softens or soothes the skin
erythema (er-i-THĒ-ma)	redness
fungus (*pl.* fungi) (FUN-gus) (FUN-jī)	organism that feeds by absorbing organic molecules from its surroundings and may cause infection by invading body tissue; single-celled fungi (yeast) reproduce by budding; multicelled fungi (mold) reproduce by spore formation
induration (in-dū-RĀ-shun)	abnormal hard spot(s)
jaundice (JAWN-dis)	condition characterized by a yellow tinge to the skin (also called **xanthoderma**)
keloid (KĒ-loyd)	overgrowth of scar tissue (Figure 4-12)
leukoplakia (lū-kō-PLĀ-kē-a)	condition characterized by white spots or patches on mucous membrane, which may be precancerous
macule (MAK-ūl)	flat, colored spot on the skin (Table 4-2)
nevus (*pl.* nevi) (NĒ-vus) (NĒ-vī)	circumscribed malformation of the skin, usually brown, black, or flesh colored. A congenital nevus is present at birth and is referred to as a birthmark (Figure 4-13) (also called a **mole**).
nodule (NOD-ūl)	a small, knotlike mass that can be felt by touch (Table 4-2)
pallor (PAL-or)	paleness
papule (PAP-ūl)	small, solid skin elevation (Table 4-2) (also called **pimple**)
petechia (*pl.* petechiae) (pe-TĒ-kē-a) (pe-TĒ-kē-ē)	a pinpoint skin hemorrhage
pressure ulcer (decub) (PRESH-ur) (UL-sir)	eroded sore on the skin caused by prolonged pressure, often occurring in bedridden patients (Figure 4-14) (also called **decubitus ulcer** or **bed sore**)
pruritus (prū-RĪ-tus)	severe itching
purpura (PER-pū-ra)	disorder characterized by hemorrhages into the tissue, giving the skin a purple-red discoloration
pustule (PUS-tūl)	elevation of skin containing pus (Table 4-2)

TABLE 4-2
Common Skin Lesions

Lesion	Definition	Cutaway Sections	Example
Macule	flat, colored spot on the skin		freckle
Papule	small, solid skin elevation		skin tag basal cell carcinoma
Nodule	a small, knotlike mass		lipoma metastatic carcinoma rheumatoid nodule
Wheal	round, itchy elevation of the skin		urticaria (hive)
Vesicle	small elevation of epidermis containing liquid		shingles (herpes zoster) Herpes simplex contact dermatitis
Pustule	elevation of the skin containing pus		impetigo acne
Cyst	a closed sac containing fluid or semisolid material		acne

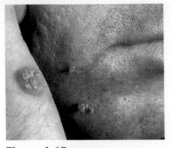

Figure 4-15
Verruca (also called **wart**).

**Dermatology, *or*
Give Me a Man
Who Calls a Spade
a Geotome**

I wish the *dermatologist*
Were less a firm apologist
For all the terminology
That's used in *dermatology*

Something you or I would
   deem a
Redness he calls *erythema;*
If it's blistered, raw and warm
   he
Has to call it multiforme
Things to him are never
   simple;
Papule is his word for pimple
What's a macule, clearly
   stated?
Just a spot that's over-rated!

Over the skin that looks
   unwell
He chants Latin like a spell;
What he's labeled and
   obscured
Looks to him as good as
   cured.

Reprinted with permission from
*The New England Journal of
Medicine,* 1977; 297(12):660.

Complementary Terms—*cont'd*
Not Built from Word Parts

Term	Definition
ulcer. (UL-ser)	eroded sore on the skin or mucous membrane (Figure 4-14)
verruca . . . . (ver-RŪ-ka)	circumscribed cutaneous elevation caused by a virus (Figure 4-15) (also called **wart**)
vesicle . . . . (VES-i-kl)	small elevation of the epidermis containing liquid (Table 4-2) (also called **blister**)
virus. . . . . (VĪ-ras)	minute microorganism, much smaller than bacterium, characterized by a lack of independent metabolism and the ability to replicate only within living host cells; may cause infection by invading body tissue
wheal. . . . . (hwēl)	transitory, itchy elevation of the skin with a white center and a red surrounding area; a wheal is an individual urticaria (hive) lesion (Table 4-2)

EXERCISE 31

Practice saying aloud each of the complementary terms not built from word parts on pp. 121-124.

 To hear the terms select Chapter 4, Chapter Exercises, Pronunciation.

☐ Place a check mark in the box when you have completed this exercise.

EXERCISE 32

Fill in the blanks with the correct terms.

1. Another name for *scar* is _____.

2. Profuse sweating is called _____.

3. The term for an agent that softens or soothes the skin is _____.

4. The medical term for *wart* is _____.

5. _____ is the name for a flat, colored skin spot.

6. A yellow skin condition is known as _____.

7. The condition of white spots or patches on mucous membrane is called _____.

8. _____ is a pinpoint hemorrhage of the skin.

9. An eroded sore is called a(n) _____.

10. A(n) _____ is an overgrowth of scar tissue.

11. Another name for paleness is _____.

12. Superficial skin discoloration caused by escaping blood is referred to as _____.

13. An eroded sore on the skin caused by prolonged pressure is a(n) _____ _____.

14. A small knotlike mass that can be felt by touch is called a(n) _____.

15. Another term for fat is _____.

16. A closed sac containing fluid or semisolid material is called a(n) _____.

17. Severe itching is called _____.

18. Another name for redness is _____.

19. The condition of tissue hemorrhages giving the skin a purple-red discoloration is known as _____.

20. _____ is another name for mole.

21. Single-celled microorganisms that reproduce by cell division and may cause infection by invading body tissue are called _____.

22. The term for loss of hair is _____.

23. Hypersensitivity to a substance is called a(n) _____.

24. A small, solid skin elevation is called a(n) _____.

25. A transitory skin elevation with a white center and a red surrounding area is a(n) _____.

26. A(n) _____ is a skin elevation containing pus.

27. A blister is also called a(n) _____.

28. An organism that feeds by absorbing organic molecules from its surroundings and may cause infection by invading body tissue is called _____.

29. _____ is a minute microorganism characterized by a lack of independent metabolism and the ability to replicate only within living host cells; it also may cause infection by invading body tissue.

30. An abnormal hard spot(s) is called _____.

31. _____ is the swelling of tissue.

32. _____ is a herpes-type virus.

EXERCISE 33

Match the words in the first column with their correct definitions in the second column.

_____ 1. adipose

_____ 2. pressure ulcer

_____ 3. allergy

_____ 4. alopecia

_____ 5. cicatrix

_____ 6. fungus

_____ 7. nodule

_____ 8. bacteria

_____ 9. diaphoresis

_____ 10. cyst

_____ 11. ecchymosis

_____ 12. emollient

_____ 13. erythema

_____ 14. jaundice

_____ 15. edema

_____ 16. induration

a. loss of hair

b. superficial discoloration caused by blood escaping into the tissues

c. yellow color to the skin

d. closed sac containing fluid

e. organism that feeds by absorbing organic molecules from its surroundings and may cause infection by invading body tissue

f. agent that softens or soothes the skin

g. profuse sweating

h. hypersensitivity to a substance

i. hard spot(s)

j. scar

k. redness

l. single-celled microorganisms that reproduce by cell division and may cause infection by invading body tissue

m. fat

n. small knot

o. eroded sore on the skin caused by prolonged pressure

p. patches

q. swelling of tissue

EXERCISE 34

Match the terms in the first column with their correct definitions in the second column.

_____ 1. keloid

_____ 2. leukoplakia

_____ 3. macule

_____ 4. nevus

_____ 5. pallor

_____ 6. papule

_____ 7. petechiae

_____ 8. pruritus

_____ 9. purpura

_____ 10. pustule

_____ 11. ulcer

_____ 12. verruca

_____ 13. vesicle

_____ 14. wheal

_____ 15. virus

_____ 16. cytomegalovirus

a. mole

b. severe itching

c. wart

d. condition of white spots or patches on mucous membranes

e. hemorrhages in tissue giving skin a red-purple color

f. skin elevation containing pus

g. overgrowth of scar tissue

h. small elevation of epidermis containing liquid

i. individual urticaria lesion

j. flat, colored spot on skin

k. small, solid skin elevation

l. paleness

m. minute microorganism characterized by a lack of independent metabolism and the ability to replicate only within living host cells that may cause infection by invading body tissue

n. pinpoint skin hemorrhages

o. eroded sore on the skin or mucous membrane

p. profuse sweating

q. herpes-type virus

EXERCISE 35

Spell each of the complementary terms not built from word parts on pp. 121-124 by having someone dictate them to you.

 To hear and spell the terms select Chapter 4, Chapter Exercises, Spelling. You may type the terms on the screen or write them below in the spaces provided.

☐ Place a check mark in the box if you have completed this exercise using your CD-ROM.

1. _____

2. _____

3. _____

4. _____

5. _____

6. _____

7. _____

8. _____

9. _____

10. _____

11. _____   22. _____

12. _____   23. _____

13. _____   24. _____

14. _____   25. _____

15. _____   26. _____

16. _____   27. _____

17. _____   28. _____

18. _____   29. _____

19. _____   30. _____

20. _____   31. _____

21. _____   32. _____

Refer to Appendix E for pharmacology terms related to the integumentary system.

Abbreviations

BCC	basal cell carcinoma
bx	biopsy
CMV	cytomegalovirus
decub.	pressure ulcer
derm	dermatology
I&D	incision and drainage
ID	intradermal
SLE	systemic lupus erythematosus
SqCCA	squamous cell carcinoma
staph	staphylococcus
strep	streptococcus
subcut	subcutaneous
TD	transdermal

Refer to Appendix D for a complete list of abbreviations.

EXERCISE 36

Write the meaning for each of the abbreviations in the following sentences.

1. The most common form of skin cancer is **BCC** _____
   _____ _____.

2. It is rare to see cutaneous **CMV** _____ infections.

3. **SLE** _____ _____ _____ is a chronic
   relapsing disease, often with long periods of remission.

4. Long-term exposure to sunlight is by far the most frequent cause of
   SqCCA _____ _____ _____.

5. The **bx** _____ results were negative.

6. The medication was administered by **subcut** _____
   injection.

7. **Staph** _____ bacterium was cultured from the abscess.

8. The culture confirmed a **strep** _____ infection of the
   throat.

9. **I&D** _____ _____ _____ is used to treat
   cutaneous abscesses, such as a furuncle.

10. Hormone replacement therapy is available in **TD** _____
    administration.

11. The tuberculin test was administered by an **ID** _____
    injection.

12. The patient visited the **derm** _____ clinic for a
    psoriasis follow-up visit.

13. Débridement may be used to treat a **decub** _____
    _____.

PRACTICAL APPLICATION

EXERCISE 37   *Interact with Medical Documents*

A. Below is an operative report. Complete the report by writing the medical terms in the blanks that correspond to the numbered definitions on the next page.

University Hospital and Medical Center

4700 North Main Street • Wellness, Arizona 54321 • (987) 555-3210

PATIENT NAME: Sandra Wharton   **CASE NUMBER:** 76548-INT

DATE OF BIRTH: 10/03/19XX   **DATE:** 07/27/20XX

OPERATIVE REPORT

CASE HISTORY: The patient is a 50-year-old white woman presenting to the 1. _____ clinic for follow-up of a 2. _____ located at the 3. _____ aspect of her left eyebrow.

The patient's medical history is also significant for 4. _____ _____, primarily of the scalp and ears, as well as chronic 5. _____, primarily of the forearms bilaterally.

INDICATIONS FOR PROCEDURE: Comparing today's exam with past medical records and photos from 10/20/20XX, the nevus shows changes that include hair loss, "crusty" surface, and some enlargement of the 6. _____. The nevus has been present for approximately 3 years. Risks, benefits, indications, and expectations were discussed with the patient regarding biopsy, and she has agreed to proceed with 7. _____.

PREOPERATIVE DIAGNOSIS: Dysplastic nevus, left eyebrow.

ANESTHESIA: Xylocaine 1% with epinephrine.

PROCEDURE: After written consent was obtained, the site was prepped with Betadine and draped in the usual sterile fashion. The skin was incised at the 8. _____ pole of the lesion. The lesion was then excised, including a margin of clinically normal dermis. Specimen was submitted to 9. _____. The superior pole was sutured. 10. _____ was used to achieve hemostasis. Two A-T flaps were then constructed on superior aspect of upper left eyelid. Flaps and upper left eyelid undermined 2 to 3 mm. Flaps sutured with 6-0 Vicryl, followed by 6-0 nylon for closure. Pressure dressing was applied.

The patient tolerated the procedure well.

POSTOPERATIVE DIAGNOSIS: 11. _____ revealed 12. _____ _____ _____, nodular, transected at base.

_____
William Hickman, MD

WH/mcm

1. study of skin
2. mole
3. pertaining to the middle
4. precancerous skin condition of horny tissue formation
5. noninfectious, inflammatory skin disease with redness, blisters, scabs, and itching
6. changes in tissue resulting from injury or disease
7. removal by cutting
8. pertaining to above
9. study of disease
10. destruction of tissue with a hot or cold instrument, electric current, or caustic substance
11. view of life
12. epithelial tumor arising from epidermis

B. Read the pathology report and answer the questions following it.

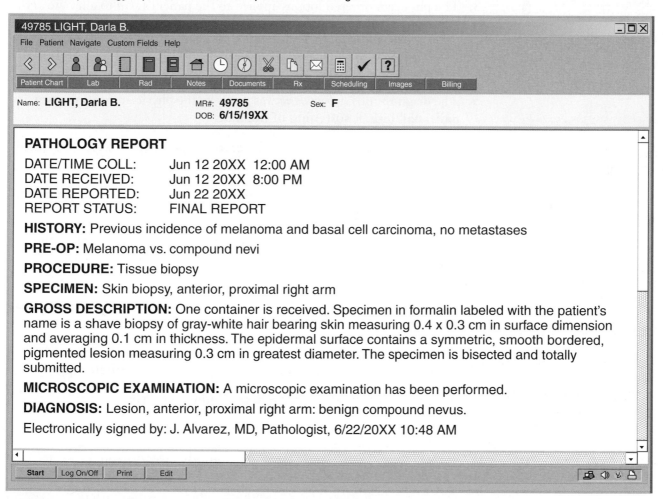

1. Identify singular and plural forms of medical terms used in the pathology report. Write "p" for plural and "s" for singular next to the terms. Refer to Table 2-2 for plural endings.
   a. melanoma _____
   b. melanomata _____
   c. nevi _____
   d. nevus _____
   e. metastasis _____
   f. metastases _____
   g. biopsy _____
   h. biopsies _____

2. The skin biopsy was obtained from:
   a. near the shoulder on the back of the right arm
   b. near the shoulder on the front of the right arm
   c. near the wrist on the back of the right arm
   d. near the wrist on the front of the right arm

3. Use your medical dictionary to find the meanings of the following terms used in the pathology report:
   a. compound _____
   b. pigmented _____
   c. bisected _____
   d. microscopic _____

EXERCISE **38** *Interpret Medical Terms*

To test your understanding of the terms introduced in this chapter, circle the words that correctly complete the sentences. The italicized words refer to the correct answer.

WEB LINK
For more information about diseases and disorders of the integumentary system and current treatments, visit the American Academy of Dermatology at www.aad.org.

1. The physician called *the injury with pain, swelling, and discoloration with no break in the skin* a (**fissure, contusion, laceration**).

2. *Berry-shaped bacteria in grapelike clusters* are (**streptococci, staphylococci, pediculosis**).

3. The physician ordered lotions applied to the patient's *skin* to alleviate *dryness,* or (**pachyderma, dermatoconiosis, xeroderma**).

4. The injection given *within the skin* is called a(n) (**intradermal, epidermal, hypodermic**) injection.

5. The diagnosis of *onychomalacia* was given by the physician for (**ingrown nails, nail biting, softening of the nails**).

6. The *pinpoint hemorrhages,* or (**nevi, verrucae, petechiae**), were distributed over the patient's entire body.

7. The primary symptom of the disease was *profuse sweating,* or (**diaphoresis, ecchymosis, pruritus**).

8. The patient had an *abnormal condition of fungus in the hair;* therefore the doctor recorded the diagnosis as (**onychocryptosis, trichomycosis, onychomycosis**).

9. The student nurse learned that the medical name for a *blister* was (**verruca, keloid, vesicle**).

10. The patient was to receive a *skin graft from her mother,* so the operation was listed as a (**dermatoplasty, dermatoautoplasty, dermatoheteroplasty**).

11. An *abnormal hard spot* is called (**edema, induration, virus**).

12. Another word for *jaundice* is (**erythroderma, leukoderma, xanthoderma**).

13. *Leiodermia* is a condition of (**striated, smooth, sweaty**) skin.

14. The *localized collection of pus* (**acne, abscess, cyst**) was incised and drained followed by débridement. A culture swab of the wound revealed methicillin-resistant *Staphylococcus aureus.*

15. *A technique of microscopically controlled serial excisions* (**cryosurgery, laser surgery, Mohs surgery**) was used to treat the patient's recurrent squamous cell carcinoma.

EXERCISE 39   *Read Medical Terms in Use*

Practice pronunciation of terms by reading aloud the following medical document. Use the pronunciation key following the medical term to assist you in saying the word.

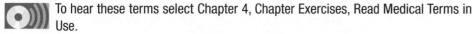 To hear these terms select Chapter 4, Chapter Exercises, Read Medical Terms in Use.

Emily visited the **dermatology** (*der*-ma-TOL-ò-jē) clinic because of **pruritus** (prū-RĪ-tus) secondary to **dermatitis** (*der*-ma-TĪ-tis) involving her scalp, arms, and legs. A diagnosis of **psoriasis** (so-RĪ-a-sis) was made. **Eczema** (EK-ze-ma), **scabies** (SKĀ-bēz), and **tinea** (TIN-ē-a) were considered in the differential diagnosis. An **emollient** (e-MOL-yent) cream was prescribed. In addition the patient showed the **dermatologist** (der-ma-TOL-o-jist) the tender, discolored, thickened nail of her right great toe. Emily learned she had **onychomycosis** (*on*-i-kō-mī-KŌ-sis), for which she was given an additional prescription for an oral antifungal drug.

EXERCISE 40   *Comprehend Medical Terms in Use*

Test your comprehension of terms in the above medical document by circling the correct answer.

1. Emily sought medical attention because of:
   a. an eroded sore and inflammation of the skin
   b. severe itching and inflammation of the skin
   c. severe itching and thickness of the skin
   d. an eroded sore and thickening of the skin

2. T   F An inflammatory disease of the skin involving sebaceous glands and hair follicles was considered in the differential diagnosis.

3. Emily was given an additional prescription for an abnormal condition of fungus in the:
   a. sudoriferous glands
   b. hair follicles
   c. sebaceous glands
   d. nails

CHAPTER REVIEW

CHAPTER REVIEW ON CD-ROM

Use the CD-ROM that accompanies this textbook to play and practice what you have learned in this chapter. The Chapter Exercises, Practice Activities, Animations, and Games allow you to hear, see, and interact with the chapter content.

Chapter Exercises

Exercises in this section of your CD-ROM correlate to exercises in your textbook. You may have completed them as you worked through the chapter.

☐ Pronunciation
☐ Spelling
☐ Read Medical Terms in Use

Practice Activities

Practice in study mode, then test your learning in assessment mode. Keep track of your scores from assessment mode if you wish.

	SCORE
☐ Picture It	___
☐ Define Word Parts	___
☐ Build Medical Terms	___
☐ Word Shop	___
☐ Define Medical Terms	___
☐ Use It	___
☐ Hear It and Type It: Clinical Vignettes	___

Animations

☐ Pressure Ulcer (decubitus ulcer)

Games

☐ Name that Word Part
☐ Term Storm
☐ Term Explorer
☐ Termbusters
☐ Medical Millionaire

REVIEW OF WORD PARTS

Can you define and spell the following word parts?

Combining Forms		Prefixes	Suffixes
aut/o	myc/o	epi-	-a
bi/o	necr/o	intra-	-coccus (*pl.* -cocci)
coni/o	onych/o	para-	-ectomy
crypt/o	pachy/o	per-	-ia
cutane/o	rhytid/o	sub-	-itis
derm/o	seb/o	trans-	-malacia
dermat/o	staphyl/o		-opsy
heter/o	strept/o		-phagia
hidr/o	trich/o		-plasty
kerat/o	ungu/o		-rrhea
	xer/o		-tome

REVIEW OF TERMS

Can you build, analyze, define, pronounce, and spell the following terms *built from word parts?*

Diseases and Disorders		Surgical	Complementary	
dermatitis	onychomycosis	biopsy (bx)	dermatologist	percutaneous
dermatoconiosis	onychophagia	dermatoautoplasty	dermatology (derm)	staphylococcus (staph)
dermatofibroma	pachyderma	dermatoheteroplasty	epidermal	(*pl.* staphylococci)
hidradenitis	paronychia	dermatome	erythroderma	streptococcus (strep)
leiodermia	seborrhea	dermatoplasty	hypodermic	(*pl.* streptococci)
onychocryptosis	trichomycosis	onychectomy	intradermal (ID)	subcutaneous (subcut)
onychomalacia	xeroderma	rhytidectomy	keratogenic	transdermal (TD)
		rhytidoplasty	leukoderma	ungual
			necrosis	xanthoderma

Can you define, pronounce, and spell the following terms *not built from word parts?*

Diseases and Disorders	Surgical	Complementary
abrasion	cauterization	adipose
abscess	cryosurgery	allergy
acne	débridement	alopecia
actinic keratosis	dermabrasion	bacteria (*s.* bacterium)
albinism	excision	cicatrix
basal cell carcinoma (BCC)	incision	cyst
candidiasis	incision and drainage (I&D)	cytomegalovirus (CMV)
carbuncle	laser surgery	diaphoresis
cellulitis	Mohs surgery	ecchymosis
contusion	suturing	edema
eczema		emollient
fissure		erythema
furuncle		fungus (*pl.* fungi)
gangrene		induration
herpes		jaundice
impetigo		keloid
Kaposi sarcoma		leukoplakia
laceration		macule
lesion		nevus (*pl.* nevi)
pediculosis		nodule
psoriasis		pallor
rosacea		papule
scabies		petechia (*pl.* petechiae)
scleroderma		pressure ulcer (decub)
shingles		pruritus
squamous cell carcinoma (SqCCA)		purpura
systemic lupus erythematosus (SLE)		pustule
tinea		ulcer
urticaria		verruca
		vesicle
		virus
		wheal

ANSWERS

Exercise Figures

Exercise Figure
A. 1. horny tissue: kerat/o
   2. hair: trich/o
   3. skin: cutane/o, dermat/o, derm/o
   4. sebum: seb/o
   5. sweat: hidr/o

Exercise Figure
B. 1. nail: onych/o, ungu/o

Exercise Figure
C. 1. onych/o/myc/osis
   2. par/onych/ia

Exercise Figure
D. 1. intra/derm/al
   2. sub/cutane/ous, hypo/derm/ic
   3. trans/dermal

Exercise Figure
E. 1. staphyl/o/cocci
   2. strept/o/cocci

Exercise 1
1. c
2. d
3. g
4. b
5. f
6. h
7. a

Exercise 2
1. sweat
2. skin
3. nail
4. hair
5. horny tissue, hard
6. skin
7. sebum (oil)
8. nail
9. skin

Exercise 3
1. trich/o
2. hidr/o
3. a. onych/o
   b. ungu/o
4. seb/o
5. a. derm/o
   b. dermat/o
   c. cutane/o
6. kerat/o

Exercise 4
1. death
2. grapelike clusters
3. hidden
4. thick
5. dust
6. fungus
7. life
8. other
9. twisted chains
10. dry
11. self
12. wrinkles

Exercise 5
1. myc/o
2. necr/o
3. heter/o
4. xer/o
5. pachy/o
6. strept/o
7. rhytid/o
8. staphyl/o
9. aut/o
10. crypt/o
11. coni/o
12. bi/o

Exercise 6
1. under, below
2. beside, beyond, around, abnormal
3. on, upon, over
4. within
5. through
6. through, across, beyond

Exercise 7
1. intra-
2. sub-
3. epi-
4. para-
5. per-
6. trans-

Exercise 8
1. c
2. e
3. a
4. j
5. i
6. h
7. d
8. b
9. f
10. k
11. l

Exercise 9
1. surgical repair
2. excision or surgical removal
3. softening
4. inflammation
5. instrument used to cut
6. eating, swallowing
7. flow, discharge
8. berry-shaped
9. view of, viewing
10. diseased or abnormal state, condition of
11. noun suffix, no meaning

Exercise 10
Pronunciation Exercise

Exercise 11
1. WR CV WR   S
   dermat/o/coni/osis
        CF
   abnormal condition of the skin caused by dust
2. WR WR   S
   hidr/aden/itis
   inflammation of the sweat glands

3. WR   S
   dermat/itis
   inflammation of the skin
4. WR WR S
   pachy/derm/a
   thickening of the skin
5. WR CV S
   onych/o/malacia
        CF
   softening of the nails
6. WR CV WR S
   trich/o/myc/osis
        CF
   abnormal condition of a fungus in the hair
7. WR CV WR S
   dermat/o/fibr/oma
        CF
   fibrous tumor of the skin
8. P WR   S
   par/onych/ia
   diseased state around the nail
9. WR CV WR   S
   onych/o/crypt/osis
        CF
   abnormal condition of a hidden nail
10. WR CV S
   seb/o/rrhea
        CF
   discharge of sebum (excessive)
11. WR CV S
   onych/o/phagia
        CF
   eating the nails, nail biting
12. WR CV WR S
   xer/o/derm/a
        CF
   dry skin
13. WR CV WR S
   lei/o/derm/ia
        CF
   condition of smooth skin

Exercise 12
1. pachy/derm/a
2. onych/o/myc/osis
3. seb/o/rrhea
4. dermat/itis
5. dermat/o/fibr/oma
6. onych/o/malacia
7. hidr/aden/itis
8. onych/o/crypt/osis
9. dermat/o/coni/osis
10. onych/o/phagia

11. par/onych/ia
12. xer/o/derm/a
13. lei/o/derm/ia

Exercise 13
Spelling Exercise; see text p. 102.

Exercise 14
Pronunciation Exercise

Exercise 15
1. systemic lupus erythematosus
2. abscess
3. fissure
4. abrasion
5. psoriasis
6. herpes
7. pediculosis
8. tinea
9. contusion
10. gangrene
11. lesion
12. Kaposi sarcoma
13. actinic keratosis
14. carbuncle
15. acne
16. laceration
17. furuncle
18. squamous cell
19. cellulitis
20. impetigo
21. eczema
22. scabies
23. urticaria
24. basal cell
25. scleroderma
26. candidiasis
27. shingles
28. rosacea
29. albinism

Exercise 16

1. f		8. k	
2. j		9. e	
3. g		10. b	
4. l		11. h	
5. n		12. a	
6. c		13. d	
7. i		14. m	

Exercise 17

1. d		9. n	
2. i		10. e	
3. f		11. b	
4. h		12. g	
5. m		13. k	
6. l		14. o	
7. c		15. j	
8. a			

Exercise 18
Spelling Exercise; see text p. 110.

Exercise 19
Pronunciation Exercise

Exercise 20
1. WR   S
   rhytid/ectomy
   excision of wrinkles
2. WR S
   bi/opsy
   view of life (removal of living tissue)
3. WR CV WR CV S
   dermat/o/aut/o/plasty
   ___ CF ___ CF
   surgical repair using one's own skin
   (for the skin graft)
4. WR   S
   onych/ectomy
   excision of a nail
5. WR CV S
   rhytid/o/plasty
   ___ CF
   surgical repair of wrinkles
6. WR   CV WR CV S
   dermat/o/heter/o/plasty
   ___ CF ___ CF
   surgical repair using skin from others
   (for the skin graft)
7. WR   S
   derma/tome
   instrument used to cut skin

Exercise 21
1. rhytid/ectomy
2. bi/opsy
3. dermat/o/heter/o/plasty
4. onych/ectomy
5. rhytid/o/plasty
6. dermat/o/plasty
7. derma/tome

Exercise 22
Spelling Exercise; see text p. 113.

Exercise 23
Pronunciation Exercise

Exercise 24
1. Mohs surgery
2. incision
3. cauterization
4. suturing
5. incision and drainage
6. débridement
7. excision
8. laser surgery
9. cryosurgery
10. dermabrasion

Exercise 25

1. i		6. e	
2. h		7. b	
3. g		8. f	
4. d		9. j	
5. a		10. c	

Exercise 26
Spelling Exercise, see text p. 115.

Exercise 27
Pronunciation Exercise

Exercise 28
1. WR S
   ungu/al
   pertaining to the nail
2. P   WR S
   trans/derm/al
   pertaining to through the skin
3. WR CV   S
   strept/o/coccus
   ___ CF
   berry-shaped (bacteria) in twisted
   chains
4. P   WR S
   hypo/derm/ic
   pertaining to under the skin
5. WR CV S
   dermat/o/logy
   ___ CF
   study of the skin (diseases)
6. P   WR   S
   sub/cutane/ous
   pertaining to under the skin
7. WR CV S
   staphyl/o/coccus
   ___ CF
   berry-shaped (bacteria) in grapelike
   clusters
8. WR CV S
   kerat/o/genic
   ___ CF
   originating in horny tissue
9. WR CV S
   dermat/o/logist
   ___ CF
   physician who studies and treats skin
   (diseases)
10. WR   S
    necr/osis
    abnormal condition of death
11. P   WR S
    epi/derm/al
    pertaining to upon the skin
12. WR CV WR S
    xanth/o/derm/a
    ___ CF
    yellow skin

13. WR CV WR S
    erythr/o/derm/a
         CF
    red skin

14. WR CV WR S
    leuk/o/derm/a
         CF
    white skin

15. P WR S
    per/cutane/ous
    pertaining to through the skin

Exercise 29
1. dermat/o/logy
2. necr/osis
3. ungu/al
4. staphyl/o/coccus
5. dermat/o/logist
6. intra/derm/al
7. epi/derm/al
8. sub/cutane/ous, hypo/derm/ic
9. strept/o/coccus
10. kerat/o/genic
11. leuk/o/derm/a
12. erythr/o/derm/a
13. xanth/o/derm/a
14. per/cutane/ous, trans/derm/al

Exercise 30
Spelling Exercise; see text pp. 120-121.

Exercise 31
Pronunciation Exercise

Exercise 32
1. cicatrix
2. diaphoresis
3. emollient
4. verruca
5. macule
6. jaundice
7. leukoplakia
8. petechia
9. ulcer
10. keloid
11. pallor
12. ecchymosis
13. pressure ulcer
14. nodule
15. adipose
16. cyst
17. pruritus

18. erythema
19. purpura
20. nevus
21. bacteria
22. alopecia
23. allergy
24. papule
25. wheal
26. pustule
27. vesicle
28. fungus
29. virus
30. induration
31. edema
32. cytomegalovirus

Exercise 33
1. m
2. o
3. h
4. a
5. j
6. e
7. n
8. l
9. g
10. d
11. b
12. f
13. k
14. c
15. q
16. i

Exercise 34
1. g
2. d
3. j
4. a
5. l
6. k
7. n
8. b
9. e
10. f
11. o
12. c
13. h
14. i
15. m
16. q

Exercise 35
Spelling Exercise; see text pp. 127-128.

Exercise 36
1. basal cell carcinoma
2. cytomegalovirus
3. systemic lupus erythematosus
4. squamous cell carcinoma
5. biopsy
6. subcutaneous
7. staphylococcus
8. streptococcus
9. incision and drainage
10. transdermal
11. intradermal
12. dermatology
13. pressure ulcer

Exercise 37
A. 1. dermatology
   2. nevus
   3. medial
   4. actinic keratosis
   5. eczema
   6. lesion
   7. excision
   8. superior
   9. pathology
   10. cauterization
   11. biopsy
   12. basal cell carcinoma

B. 1. a. s
      b. p
      c. p
      d. s
      e. s
      f. p
      g. s
      h. p
   2. b
   3. dictionary exercise

Exercise 38
1. contusion
2. staphylococci
3. xeroderma
4. intradermal
5. softening of the nails
6. petechiae
7. diaphoresis
8. trichomycosis
9. vesicle
10. dermatoheteroplasty
11. induration
12. xanthoderma
13. smooth
14. abscess
15. Mohs surgery

Exercise 39
Reading Exercise

Exercise 40
1. b
2. F, acne is the condition described in the sentence.
3. d

NOTES

CHAPTER 5
Respiratory System

OUTLINE

ANATOMY, 142

WORD PARTS, 145
Combining Forms, 145
Prefixes, 149
Suffixes, 150

MEDICAL TERMS, 152
Disease and Disorder Terms, 152
　　Built from Word Parts, 152
　　Not Built from Word Parts, 159
Surgical Terms, 165
　　Built from Word Parts, 165
Diagnostic Terms, 171
　　Built from Word Parts, 171
　　Not Built from Word Parts, 179
Complementary Terms, 181
　　Built from Word Parts, 181
　　Not Built from Word Parts, 187
Abbreviations, 191

PRACTICAL APPLICATION, 193
Interact with Medical Documents, 193
Interpret Medical Terms, 196
Read Medical Terms in Use, 197
Comprehend Medical Terms in Use, 197

CHAPTER REVIEW, 198

TABLE 5-1 TYPES OF DIAGNOSTIC PROCEDURES, 174

OBJECTIVES

Upon completion of this chapter you will be able to:

1. Identify organs and structures of the respiratory system.

2. Define and spell word parts related to the respiratory system.

3. Define, pronounce, and spell disease and disorder terms related to the respiratory system.

4. Define, pronounce, and spell surgical terms related to the respiratory system.

5. Define, pronounce, and spell diagnostic terms related to the respiratory system.

6. Define, pronounce, and spell complementary terms related to the respiratory system.

7. Interpret the meaning of abbreviations related to the respiratory system.

8. Interpret, read, and comprehend medical language in simulated medical statements and documents.

ANATOMY

Function

The function of the respiratory system is the exchange of oxygen (O_2) and carbon dioxide (CO_2) between the atmosphere and body cells. The process is called *respiration*. During external respiration, or breathing, oxygen passes from the lungs to the blood in the capillaries. Carbon dioxide also passes from the capillaries back into the lungs to be expelled. During internal respiration the body cells take on oxygen from the blood and give back carbon dioxide, which is transported back to the lungs. The process of inhalation brings air into the lungs. Exhalation expels air from the lungs. Respiration, or breathing, normally occurs every 3 to 5 seconds. See Figure 5-1 to identify the organs of respiration.

> **RESPIRATION**
> is also called **breathing**, or **ventilation**.

Organs of the Respiratory System

Term	Definition
nose	lined with mucous membrane and fine hairs. It acts as a filter to moisten and warm the entering air.
nasal septum	partition separating the right and left nasal cavities
paranasal sinuses	air cavities within the cranial bones that open into the nasal cavities
pharynx	serves as a food and air passageway. Air enters from the nasal cavities and passes through the pharynx to the larynx. Food enters the pharynx from the mouth and passes into the esophagus (also called the **throat**).
adenoids	lymphoid tissue located behind the nasal cavity
tonsils	lymphoid tissue located behind the mouth
larynx	location of the vocal cords. Air enters from the pharynx (also called the **voice box**).
epiglottis	flap of cartilage that automatically covers the opening of and keeps food from entering the larynx during swallowing
trachea	passageway for air to the bronchi (also called the **windpipe**)
bronchus (*pl.* bronchi)	one of two branches from the trachea that conducts air into the lungs, where it divides and subdivides. The branchings resemble a tree; therefore, they are referred to as a **bronchial tree.**
bronchioles	smallest subdivision of the bronchial tree

>
> **ADAM'S APPLE**
> is the largest ring of cartilage in the larynx and is also known as the **thyroid cartilage.** The name came from the belief that Adam, realizing he had sinned when he ate the forbidden fruit, was unable to swallow the apple lodged in his throat.

> **BRONCHI**
> originated from the Greek **brecho,** meaning **to pour** or **wet.** An ancient belief was that the esophagus carried solid food to the stomach and the bronchi carried liquids.

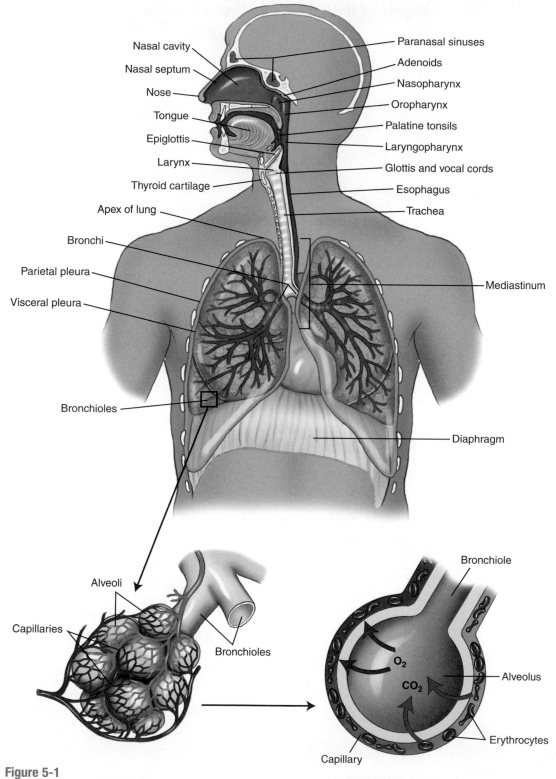

Nasal cavity
Nasal septum
Nose
Tongue
Epiglottis
Larynx
Thyroid cartilage
Apex of lung
Bronchi
Parietal pleura
Visceral pleura
Bronchioles

Paranasal sinuses
Adenoids
Nasopharynx
Oropharynx
Palatine tonsils
Laryngopharynx
Glottis and vocal cords
Esophagus
Trachea
Mediastinum
Diaphragm

Alveoli
Capillaries
Bronchioles

Bronchiole
O₂
CO₂
Alveolus
Erythrocytes
Capillary

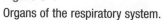

Figure 5-1
Organs of the respiratory system.

Organs of the Respiratory System—*cont'd*

Term	Definition
alveolus (*pl.* alveoli).......	air sacs at the end of the bronchioles. Oxygen and carbon dioxide are exchanged through the alveolar walls and the capillaries.
lungs	two spongelike organs in the thoracic cavity. The right lung consists of three lobes, and the left lung has two lobes.
pleura	double-folded serous membrane covering each lung and lining the thoracic cavity with a small space between, called the pleural cavity, which contains serous fluid
diaphragm	muscular partition that separates the thoracic cavity from the abdominal cavity. It aids in the breathing process by contracting and pulling air in, then relaxing and pushing air out.
mediastinum	space between the lungs. It contains the heart, esophagus, trachea, great blood vessels, and other structures.

MEDIASTINUM literally means **to stand in the middle** because it is derived from the Latin **medius,** meaning **middle,** and **stare,** meaning **to stand.**

EXERCISE 1

Match the anatomic terms in the first column with the correct definitions in the second column.

_____ 1. alveoli
_____ 2. bronchi
_____ 3. larynx
_____ 4. lungs
_____ 5. pharynx
_____ 6. pleura
_____ 7. adenoids
_____ 8. trachea

a. tubes carrying air between the trachea and lungs
b. passageway for air to the bronchi
c. located in the thoracic cavity
d. membrane covering the lung
e. lymphoid tissue behind the nasal cavity
f. acts as food and air passageway
g. location of the vocal cords
h. air sacs at the end of the bronchioles
i. keeps food out of the trachea and larynx

EXERCISE 2

Fill in the blanks with the correct terms.

1. The partition that separates the right and left nasal cavities is called the _____ _____.

2. The _____ is a flap of cartilage that prevents food from entering the larynx.

3. The smallest subdivisions of the bronchial tree are the _____.

4. The _____ serves as a filter to moisten and warm air entering the body.

5. The thoracic cavity is separated from the abdominal cavity by the _____.

6. The space between the lungs is called the _____.

7. The lymphoid tissues located in the pharynx behind the mouth are called the _____.

WORD PARTS

Combining Forms of the Respiratory System

Words you need to learn to complete this chapter are listed on the following pages. The exercises at the end of each list will help you learn their definitions and spelling.

Combining Form	Definition
adenoid/o	adenoids
alveol/o	alveolus
bronchi/o, bronch/o	bronchus
diaphragmat/o, phren/o	diaphragm
epiglott/o	epiglottis
laryng/o	larynx
lob/o	lobe
nas/o, rhin/o	nose
pharyng/o	pharynx
pleur/o	pleura
pneum/o, pneumat/o, pneumon/o	lung, air
pulmon/o	lung
sept/o	septum (wall off, fence)
sinus/o	sinus
thorac/o	thorax (chest)
tonsill/o	tonsil
(NOTE: tonsil has one *l*, and the combining form has two *l*s.)	
trache/o	trachea

ADENOID
is derived from the Greek **aden**, meaning **gland**, and **eidos**, meaning **like**. The word was once used for the prostate gland. The first adenoid surgery was performed in 1868.

LOBE
literally means **the part that hangs down**, although it comes from the Greek **lobos**, meaning **capsule** or **pod**. Also applied to the lobe of an ear, liver, or brain.

 Do not be concerned at this time about which word root to use for terms such as *lung* or *nose*, which have more than one word root. As you continue to study and use medical terms you will become familiar with common usage of each word part.

EXERCISE FIGURE A

Fill in the blanks with combining forms in this diagram of the respiratory system.

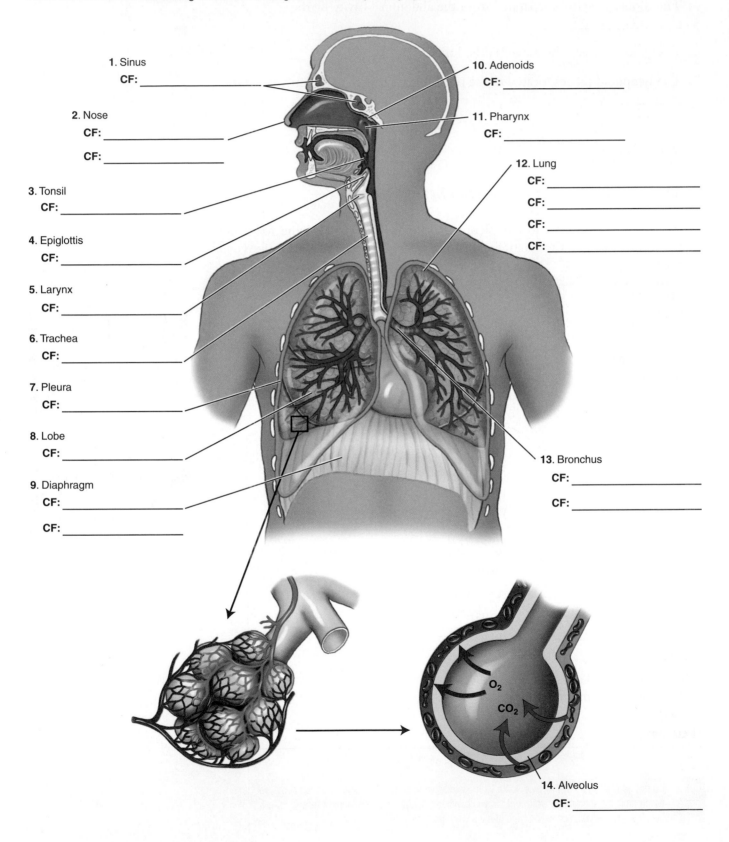

1. Sinus
   CF: _____

2. Nose
   CF: _____
   CF: _____

3. Tonsil
   CF: _____

4. Epiglottis
   CF: _____

5. Larynx
   CF: _____

6. Trachea
   CF: _____

7. Pleura
   CF: _____

8. Lobe
   CF: _____

9. Diaphragm
   CF: _____
   CF: _____

10. Adenoids
    CF: _____

11. Pharynx
    CF: _____

12. Lung
    CF: _____
    CF: _____
    CF: _____
    CF: _____

13. Bronchus
    CF: _____
    CF: _____

14. Alveolus
    CF: _____

EXERCISE 3

Write the definitions of the following combining forms.

1. laryng/o _____

2. bronchi/o,
   bronch/o _____

3. pleur/o _____

4. pneum/o _____

5. tonsill/o _____

6. pulmon/o _____

7. diaphragmat/o _____

8. trache/o _____

9. alveol/o _____

10. pneumon/o _____

11. thorac/o _____

12. adenoid/o _____

13. pharyng/o _____

14. rhin/o _____

15. sinus/o _____

16. lob/o _____

17. epiglott/o _____

18. pneumat/o _____

19. nas/o _____

20. sept/o _____

21. phren/o _____

EXERCISE 4

Write the combining form for each of the following terms.

1. nose   a. _____
               b. _____

2. larynx   _____

3. lung, air   a. _____
               b. _____
               c. _____

4. lung   _____

5. tonsils   _____

6. trachea   _____

7. adenoids   _____

8. pleura   _____

9. diaphragm   a. _____
               b. _____

10. sinus   _____

11. thorax   _____

12. alveolus   _____

13. pharynx   _____

14. bronchus   a. _____
               b. _____

15. lobe   _____

16. epiglottis _____

17. septum   _____

Combining Forms Commonly Used with Respiratory System Terms

Combining Form	Definition
atel/o	imperfect, incomplete
capn/o	carbon dioxide
hem/o, hemat/o	blood
muc/o	mucus
orth/o.	straight
ox/o, ox/i	oxygen
(NOTE: the combining vowels *o* and *i* are used with the word root *ox*.)	
phon/o	sound, voice
py/o	pus
somn/o.	sleep
spir/o	breathe, breathing

OXYGEN was discovered in 1774 by Joseph Priestley. In 1775 Antoine-Laurent Lavoisier, a French chemist, noted that all the acids he knew contained oxygen. Because he thought it was an acid producer, he named it using the Greek **oxys,** meaning **sour,** and the suffix **gen,** meaning **to produce.**

EXERCISE 5

Write the definition of the following combining forms.

1. ox/o, ox/i _____

2. spir/o _____

3. muc/o _____

4. atel/o _____

5. orth/o _____

6. py/o _____

7. hem/o, hemat/o _____

8. somn/o _____

9. capn/o _____

10. phon/o _____

EXERCISE 6

Write the combining form for each of the following.

1. breathe, breathing _____

2. oxygen a. _____
          b. _____

3. imperfect, incomplete _____

4. straight _____

5. pus _____

6. mucus _____

7. blood a. _____
         b. _____

8. sleep _____

9. sound, voice _____

10. carbon dioxide _____

Prefixes

Prefix	Definition
a-, an-	without or absence of
(NOTE: *an-* is used when the word root begins with a vowel.)	
endo-	within
(NOTE: the prefix *intra-*, introduced in Chapter 4, also means *within*.)	
eu-	normal, good
pan-	all, total
poly-	many, much
tachy-	fast, rapid

EXERCISE 7

Write the definitions of the following prefixes.

1. endo- _____

2. a-, an- _____

3. pan- _____

4. eu- _____

5. poly- _____

6. tachy- _____

EXERCISE 8

Write the prefix for each of the following.

1. within _____

2. normal, good _____

3. without or absence of   a. _____

   b. _____

4. all, total _____

5. many, much _____

6. fast, rapid _____

Suffixes

Suffix	Definition
-algia	pain
-ar, -ary, -eal	pertaining to
-cele	hernia or protrusion
-centesis	surgical puncture to aspirate fluid (with a sterile needle)
-ectasis	stretching out, dilatation, expansion
-emia	blood condition
-graphy	process of recording, radiographic imaging
-meter	instrument used to measure
-metry	measurement
-pexy	surgical fixation, suspension
-pnea	breathing
-rrhagia	rapid flow of blood
-scope	instrument used for visual examination
-scopic	pertaining to visual examination
-scopy	visual examination
-spasm	sudden, involuntary muscle contraction (spasmodic contraction)
-stenosis	constriction or narrowing
-stomy	creation of an artificial opening
-thorax	chest
-tomy	cut into or incision

Refer to Appendix A and Appendix B for alphabetical lists of word parts and their meanings.

EXERCISE 9

Match the suffixes in the first column with their correct definitions in the second column.

_____	1. -algia	a. process of recording, radiographic imaging
_____	2. -ar, -ary, -eal	b. stretching out, dilatation, expansion
_____	3. -cele	c. surgical puncture to aspirate fluid
_____	4. -centesis	d. measurement
_____	5. -ectasis	e. pertaining to visual examination
_____	6. -emia	f. pertaining to
_____	7. -graphy	g. hernia or protrusion
_____	8. -meter	h. instrument used to measure
_____	9. -metry	i. rapid flow of blood
_____	10. -scopic	j. blood condition
		k. pain

EXERCISE 10

Match the suffixes in the first column with their correct definitions in the second column.

_____ 1. -rrhagia   a. cut into or incision

_____ 2. -stomy   b. instrument used for visual examination

_____ 3. -tomy   c. rapid flow of blood

_____ 4. -pexy   d. constriction, narrowing

_____ 5. -scope   e. creation of an artificial opening

_____ 6. -scopy   f. sudden, involuntary muscle contraction

_____ 7. -spasm   g. chest

_____ 8. -stenosis   h. surgical fixation, suspension

_____ 9. –thorax   i. visual examination

_____ 10. -pnea   j. breathing

EXERCISE 11

Write the definitions of the following suffixes.

1. -thorax _____

2. -ar, -ary, -eal _____

3. -stenosis _____

4. -cele _____

5. -stomy _____

6. -pexy _____

7. -meter _____

8. -spasm _____

9. -algia _____

10. -scopy _____

11. -centesis _____

12. -tomy _____

13. -scope _____

14. -rrhagia _____

15. -ectasis _____

16. -graphy _____

17. -metry _____

18. -emia _____

19. -scopic _____

20. -pnea _____

MEDICAL TERMS

The terms you need to learn to complete this chapter are listed below. The exercises following each list will help you learn the definition and the spelling of each word.

Disease and Disorder Terms

Built from Word Parts

The following terms are built from word parts you have already learned and can be translated literally to find their meanings. Further explanation of terms beyond the definition of their word parts, if needed, is included in parentheses.

Term	Definition
adenoiditis . . . . (*ad*-e-noyd-Ī-tis)	inflammation of the adenoids
atelectasis . . . . (at-e-LEK-ta-sis)	incomplete expansion (of the lung of a newborn or collapsed lung) (Figure 5-2)
bronchiectasis . . . . (*bron*-kē-EK-ta-sis)	dilation of the bronchi (Exercise Figure B)
bronchitis . . . . (bron-KĪ-tis)	inflammation of the bronchi (see Figure 5-5)
bronchogenic carcinoma . . . . . (bron-kō-JEN-ik) (kar-si-NŌ-ma)	cancerous tumor originating in a bronchus
bronchopneumonia . . . . (*bron*-kō-nū-MŌ-nē-a)	diseased state of the bronchi and lungs, usually caused by infection

> **ATELECTASIS**
> is derived from the Greek **ateles,** meaning **not perfect,** and **ektasis,** meaning **expansion.** It denotes an incomplete expansion of the lungs, especially at birth.

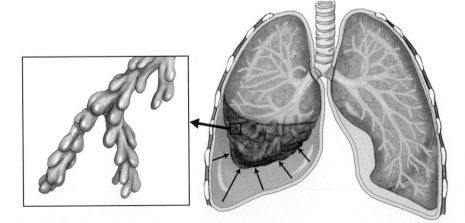

Figure 5-2
Atelectasis showing the collapsed alveoli.

Fill in the blanks to complete labeling of the diagram.

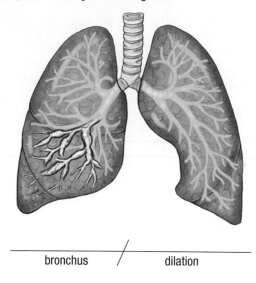

_____ / _____
bronchus   dilation

Term	Definition
diaphragmatocele . . . . (*dī*-a-frag-MAT-ō-sēl)	hernia of the diaphragm
epiglottitis . . . . (*ep*-i-glo-TĪ-tis)	inflammation of the epiglottis
hemothorax . . . . (hē-mō-THOR-aks)	blood in the chest (pleural space) (Exercise Figure C)
laryngitis . . . . (*lar*-in-JĪ-tis)	inflammation of the larynx
laryngotracheobronchitis (LTB). . . . . (la-*ring*-gō-*trā*-kē-ō-bron-KĪ-tis)	inflammation of the larynx, trachea, and bronchi (the acute form is called **croup**)
lobar pneumonia . . . . (LŌ-bar) (nū-MŌ-nē-a)	pertaining to the lobe(s); diseased state of the lung (infection of one or more lobes of the lung)
nasopharyngitis. . . . . (nā-zō-far-in-JĪ-tis)	inflammation of the nose and pharynx
pansinusitis . . . . (*pan*-sī-nu-SĪ-tis)	inflammation of all sinuses
pharyngitis. . . . . (far-in-JĪ-tis)	inflammation of the pharynx
pleuritis . . . . (plū-RĪ-tis)	inflammation of the pleura (also called **pleurisy**) (Figure 5-3)
pneumatocele . . . . (nū-MAT-ō-sēl)	hernia of the lung (lung tissue protrudes through an opening in the chest)
pneumoconiosis . . . . (nū-mō-*kō*-nē-Ō-sis)	abnormal condition of dust in the lungs

PNEUMOCONIOSIS is the general name given for chronic inflammatory disease of the lung caused by excessive inhalation of mineral dust. When the disease is caused by a specific dust, it is named for the dust. For example, the disease caused by silica dust is called **silicosis.**

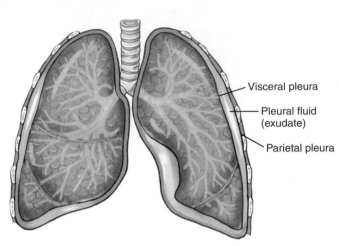

Figure 5-3
Pleuritis, also called pleurisy.

Figure 5-4
Chest radiograph revealing pneumonia of the right lung.

Disease and Disorder Terms—*cont'd*

Built from Word Parts

PNEUMOCYSTIS CARINII PNEUMONIA (PCP)
has officially been renamed *Pneumocystis jiroveci* pneumonia. Before the 1980s, PCP was rare. During the 1980s it became the most common opportunistic infection of patients with HIV or AIDS. Since the introduction of HAART (highly active antiretroviral therapy) for HIV infection, this infection is most commonly seen in newly diagnosed patients or those who do not follow the HAART regimen.

EPISTAXIS
and rhinorrhagia are both medical terms for **nosebleed.**

Term	Definition
pneumonia.............. (nū-MŌ-nē-a)	diseased state of the lung (the infection and inflammation are caused by bacteria such as *Pneumococcus, Staphylococcus, Streptococcus,* and *Haemophilus;* viruses; and fungi)
pneumonitis............. (*nū*-mō-NĪ-tis)	inflammation of the lung (Figure 5-4)
pneumothorax............ (*nū*-mō-THOR-aks)	air in the chest (pleural space), which causes collapse of the lung (Exercise Figure C)
pulmonary neoplasm........ (PUL-mō-nar-ē) (NĒ-ō-plazm)	pertaining to (in) the lung, new growth (tumor)
pyothorax................ (pī-ō-THOR-aks)	pus in the chest (pleural space) (also called **empyema**)
rhinitis.................. (rī-NĪ-tis)	inflammation of the (mucous membranes) nose
rhinomycosis............. (*rī*-nō-mī-KŌ-sis)	abnormal condition of fungus in the nose
rhinorrhagia.............. (rī-nō-RĀ-ja)	rapid flow of blood from the nose (also called **epistaxis**)
thoracalgia............... (thor-a-KAL-ja)	pain in the chest
tonsillitis................ (*ton*-sil-Ī-tis)	inflammation of the tonsils
tracheitis................ (trā-kē-Ī-tis)	inflammation of the trachea
tracheostenosis............ (trā-kē-ō-sten-Ō-sis)	narrowing of the trachea

| EXERCISE FIGURE **C** |

Fill in the blanks to label the diagram.

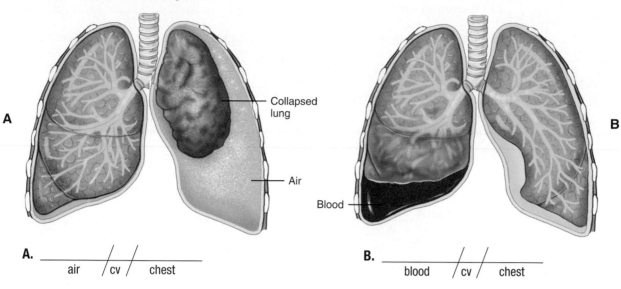

Collapsed
lung

Air

Blood

A

B

A. _____ / ____ / _____
     air   / cv /   chest

B. _____ / ____ / _____
     blood / cv /   chest

| EXERCISE **12** |

Practice saying aloud each of the disease and disorder terms built from word parts on
pp. 152-154.

To hear the terms select Chapter 5, Chapter Exercises, Pronunciation.

☐ Place a check mark in the box when you have completed this exercise.

| EXERCISE **13** |

Analyze and define the following terms.

                 WR   CV S

Example: diaphragmat / o / cele   *hernia of the diaphragm* _____

                  CF

1. pleuritis _____

2. nasopharyngitis _____

3. pneumothorax _____

4. pansinusitis _____

5. atelectasis _____

6. rhinomycosis _____

7. tracheostenosis _____

8. epiglottitis _____

9. thoracalgia _____

10. pulmonary neoplasm _____

11. bronchiectasis _____

12. tonsillitis _____

13. pneumoconiosis _____

14. bronchopneumonia _____

15. pneumonitis _____

16. laryngitis _____

17. pneumatocele _____

18. pyothorax _____

19. rhinorrhagia _____

20. bronchitis _____

21. pharyngitis _____

22. tracheitis _____

23. laryngotracheobronchitis _____

24. adenoiditis _____

25. hemothorax _____

26. lobar pneumonia _____

27. rhinitis _____

28. bronchogenic carcinoma _____

29. pneumonia _____

EXERCISE 14

Build disease and disorder terms for the following definitions with the word parts you have learned.

Example: inflammation of the tonsils   <u>tonsill / itis</u>
                                                WR   S

1. pain in the chest

   _____ / _____
       WR   /   S

2. abnormal condition
   of fungus (infection)
   in the nose

   _____ / ___ / _____ / ___
     WR   / CV /   WR   / S

3. hernia of the lung

   _____ / ___ / ___
     WR   / CV /   S

4. pertaining to the
   lung; new growth (tumor)

   _____ / ___   _____ / _____
     WR   / S   P   / S(WR)

5. inflammation of the larynx

    _____ / _____
         WR   S

6. incomplete expansion (of the lung)

    _____ / _____
         WR   S

7. inflammation of the adenoids

    _____ / _____
         WR   S

8. inflammation of the larynx, trachea, and bronchi

    _____ / CV / _____ / CV / _____ / _____
    WR   WR   WR   S

9. dilation of the bronchi

    _____ / _____
         WR   S

10. inflammation of the pleura

    _____ / _____
         WR   S

11. abnormal condition of dust in the lung

    _____ / CV / _____ / _____
    WR   WR   S

12. inflammation of the lung

    _____ / _____
         WR   S

13. inflammation of all sinuses

    _____ / _____ / _____
    P   WR   S

14. narrowing of the trachea

    _____ / CV / _____
         WR   S

15. inflammation of the nose and pharynx

    _____ / CV / _____ / _____
    WR   WR   S

16. pus in the chest (pleural space)

    _____ / CV / _____
         WR   S

17. inflammation of the epiglottis

    _____ / _____
         WR   S

18. hernia of the diaphragm

    _____ / CV / _____
         WR   S

19. air in the chest (pleural space)

    _____ / CV / _____
         WR   S

20. diseased state of the bronchi and the lungs

    _____ / CV / _____ / _____
    WR   WR   S

21. rapid flow of blood from the nose

    _____ / CV / _____
         WR   S

22. inflammation of the pharynx

    _____ / _____
         WR   S

23. blood in the chest (pleural space)

    _____ / CV / _____
         WR   S

24. inflammation of the trachea

    _____ / _____
    WR   S

25. inflammation of the bronchi

    _____ / _____
    WR   S

26. pertaining to the lobe(s);
    diseased state of the lung(s)

    _____ / _____   _____ / _____
    WR   S   WR   S

27. inflammation of the
    (mucous membranes) nose

    _____ / _____
    WR   S

28. cancerous tumor originating
    in a bronchus

    _____ / CV / _____
    WR   S

    _____ / _____
    WR   S

29. diseased state of the lung

    _____ / _____
    WR   S

EXERCISE 15

Spell each of the disease and disorder terms built from word parts on pp. 152-154 by having someone dictate them to you.

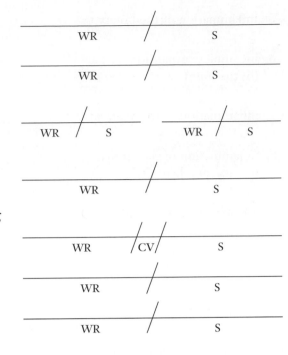 To hear and spell the terms select Chapter 5, Chapter Exercises, Spelling. You may type the terms on the screen or write them below in the spaces provided.

☐ Place a check mark in the box when you have completed this exercise using your CD-ROM.

1. _____   16. _____

2. _____   17. _____

3. _____   18. _____

4. _____   19. _____

5. _____   20. _____

6. _____   21. _____

7. _____   22. _____

8. _____   23. _____

9. _____   24. _____

10. _____   25. _____

11. _____   26. _____

12. _____   27. _____

13. _____   28. _____

14. _____   29. _____

15. _____   30. _____

Disease and Disorder Terms

Not Built from Word Parts

In some of the following terms, you may recognize word parts; however, the terms cannot be translated literally to find their meanings.

Term	Definition
adult respiratory distress syndrome (ARDS) . . . . (a-DULT) (RES-pi-ra-*tor*-ē) (di-STRES) (SIN-drōm)	respiratory failure in an adult as a result of disease or injury. Symptoms include dyspnea, rapid breathing, and cyanosis (also called **acute respiratory distress syndrome**).
asthma . . . . (AZ-ma)	respiratory disease characterized by paroxysms of coughing, wheezing, shortness of breath, and constriction of airways
chronic obstructive pulmonary disease (COPD) . . . . (KRON-ik) (ob-STRUK-tiv) (PUL-mō-nar-ē) (di-ZĒZ)	a group of disorders that are almost always a result of smoking that obstructs bronchial flow. One or more of the following is present in COPD in varying degrees: emphysema, chronic bronchitis, bronchospasm, and bronchiolitis.
coccidioidomycosis . . . . (kok-*sid*-ē-oyd-ō-mī-KŌ-sis)	fungal disease affecting the lungs and sometimes other organs of the body (also called **valley fever** or **cocci**)
cor pulmonale . . . . (kōr) (pul-mō-NAL-ē)	serious cardiac disease associated with chronic lung disorders, such as emphysema
croup . . . . (krūp)	condition resulting from acute obstruction of the larynx, characterized by a barking cough, hoarseness, and stridor. It may be caused by viral or bacterial infection, allergy, or foreign body. Occurs mainly in children.
cystic fibrosis (CF) . . . . (SIS-tik) (fī-BRŌ-sis)	hereditary disorder of the exocrine glands characterized by excess mucus production in the respiratory tract, pancreatic deficiency, and other symptoms.
deviated septum . . . . (DĒ-vē-āt-ed) (SEP-tum)	one part of the nasal cavity is smaller because of malformation or injury of the nasal septum
emphysema . . . . (em-fi-SĒ-ma)	stretching of lung tissue caused by the alveoli becoming distended and losing elasticity (Figure 5-5)
epistaxis . . . . (ep-i-STAK-sis)	nosebleed (synonymous with **rhinorrhagia**)
influenza . . . . (in-flū-EN-za)	highly infectious respiratory disease caused by a virus (also called **flu**)
Legionnaire disease . . . . (lē-je-NĀR) (di-ZĒZ)	a lobar pneumonia caused by the bacterium *Legionella pneumophila*

ADULT RESPIRATORY DISTRESS SYNDROME (ARDS) is respiratory failure in an adult. In newborns the condition is referred to as **infant respiratory distress syndrome of newborn (IRDS)** or **hyaline membrane disease.**

ASTHMA is derived from the Greek **astma,** meaning **to pant.**

 CAM TERM Vitamin therapy is the use of nutrition, through diet and supplements, to decrease the incidence of disease and symptoms and support wellness. Coenzyme Q10 supplementation has demonstrated efficacy in reducing the dosage of corticosteroids required by patients with bronchial asthma.

OBSTRUCTIVE SLEEP APNEA (OSA) is becoming increasingly common. It is characterized by episodes of apnea during sleep that cause hypoxia. OSA can produce excessive daytime drowsiness and fatigue and is associated with increased risk for elevated blood pressure, cardiovascular disease, diabetes, and stroke. **Polysomnography** is used to diagnose OSA. Obesity is a major risk factor and significant weight loss can be an effective treatment. **CPAP** (continuous positive airway pressure), a type of ventilator, may be prescribed for use during sleep. See Figure 5-6 and 5-13. **Uvulopalatopharyngoplasty (UPPP)** is a surgical procedure used to treat OSA.

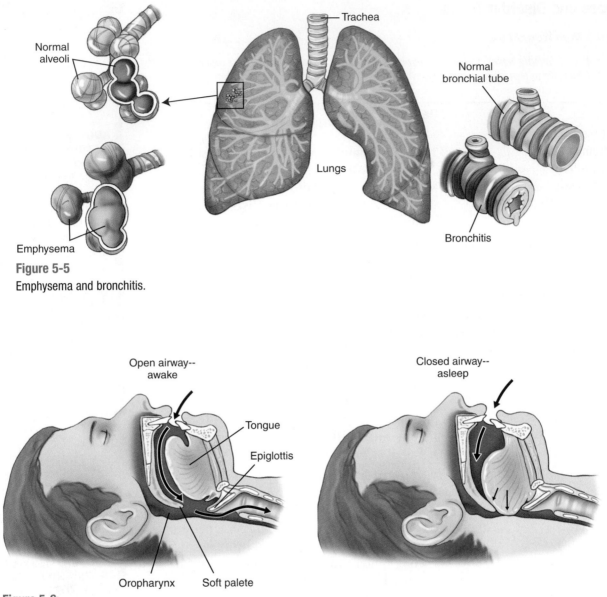

Figure 5-5
Emphysema and bronchitis.

Figure 5-6
Obstructive sleep apnea. During sleep the absence of activity of the pharyngeal muscle structure allows the airway to close.

Disease and Disorder Terms—*cont'd*

Not Built from Word Parts

Term	Definition
obstructive sleep apnea (OSA) . . . . (ob-STRUK-tiv) (slēp) (AP-nē-a)	repetitive pharyngeal collapse during sleep, which leads to absence of breathing; can produce daytime drowsiness and elevated blood pressure (Figure 5-6)
pertussis . . . . (per-TUS-sis)	highly contagious bacterial infection of the respiratory tract characterized by an acute crowing inspiration, or whoop (also called **whooping cough**)

Term	Definition
pleural effusion . . . . (PLŪ-ral) (e-FŪ-zhun)	escape of fluid into the pleural space as a result of inflammation
pulmonary edema . . . . (PUL-mō-nar-ē) (e-DĒ-ma)	fluid accumulation in the alveoli and bronchioles
pulmonary embolism (*pl.* emboli) (PE) . . . . (PUL-mō-nar-ē) (EM-bo-lizm)	foreign matter, such as a blood clot, air, or fat clot, carried in the circulation to the pulmonary artery, where it blocks circulation (Figure 5-7)
tuberculosis (TB) . . . . (tū-ber-kū-LŌ-sis)	an infectious disease, caused by an acid-fast bacillus, most commonly spread by inhalation of small particles and usually affecting the lungs
upper respiratory infection (URI) . . . . (UP-er) (RES-pi-ra-*tor*-ē) (in-FEK-shun)	infection of the nasal cavity, pharynx, or larynx (Figure 5-8)

REACTIVE AIRWAY DISEASE (RAD)
Is a general term and not a specific diagnosis. It is used to describe a history of wheezing, coughing, and shortness of breath. In some people RAD may lead to asthma.

TUBERCULOSIS (TB)
causes more deaths worldwide than any other infectious disease even though it is preventable and curable. The risk for active TB is higher in HIV-infected persons and drug users. The development of multidrug–resistant TB is becoming a problem in treatment of the disease.

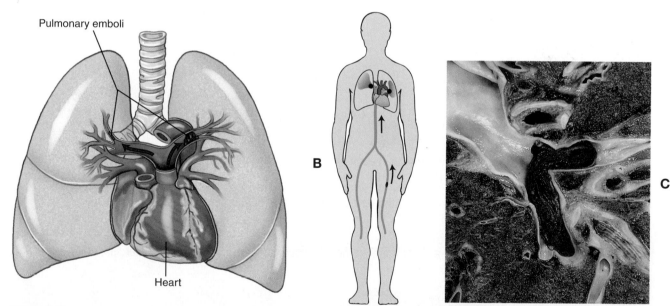

Figure 5-7

A, Bilateral pulmonary emboli. **B,** Pulmonary emboli usually originate in the deep veins of the lower extremities. **C,** Necropsy specimen of the lung showing a large embolus.

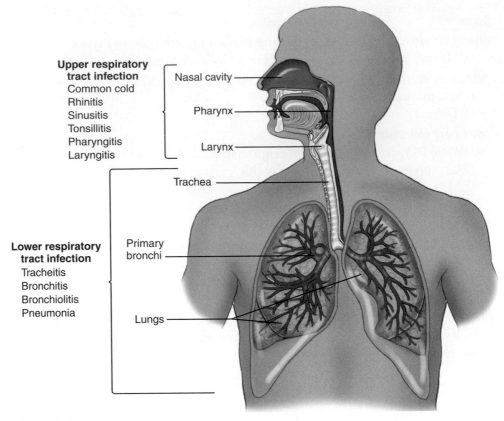

Figure 5-8
Upper and lower respiratory tract infections.

EXERCISE 16

Practice saying aloud each of the disease and disorder terms not built from word parts on pp. 159-161.

 To hear the terms select Chapter 5, Chapter Exercises, Pronunciation.

☐ Place a check mark in the box when you have completed this exercise.

EXERCISE 17

Fill in the blanks with the correct terms.

1. A disease characterized by lung tissue stretching that results from the alveoli losing elasticity and becoming distended is called _____.

2. _____ _____ is the name given to the escape of fluid into the pleural space as a result of inflammation.

3. A cardiac condition that is associated with chronic lung disorders is called
   _____ _____.

4. A fungal disease affecting the lungs is called _____.

5. _____ _____ is a hereditary disorder
   characterized by excess mucus production in the respiratory tract.

6. The medical name of the infectious respiratory disease commonly referred
   to as *flu* is _____.

7. A group of disorders that obstruct the bronchial airflow is known as
   _____ _____ _____ _____.

8. The medical name for the disease characterized by an acute crowing
   inspiration is _____.

9. _____ is a condition resulting from an acute obstruction
   of the larynx.

10. A chronic respiratory disease characterized by shortness of breath,
    wheezing, and paroxysmal coughing is called _____.

11. A condition in which fluid accumulates in the alveoli and bronchioles is
    _____ _____.

12. A(n) _____ _____ _____ generally
    refers to an infection involving the nasal cavity, pharynx, or larynx.

13. Foreign matter, such as a clot, air, or fat carried in the circulation to
    the pulmonary artery, where it blocks circulation, is called a(n)
    _____ _____.

14. _____ is another name for nosebleed.

15. A lobar pneumonia caused by the *Legionella pneumophila* bacterium is
    commonly called _____ _____.

16. _____ _____ is one part of the nasal cavity that is
    smaller than the other because of malformation or injury.

17. The diagnosis for repetitive pharyngeal collapse is _____
    _____ _____.

18. An infectious disease usually affecting the lungs and caused by inhaling
    infected small particles is _____.

19. _____ _____ _____ _____ occurs in
    adults as a result of disease or injury.

EXERCISE 18

Match the terms in the first column with the correct definitions in the second column.

_____ 1. asthma

_____ 2. chronic obstructive pulmonary disease

_____ 3. coccidioidomycosis

_____ 4. cor pulmonale

_____ 5. croup

_____ 6. cystic fibrosis

_____ 7. emphysema

_____ 8. epistaxis

_____ 9. influenza

_____ 10. Legionnaire disease

a. alveoli become distended and lose elasticity

b. caused by a virus (commonly called *flu*)

c. hereditary disorder characterized by excess mucus in the respiratory system

d. characterized by wheezing, paroxysmal coughing, and shortness of breath

e. nosebleed

f. cardiac disease associated with chronic lung disorders

g. condition resulting from obstruction of the larynx

h. also called *valley fever*

i. lobar pneumonia caused by the bacterium *Legionella pneumophila*

j. lung disorder that obstructs the bronchial airflow

EXERCISE 19

Match the terms in the first column with the correct definitions in the second column.

_____ 1. pertussis

_____ 2. pleural effusion

_____ 3. pulmonary edema

_____ 4. pulmonary embolism

_____ 5. upper respiratory infection

_____ 6. deviated septum

_____ 7. obstructive sleep apnea

_____ 8. tuberculosis

_____ 9. adult respiratory distress syndrome

a. respiratory failure in an adult

b. escape of fluid into pleural cavity

c. fluid accumulation in alveoli and bronchioles

d. whooping cough

e. foreign material, moved by circulation, that blocks the pulmonary artery

f. infection of the nasal cavity, pharynx, or larynx

g. unequal size of nasal cavities

h. repetitive pharyngeal collapse

i. an infectious disease usually affecting the lungs

EXERCISE 20

Spell each of the disease and disorder terms not built from word parts on pp. 159-161 by having someone dictate them to you.

To hear and spell the terms select Chapter 5, Chapter Exercises, Spelling. You may type the terms on the screen or write them below in the spaces provided.

☐ Place a check mark in the box when you have completed this exercise using your CD-ROM.

1. _____   11. _____

2. _____   12. _____

3. _____   13. _____

4. _____   14. _____

5. _____   15. _____

6. _____   16. _____

7. _____   17. _____

8. _____   18. _____

9. _____   19. _____

10. _____

Surgical Terms

Built from Word Parts

The following terms are built from word parts you have already learned and can be translated literally to find their meanings. Further explanation of terms beyond the definition of their word parts, if needed, is included in parentheses.

Term	Definition
adenoidectomy . . . . (*ad*-e-noyd-EK-to-mē)	excision of the adenoids (Exercise Figure D)
adenotome. . . . . (AD-e-nō-tōm) (NOTE: the *oid* is missing from the word root *ade-noid* in this term.)	surgical instrument used to cut the adenoids (Exercise Figure D)
bronchoplasty . . . . (BRON-kō-*plas*-tē)	surgical repair of a bronchus
laryngectomy. . . . . (lār-in-JEK-to-mē)	excision of the larynx
laryngoplasty. . . . . (la-RING-gō-*plas*-tē)	surgical repair of the larynx

Fill in the blanks to complete labeling of the diagram.

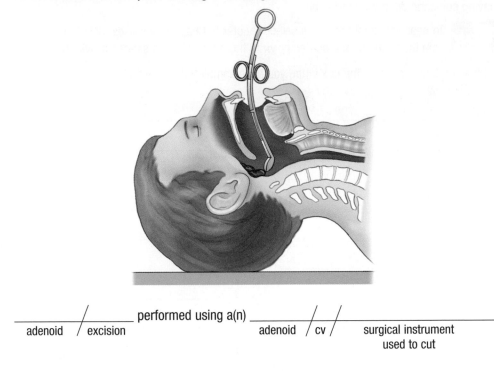

_____ / _____ performed using a(n) _____ / cv / _____
  adenoid   / excision   adenoid /   / surgical instrument
                                                                          used to cut

Surgical Terms—*cont'd*

Built from Word Parts

Term	Definition
laryngostomy . . . . (lar-in-GOS-to-mē)	creation of an artificial opening into the larynx
laryngotracheotomy . . . . (la-ring-gō-*trā*-ke-OT-o-mē)	incision of the larynx and trachea
lobectomy . . . . (lō-BEK-to-mē)	excision of a lobe (of the lung) (Figure 5-9)
pleuropexy . . . . (plū-rō-PEK-sē)	surgical fixation of the pleura
pneumobronchotomy . . . . (*nū*-mō-bron-KOT-o-mē)	incision of lung and bronchus
pneumonectomy . . . . (*nū*-mō-NEK-to-mē)	excision of a lung (see Figure 5-9)
rhinoplasty . . . . (RĪ-nō-*plas*-tē)	surgical repair of the nose
septoplasty . . . . (SEP-tō-*plas*-tē)	surgical repair of the (nasal) septum
septotomy . . . . (*sep*-TOT-o-mē)	incision into the (nasal) septum
sinusotomy . . . . (*sī*-nū-SOT-o-mē)	incision of a sinus

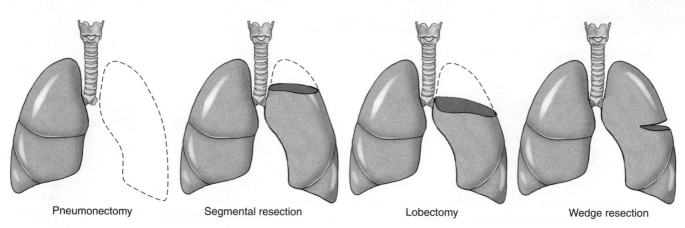

Pneumonectomy   Segmental resection   Lobectomy   Wedge resection

Figure 5-9
Types of lung resection. The diagram illustrates the amount of lung tissue removed with each type of surgery.

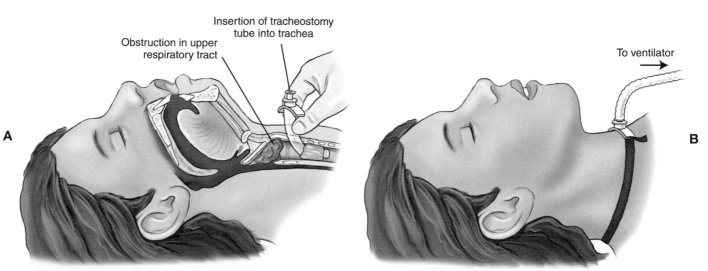

Figure 5-10
Tracheostomy. **A,** A tracheotomy is performed to establish an airway when normal breathing is blocked from choking or other causes. **B,** If the opening needs to be maintained, a tube is inserted, creating a tracheostomy. A tracheostomy may be temporary, as for prolonged mechanical ventilation to support breathing or it may be permanent, as in airway reconstruction after laryngeal cancer surgery.

Term	Definition
thoracocentesis .... (*thor*-a-kō-sen-TĒ-sis)	surgical puncture to aspirate fluid from the chest cavity (also called **thoracentesis**) (Exercise Figure E)
thoracotomy .... (*thor*-a-KOT-o-mē)	incision into the chest cavity
tonsillectomy .... (*ton*-sil-EK-to-mē)	excision of the tonsils
tracheoplasty .... (TRĀ-kē-ō-*plas*-tē)	surgical repair of the trachea
tracheostomy .... (*trā*-kē-OS-to-mē)	creation of an artificial opening into the trachea (Figure 5-10)
tracheotomy .... (*trā*-kē-OT-o-mē)	incision of the trachea (Figure 5-10)

VIDEO-ASSISTED THORACIC SURGERY (VATS)
is the use of a thoracoscope and video equipment for an endoscopic approach to diagnose and treat thoracic conditions. It replaces the traditional thoracotomy, which required a large incision and greater recovery time.

Fill in the blanks to complete labeling of the diagram.

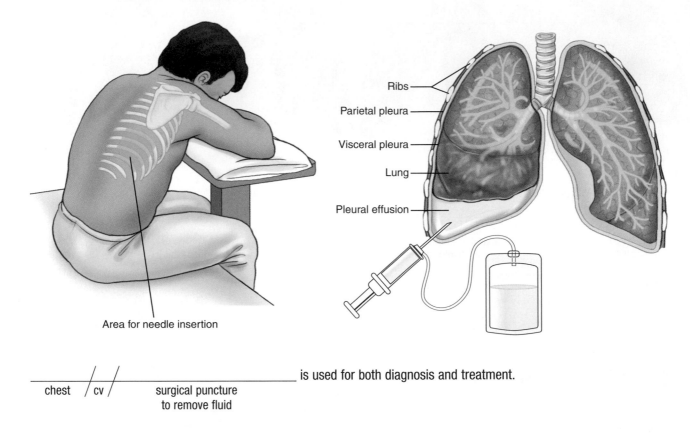

Ribs

Parietal pleura

Visceral pleura

Lung

Pleural effusion

Area for needle insertion

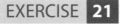 _____ is used for both diagnosis and treatment.

chest / cv / surgical puncture
to remove fluid

EXERCISE 21

Practice saying aloud each of the surgical term built from word parts on pp. 165-167.

 To hear the terms select Chapter 5, Chapter Exercises, Pronunciation.

☐ Place a check mark in the box when you have completed this exercise.

EXERCISE 22

Analyze and define the following surgical terms.

WR   S
Example: pneumon/ectomy   _excision of lung_____

1. tracheotomy _____

2. laryngostomy _____

3. adenoidectomy _____

4. rhinoplasty _____

5. adenotome _____

6. tracheostomy _____

7. sinusotomy _____

8. laryngoplasty_____

9. pneumobronchotomy _____

10. bronchoplasty_____

11. lobectomy _____

12. laryngotracheotomy_____

13. tracheoplasty _____

14. thoracotomy _____

15. laryngectomy _____

16. thoracocentesis_____

17. tonsillectomy _____

18. pleuropexy_____

19. septoplasty_____

20. septotomy _____

EXERCISE 23

Build surgical terms for the following definitions by using the word parts you have learned.

Example: surgical fixation of the pleura   pleur / o / pexy
                                                WR / CV / S

1. surgical repair of the trachea   _____ / ___ / _____
                                      WR   /CV/   S

2. incision of larynx and trachea   ___ / ___ / ___ / ___ / ___
                                      WR /CV/ WR /CV/ S

3. surgical instrument used to
   cut the adenoids   _____ / ___ / ___
                                      WR   /CV/   S

4. incision into the chest cavity   _____ / ___ / ___
                                      WR   /CV/   S

5. creation of an artificial opening
   into the trachea   _____ / ___ / ___
                                      WR   /CV/   S

6. excision of the tonsils

_____ / _____
WR   S

7. incision of the trachea

_____ / CV / _____
WR   CV   S

8. surgical repair of a bronchus

_____ / CV / _____
WR   CV   S

9. excision of the larynx

_____ / _____
WR   S

10. surgical repair of the nose

_____ / CV / _____
WR   CV   S

11. incision of a sinus

_____ / CV / _____
WR   CV   S

12. surgical puncture to aspirate fluid from the chest cavity

_____ / CV / _____
WR   CV   S

or

_____ / _____
WR   S

13. excision of the adenoids

_____ / _____
WR   S

14. surgical repair of the larynx

_____ / CV / _____
WR   CV   S

15. excision of a lobe (of the lung)

_____ / _____
WR   S

16. incision of a lung and bronchus

_____ / CV / _____ / CV / _____
WR   CV   WR   CV   S

17. creation of an artificial opening into the larynx

_____ / CV / _____
WR   CV   S

18. excision of a lung

_____ / _____
WR   S

19. incision into the septum

_____ / CV / _____
WR   CV   S

20. surgical repair of the septum

_____ / CV / _____
WR   CV   S

EXERCISE 24

Spell each of the surgical terms built from word parts on pp. 165-167 by having someone dictate them to you.

To hear and spell the terms select Chapter 5, Chapter Exercises, Spelling. You may type the terms on the screen or write them below in the spaces provided.

☐ Place a check mark in the box when you have completed this exercise using your CD-Rom.

1. _____   12. _____

2. _____   13. _____

3. _____   14. _____

4. _____   15. _____

5. _____   16. _____

6. _____   17. _____

7. _____   18. _____

8. _____   19. _____

9. _____   20. _____

10. _____   21. _____

11. _____

Diagnostic Terms

Built from Word Parts

The following terms are built from word parts you have already learned and can be translated literally to find their meanings. Further explanation of terms beyond the definition of their word parts, if needed, is included in parentheses.

Term	Definition
ENDOSCOPY	
bronchoscope . . . . (BRON-kō-skōp)	instrument used for visual examination of the bronchi (Table 5-1 and Exercise Figure F)
bronchoscopy . . . . (bron-KOS-ko-pē)	visual examination of the bronchi (Exercise Figure F)
endoscope . . . . (EN-dō-skōp)	instrument used for visual examination within (a hollow organ or body cavity). (Current trend is to use endoscopes for surgical procedures as well as for viewing.) (Table 5-1)
endoscopic . . . . (en-dō-SKOP-ik)	pertaining to visual examination within (a hollow organ or body cavity) (used to describe the practice of performing surgeries that use endoscopes)

EXERCISE FIGURE **F**

Fill in the blanks to complete labeling of the diagram.

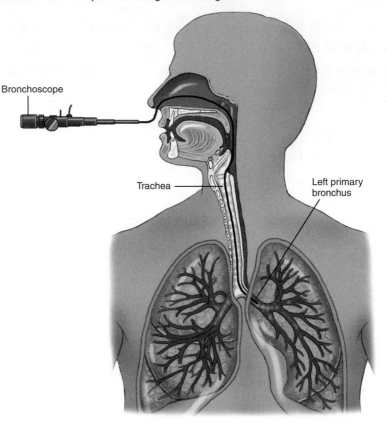

Bronchoscope

Trachea

Left primary bronchus

A bronchoscope is inserted through the nostril and passed through the throat, larynx, and trachea into the bronchus.

bronchi	/ cv /	visual examination

SCOPE

is taken from the Greek **skopein,** which means to **see** or to **view.** It also means **observing for a purpose.** To the ancient Greeks it meant "to look out for, to monitor, or to examine."

Today the following suffixes commonly are used:

- **-scope** describes the **instrument used to view or to examine,** such as in the term **endoscope** (means **instrument used for visual examination within** a hollow organ or body cavity).
- **-scopy** means **visual examination,** such as in the term **endoscopy** (**visual examination within** a hollow organ or body cavity).
- **-scopic** means **pertaining to visual examination,** such as in the term **endoscopic (pertaining to visual examination within** a hollow organ or body cavity).

Endoscopic surgery is now a common term used to describe modern surgery performed with the use of endoscopes. Most often the suffixes **-scope, -scopy,** and **-scopic** mean to **examine visually,** and that is the definition given in this text. However, a term included in a subsequent chapter, **stethoscope,** is an **instrument used for listening** to body sounds.

Diagnostic Terms—*cont'd*

Built from Word Parts

Term	Definition
endoscopy................. (en-DOS-ko-pē)	visual examination within (a hollow organ or body cavity) (Table 5-1)
laryngoscope............... (la-RING-go-skōp)	instrument used for visual examination of the larynx (Exercise Figure G)
laryngoscopy............... (lar-in-GOS-ko-pē)	visual examination of the larynx
thoracoscope............... (tho-RAK-o-skōp)	instrument used for visual examination of the thorax) (Table 5-1)
thoracoscopy............... (thor-a-KOS-ko-pē)	visual examination of the thorax (Table 5-1)

Term	Definition
PULMONARY FUNCTION	
capnometer . . . . (kap-NOM-e-ter)	instrument used to measure carbon dioxide (levels in expired gas) (Figure 5-11, *A*)
oximeter . . . . (ok-SIM-e-ter) (NOTE: the combining vowel is *i*.)	instrument used to measure oxygen (saturation in the blood) (Table 5-1)
spirometer . . . . (spī-ROM-e-ter)	instrument used to measure breathing (or lung volumes) (Figure 5-11, *B*)
spirometry . . . . (spī-ROM-e-trē)	a measurement of breathing (or lung volumes) (Figure 5-11, *B*)
Sleep Studies	
polysomnography (PSG) . . . . . . (*pol*-ē-som-NOG-rah-fē)	process of recording many (tests) during sleep (performed to diagnose obstructive sleep apnea [see Figure 5-6]). Tests include electrocardiography, electromyography, electroencephalography, air flow monitoring, and oximetry.

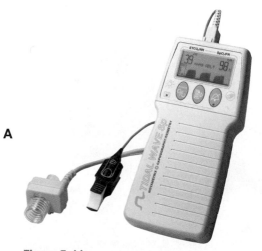

A

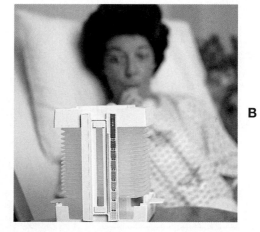

B

Figure 5-11
A, Capnometer; **B,** Spirometer.

TABLE 5-1

Types of Diagnostic Procedures

The following table illustrates the types of diagnostic procedures included in the **diagnostic term word lists** in this and subsequent chapters of this text.

Diagnostic Imaging

Diagnostic imaging is a generic term that covers radiology, ultrasonography, nuclear medicine, computed tomography, and magnetic resonance imaging.

Radiography produces images of internal organs by using ionizing radiation.

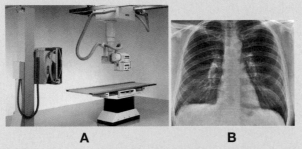

A   B

A, Radiograpic table with chest unit; **B,** chest radiograph.

Nuclear medicine produces scans by using radioactive material.

A

B

Posterior   RPO   Rt. lateral   LPO
                       Perfusion lung scan   Hx: 46-year-old
                                                female;
                                                history of
                                                shortness of
                                                breath
Lt. lateral   Anterior   Diacam   Dx: Normal lung
                         Matrix: 128×128   study
                         Dose: 3mCi 99mTc-MPA
                         Counts: 500K/view

A, Nuclear medicine scanner; **B,** lung scan.

Ultrasonography produces scans by using high-frequency sound waves.

A   B

A, Ultrasound scanner; **B,** ultrasound image of the kidney.

Computed tomography produces scans of computerized images of body organs in sectional slices.

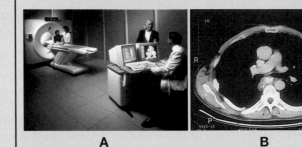

A   B

A, Computed tomography scanner; **B,** scan of the chest with intravenous contrast media.

Magnetic resonance imaging produces scans that give information about the body's anatomy by placing the patient in a magnetic field.

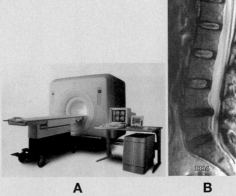

A   B

A, Magnetic resonance scanner; **B,** sagittal scan of the lumbar spine with herniated disk.

TABLE 5-1
Types of Diagnostic Procedures—*cont'd*

Endoscopy
Endoscopy uses endoscopes, which are lighted, flexible instruments, to visually examine a hollow organ or body cavity, such as the bronchus.

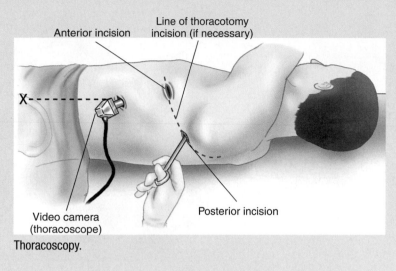

Thoracoscopy.

Laboratory
Laboratory procedures are performed on specimens such as blood, tissue, and urine.

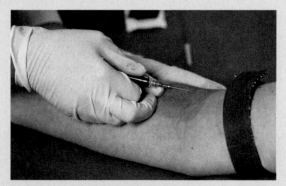

Drawing blood for laboratory test.

Pulmonary Function
Pulmonary function tests are performed in a variety of methods to determine lung function.

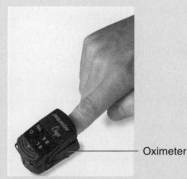

Pulse oximetry measures oxygen saturation of the blood.

EXERCISE FIGURE **G**

Fill in the blanks to complete labeling of the diagram.

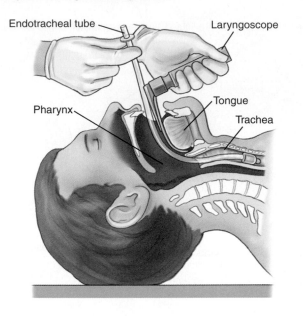

Endotracheal tube   Laryngoscope

Pharynx   Tongue   Trachea

The physician is inserting a(an) _____ / _____ / _____ tube,

within / trachea / pertaining to

using a(an) _____ / __ / _____ to

larynx / cv / instrument used for visual examination

guide the tube into place.

EXERCISE **25**

Practice saying aloud each of the diagnostic terms built from word parts on pp. 171-173.

 To hear the terms select Chapter 5, Chapter Exercises, Pronunciation.

☐ Place a check mark in the box when you have completed this exercise.

EXERCISE **26**

Analyze and define the following procedural terms.

> WR CV S
> **Example:** bronch/o/scopy   _visual examination of the bronchi_
> CF

1. spirometer _____

2. laryngoscope _____

3. capnometer _____

4. spirometry _____

5. oximeter _____

6. laryngoscopy _____

7. bronchoscope _____

8. thoracoscope _____

9. endoscope _____

10. thoracoscopy _____

11. endoscopic _____

12. endoscopy _____

13. polysomnography _____

EXERCISE 27

Build diagnostic terms that correspond to the following definitions by using the word parts you have learned.

Example: instrument used to measure oxygen   _ox_ / _i_ / _meter_
WR CV S

1. visual examination of the
   larynx
   _____ / _____ / _____
   WR   CV   S

2. instrument used to measure
   breathing
   _____ / _____ / _____
   WR   CV   S

3. instrument used to measure
   carbon dioxide
   _____ / _____ / _____
   WR   CV   S

4. instrument used for visual
   examination of the larynx
   _____ / _____ / _____
   WR   CV   S

5. visual examination of the
   bronchi
   _____ / _____ / _____
   WR   CV   S

6. measurement of breathing   _____ / _____ / _____
   WR   CV   S

7. instrument used for visual
   examination of the bronchi
   _____ / _____ / _____
   WR   CV   S

8. visual examination of a
   hollow organ or body cavity
   _____ / _____ / _____
   P   S(WR)

9. instrument used for visual
   examination of the thorax
   _____ / _____ / _____
   WR   CV   S

10. instrument used for visual
    examination of a hollow
    organ or body cavity

    _____
           P   /   S(WR)

11. visual examination of
    the thorax

    _____
           WR   /CV/   S

12. pertaining to visual
    examination of a hollow
    organ or body cavity

    _____
           P   /   S(WR)

13. process of recording
    of many (tests) during
    sleep

    _____
        P /   WR   /CV/   S

EXERCISE 28

Spell each of the diagnostic terms built from word parts on pp. 171-173 by having someone dictate them to you.

 To hear and spell the terms select Chapter 5, Chapter Exercises, Spelling. You may type the terms on the screen or write them below in the spaces provided.

☐ Place a check mark in the box when you have completed this exercise using your CD-ROM.

1._____   8._____

2._____   9._____

3._____   10._____

4._____   11._____

5._____   12._____

6._____   13._____

7._____   14._____

Diagnostic Terms

Not Built from Word Parts

In some of the following terms, you may recognize word parts; however, the terms cannot be translated literally to find their meanings.

Term	Definition
DIAGNOSTIC IMAGING	
chest computed tomography (CT) scan . . . . (chest) (kom-PŪ-ted) (tō-MOG-ra-fē-) (skan)	computerized images of the chest created in sections sliced from front to back. Used to diagnose tumors, abscesses, and pleural effusion. Computed tomography is used to visualize other body parts such as the abdomen and the brain (see Table 5-1).
chest radiograph (CXR) . . . . (chest) (RĀ-dē-ō-*graf*)	a radiographic image of the chest used to evaluate the lungs and the heart (also called a **chest x-ray**) (see Table 5-1)
ventilation-perfusion scanning (VPS) . . . . (ven-ti-LĀ-shun) (per-FŪ-zhun)	a nuclear medicine procedure used to diagnose pulmonary embolism and other conditions (also called a **lung scan**) (see Table 5-1)
LABORATORY	
acid-fast bacilli (AFB) smear . . . . (AS-id-fast) (bah-SIL-ī) (smēr)	a test performed on sputum to determine the presence of acid-fast bacilli, which cause tuberculosis
Pulmonary Function	
arterial blood gases (ABGs) . . . . (ar-TĒ-rē-al) (blud) (GAS-es)	a test performed on arterial blood to determine levels of oxygen, carbon dioxide, and other gases present
pulmonary function tests (PFTs) . . . . (PUL-mō-ner-ē) (FUNK-shun) (tests)	a group of tests performed to measure breathing, which is used to determine respiratory function or abnormalities and is useful in distinguishing chronic obstructive pulmonary disease from asthma
pulse oximetry . . . . (puls) (ok-SIM-e-trē)	a noninvasive method of measuring oxygen in the blood by using a device that attaches to the fingertip (see Table 5-1)
OTHER	
PPD (purified protein derivative) skin test	a test performed on individuals who have recently been exposed to tuberculosis. PPD of the tuberculin bacillus is injected intradermally. Positive tests indicate previous exposure, not necessarily active tuberculosis (also called **TB skin test**)

HELICAL COMPUTED TOMOGRAPHY (CT) SCAN of the chest, also called **spiral CT scan,** is an improvement over standard CT and is the preferred study to identify pulmonary embolism. Images are continually obtained as the patient passes through the gantry, which is part of the scanner. It produces a more concise and faster image, which can be performed with one breath hold.

X-RAY FILM AND RADIOGRAPH are terms used interchangeably; however, they have different meanings. **X-ray film** is the material on which the image is exposed, whereas **radiograph** refers to the film and image. **Radiographic images,** referred to as **x-ray images** in former editions of this text, can be obtained as hard copy on x-ray film (radiograph) or as digital images stored electronically and viewed on a monitor.

EXERCISE 29

Practice saying aloud each of the diagnostic terms not built from word parts on p. 179.

 To hear the terms select Chapter 5, Chapter Exercises, Pronunciation.

☐ Place a check mark in the box when you have completed this exercise.

EXERCISE 30

Fill in the blanks with the correct terms.

1. _____ _____ _____ is a nuclear medicine procedure used to diagnose pulmonary embolism and other conditions.

2. Computerized images of the chest, created in sections sliced from front to back, are called a(n) _____ _____ _____ scan.

3. _____ _____ is used to evaluate the lungs and the heart.

4. The test performed on arterial blood to determine levels of oxygen, carbon dioxide, and other gases present is called _____ _____ _____.

5. A noninvasive test to measure oxygen in the blood is called _____ _____.

6. A test performed on sputum to diagnose tuberculosis is called _____ _____ _____ _____.

7. _____ _____ _____ is the name of a group of tests performed on breathing to determine respiratory function or abnormalities.

8. _____ _____ _____ is a test that, when positive, indicates an individual has been exposed to tuberculosis.

EXERCISE 31

Match the terms in the first column with their correct definitions in the second column.

_____ 1. ventilation-perfusion scanning

_____ 2. chest radiograph

_____ 3. chest CT scan

_____ 4. acid-fast bacilli smear

_____ 5. pulse oximetry

_____ 6. arterial blood gases

_____ 7. pulmonary function tests

_____ 8. PPD skin test

a. computerized images of the chest

b. a noninvasive method used to measure oxygen in the blood

c. a blood test used to determine oxygen and other gases in the blood

d. a test for tuberculosis

e. chest x-ray

f. a nuclear medicine procedure used to diagnose pulmonary conditions

g. injected intradermally

h. tests performed on breathing

i. an instrument to measure pulse waves

EXERCISE 32

Spell each of the diagnostic terms not built from word parts on p. 179 by having someone dictate them to you.

To hear and spell the terms select Chapter 5, Chapter Exercises, Spelling. You may type the terms on the screen or write them below in the spaces provided.

☐ Place a check mark in the box if you have completed this exercise using your CD-ROM.

1._____   5._____

2._____   6._____

3._____   7._____

4._____   8._____

Complementary Terms

Built from Word Parts

The following terms are built from word parts you have already learned and can be translated literally to find their meanings. Further explanation of terms beyond the definition of their word parts, if needed, is included in parentheses.

Term	Definition
acapnia . . . . (a-CAP-nē-a)	condition of absence (less than normal level) of carbon dioxide (in the blood)
anoxia . . . . (a-NOK-sē-a)	condition of absence (deficiency) of oxygen
aphonia . . . . (ā-FŌ-nē-a)	condition of absence of voice
apnea . . . . (AP-nē-a)	absence of breathing
bronchoalveolar . . . . (*bron*-kō-al-VĒ-o-lar)	pertaining to the bronchi and alveoli
bronchospasm . . . . (BRON-kō-spazm)	spasmodic contraction in the bronchi
diaphragmatic . . . . (*dī*-a-frag-MAT-ik)	pertaining to the diaphragm (also called **phrenic**)
dysphonia . . . . (dis-FŌ-nē-a)	condition of difficult speaking (voice)
dyspnea . . . . (DISP-nē-a)	difficult breathing
endotracheal . . . . (*en*-dō-TRĀ-kē-al)	pertaining to within the trachea (see Exercise Figure G)
eupnea . . . . (ŪP-nē-a)	normal breathing
hypercapnia . . . . (hī-per-KAP-nē-a)	condition of excessive carbon dioxide (in the blood)

ANOXIA
literally means **without oxygen** or **absence of oxygen.** The term actually denotes an oxygen deficiency in the body tissues.

Complementary Terms—*cont'd*
Built from Word Parts

Term	Definition
hyperpnea (hī-perp-NĒ-a)	excessive breathing
hypocapnia (hī-pō-KAP-nē-a)	condition of deficient carbon dioxide (in the blood)
hypopnea (hī-POP-nēa)	deficient breathing
hypoxemia (hī-pok-SĒ-mē-a) (NOTE: the *o* from *hypo* has been dropped. The final vowel in a prefix may be dropped when the word to which it is added begins with a vowel.)	condition of deficient oxygen (in the blood)
hypoxia (hī-POK-sē-a) (NOTE: see note for hypoxemia.)	condition of deficient oxygen (to the tissues)
intrapleural (in-tra-PLUR-al)	pertaining to within the pleura (space between the two pleural membranes)
laryngeal (lar-IN-jē-al)	pertaining to the larynx
laryngospasm (la-RING-gō-spazm)	spasmodic contraction of the larynx
mucoid (MŪ-koyd)	resembling mucus
mucous (MŪ-kus)	pertaining to mucus
nasopharyngeal (*nā*-zō-fa-RIN-jē-al)	pertaining to the nose and pharynx
orthopnea (or-THOP-nē-a)	able to breathe easier in an upright position
phrenalgia (fre-NAL-ja)	pain in the diaphragm (also called **diaphragmalgia**)
phrenospasm (FREN-ō-spazm)	spasm of the diaphragm
pulmonary (PUL-mō-ner-ē)	pertaining to the lungs
pulmonologist (pul-mon-OL-o-jist)	a physician who studies and treats diseases of the lung
pulmonology (pul-mon-OL-o-jē)	study of the lung (a branch of medicine dealing with diseases of the lung)
rhinorrhea (rī-nō-RĒ-a)	discharge from the nose (as in a cold)

MUCUS
is the noun that means the slimy fluid secreted by the mucous membrane. **Mucous** is the adjective that means pertaining to the mucous membrane. Pronunciation is the same for both terms.

Term	Definition
tachypnea . . . . (tak-IP-nē-a)	rapid breathing
thoracic . . . . (thō-RAS-ik)	pertaining to the chest

EXERCISE 33

Practice saying aloud each of the complementary terms built from word parts on pp. 181-183.

To hear the terms select Chapter 5, Chapter Exercises, Pronunciation.

☐ Place a check mark in the box when you have completed this exercise.

EXERCISE 34

Analyze and define the following complementary terms.

             P   WR S

Example: hyper/capn/ia   *condition of excessive carbon dioxide (in the blood)*

1. laryngeal _____

2. eupnea _____

3. mucoid_____

4. apnea _____

5. hypoxia _____

6. laryngospasm _____

7. endotracheal _____

8. anoxia _____

9. dysphonia _____

10. bronchoalveolar _____

11. dyspnea _____

12. hypocapnia _____

13. bronchospasm_____

14. orthopnea _____

15. hyperpnea _____

16. acapnia_____

17. hypopnea_____

18. hypoxemia_____

19. aphonia _____

20. rhinorrhea _____

21. thoracic _____

22. mucous _____

23. nasopharyngeal _____

24. diaphragmatic _____

25. intrapleural _____

26. pulmonary _____

27. phrenalgia _____

28. tachypnea _____

29. phrenospasm _____

30. pulmonologist _____

31. pulmonology _____

EXERCISE 35

Build the complementary terms for the following definitions by using the word parts you have learned.

Example: pertaining to bronchi and alveoli   <u>bronch / o / alveol / ar</u>
                                                      WR /CV/ WR / S

1. condition of deficient oxygen   _____/_____/_____
                                      P / WR / S

2. resembling mucus   _____/_____
                        WR / S

3. able to breathe easier
   an upright position   _____/_____/_____
                           WR /CV/ S

4. pertaining to within
   the trachea   _____/_____/_____
                   P / WR / S

5. condition of absence
   of oxygen   _____/_____/_____
                 P / WR / S

6. difficult breathing   _____/_____
                           P / S(WR)

7. pertaining to the larynx   _____/_____
                                WR / S

8. condition of excessive
   carbon dioxide (in the blood)   _____/_____/_____
                                     P / WR / S

9. normal breathing

_____ / _____
P   S(WR)

10. condition of absence of voice

_____ / _____ / _____
P   WR   S

11. spasmodic contraction
    of the larynx

_____ /CV/ _____
WR   S

12. condition of deficient
    carbon dioxide (in the blood)

_____ / _____ / _____
P   WR   S

13. pertaining to the nose
    and pharynx

_____ /CV/ _____ / _____
WR   WR   S

14. pertaining to the diaphragm

_____ / _____
WR   S

15. condition of absence
    of breathing

_____ / _____
P   S(WR)

16. condition of deficient
    oxygen in the blood

_____ / _____ / _____
P   WR   S

17. excessive breathing

_____ / _____
P   S(WR)

18. spasmodic contraction
    in the bronchi

_____ /CV/ _____
WR   S

19. deficient breathing

_____ / _____
P   S(WR)

20. condition of absence
    of carbon dioxide
    (in the blood)

_____ / _____ / _____
P   WR   S

21. condition of difficulty
    in speaking (voice)

_____ / _____ / _____
P   WR   S

22. discharge from the nose

_____ /CV/ _____
WR   S

23. pertaining to mucus

_____ / _____
WR   S

24. pertaining to the chest

_____ / _____
WR   S

25. pertaining to within the pleura

_____ / _____ / _____
P   WR   S

26. pertaining to the lungs

_____ / _____
WR   S

27. spasm of the diaphragm

_____ /___/ ___
WR   /CV/   S

28. rapid breathing

_____ /___
P   /   S(WR)

29. pain in the diaphragm

_____ /___
WR   /   S

30. study of the lung

_____ /___/ ___
WR   /CV/   S

31. a physician who studies and
    treats diseases of the lung

_____ /___/ ___
WR   /CV/   S

EXERCISE 36

Spell each of the complementary terms built from word parts on pp. 181-183 by having someone dictate them to you.

 To hear and spell the terms select Chapter 5, Chapter Exercises, Spelling. You may type the terms on the screen or write them below in the spaces provided.

☐ Place a check mark in the box if you have completed this exercise using your CD-ROM.

1. _____
2. _____
3. _____
4. _____
5. _____
6. _____
7. _____
8. _____
9. _____
10. _____
11. _____
12. _____
13. _____
14. _____
15. _____
16. _____

17. _____
18. _____
19. _____
20. _____
21. _____
22. _____
23. _____
24. _____
25. _____
26. _____
27. _____
28. _____
29. _____
30. _____
31. _____

Complementary Terms

Not Built from Word Parts

In some of the following terms, you may recognize word parts; however, the terms cannot be translated literally to find their meanings.

Term	Definition
airway (AR-wā)	passageway by which air enters and leaves the lungs as well as a mechanical device used to keep the air passageway unobstructed
asphyxia (as-FIK-sē-a)	deprivation of oxygen for tissue use; suffocation
aspirate (AS-per-āt)	to withdraw fluid or to suction as well as to draw foreign material into the respiratory tract
bronchoconstrictor (*bron*-kō-kon-STRIK-tor)	agent causing narrowing of the bronchi
bronchodilator (*bron*-kō-dī-LĀ-tor)	agent causing the bronchi to widen
cough (kawf)	sudden, noisy expulsion of air from the lungs
hiccup (HIK-up)	sudden catching of breath with a spasmodic contraction of the diaphragm (also called **hiccough** and **singultus**)
hyperventilation (*hī*-per-ven-ti-LĀ-shun)	ventilation of the lungs beyond normal body needs
hypoventilation (*hī*-pō-ven-ti-LĀ-shun)	ventilation of the lungs that does not fulfill the body's gas exchange needs
mucopurulent (*mū*-kō-PŪR-ū-lent)	containing both mucus and pus
mucus (MŪ-kus)	slimy fluid secreted by the mucous membranes
nebulizer (NEB-ū-lī-zer)	device that creates a mist used to deliver medication for giving respiratory treatment (Figure 5-12)
nosocomial infection (nos-ō-KŌ-mē-al) (in-FEK-shun)	an infection acquired during hospitalization
paroxysm (PAR-ok-sizm)	periodic, sudden attack
patent (PĀ-tent)	open (an airway must be patent)
sputum (SPŪ-tum)	mucous secretion from the lungs, bronchi, and trachea expelled through the mouth
ventilator (VEN-ti-lā-tor)	mechanical device used to assist with or substitute for breathing when a patient cannot breathe unassisted (Figure 5-13)

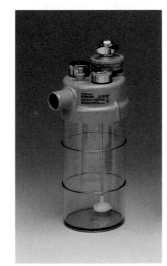

FIGURE 5-12
Nebulizer.

SPUTUM
is derived from the Latin *spuere*, meaning **to spit.** In a 1693 dictionary it is defined as a "secretion thicker than ordinary spittle."

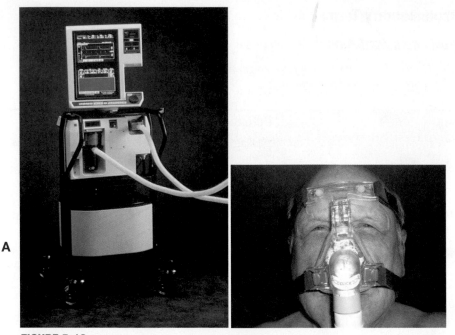

FIGURE 5-13
A, Positive pressure ventilator is applied to the patient's airway through an endotracheal or tracheostomy tube and is used when spontaneous breathing is inadequate to sustain life.
B, CPAP (continuous positive airway pressure) is a type of ventilator used for patients who can initiate their own breathing and is often used to treat obstructive sleep apnea.

EXERCISE 37

Practice saying aloud each of the complementary terms not built from word parts on p. 187.

 To hear the terms select Chapter 5, Chapter Exercises, Pronunciation.

☐ Place a check mark in the box when you have completed this exercise.

EXERCISE 38

Fill in the blanks with the correct terms.

1. Another term for ventilation of the lungs beyond normal body needs is _____.

2. A device that creates a mist used to deliver medication for giving respiratory treatment is a(n) _____.

3. A(n) _____ is an agent that causes the air passages to widen.

4. A patient who has difficulty breathing can be attached to a mechanical breathing device called a(n) _____.

5. Another term for suffocation is _____.

6. Material made up of mucous secretions from the lungs, bronchi, and trachea is called _____.

7. To suction or withdraw fluid is to _____.

8. A(n) _____ is a mechanical device that keeps the air passageway unobstructed.

9. A sudden catching of breath with spasmodic contraction of the diaphragm is called a(n) _____.

10. A sudden, noisy expulsion of air from the lung is a(n) _____.

11. Material containing both mucus and pus is referred to as being

    _____.

12. _____ is the name given to ventilation of the lungs that does not fulfill the body's gas exchange needs.

13. An infection acquired during hospitalization is called _____.

14. The term that applies to a periodic sudden attack is _____.

15. An airway must be kept _____ (open) for the patient to breathe.

16. An agent that causes bronchi to narrow is called a(n) _____.

17. _____ is the name given to the slimy fluid secreted by the mucous membranes.

EXERCISE 39

Match the terms in the first column with their correct definitions in the second column.

_____ 1. airway

_____ 2. aspirate

_____ 3. bronchoconstrictor

_____ 4. bronchodilator

_____ 5. cough

_____ 6. hiccup

_____ 7. hyperventilation

_____ 8. asphyxia

a. sudden, noisy expulsion of air from the lungs

b. mechanical device used to keep the air passageway unobstructed

c. agent that narrows the bronchi

d. catching of breath with spasmodic contraction of diaphragm

e. mucus from throat and lungs

f. suffocation

g. ventilation of the lungs beyond normal body needs

h. to draw foreign material into the respiratory tract

i. agent that widens the bronchi

EXERCISE 40

Match the terms in the first column with their correct definitions in the second column.

_____ 1. hypoventilation

_____ 2. mucopurulent

_____ 3. mucus

_____ 4. nebulizer

_____ 5. nosocomial

_____ 6. patent

_____ 7. sputum

_____ 8. ventilator

_____ 9. paroxysm

a. open

b. mucous secretion from lungs, bronchi, and trachea, expelled through the mouth

c. respiratory treatment device that sends a mist

d. mechanical breathing device

e. ventilation of the lungs that does not fulfill the body's gas exchange needs

f. periodic, sudden attack

g. agent that widens air passages

h. containing both mucus and pus

i. slimy fluid secreted by mucous membranes

j. hospital-acquired infection

EXERCISE 41

Spell each of the complementary terms not built from word parts on p. 187 by having someone dictate them to you.

To hear and spell the terms select Chapter 5, Chapter Exercises, Spelling. You may type the terms on the screen or write them below in the spaces provided.

☐ Place a check mark in the box if you have completed this exercise using your CD-ROM.

1. _____

2. _____

3. _____

4. _____

5. _____

6. _____

7. _____

8. _____

9. _____

10. _____

11. _____

12. _____

13. _____

14. _____

15. _____

16. _____

17. _____

Refer to Appendix E for pharmacology terms related to the respiratory system.

Abbreviations

ABGs	arterial blood gases
AFB	acid-fast bacilli
ARDS	adult respiratory distress syndrome
CF	cystic fibrosis
CO_2	carbon dioxide
COPD	chronic obstructive pulmonary disease
CT	computed tomography
CXR	chest radiograph (chest x-ray)
flu	influenza
LLL	left lower lobe
LTB	laryngotracheobronchitis
LUL	left upper lobe
O_2	oxygen
OSA	obstructive sleep apnea
PE	pulmonary embolism
PFTs	pulmonary function tests
PSG	polysomnography
RLL	right lower lobe
RML	right middle lobe
RUL	right upper lobe
TB	tuberculosis
URI	upper respiratory infection
VPS	ventilation-perfusion scanning

Refer to Appendix D for a complete list of abbreviations.

EXERCISE 42

Write the meaning of the abbreviations in the following sentences.

1. A variety of tests are used to diagnose **COPD** _____ _____ _____ _____, including **PFTs** _____ _____ _____, **CXR** _____ _____, **ABGs** _____ _____ _____, and chest **CT** _____ _____ scan.

2. **VPS** _____ _____ _____ is very helpful in diagnosing **PE** _____ _____.

3. The lobes of the left lung are **LUL** _____ _____ _____ and **LLL** _____ _____ _____; the lobes of the right lung are **RUL** _____ _____ _____, **RML** _____ _____ _____, and **RLL** _____ _____ _____.

4. **AFB** _____ _____ _____ smear is used to support the diagnosis of **TB** _____.

5. **PSG** _____ is used to confirm the diagnosis of OSA _____ _____ _____.

6. Respiration is the exchange of **O₂** _____ and **CO₂** _____ _____ between the atmosphere and body cells.

EXERCISE 43

Write the definition for the following abbreviations.

1. ARDS _____ _____ _____ _____

2. CF _____ _____

3. flu _____

4. LTB _____

5. URI _____ _____ _____

Common Abbreviations used in Respiratory Care

BiPAP	bilevel positive airway pressure
CPT	chest physiotherapy
CPAP	continuous positive airway pressure
DPI	dry powder inhaler
MDI	metered-dose inhaler
PEP	positive expiratory pressure
SVN	small-volume nebulizer
VAP	ventilator-associated pneumonia

PRACTICAL APPLICATION

EXERCISE **44**   *Interact with Medical Documents*

A. Complete the medical consultation report by writing the medical terms in the blanks. Use the list of definitions with the corresponding numbers following it.

University Hospital and Medical Center
4700 North Main Street • Wellness, Arizona 54321 • (987) 555-3210

PATIENT NAME: Victor Marquez   **CASE NUMBER:** 516987-RSP
DATE OF BIRTH: 02/01/19XX   **DATE:** 02/16/20XX

MEDICAL CONSULT REPORT

HISTORY: Victor Marquez is a 55-year-old Mexican-American man who came to the Emergency Department on 02/16/XX because of recent onset of 1. _____ and 2. _____. He has also had weight loss and cough for the past 6 months. He denies hemoptysis, chest pain, fever, or night sweats. He has a history of smoking two packs of cigarettes a day for 40 years. It was decided that he should be admitted and scheduled for a 3. _____ consultation.

PHYSICAL EXAMINATION: VITAL SIGNS: Blood pressure, 148/82. Temperature, 98.2. Pulse, 60. Respirations, 18. The chest is clear except for scattered rhonchi over left posterior lung. The heart is regular rhythm without murmur. He is in no acute distress. Pulses are full and equal throughout. There is mild clubbing of the fingers.

PULMONARY EXAM: 4. _____ reveals a suspicious lesion in the left upper lobe of the lung with diffuse interstitial fibrotic lesions. Fiberoptic 5. _____ shows edematous vocal cords with no obvious nodules. However, at the entry of the left bronchus, a lesion is observed that partially obstructs the opening. A biopsy and brush cytology of the specimen were obtained. 6. _____ _____ _____ shows mild 7. _____ .

IMPRESSION: It is my impression that the patient has 8. _____ _____ .

DISPOSITION:
1. Obtain 9. _____ _____ _____ to include lung volumes and diffusing capacity.
2. Obtain a CT scan of the chest and a 10. _____ surgery consultation.

_____
Miguel Valdez, MD

MV/mcm

---

1. sudden noisy expulsion of air from the lungs
2. difficult breathing
3. pertaining to the lungs
4. radiographic image used to evaluate the lungs and heart
5. visual examination of the bronchi

6. test performed on arterial blood to determine the presence of oxygen, carbon dioxide, and other gases
7. condition of deficient oxygen in the blood
8. cancerous tumor originating in the bronchus
9. a group of tests performed on breathing
10. pertaining to the chest

EXERCISE **44**   *Interact with Medical Documents—cont'd*

B. Read the clinical case study and answer the questions following it.

Medical History: A 65-year-old man who has a history of nonproductive cough and shortness of breath of 3 weeks' duration was admitted to the hospital. He has smoked one pack of cigarettes daily for nearly 40 years.

Physical Examination: The patient is thin, has tachypnea, and is mildly cyanotic with a barrel chest. He uses accessory muscles of inspiration and pursed-lip breathing. Expiration is prolonged, breath sounds are diminished, and wheezing is present. Respiratory rate: 30 breaths/min, heart rate: 100 beats/min, blood pressure: 110/70, temperature: 38.2.

Diagnostic Studies: PA and lateral chest radiographs reveal pulmonary hyperinflation, a widened anteroposterior diameter, increased depth of the retrosternal air space, and a right lobe infiltrate consistent with pneumonia.

Arterial blood gases: PaO_2, 52 mm Hg; $PaCO_2$, 68 mm Hg; pH, 7.30

O_2 saturation measured by pulse oximetry at room air is 87%.

Diagnosis: Chronic obstructive pulmonary disease with respiratory insufficiency, pneumonia, hypoxia, hypercapnia, and respiratory acidosis.

---

1. Three tests used to determine the diagnosis are

   _____ _____;

   _____ _____ _____;

   _____ _____.

2. The patient was experiencing (excessive, deficient) carbon dioxide and (excessive, deficient) oxygen in the blood.

3. a. T F   On physical examination the patient was experiencing rapid breathing.

   b. T F   The patient was diagnosed as having COPD.

   c. T F   A CXR was performed as one of the diagnostic studies.

EXERCISE **44**   *Interact with Medical Documents—cont'd*

C. Below is a printed report of a CT scan of the chest. Refer to Table 5-1 for illustrations of a CT scanner and images.

Terms you have studied thus far are in bold. Note how they are used within a medical record.

NAME: Abigail Frank   **MR #:** 7463802   **ACCESSION #:** 1503132
DATE OF EXAM: 11/16/20XX   **PHYSICIAN:** Irene Buchanan, MD

CT CHEST W/CONTRAST AT 1117 HOURS

EXAM: **CT OF THE CHEST**

History: Cervical **cancer**

TECHNIQUE: Multiple contiguous axial images were obtained to the chest during the uneventful infusion of **intravenous** contrast.

FINDINGS: There has been interval decrease in size of **bilateral pulmonary metastases.** Again the largest is noted within the left lower **lobe** and measures 4.8 × 3.9 cm compared to 6.5 × 5.0 cm previously when measured at the same weight. Multiple smaller **lesions** within both **lungs** have decreased in size.

No significant **adenopathy** is identified. Postsurgical changes centrally within the right lower lobe are again noted with a surgical staple line in place.

There has been interval development of several patchy probably interstitial opacities within both lungs. Some are located adjacent to **metastases** which have decreased in size.

No new masses are noted. There is no **pleural** or pericardial **effusion.** The osseous structures remain within normal limits.

A left adrenal **nodule** remains essentially unchanged measuring approximately 2 cm in greatest dimension.

IMPRESSION: Interval decrease in size of **bilateral pulmonary metastases** as described following **chemotherapy** and **radiation therapy.**

Development of occasional patchy predominately interstitial opacities. Given the history of **chemotherapy** and **radiation therapy** this likely reflects a postradiation or post-therapeutic **pneumonitis** or hypersensitivity. Additional considerations are an infectious **pneumonitis** or hemorrhage. Continued follow-up is recommended. Stable small left adrenal **nodule.**

Transcribed By: MCM 11/16/20XX: 1641

Approved By: Radiologist: Brian Benson, MD

To test your understanding of the terms introduced in this chapter, circle the words that correctly complete the sentences. The italicized words refer to the correct answer.

1. The patient in the emergency room was admitted with a *severe nosebleed*, or (**rhinomycosis, epistaxis, nasopharyngitis**).

2. The accident caused damage to the *larynx*, necessitating a *surgical repair*, or a (**laryngectomy, laryngostomy, laryngoplasty**).

3. Mr. Prince was *able to breathe easier in an upright position*, so the nurse recorded that he had (**orthopnea, eupnea, dyspnea**).

4. The *test on arterial blood to determine oxygen and carbon dioxide levels* (**pulse oximetry, pulmonary function tests, arterial blood gases**) indicated that the patient was *deficient in oxygen*, or had (**dysphonia, hypoxia, hypocapnia**).

5. The physician informed the patient that a heart attack was not the cause of the *chest pain*, or (**thoracalgia, pneumothorax, thoracentesis**).

6. The patient reported dizziness brought on by *ventilation of the lungs beyond normal body needs*, or (**hyperventilation, hypoventilation, dysphonia**).

7. The physician wished the patient to have the medication given by *a device that delivers mist*, so he ordered that the treatment be given by (**airway, nebulizer, ventilator**).

8. The patient with *blood in the chest* was diagnosed as having a (**pneumothorax, pleuritis, hemothorax**).

9. After surgery, the patient had a *block in the circulation to the pulmonary artery* or (**pleural effusion, pulmonary edema, pulmonary embolism**).

10. The patient was diagnosed as having *a fungal disease affecting the lung*, or (**obstructive sleep apnea, tuberculosis, coccidioidomycosis**).

11. The physician ordered a *radiographic image of the chest* (**chest radiograph, chest CT scan, bronchoscopy**) because she suspected *an infection acquired during hospitalization*, or (**patent, nosocomial, paroxysm**) pneumonia.

12. The patient received an *intradermal injection* (**AFB, ABGs, PPD skin test**) *to determine if she had been exposed to TB*.

13. The patient was experiencing *rapid breathing* or (**phrenospasm, tachypnea, phrenalgia**).

EXERCISE **46**   *Read Medical Terms in Use*

Practice pronouncing the terms by reading the following medical document. Use the pronunciation key following the medical terms to assist you in saying the word.

To hear these terms select Chapter 5, Chapter Exercises, Read Medical Terms in Use.

A 24-year-old man visited the emergency department because of **dyspnea** (DISP-nē-a), **hyperpnea** (hī-perp-NĒ-a), **paroxysms** (PAR-ok-sizms) of **cough** (kawf), and the presence of thick, tenacious **mucus** (MŪ-kus). He had a history of **asthma** (AZ-ma) since the age of 12 years. A chest radiograph was negative for **pneumonia** (nū-MŌ-nē-a). **Arterial blood gases** (ar-TĒ-rē-al) (blud) (GAS-es) showed **hypoxemia** (hī-pok-SĒ mē-a) but no **hypercapnia** (hī-per-KAP-nē–a). **Pulmonary function tests** (PUL-mō-ner-ē) (FUNK-shun) (tests) disclosed bronchoconstriction, which was corrected by a **bronchodilator** (*bron*-kō–dī-LĀ-tor). A **nebulizer** (NEB-ū-lī-zer) was prescribed for treatment. The asthma attack was probably precipitated by an episode of **bronchitis** (bron-KĪ-tis).

EXERCISE **47**   *Comprehend Medical Terms in Use*

Test your comprehension of terms in the previous medical document by answering *T* for true and *F* for false.

_____ 1. The patient visited the emergency department because of many symptoms, one of which was sudden, periodic coughing.

_____ 2. Diagnostic procedures were performed to assist with the diagnosis. ABGs showed increased O_2 and decreased CO_2.

_____ 3. An agent that causes the bronchi to widen was used to treat the condition diagnosed with the PFTs.

_____ 4. The asthma attack was precipitated by narrowing of the bronchi.

WEB LINK
For additional information on diseases of the lung, visit the American Lung Association at www.lungusa.org.

CHAPTER REVIEW

CHAPTER REVIEW ON CD-ROM

Use the CD-ROM that accompanies this textbook to play and practice what you have learned in this chapter. The Chapter Exercises, Practice Activities, Animations, and Games allow you to hear, see, and interact with the chapter content.

Chapter Exercises

Exercises in this section of your CD-ROM correlate to exercises in your textbook. You may have completed them as you worked through the chapter.
- ☐ Pronunciation
- ☐ Spelling
- ☐ Read Medical Terms in Use

Practice Activities

Practice in study mode, then test your learning in assessment mode. Keep track of your scores from assessment mode if you wish.

SCORE

- ☐ Picture It   _____
- ☐ Define Word Parts   _____
- ☐ Build Medical Terms _____
- ☐ Word Shop   _____
- ☐ Define Medical Terms _____
- ☐ Use It   _____
- ☐ Hear It and Type It: _____
  Clinical Vignettes

Animations
- ☐ Atelectasis
- ☐ Asthma
- ☐ Pneumothorax

Games
- ☐ Name that Word Part
- ☐ Term Storm
- ☐ Term Explorer
- ☐ Termbusters
- ☐ Medical Millionaire

REVIEW OF WORD PARTS

Can you define and spell the following word parts?

Combining Forms		Prefixes	Suffixes	
adenoid/o	pharyng/o	a-	-algia	-pexy
alveol/o	phon/o	an-	-ar	-pnea
atel/o	phren/o	endo-	-ary	-rrhagia
bronchi/o	pleur/o	eu-	-cele	-scope
bronch/o	pneumat/o	pan-	-centesis	-scopic
capn/o	pneum/o	poly-	-eal	-scopy
diaphragmat/o	pneumon/o	tachy-	-ectasis	-spasm
epiglott/o	pulmon/o		-emia	-stenosis
hemat/o	py/o		-graphy	-stomy
hem/o	rhin/o		-meter	-thorax
laryng/o	sept/o		-metry	-tomy
lob/o	sinus/o			
muc/o	somn/o			
nas/o	spir/o			
orth/o	thorac/o			
ox/i	tonsill/o			
ox/o	trache/o			

REVIEW OF TERMS

Can you build, analyze, define, pronounce, and spell the following terms *built from word parts?*

Diseases and Disorders	Surgical	Diagnostic	Complementary
adenoiditis	adenoidectomy	bronchoscope	acapnia
atelectasis	adenotome	bronchoscopy	anoxia
bronchiectasis	bronchoplasty	capnometer	aphonia
bronchitis	laryngectomy	endoscope	apnea
bronchogenic carcinoma	laryngoplasty	endoscopic	bronchoalveolar
bronchopneumonia	laryngostomy	endoscopy	bronchospasm
diaphragmatocele	laryngotracheotomy	laryngoscope	diaphragmatic
epiglottitis	lobectomy	laryngoscopy	dysphonia
hemothorax	pleuropexy	oximeter	dyspnea
laryngitis	pneumobronchotomy	polysomnography (PSG)	endotracheal
laryngotracheobronchitis (LTB)	pneumonectomy	spirometer	eupnea
lobar pneumonia	rhinoplasty	spirometry	hypercapnia
nasopharyngitis	septoplasty	thoracoscope	hyperpnea
pansinusitis	septotomy	thoracoscopy	hypocapnia
pharyngitis	sinusotomy		hypopnea
pleuritis	thoracocentesis		hypoxemia
pneumatocele	thoracotomy		hypoxia
pneumoconiosis	tonsillectomy		intrapleural
pneumonia	tracheoplasty		laryngeal
pneumonitis	tracheostomy		laryngospasm
pneumothorax	tracheotomy		mucoid
pulmonary neoplasm			mucous
pyothorax			nasopharyngeal
rhinitis			orthopnea
rhinomycosis			phrenalgia
rhinorrhagia			phrenospasm
thoracalgia			pulmonary
tonsillitis			pulmonologist
tracheitis			pulmonology
tracheostenosis			rhinorrhea
			tachypnea
			thoracic

REVIEW OF TERMS—*cont'd*

Can you define, pronounce, and spell the following terms *not built from word parts?*

Diseases and Disorders	**Diagnostic**	**Complementary**
adult respiratory distress syndrome (ARDS)	acid-fast bacilli smear (AFB)	airway
asthma	arterial blood gases (ABGs)	asphyxia
chronic obstructive pulmonary disease (COPD)	chest computed tomography (CT) scan	aspirate
		bronchoconstrictor
coccidioidomycosis	chest radiograph (CXR)	bronchodilator
cor pulmonale	PPD skin test	cough
croup	pulmonary function tests (PFTs)	hiccup
cystic fibrosis (CF)	pulse oximetry	hyperventilation
deviated septum	ventilation-perfusion scanning (VPS)	hypoventilation
emphysema		mucopurulent
epistaxis		mucus
influenza (flu)		nebulizer
Legionnaire disease		nosocomial infection
obstructive sleep apnea (OSA)		paroxysm
pertussis		patent
pleural effusion		sputum
pulmonary edema		ventilator
pulmonary embolism (PE)		
tuberculosis (TB)		
upper respiratory infection (URI)		

ANSWERS

Exercise Figures

Exercise Figure

A.
1. sinus: sinus/o
2. nose: nas/o, rhin/o
3. tonsils: tonsill/o
4. epiglottis: epiglott/o
5. larynx: laryng/o
6. trachea: trache/o
7. pleura: pleur/o
8. lobe: lob/o
9. diaphragm: diaphragmat/o, phren/o
10. adenoids: adenoid/o
11. pharynx: pharyng/o
12. lung: pneum/o, pneumat/o, pneumon/o, pulmon/o
13. bronchus: bronch/o, bronchi/o
14. alveolus: alveol/o

Exercise Figure

B. bronchi/ectasis

Exercise Figure

C. A. pneum/o/thorax,
B. hem/o/thorax

Exercise Figure

D. adenoid/ectomy, aden/o/tome

Exercise Figure

E. thorac/o/centesis

Exercise Figure

F. bronch/o/scopy

Exercise Figure

G. endo/trache/al, laryng/o/scope

Exercise 1
1. h
2. a
3. g
4. c
5. f
6. d
7. e
8. b

Exercise 2
1. nasal septum
2. epiglottis
3. bronchioles
4. nose
5. diaphragm
6. mediastinum
7. tonsils

Exercise 3
1. larynx
2. bronchus
3. pleura
4. air, lung
5. tonsil
6. lung
7. diaphragm
8. trachea
9. alveolus
10. air, lung
11. thorax (chest)
12. adenoids
13. pharynx
14. nose
15. sinus
16. lobe
17. epiglottis
18. lung, air
19. nose
20. septum
21. diaphragm

Exercise 4
1. a. nas/o
   b. rhin/o
2. laryng/o
3. a. pneum/o
   b. pneumat/o
   c. pneumon/o
4. pulmon/o
5. tonsill/o
6. trache/o
7. adenoid/o
8. pleur/o
9. a. diaphragmat/o
   b. phren/o
10. sinus/o
11. thorac/o
12. alveol/o
13. pharyng/o
14. a. bronchi/o
    b. bronch/i
15. lob/o
16. epiglott/o
17. sept/o

Exercise 5
1. oxygen
2. breathe, breathing
3. mucus
4. imperfect, incomplete
5. straight
6. pus
7. blood
8. sleep

9. carbon dioxide
10. sound, voice

Exercise 6
1. spir/o
2. a. ox/o
   b. ox/i
3. atel/o
4. orth/o
5. py/o
6. muc/o
7. a. hem/o
   b. hemat/o
8. somn/o
9. phon/o
10. capn/o

Exercise 7
1. within
2. without, absence of
3. all, total
4. normal, good
5. many, much
6. fast, rapid

Exercise 8
1. endo-
2. eu-
3. a. a-
   b. an-
4. pan-
5. poly-
6. tachy-

Exercise 9
1. k
2. f
3. g
4. c
5. b
6. j
7. a
8. h
9. d
10. e

Exercise 10
1. c
2. e
3. a
4. h
5. b
6. i
7. f
8. d
9. g
10. j

Exercise 11
1. chest
2. pertaining to
3. constriction, narrowing
4. hernia, protrusion
5. creation of an artificial opening
6. surgical fixation or suspension
7. instrument used to measure
8. sudden, involuntary muscle contraction
9. pain
10. visual examination
11. surgical puncture to aspirate fluid
12. cut into, incision
13. instrument used for visual examination
14. rapid flow of blood
15. stretching out, dilatation, expansion
16. process of recording, radiographic imaging
17. measurement
18. blood condition
19. pertaining to visual examination
20. breathing

Exercise 12
Pronunciation Exercise

Exercise 13
1. WR S
   pleur/itis
   inflammation of the pleura
2. WR CV WR   S
   nas/o/pharyng/itis
   ___
   CF
   inflammation of the nose and pharynx
3. WR   CV S
   pneum/o/thorax
   ___
   CF
   air in the chest
4. P WR S
   pan/sinus/itis
   inflammation of all sinuses
5. WR   S
   atel/ectasis
   incomplete expansion (or collapsed lung)
6. WR CV WR S
   rhin/o/myc/osis
   ___
   CF
   abnormal condition of fungus in the nose
7. WR CV S
   trache/o/stenosis
   ___
   CF
   narrowing of the trachea
8. WR   S
   epiglott/itis
   inflammation of the epiglottis

9. WR   S
   thorac/algia
   pain in the chest
10. WR   S P   S(WR)
    pulmon/ary neo/plasm
    pertaining to (in) the lung new growth (tumor)
11. WR   S
    bronchi/ectasis
    dilation of the bronchi
12. WR   S
    tonsill/itis
    inflammation of the tonsils
13. WR CV WR S
    pneum/o/coni/osis
    ___
    CF
    abnormal condition of dust in the lungs
14. WR CV WR   S
    bronch/o/pneumon/ia
    ___
    CF
    diseased state of bronchi and lungs
15. WR   S
    pneumon/itis
    inflammation of the lung
16. WR   S
    laryng/itis
    inflammation of the larynx
17. WR   CV S
    pneumat/o/cele
    ___
    CF
    hernia of the lung
18. WR CV S
    py/o/thorax
    ___
    CF
    pus in the chest (pleural space)
19. WR CV   S
    rhin/o/rrhagia
    ___
    CF
    rapid flow of blood from the nose
20. WR   S
    bronch/itis
    inflammation of the bronchi
21. WR   S
    pharyng/itis
    inflammation of the pharynx
22. WR   S
    trache/itis
    inflammation of the trachea
23. WR CV WR CV WR   S
    laryng/o/trache/o/bronch/itis
    ___   ___
    CF   CF
    inflammation of the larynx, trachea, and bronchi
24. WR   S
    adenoid/itis
    inflammation of the adenoids

25. WR CV S
    hem/o/thorax
    ___
    CF
    blood in the chest (pleural space)
26. WR S   WR   S
    lob/ar pneumon/ia
    pertaining to the lobe, diseased state of a lung
27. WR S
    rhin/itis
    inflammation of the nose
28. WR CV S   WR   S
    bronch/o/genic carcin/oma
    ___
    CF
    cancerous tumor originating in a bronchus
29. WR   S
    pneumon/ia
    diseased state of the lung

Exercise 14
1. thorac/algia
2. rhin/o/myc/osis
3. pneumat/o/cele
4. pulmon/ary neo/plasm
5. laryng/itis
6. atel/ectasis
7. adenoid/itis
8. laryng/o/trache/o/bronch/itis
9. bronchi/ectasis
10. pleur/itis
11. pneum/o/coni/osis
12. pneumon/itis
13. pan/sinus/itis
14. trache/o/stenosis
15. nas/o/pharyng/itis
16. py/o/thorax
17. epiglott/itis
18. diaphragmat/o/cele
19. pneum/o/thorax
20. bronch/o/pneumon/ia
21. rhin/o/rrhagia
22. pharyng/itis
23. hem/o/thorax
24. trache/itis
25. bronch/itis
26. lob/ar pneumon/ia
27. rhin/itis
28. bronch/o/genic carcin/oma
29. pneumon/ia

Exercise 15
Spelling Exercise; see text p. 158.

Exercise 16
Pronunciation Exercise

Exercise 17
1. emphysema
2. pleural effusion

3. cor pulmonale
4. coccidioidomycosis
5. cystic fibrosis
6. influenza
7. chronic obstructive pulmonary disease
8. pertussis
9. croup
10. asthma
11. pulmonary edema
12. upper respiratory infection
13. pulmonary embolism
14. epistaxis
15. Legionnaire disease
16. deviated septum
17. obstructive sleep apnea
18. tuberculosis
19. adult respiratory distress syndrome

Exercise 18
1. d
2. j
3. h
4. f
5. g
6. c
7. a
8. e
9. b
10. i

Exercise 19
1. d
2. b
3. c
4. e
5. f
6. g
7. h
8. i
9. a

Exercise 20
Spelling Exercise; see text p. 165.

Exercise 21
Pronunciation Exercise

Exercise 22
1. WR CV S
    trache/o/tomy
       CF
    incision of the trachea
2. WR CV S
    laryng/o/stomy
       CF
    creation of an artificial opening into the larynx

3. WR   S
    adenoid/ectomy
    excision of the adenoids
4. WR CV S
    rhin/o/plasty
       CF
    surgical repair of the nose
5. WR CV S
    aden/o/tome
       CF
    surgical instrument used to cut the adenoids
6. WR   CV S
    trache/o/stomy
        CF
    creation of an artificial opening into the trachea
7. WR CV S
    sinus/o/tomy
       CF
    incision of a sinus
8. WR CV S
    laryng/o/plasty
        CF
    surgical repair of the larynx
9. WR CV WR CV S
    pneum/o/bronch/o/tomy
       CF   CF
    incision of lung and bronchus
10. WR   CV S
     bronch/o/plasty
         CF
     surgical repair of a bronchus
11. WR   S
    lob/ectomy
    excision of a lobe (of the lung)
12. WR CV WR CV S
     laryng/o/trache/o/tomy
        CF   CF
     incision of larynx and trachea
13. WR CV S
     trache/o/plasty
         CF
     surgical repair of the trachea
14. WR CV S
     thorac/o/tomy
         CF
     incision into the chest cavity
15. WR   S
     laryng/ectomy
     excision of the larynx
16. WR CV S
     thorac/o/centesis
         CF
     surgical puncture to aspirate fluid from the chest cavity

17. WR   S
     tonsill/ectomy
     excision of the tonsils
18. WR CV S
     pleur/o/pexy
         CF
     surgical fixation of the pleura
19. WR CV S
     sept/o/plasty
         CF
     surgical repair of the septum
20. WR CV S
     sept/o/tomy
         CF
     incision into the septum

Exercise 23
1. trache/o/plasty
2. laryng/o/trache/o/tomy
3. aden/o/tome
4. thorac/o/tomy
5. trache/o/stomy
6. tonsill/ectomy
7. trache/o/tomy
8. bronch/o/plasty
9. laryng/ectomy
10. rhin/o/plasty
11. sinus/o/tomy
12. thorac/o/centesis or thora/centesis
13. adenoid/ectomy
14. laryng/o/plasty
15. lob/ectomy
16. pneum/o/bronch/o/tomy
17. laryng/o/stomy
18. pneumon/ectomy
19. sept/o/tomy
20. sept/o/plasty

Exercise 24
Spelling Exercise; see text p. 171.

Exercise 25
Pronunciation Exercise

Exercise 26
1. WR CV S
    spir/o/meter
        CF
    instrument used to measure breathing
2. WR CV S
    laryng/o/scope
         CF
    instrument used for visual examination of the larynx
3. WR CV S
    capn/o/meter
        CF
    instrument used to measure carbon dioxide

4. WR CV S
spir/o/metry
CF
measurement of breathing

5. WR CV S
ox/i/meter
CF
instrument used to measure oxygen

6. WR CV S
laryng/o/scopy
CF
visual examination of the larynx

7. WR CV S
bronch/o/scope
CF
instrument used for visual
examination of the bronchi

8. WR CV S
thorac/o/scope
CF
instrument used for visual
examination of the thorax

9. P S(WR)
endo/scope
instrument used for visual examination
of a hollow organ or body cavity

10. WR CV S
thorac/o/scopy
CF
visual examination of the thorax

11. P S(WR)
endo/scopic
pertaining to visual examination of a
hollow organ or body cavity

12. P S(WR)
endo/scopy
visual examination of a hollow organ
or body cavity

13. P WR CV S
poly/somn/o/graphy
CF
process of recording many (tests)
during sleep

Exercise 27
1. laryng/o/scopy
2. spir/o/meter
3. capn/o/meter
4. laryng/o/scope
5. bronch/o/scopy
6. spir/o/metry
7. bronch/o/scope
8. endo/scopy
9. thorac/o/scope
10. endo/scope
11. thorac/o/scopy
12. endo/scopic
13. poly/somn/o/graphy

Exercise 28
Spelling Exercise; see text p. 178.

Exercise 29
Pronunciation Exercise

Exercise 30
1. ventilation-perfusion scanning
2. chest computed tomography
3. chest radiograph
4. arterial blood gases
5. pulse oximetry
6. acid-fast bacilli smear
7. pulmonary function tests
8. PPD skin test

Exercise 31
1. f   5. b
2. e   6. c
3. a   7. h
4. d   8. g

Exercise 32
Spelling Exercise; see text p. 181.

Exercise 33
Pronunciation Exercise

Exercise 34
1. WR S
laryng/eal
pertaining to the larynx

2. P S(WR)
eu/pnea
normal breathing

3. WR S
muc/oid
resembling mucus

4. P S(WR)
a/pnea
absence of breathing

5. P WR S
hyp/ox/ia
condition of deficient oxygen
(to tissues)

6. WR CV S
laryng/o/spasm
CF
spasmodic contraction of the larynx

7. P WR S
endo/trache/al
pertaining to within the trachea

8. P WR S
an/ox/ia
condition of absence of oxygen

9. P WR S
dys/phon/ia
condition of difficulty in speaking
(voice)

10. WR CV WR S
bronch/o/alveol/ar
CF
pertaining to the bronchi and alveoli

11. P S(WR)
dys/pnea
difficult breathing

12. P WR S
hypo/capn/ia
condition of deficient in carbon
dioxide (in the blood)

13. WR CV S
bronch/o/spasm
CF
spasmodic contraction in the
bronchus(i)

14. WR CV S
orth/o/pnea
CF
able to breathe easier in a straight
position

15. P S(WR)
hyper/pnea
excessive breathing

16. P WR S
a/capn/ia
condition of absence of carbon
dioxide (in the blood)

17. P S(WR)
hypo/pnea
deficient breathing

18. P WR WR S
hyp/ox/em/ia
condition of deficient oxygen (in the
blood)

19. P WR S
a/phon/ia
condition of absence of voice

20. WR CV S
rhin/o/rrhea
CF
discharge from the nose

21. WR S
thorac/ic
pertaining to the chest

22. WR S
muc/ous
pertaining to mucus

23. WR CV WR S
nas/o/pharyng/eal
CF
pertaining to the nose and pharynx

24. WR S
diaphragmat/ic
pertaining to the diaphragm

25. P WR S
intra/pleur/al
pertaining to within the pleura

26. WR   S
pulmon/ary
pertaining to the lungs
27. WR   S
phren/algia
pain in the diaphragm
28. P   S(WR)
tachy/pnea
rapid breathing
29. WR   CV   S
phren/o/spasm
spasm of the diaphragm
30. WR   CV   S
pulmon/o/logist
　　　CF
a physician who studies and treats
diseases of the lung
31. WR   CV   S
pulmon/o/logy
　　　CF
study of the lung

Exercise 35
1. hyp/ox/ia
2. muc/oid
3. orth/o/pnea
4. endo/trache/al
5. an/ox/ia
6. dys/pnea
7. laryng/eal
8. hyper/capn/ia
9. eu/pnea
10. a/phon/ia
11. laryng/o/spasm
12. hypo/capn/ia
13. nas/o/pharyng/eal
14. diaphragmat/ic
15. a/pnea
16. hyp/ox/emia
17. hyper/pnea
18. bronch/o/spasm
19. hypo/pnea
20. a/capn/ia
21. dys/phon/ia
22. rhin/o/rrhea
23. muc/ous
24. thorac/ic
25. intra/pleur/al
26. pulmon/ary
27. phren/o/spasm
28. tachy/pnea
29. phren/algia
30. pulmon/o/logy
31. pulmon/o/logist

Exercise 36
Spelling Exercise; see text p. 186.

Exercise 37
Pronunciation Exercise

Exercise 38
1. hyperventilation
2. nebulizer
3. bronchodilator
4. ventilator
5. asphyxia
6. sputum
7. aspirate
8. airway
9. hiccup (hiccough)
10. cough
11. mucopurulent
12. hypoventilation
13. nosocomial
14. paroxysm
15. patent
16. bronchoconstrictor
17. mucus

Exercise 39
1. b
2. h
3. c
4. i
5. a
6. d
7. g
8. f

Exercise 40
1. e
2. h
3. i
4. c
5. j
6. a
7. b
8. d
9. f

Exercise 41
Spelling Exercise; see text p. 190.

Exercise 42
1. chronic obstructive pulmonary disease;
pulmonary function tests, chest x-ray,
arterial blood gases, computed
tomography
2. ventilation-perfusion scanning;
pulmonary embolism
3. left upper lobe; left lower lobe; right
upper lobe, right middle lobe, right
lower lobe
4. acid-fast bacilli; tuberculosis
5. polysomnography; obstructive sleep
apnea
6. oxygen; carbon dioxide

Exercise 43
1. adult respiratory distress syndrome
2. cystic fibrosis

3. influenza
4. laryngotracheobronchitis
5. upper respiratory infection

Exercise 44
A. 1. cough
2. dyspnea
3. pulmonary
4. chest radiograph
5. bronchoscopy
6. arterial blood gases
7. hypoxemia
8. bronchogenic carcinoma
9. pulmonary function tests
10. thoracic

B. 1. chest radiograph
arterial blood gases
pulse oximetry
2. excessive, deficient
3. a. T
b. T
c. T

Exercise 45
1. epistaxis
2. laryngoplasty
3. orthopnea
4. arterial blood gases, hypoxia
5. thoracalgia
6. hyperventilation
7. nebulizer
8. hemothorax
9. pulmonary embolism
10. coccidioidomycosis
11. chest radiograph, nosocomial
12. PPD skin test
13. tachypnea

Exercise 46
Reading Exercise

Exercise 47
1. *T*
2. *F*, "hypoxemia" means deficient oxygen in the blood; "hypercapnia" means
excessive carbon dioxide in the blood.
3. *T*
4. *F*, "bronchitis" means inflammation of
the bronchi

CHAPTER 6
Urinary System

OUTLINE

ANATOMY, 208

WORD PARTS, 211
Combining Forms, 211
Suffixes, 214

MEDICAL TERMS, 216
Disease and Disorder Terms, 216
    Built from Word Parts, 216
    Not Built from Word Parts, 220
Surgical Terms, 223
    Built from Word Parts, 223
    Not Built from Word Parts, 228
Diagnostic Terms, 230
    Built from Word Parts, 230
    Not Built from Word Parts, 236
Complementary Terms, 238
    Built from Word Parts, 238
    Not Built from Word Parts, 241
Abbreviations, 245

PRACTICAL APPLICATION, 247
Interact with Medical Documents, 247
Interpret Medical Terms, 248
Read Medical Terms in Use, 249
Comprehend Medical Terms in Use, 250

CHAPTER REVIEW, 250

OBJECTIVES

Upon completion of this chapter you will be able to:

1. Identify organs and structures of the urinary system.

2. Define and spell word parts related to the urinary system.

3. Define, pronounce, and spell disease and disorder terms related to the urinary system.

4. Define, pronounce, and spell surgical terms related to the urinary system.

5. Define, pronounce, and spell diagnostic terms related to the urinary system.

6. Define, pronounce, and spell complementary terms related to the urinary system.

7. Interpret the meaning of abbreviations related to the urinary system.

8. Interpret, read, and comprehend medical language in simulated medical statements and documents.

ANATOMY

Function

The urinary system removes waste material from the body, regulates fluid volume, and maintains electrolyte concentration in the body fluid. Organs of the urinary system are the kidneys, ureters, bladder, and urethra (Figures 6-1, 6-2, and 6-3).

Organs of the Urinary System

Term	Definition
kidneys	two bean-shaped organs located on each side of the vertebral column on the posterior wall of the abdominal cavity behind the parietal peritoneum. Their function is to remove waste products from the blood and to aid in maintaining water and electrolyte balances.
nephron	urine-producing microscopic structure. Approximately 1 million nephrons are located in each kidney.
glomerulus (*pl.* glomeruli)	cluster of capillaries at the entrance of the nephron. The process of filtering the blood, thereby forming urine, begins here.
renal pelvis	funnel-shaped reservoir that collects the urine and passes it to the ureter
hilum	indentation on the medial side of the kidney where the ureter leaves the kidney
ureters	two slender tubes, approximately 10 to 13 inches (26 to 33 cm) long, that receive the urine from the kidneys and carry it to the posterior portion of the bladder
urinary bladder	muscular, hollow organ that temporarily holds the urine. As it fills, the thick, muscular wall becomes thinner, and the organ increases in size.
urethra	lowest part of the urinary tract, through which the urine passes from the urinary bladder to the outside of the body. This narrow tube varies in length by sex. It is approximately 1.5 inches (3.8 cm) long in the female and approximately 8 inches (20 cm) in the male, in whom it is also part of the reproductive system. It carries seminal fluid (semen) at the time of ejaculation.
urinary meatus	opening through which the urine passes to the outside

BLADDER is a derivative of the Anglo-Saxon **blaeddre,** meaning a **blister** or **windbag.**

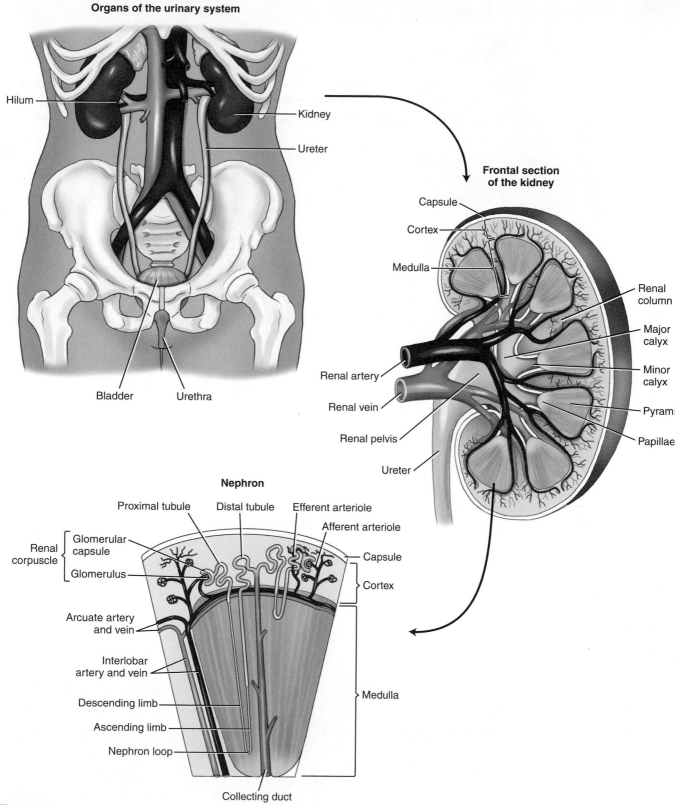

Figure 6-1

The urinary system.

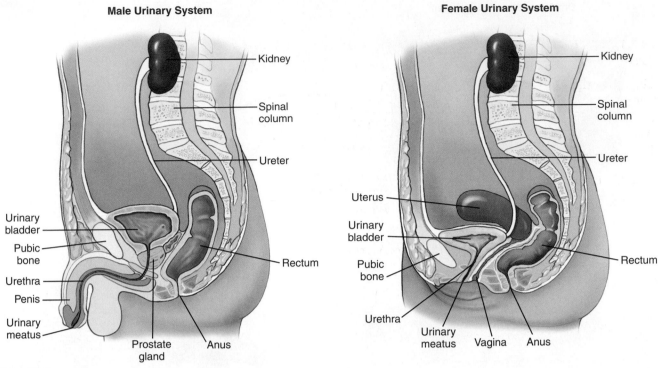

Figure 6-2

Male and female urinary systems, sagittal view. The male urethra is approximately 8 inches (20 cm) in length compared with female urethra, which is approximately 1.5 inches (3.8 cm) in length.

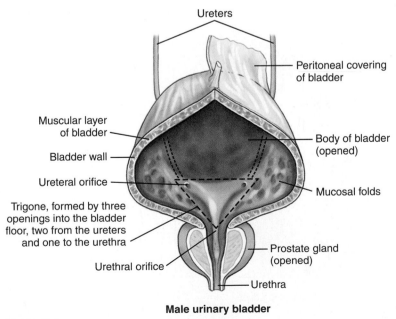

Male urinary bladder

Figure 6-3

Male urinary bladder.

EXERCISE 1

Match the anatomic terms in the first column with the correct definitions in the second column.

_G_   1. kidney(s)

_D_   2. glomerulus

_F_   3. nephron

_C_   4. ureters

_A_   5. urinary bladder

_B_   6. urinary meatus

_E_   7. urethra

a. stores urine

b. outside opening through which the urine passes

c. carry urine from the kidney to the urinary bladder

d. cluster of capillaries in the kidney where the urine begins to form

e. carries urine from the bladder to the urinary meatus

f. kidney's urine-producing unit

g. organs that remove waste products from the blood

WORD PARTS

Word parts you need to know to complete this chapter are listed on the following pages. The exercises at the end of each list will help you learn their definitions and spellings.

Combining Forms of the Urinary System

Combining Form	Definition
cyst/o, vesic/o . . . . (NOTE: these refer to the _urinary bladder_ unless otherwise identified.)	bladder, sac
glomerul/o	glomerulus
meat/o	meatus (opening)
nephr/o, ren/o	kidney
pyel/o	renal pelvis
ureter/o	ureter
urethr/o	urethra

GLOMERULUS is derived from the Latin **glomus,** which means **ball of thread.** It was thought that the rounded cluster of capillary loops at the nephron's entrance resembled thread in a ball.

MEATUS is derived from the Latin **meare,** meaning **to pass** or **to go.** Other anatomic passages share the same name, such as the auditory meatus.

PYELOS is the Greek word for **tub-shaped vessel,** which describes the kidney's shape.

EXERCISE FIGURE A

Fill in the blanks with combining forms for the diagram of the urinary system.

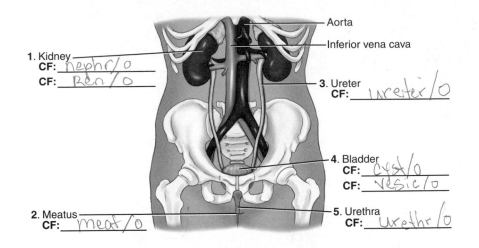

Aorta

Inferior vena cava

1. Kidney
   CF: _nephr/o_
   CF: _Ren/o_

3. Ureter
   CF: _ureter/o_

4. Bladder
   CF: _cyst/o_
   CF: _vesic/o_

2. Meatus
   CF: _meat/o_

5. Urethra
   CF: _urethr/o_

EXERCISE FIGURE B

Fill in the blanks to label the diagram of the internal kidney structure.

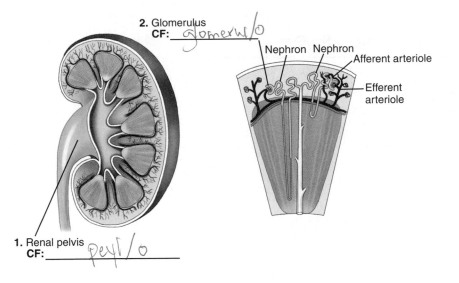

2. Glomerulus
   CF: _glomerul/o_

Nephron   Nephron

Afferent arteriole

Efferent arteriole

1. Renal pelvis
   CF: _pyel/o_

EXERCISE 2

Write the definitions of the following combining forms.

1. glomerul/o _Glomerulus_
2. vesic/o _bladder_
3. nephr/o _Kidney_
4. pyel/o _Renal Pelvis_
5. ureter/o _ureter_
6. cyst/o _bladder_
7. urethr/o _Urethra_
8. ren/o _Kidney_
9. meat/o _meatus_

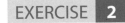

EXERCISE 3

Write the combining form for each of the following terms.

1. kidney   a. _nephr/o_   4. renal pelvis   _pyel/o_

           b. _Ren/o_   5. glomerulus   _glomerul/o_

2. bladder, sac a. _cysto_   6. urethra   _urethr/o_

              b. _vesic/o_   7. meatus   _meat/o_

3. ureter   _ureter/o_

Combining Forms Commonly Used with Urinary System Terms

Combining Form	Definition
albumin/o...............	albumin
azot/o..................	urea, nitrogen
blast/o.................	developing cell, germ cell
glyc/o, glycos/o...........	sugar
hydr/o.................	water
lith/o.................	stone, calculus
noct/i................. (NOTE: the combining vowel is i.)	night
olig/o.................	scanty, few
son/o.................	sound
tom/o.................	cut, section
urin/o, ur/o..............	urine, urinary tract

EXERCISE 4

Write the definitions of the following combining forms.

1. hydr/o _Water_

2. azot/o _urea, nitrogen_

3. noct/i _night_

4. lith/o _Stone, calculus_

5. tom/o _Cut, section_

6. albumin/o _albumin_

7. urin/o _Urine_

8. son/o _Sound_

9. glyc/o _sugar_

10. blast/o _developing cell, germ cell_

11. olig/o _scanty, few_

12. ur/o _urinary tract_

13. glycos/o _sugar_

EXERCISE 5

Write the combining form for each of the following.

1. sugar
   a. _Glyc/o_
   b. _glycos/o_

2. sound
   son/o

3. urine, urinary tract
   a. _urin/o_
   b. _ur/o_

4. water
   hydr/o

5. developing cell, germ cell
   blast/o

6. cut, section   _tom/o_

7. albumin   _albumin/o_

8. night   _noct/i_

9. urea, nitrogen   _azot/o_

10. stone, calculus   _lith/o_

11. scanty, few   _olig/o_

Suffixes

Suffix	Definition
-iasis, -esis	condition
-gram	record, radiographic image
-lysis	loosening, dissolution, separating
-megaly	enlargement
-ptosis	drooping, sagging, prolapse
-rrhaphy	suturing, repairing
-tripsy	surgical crushing
-trophy	nourishment, development
-uria	urine, urination

Refer to Appendix A and Appendix B for alphabetized lists of word parts and their meanings.

EXERCISE 6

Match the suffixes in the first column with their correct definitions in the second column.

_C_   1. -iasis, -esis   a. nourishment, development

_I_   2. -lysis   b. urine, urination

_D_   3. -megaly   c. condition

_F_   4. -rrhaphy   d. enlargement

_G_   5. -ptosis   e. surgical crushing

_E_   6. -tripsy   f. suturing, repairing

_A_   7. -trophy   g. drooping, sagging, prolapse

_B_   8. -uria   h. record, radiographic image

_H_   9. -gram   i. loosening, dissolution, separating

EXERCISE 7

Write the definitions of the following suffixes.

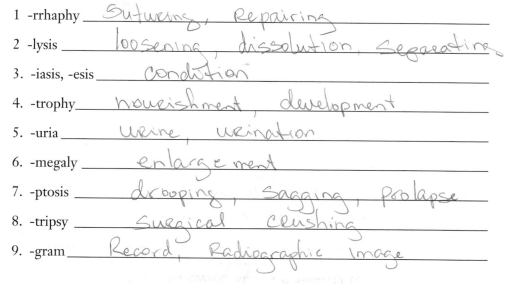

1 -rrhaphy ___Suturing, Repairing___

2 -lysis ___loosening, dissolution, separating___

3. -iasis, -esis ___Condition___

4. -trophy ___nourishment, development___

5. -uria ___urine, urination___

6. -megaly ___enlargement___

7. -ptosis ___drooping, sagging, prolapse___

8. -tripsy ___Surgical crushing___

9. -gram ___Record, Radiographic Image___

MEDICAL TERMS

The terms you need to learn to complete this chapter are listed next. The exercises following each list will help you learn the definition and the spelling of each word.

Disease and Disorder Terms

Built from Word Parts

The following terms are built from word parts you have already learned and can be translated literally to find their meanings. Further explanation of terms beyond the definition of their word parts, if needed, is included in parentheses.

Term	Definition
cystitis................... (sis-TĪ-tis)	inflammation of the bladder (Figure 6-4)
cystocele.................. (SIS-tō-sēl)	protrusion of the bladder
cystolith.................. (SIS-tō-lith)	stone in the bladder (Exercise Figure C)
glomerulonephritis .... (glō-*mer*-ū-lō-ne-FRĪ-tis)	inflammation of the glomeruli of the kidney
hydronephrosis .... (*hī*-dro-ne-FRŌ-sis)	abnormal condition of water in the kidney (distension of the renal pelvis with urine because of an obstruction)
nephritis.................. (ne-FRĪ-tis)	inflammation of a kidney
nephroblastoma............. (*nef*-rō-blas-TŌ-ma)	kidney tumor containing developing cell (malignant tumor) (also called **Wilms' tumor**)
nephrohypertrophy .... (*nef*-rō-hī-PER-tro-fē) (NOTE: the prefix *hyper-* appears in the middle of this term.)	excessive development (increase in size) of the kidney
nephrolithiasis............. (*nef*-rō-lith-Ī-a-sis)	condition of stone(s) in the kidney
nephroma .... (nef-RŌ-ma)	tumor of the kidney
nephromegaly .... (*nef*-rō-MEG-a-lē)	enlargement of a kidney
nephroptosis .... (*nef*-rop-TŌ-sis)	drooping kidney
pyelitis................... (*pī*-e-LĪ-tis)	inflammation of the renal pelvis
pyelonephritis .... (*pī*-e-lō-ne-FRĪ-tis)	inflammation of the renal pelvis and the kidney (Figures 6-4 and 6-5)
uremia................... (ū-RĒ-mē-a)	condition of urine (urea) in the blood (toxic condition resulting from retention of by-products of the kidney in the blood)

NEPHROPTOSIS
is also known as a **floating kidney** and occurs when the kidney is no longer held in place and drops out of its normal position. The kidney is normally held in position by connective and adipose tissue, so it is prone to injury and also may cause the ureter to twist. Truck drivers and horseback riders are prone to this condition.

Term	Definition
ureteritis .... (ū-rē-ter-Ī-tis)	inflammation of a ureter
ureterocele .... (ū-RĒ-ter-ō-*sēl*)	protrusion of a ureter
ureterolithiasis............. (ū-*rē*-ter-ō-lith-Ī-a-sis)	condition of stones in the ureters
ureterostenosis .... (ū-*rē*-ter-ō-sten-Ō-sis)	narrowing of the ureter
urethrocystitis .... (ū-*rē*-thrō-sis-TĪ-tis)	inflammation of the urethra and the bladder

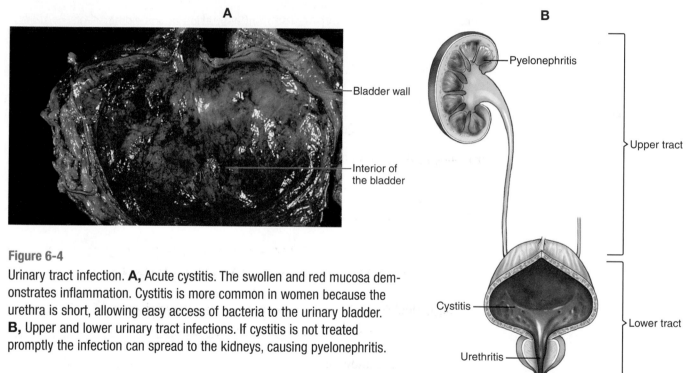

A

B

Bladder wall

Interior of the bladder

Pyelonephritis

Upper tract

Cystitis

Urethritis

Lower tract

Figure 6-4

Urinary tract infection. **A,** Acute cystitis. The swollen and red mucosa demonstrates inflammation. Cystitis is more common in women because the urethra is short, allowing easy access of bacteria to the urinary bladder. **B,** Upper and lower urinary tract infections. If cystitis is not treated promptly the infection can spread to the kidneys, causing pyelonephritis.

EXERCISE FIGURE C

Fill in the blanks to label the diagram.

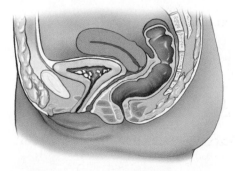

_____ / ____ / _____
  bladder   / cv /   stone

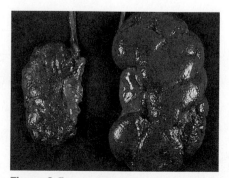

Figure 6-5

Left kidney, chronic pyelonephritis.
Right kidney, normal size with some scarring.

EXERCISE 8

Practice saying aloud each of the disease and disorder terms built from word parts on pp. 216-217.

To hear the terms select Chapter 6, Chapter Exercises, Pronunciation.

☐ Place a check mark in the box when you have completed this exercise.

EXERCISE 9

Analyze and define the following terms.

Example: glomerul/o/nephr/itis   _inflammation of the glomeruli of the kidney_

1. nephroma _tumor of kidney_
2. cystolith _stone in the bladder_
3. nephrolithiasis _condition of stones in kidney_
4. uremia _condition of urine in the blood_
5. nephroptosis _drooping kidney_
6. cystocele _protrusion of the bladder_
7. nephrohypertrophy _excessive development of kidney_
8. cystitis _inflammation of the bladder_
9. pyelitis _inflammation of the renal pelvis_
10. ureterocele _protrusion of a ureter_
11. hydronephrosis _abnormal condition of water in kidney_
12. nephromegaly _enlargement of kidney_
13. ureterolithiasis _condition of stones in ureter_
14. pyelonephritis _inflammation of renal pelvis and kidney_
15. ureteritis _inflammation of ureter_
16. nephritis _inflammation of a kidney_
17. urethrocystitis _inflammation of the urethra and kidney_
18. ureterostenosis _narrowing of the ureter_
19. nephroblastoma _kidney tumor containing developing cell_

EXERCISE 10

Build disease and disorder terms for the following definitions with the word parts you have learned.

Example: inflammation of the ureter <u>ureter/itis</u>
                                              WR / S

1. enlargement of the kidney <u>nephr /o/ megaly</u>
                                 WR / CV /   S

2. inflammation of the bladder <u>cyst / itis</u>
                                   WR /   S

3. excessive development of the kidney <u>nephr /o /hyper/ trophy</u>
                                           WR / CV / P / S

4. inflammation of the urethra and bladder <u>urethr/o/ cyst / itis</u>
                                               WR / CV / WR / S

5. protrusion of the bladder <u>cyst /o/ cele</u>
                                 WR / CV / S

6. abnormal condition of water in the kidney <u>hydr /o/ nephr /osis</u>
                                                 WR / CV / WR / S

7. stone in the bladder <u>cyst /o/ lith</u>
                            WR / CV / WR

8. inflammation of the glomeruli of the kidney <u>glomerul/o/ nephr /itis</u>
                                                   WR / CV / WR / S

9. tumor of the kidney <u>nephr / oma</u>
                           WR /   S

10. a drooping kidney <u>nephr /o/ ptosis</u>
                          WR / CV / S

11. inflammation of a kidney <u>nephr / itis</u>
                                 WR /   S

12. condition of stones in the kidney <u>nephr /o/ lithia/iasis</u>
                                          WR / CV / WR / S

13. protrusion of a ureter <u>ureter /o/ cele</u>
                               WR / CV / S

14. inflammation of the renal pelvis <u>pyel/ itis</u>
                                         WR / S

15. condition of urine (urea) in the blood <u>urem /emia</u>
                                               WR /   S

16. narrowing of the ureter <u>ureter /o/ stenosis</u>
                                WR / CV / S

17. inflammation of the renal pelvis and the kidney

Pyel / o / nephr / itis
WR / CV / WR / S

18. condition of stones in the ureters

ureter / o / lith / iasis
WR / CV / WR / S

19. kidney tumor containing developing cells

nephr / o / blast / oma
WR / CV / WR / S

EXERCISE 11

Spell each of the disease and disorder terms built from word parts on pp. 216-217 by having someone dictate them to you.

 To hear and spell the terms select Chapter 6, Chapter Exercises, Spelling. You may type the terms on the screen or write them below in the spaces provided.

☐ Place a check mark in the box if you have completed this exercise using your CD-ROM.

1. _____   11. _____
2. _____   12. _____
3. _____   13. _____
4. _____   14. _____
5. _____   15. _____
6. _____   16. _____
7. _____   17. _____
8. _____   18. _____
9. _____   19. _____
10. _____   20. _____

Disease and Disorder Terms

Not Built from Word Parts

In some of the following terms, you may recognize word parts you have already learned; however, the full meaning of the terms cannot be discerned by the definition of their word parts.

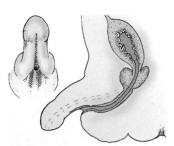

Figure 6-6
Hypospadias.

Term	Definition
epispadias . . . . (*ep*-i-SPĀ-dē-as)	congenital defect in which the urinary meatus is located on the upper surface of the penis
hypospadias . . . . (*hī*-pō-SPĀ-dē-as)	congenital defect in which the urinary meatus is located on the underside of the penis; a similar defect can occur in the female (Figure 6-6)

Term	Definition
polycystic kidney disease . . . . . (*pol*-ē-SIS-tik) (KID-nē) (di-ZĒZ)	condition in which the kidney contains many cysts and is enlarged (Figure 6-7)
renal calculus (*pl.* **calculi**) . . . . . (RĒ-nal) KAL-kū-lus (KAL-kū-lī)	stone in the kidney
renal hypertension . . . . (RĒ-nal) (hī-per-TEN- shun)	elevated blood pressure resulting from kidney disease
sepsis . . . . (SEP-sis)	a condition in which pathogenic microorganisms, usually bacteria, enter the bloodstream, causing a systemic inflammatory response to the infection (also called **septicemia**)
urinary retention . . . . (Ū-rin-*ār*-ē) (rē-TEN- shun)	abnormal accumulation of urine in the bladder because of an inability to urinate
urinary suppression . . . . (Ū-rin-*ār*-ē) (sū-PRESH-un)	sudden stoppage of urine formation
urinary tract infection (UTI) . . . . (Ū-rin-*ār*-ē) (trakt) (in-FEK-shun)	infection of one or more organs of the urinary tract (see Figure 6-4)

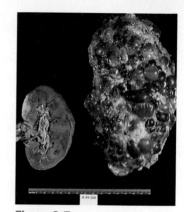

Figure 6-7
Polycystic kidney disease.

SEPSIS OR SEPTICEMIA
can result when local infections such as pneumonia or bladder infections are untreated or treated with incomplete antibiotic therapy; the microorganism can enter the bloodstream, causing sepsis. Sepsis is the tenth most common cause of death in the United States. Patients in intensive care units or patients with impaired immune function are vulnerable to developing septicemia.

RENAL FAILURE
Acute renal failure (ARF)
is a sudden and severe reduction in renal function resulting in a collection of metabolic waste in the body. Prompt treatment can reverse the condition and recovery can occur.
Chronic renal failure (CRF),
unlike ARF, is a progresive, irreversible, loss of renal function and the onset of uremia.
End-stage renal disease (ESRD) is what chronic renal failure is called when kidney function is too poor to sustain life.

CAM TERM
Acupuncture is the ancient practice of inserting very thin needles into points just under the skin to treat disease, increase immune response, relieve pain, and restore health. Studies have demonstrated that acupuncture can reduce urinary incontinence and increase ureter functions and urodynamic measurements of bladder capacity.

EXERCISE 12

Practice saying aloud each of the disease and disorder terms not built from word parts on pp. 220-221.

 To hear the terms select Chapter 6, Chapter Exercises, Pronunciation.

☐ Place a check mark in the box when you have completed this exercise.

EXERCISE 13

Fill in the blanks with the correct terms.

1. Stones in the kidney are also called _Renal_ _calculus_.

2. The inability to urinate, which results in an abnormal amount of urine in the bladder, is known as _Urinary_ _Retention_.

3. The name given to a condition in which a kidney is enlarged and contains many cysts is _Polycystic_ _Kidney_ _disease_.

4. The condition in which the urinary meatus is located on the underside of the penis is called _hypospadias_.

5. Elevated blood pressure resulting from kidney disease is _Renal_ _hypertension_.

6. Sudden stoppage of urine formation is referred to as ___Urinary___ ___Suppression___.

7. ___epispadias___ is a condition in which the urinary meatus is located on the upper surface of the penis.

8. Infection of one or more organs of the urinary system is called ___Urinary___ ___tract___ ___infection___.

9. ___Sepsis___ is a condition in which pathogenic microorganisms enter the bloodstream.

EXERCISE 14

Match the terms in the first column with the correct definitions in the second column.

___C___ 1. epispadias

___F___ 2. hypospadias

___D___ 3. renal calculus

___H___ 4. renal hypertension

___A___ 5. polycystic kidney disease

___E___ 6. urinary retention

___B___ 7. urinary suppression

___G___ 8. urinary tract infection

___I___ 9. sepsis

a. enlarged kidney with many cysts

b. sudden stoppage of urine formation

c. urinary meatus on the upper surface of the penis

d. kidney stone

e. inability to urinate

f. urinary meatus on the underside of the penis

g. infection of one or more organs of the urinary system

h. characterized by elevated blood pressure

i. causes a systemic inflammatory response to infection

j. excessive amount of urine

EXERCISE 15

Spell each of the disease and disorder terms not built from word parts on pp. 220-221 by having someone dictate them to you.

 To hear and spell the terms select Chapter 6, Chapter Exercises, Spelling. You may type the terms on the screen or write them below in the spaces provided.

☐ Place a check mark in the box if you have completed this exercise using your CD-ROM.

1. _____

2. _____

3. _____

4. _____

5. _____

6. _____

7. _____

8. _____

9. _____

Surgical Terms

Built from Word Parts

The following terms are built from word parts you have already learned and can be translated literally to find their meanings. Further explanation of terms beyond the definition of their word parts, if needed, is included in parentheses.

Term	Definition
cystectomy . . . . (sis-TEK-to-mē)	excision of the bladder
cystolithotomy . . . . (*sis*-tō-li-THOT-o-mē)	incision of the bladder to remove a stone
cystorrhaphy . . . . (sist-OR-a-fē)	suturing the bladder
cystostomy . . . . (sis-TOS-to-mē)	creating an artificial opening into the bladder (Exercise Figure D)
cystotomy, vesicotomy . . . . (sis-TOT-o-mē) (*ves*-i-KOT-o-mē)	incision of the bladder
lithotripsy . . . . (LITH-ō-trip-sē)	surgical crushing of a stone (Exercise Figure E)
meatotomy . . . . (*mē*-a-TOT-o-mē)	incision of the meatus
nephrectomy . . . . (ne-FREK-to-mē)	excision of a kidney
nephrolysis . . . . (ne-FROL-i-sis)	separating the kidney (from other body structures)
nephropexy . . . . (NEF-rō-*peks*-ē)	surgical fixation of the kidney
nephropyelolithotomy . . . . (*nef*-rō-pī-e-lō-li- THOT-o-mē)	incision through the kidney to the renal pelvis to remove a stone
nephrostomy . . . . (nef-ROS-to-mē)	creation of an artificial opening into the kidney (Exercise Figure F)
pyelolithotomy . . . . (*pī*-el-ō-lith-OT-o-mē)	incision of the renal pelvis to remove a stone (Exercise Figure G)
pyeloplasty . . . . (PĪ-el-ō-*plas*-tē)	surgical repair of the renal pelvis
ureterectomy . . . . (ū-*rē*-ter-EK-to-mē)	excision of a ureter
ureterostomy . . . . (ū-*rē*-ter-OS-to-mē)	creation of an artificial opening into the ureter
urethroplasty . . . . (ū-RĒ-thrō-*plas*-tē)	surgical repair of the urethra
vesicourethral suspension . . . . . (ves-i-kō-ū-RĒ-thral) (*sus*-PEN-shun)	suspension pertaining to the bladder and urethra

EXERCISE FIGURE D

Fill in the blanks to label the diagram.

_____ / _____ /
bladder   cv

_____
creation of an artificial opening

STRESS INCONTINENCE
is the involuntary intermittent leakage of urine as a result of pressure, from a cough or a sneeze, on the weakened area around the urethra and bladder. The Marshall-Marchetti Krantz technique, or **vesicourethral suspension** with a midurethral sling is a suspension surgery performed on patients with stress incontinence.

Fill in the blanks to complete the labeling of the diagram.

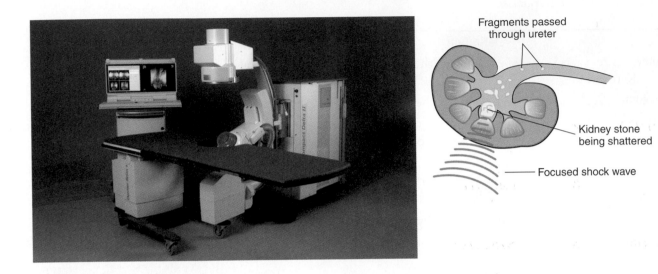

Fragments passed
through ureter

Kidney stone
being shattered

Focused shock wave

Extracorporeal shock wave _____lith____ / _O_ / _tripsy_____

  stone / cv / surgical crushing

ESWL breaks down the kidney stone into fragments by shock waves from outside
the body. The broken fragments are eliminated from the body with the passing of
urine.

Fill in the blanks to label the diagram.

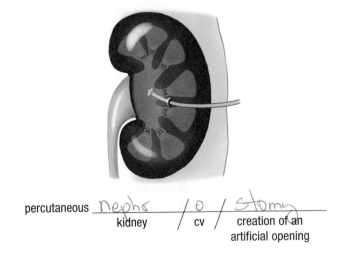

percutaneous __nephr__ / _O_ / _stomy___

   kidney / cv / creation of an
     artificial opening

Fill in the blanks to label the diagram.

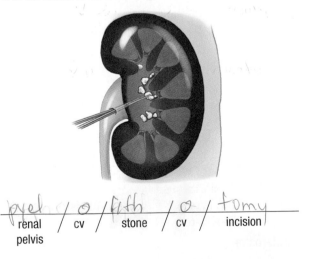

__pyel_ / _O_ /_lith_ / _O_ / _tomy___

  renal / cv / stone / cv / incision
  pelvis

EXERCISE 16

Practice saying aloud each of the surgical terms built from word parts on p. 223.

To hear the terms select Chapter 6, Chapter Exercises, Pronunciation.

☐ Place a check mark in the box when you have completed this exercise.

EXERCISE 17

Analyze and define the following surgical terms.

1. vesicotomy _incision of the bladder_
2. cystotomy _incision of the bladder_
3. nephrostomy _creation of an artifical opening into the kidney_
4. nephrolysis _separating the kidney from other body structures_
5. cystectomy _excision of the bladder_
6. pyelolithotomy _incision of the renal pelvis to remove a stone_
7. nephropexy _surgical fixation of the kidney_
8. cystolithotomy _incision of the bladder to remove a stone_
9. nephrectomy _excision of a kidney_
10. ureterectomy _excision of ureter_
11. cystostomy _creating an artificle opening in bladder_
12. pyeloplasty _incision of the renal pelvis to remove a stone_
13. cystorrhaphy _suturing the bladder_
14. meatotomy _incision of the meatus_
15. lithotripsy _surgical crushing of a stone_
16. urethroplasty _surgical repair of the urethra_
17. vesicourethral (suspension) _pertaining to the bladder and urethra_
18. nephropyelolithotomy _insicion through the kidney to renal pelvis to remove a stone_
19. ureterostomy _creation of an artificle opening in urethra_

EXERCISE 18

Build surgical terms for the following definitions by using the word parts you have learned.

1. creation of an artificial opening into the ureter

    ureter / _o_ / _stomy_
    WR / CV / S

2. excision of a kidney

    nephrea / _tomy_
    WR / S

3. incision of the renal pelvis to remove a stone

    pyel / _o_ / _lith_ / _o_ / _tomy_
    WR / CV / WR / CV / S

4. suturing of the bladder

    cyst / _o_ / _rrhaphy_
    WR / CV / S

5. separating the kidney (from other structures)

    nephr / _o_ / _lysis_
    WR / CV / S

6. creation of an artificial opening into the kidney

    nephr / _o_ / _stomy_
    WR / CV / S

7. surgical repair of the urethra

    urethr / _o_ / _plasty_
    WR / CV / S

8. excision of the bladder

    cystec / _tomy_
    WR / S

9. incision of the meatus

    meat / _o_ / _tomy_
    WR / CV / S

10. incision of the bladder

    a. _cyst_ / _o_ / _tomy_
       WR / CV / S

    b. _vesic_ / _o_ / _tomy_
       WR / CV / S

11. surgical repair of the renal pelvis

    pyel / _o_ / _plasty_
    WR / CV / S

12. excision of the ureter

     ureter / ectomy
      WR   S

13. surgical fixation of the kidney

     nephr / o / pexy
      WR   CV   S

14. incision into the bladder
    to remove a stone

     cyst / o / lith / o / tomy
      WR   CV   WR   CV   S

15. surgical crushing of a stone

     lith / o / tripsy
      WR   CV   S

16. (suspension) pertaining to
    the bladder and urethra

     vesic / o / urethr / al   suspension
      WR   CV   WR   S

17. creation of an artificial
    opening into the bladder

     cyst / o / stomy
      WR   CV   S

18. incision through the
    kidney into the renal pelvis
    to remove a stone

     nephr / o / pyel / o / lith / o / tomy
      WR / CV / WR / CV / WR / CV / S

EXERCISE 19

Spell each of the surgical terms built from word parts on p. 223 by having someone dictate them to you.

To hear and spell the terms select Chapter 6, Chapter Exercises, Spelling. You may type the terms on the screen or write them below in the spaces provided.

☐ Place a check mark in the box if you have completed this exercise using your CD-ROM.

1. _____
2. _____
3. _____
4. _____
5. _____
6. _____
7. _____
8. _____
9. _____
10. _____

11. _____
12. _____
13. _____
14. _____
15. _____
16. _____
17. _____
18. _____
19. _____

Surgical Terms

Not Built from Word Parts

In some of the following terms, you may recognize word parts you have already learned; however, the full meaning of the terms cannot be discerned by the definition of their word parts.

Term	Definition
extracorporeal shock wave lithotripsy (ESWL) . . . . (eks-tra-kor-POR-ē-al) (LITH-ō-trip-sē)	a noninvasive treatment for removal of kidney or ureteral stone(s). By using ultrasound and fluoroscopic imaging, the stone is positioned at a focal point. Repeated firing of shock waves renders the stone into fragments that pass from the body in the urine (also called **shock wave lithotripsy [SWL]**) (see Exercise Figure E).
fulguration . . . . (ful-gū-RĀ-shun)	destruction of living tissue with an electric spark (a method commonly used to remove bladder growths) (Figure 6-8)
renal transplant . . . . (RĒ-nal) (TRANS-plant)	surgical implantation of a donor kidney to replace a nonfunctioning kidney (Figure 6-9)

EXTRACORPOREAL means occurring **outside the body.**

RENAL REPLACEMENT THERAPIES
- Hemodialysis
- Peritoneal dialysis
- Kidney transplant

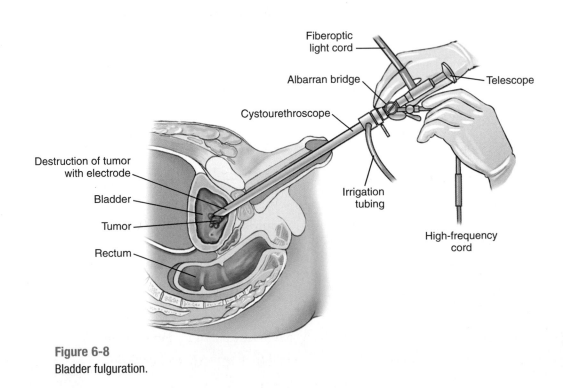

Figure 6-8
Bladder fulguration.

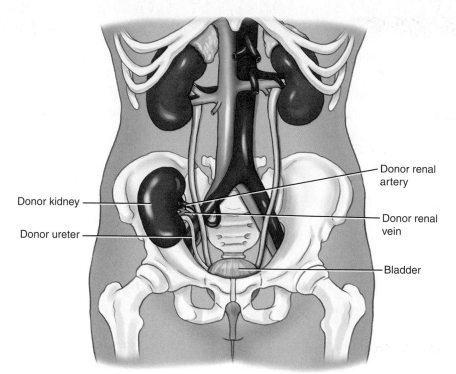

- Donor renal artery
- Donor kidney
- Donor renal vein
- Donor ureter
- Bladder

Figure 6-9
Renal transplant showing donor kidney and blood vessels in place. Recipient's kidney is not always removed unless it is infected or is a cause of hypertension.

EXERCISE 20

Practice saying aloud each of the surgical terms not built from word parts on p. 228.

To hear the terms select Chapter 6, Chapter Exercises, Pronunciation.

☐ Place a check mark in the box when you have completed this exercise.

EXERCISE 21

1. The surgical implantation of a donor kidney to replace a nonfunctioning kidney is called ____Renal_____ _____transplant____.

2. The destruction of living tissue with an electric spark is ___fulgueation___.

3. ___extracorporeal____ ____shock____ ____wave____
   ____lithotripsy____ is a noninvasive treatment for removal of kidney or ureteral stones.

EXERCISE 22

Match the terms in the first column with their correct definitions in the second column.

__B__ 1. fulguration   a. used to replace a nonfunctioning kidney

__A__ 2. renal transplant b. used to remove bladder growths

__D__ 3. ESWL   c. used to remove tumors

                          d. also called *shock wave lithotripsy*

Spell each of the surgical terms not built from word parts on p. 228 by having someone dictate them to you.

To hear and spell the terms select Chapter 6, Chapter Exercises, Spelling. You may type the terms on the screen or write them below in the spaces provided.

☐ Place a check mark in the box if you have completed this exercise using your CD-ROM.

1. _____   3. _____

2. _____

Diagnostic Terms

Built from Word Parts

The following terms are built from word parts you have already learned and can be translated literally to find their meanings. Further explanation of terms beyond the definition of their word parts, if needed, is included in parentheses.

Review Table 5-1, Types of Diagnostic Procedures, p. 174 before proceeding.

Term	Definition
DIAGNOSTIC IMAGING	
cystogram (SIS-tō-gram)	radiographic image of the bladder (Figure 6-10)
cystography (sis-TOG-ra-fē)	radiographic imaging of the bladder
intravenous urogram (IVU) (in-tra-VĒ-nus) (Ū-rō-gram)	radiographic image of the urinary tract (with contrast medium injected intravenously) (also called **intravenous pyelogram [IVP]**)
nephrogram (NEF-rō-gram)	radiographic image of the kidney
nephrography (ne-FROG-ra-fē)	radiographic imaging of the kidney
nephrosonography (*nef*-rō-so-NOG-ra-fē)	process of recording the kidney using sound (an ultrasound test) (Figure 6-11)
nephrotomogram (*nef*-rō-TŌ-mō-gram)	sectional radiographic image of the kidney (Figure 6-12)
renogram (RĒ-nō-gram)	(graphic) record of the kidney (produced by radioactivity after injecting a radiopharmaceutical, or radioactive material, into the blood) (a nuclear medicine test)
retrograde urogram (RET-rō-grād) (Ū-ro-gram)	radiographic image of the urinary tract (retrograde means to move in a direction opposite from normal) with contrast medium instilled through urethral catheters by a cystoscope (Exercise Figure H)

SPIRAL/HELICAL CT scans are replacing intravenous urograms to detect urinary tract stones and perirenal infections. Intravenous contrast media is not required.

Term	Definition
voiding cystourethrography (VCUG) .... (VOID-ing) (*sis*-tō-ū-rē-THROG-ro-fe)	radiographic imaging of the bladder and the urethra (Figure 6-13). Radiopaque dye is instilled in the bladder. Radiographic images called cystourethrograms are taken of the bladder and during urination of the dye.

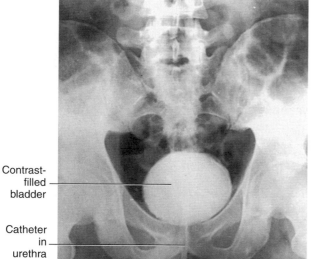

Contrast-filled bladder

Catheter in urethra

Figure 6-10
Cystogram.

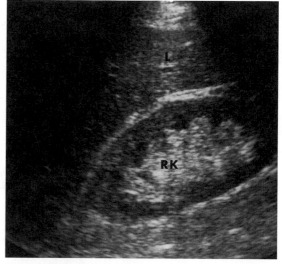

Figure 6-11
Nephrosonogram (ultrasound) of the right kidney, sagittal view.

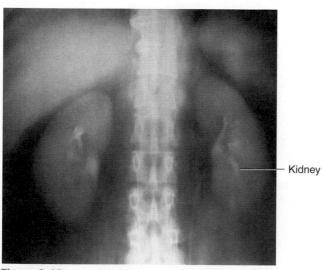

Kidney

Figure 6-12
Nephrotomogram.

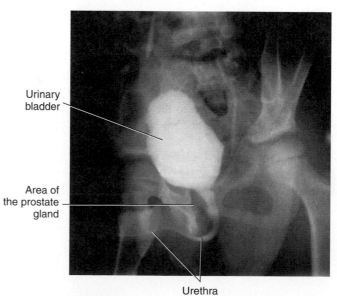

Urinary bladder

Area of the prostate gland

Urethra

Figure 6-13
Voiding cystourethrogram, male.

Diagnostic Terms—cont'd
Built from Word Parts

Term	Definition
ENDOSCOPY	
cystoscope................. (SIS-tō-skōp)	instrument used for visual examination of the bladder
cystoscopy................ (sis-TOS-ko-pē)	visual examination of the bladder (Figure 6-14)
meatoscope............... (mē-ĀT-ō-skōp)	instrument used for visual examination of the meatus
meatoscopy............... (mē-a-TOS-ko-pē)	visual examination of the meatus
nephroscopy .... (ne-FROS-ko-pē)	visual examination of the kidney (Figure 6-15)
ureteroscopy .... (ū-rē-ter-OS-ko-pē)	visual examination of the ureter
urethroscope.............. (ū-RĒ-thrō-skōp)	instrument used for visual examination of the urethra
OTHER	
urinometer................ (ū-ri-NOM-e-ter)	instrument used to measure (the specific gravity of) urine (Exercise Figure I)

 Ultrasonography (US), computed tomography (CT), and **magnetic resonance imaging (MRI)** can be used in evaluating structure and function of the urinary system organs. See Table 5-1.

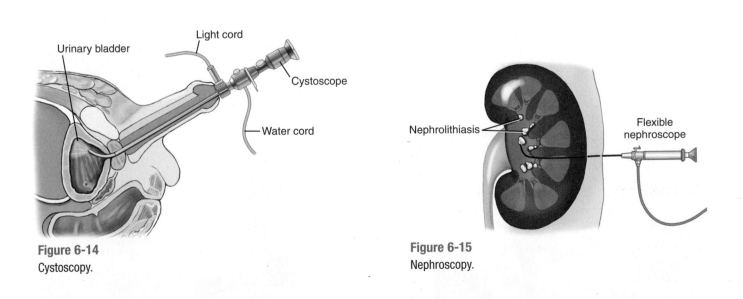

Figure 6-14
Cystoscopy.

Figure 6-15
Nephroscopy.

EXERCISE FIGURE H

Fill in the blanks to label the diagram.

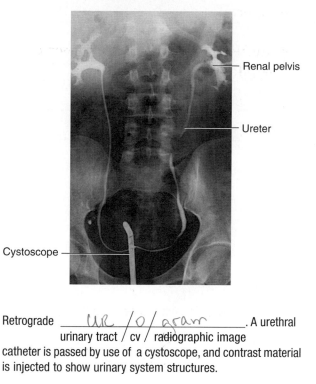

— Renal pelvis

— Ureter

Cystoscope —

Retrograde ___UR / O / gram___. A urethral
     urinary tract / cv / radiographic image
catheter is passed by use of a cystoscope, and contrast material
is injected to show urinary system structures.

EXERCISE FIGURE I

Fill in the blanks to label the diagram.

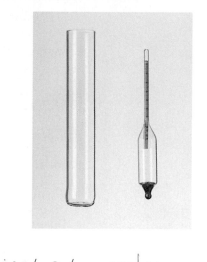

___urin / o / meter___
urine / cv / instrument used to measure

is used to measure the specific gravity of urine.

EXERCISE 24

Practice saying aloud each of the diagnostic terms built from word parts on pp. 230-232.

To hear the terms select Chapter 6, Chapter Exercises, Pronunciation.

☐ Place a check mark in the box when you have completed this exercise.

EXERCISE 25

Analyze and define the following diagnostic terms.

1. voiding cyst/o/urethr/o/graphy _Radio active imagining of the bladder_
2. meat/o/scope _Instrument used for visual exam of the meatus_
3. cyst/o/graphy _Radiographic imaging of the bladder_
4. urethr/o/scope _Instrument used for visual examination of urethra_
5. nephr/o/son/o/graphy _process of recording the kidney using sound_
6. cyst/o/scope _Instrument used for visual exam of bladder_
7. nephr/o/tom/o/gram _Sectional radiographic image of the kidney_
8. cyst/o/gram _Radiographic image of the bladder_

9. meatoscopy _Visual examination of the meatus_

10. nephrogram _Radiographic image of the Kidney_

11. cystoscopy _Visual examination of the bladder_

12. nephrography _Radiographic imagining of the Kidney_

13. urinometer _Instrument used to measure urine_

14. (intravenous) urogram _____

15. (retrograde) urogram _____

16. renogram _____

17. nephroscopy _____

18. ureteroscopy _____

EXERCISE 26

Build diagnostic terms that correspond to the following definitions by using the word parts you have learned.

1. visual examination of the bladder

   WR / CV / S

2. sectional radiographic image
   of the kidney

   WR / CV / WR / CV / S

3. radiographic image of the
   urinary tract (with contrast
   medium injected intravenously)

   intravenous

   WR / CV / S

4. instrument used for visual
   examination of the meatus

   WR / CV / S

5. instrument used for visual
   examination of the urethra

   WR / CV / S

6. process of radiographic
   recording the kidney using
   sound

   WR / CV / WR / CV / S

7. radiographic image of
   the bladder

   WR / CV / S

8. visual examination of
   the meatus

   _____
   WR   / CV /   S

9. instrument used for visual
   examination of the bladder

   _____
   WR   / CV /   S

10. radiographic imaging of
    the bladder and the urethra

    voiding _____
            WR / CV /   WR   / CV / S

11. radiographic imaging
    of the bladder

    _____
    WR   / CV /   S

12. radiographic image
    of the kidney

    _____
    WR   / CV /   S

13. instrument used to
    measure (the specific
    gravity of) urine

    _____
    WR   / CV /   S

14. (graphic) record of the
    kidney (produced by
    radioactivity after injecting
    a radio-pharmaceutical
    material into the blood)

    _____
    WR   / CV /   S

15. radiographic imaging
    of the kidney

    _____
    WR   / CV /   S

16. radiographic image of
    the urinary tract (with
    contrast medium instilled
    through the urethral
    catheters in a direction
    opposite from normal)

    retrograde _____
               WR   / CV /   S

17. visual examination
    of the kidney

    _____
    WR   / CV /   S

18. visual examination
    of the ureter

    _____
    WR   / CV /   S

EXERCISE 27

Spell each of the diagnostic terms built from word parts on pp. 230-232 by having someone dictate them to you.

 To hear and spell the terms select Chapter 6, Chapter Exercises, Spelling. You may type the terms on the screen or write them below in the spaces provided.

☐ Place a check mark in the box when if you have completed this exercise using your CD-ROM.

1. _____

2. _____

3. _____

4. _____

5. _____

6. _____

7. _____

8. _____

9. _____

10. _____

11. _____

12. _____

13. _____

14. _____

15. _____

16. _____

17. _____

18. _____

Diagnostic Terms

Not Built from Word Parts

In some of the following terms, you may recognize word parts you have already learned; however, the full meaning of the terms cannot be discerned by the definition of their word parts.

Term	Definition
DIAGNOSTIC IMAGING	
KUB (kidney, ureter, and bladder)	a simple radiographic image of the abdomen. It is often used to view the kidneys, ureters, and bladder to determine size, shape, and location. Also used to identify calculi in the kidney, ureters, or bladder, or to diagnose intestinal obstruction.
LABORATORY	
blood urea nitrogen (BUN) . . . . (ū-RĒ-a) (NĪ-trō-jen)	a blood test that measures the amount of urea in the blood; used to determine kidney function. An increased BUN indicates renal dysfunction.
creatinine . . . . (crē-AT-i-nin)	a blood test that measures the amount of creatinine in the blood. An elevated amount indicates impaired kidney function.

Term	Definition
specific gravity (SG). . . . . (spe-SIF-ik) (GRAV-i-tē)	a test performed on a urine specimen to measure the concentrating or diluting ability of the kidneys
urinalysis (UA) . . . . (ū-rin-AL-is-is)	multiple routine tests performed on a urine specimen

EXERCISE 28

Practice saying aloud each of the diagnostic terms not built from word parts on pp. 236-237.

 To hear terms select Chapter 6, Chapter Exercises, Pronunciation.

☐ Place a check mark in the box when you have completed this exercise.

EXERCISE 29

Fill in the blanks with the correct terms.

1. The radiographic image of the abdomen used to view the kidneys, ureters, and bladder to determine size, shape, and location is called _____.

2. A test performed on a urine specimen to measure concentrating and diluting ability of the kidneys is called _____ _____.

3. _____ _____ _____ measures the amount of urea in the blood.

4. Multiple routine tests performed on a urine specimen are referred to as a(n) _____.

5. _____ is a blood test that measures the amount of creatinine in the blood.

EXERCISE 30

Match the terms in the first column with their correct definitions in the second column.

_____ 1. specific gravity	a. a radiographic image of the kidneys, ureters, and bladder
_____ 2. blood urea nitrogen	b. a blood test that measures the amount of urea in the blood
_____ 3. urinalysis	c. a urine test to measure concentrating or diluting abilities of the kidneys
_____ 4. KUB	d. multiple routine tests performed on a urine sample
_____ 5. creatinine	e. a radiographic image of the kidneys, urethra, and bladder
	f. a test on blood that if elevated indicates impaired kidney function

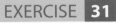

EXERCISE **31**

Spell each of the diagnostic terms not built from word parts on pp. 236-237 by having someone dictate them to you.

 To hear and spell the terms select Chapter 6, Chapter Exercises, Spelling. You may type the terms on the screen or write them below in the spaces provided.

☐ Place a check mark in the box when you have completed this exercise using your CD-ROM.

1. _____   4. _____

2. _____   5. _____

3. _____

Complementary Terms

Built from Word Parts

The following terms are built from word parts you have already learned and can be translated literally to find their meanings. Further explanation of terms beyond the definition of their word parts, if needed, is included in parentheses.

Term	Definition
albuminuria . . . . (*al*-bū-min-Ū-rē-a)	albumin in the urine (albumin is an important protein in the blood, but when found in the urine, it indicates a kidney problem)
anuria . . . . (an-Ū-rē-a)	absence of urine (failure of the kidney to produce urine)
azotemia . . . . (az-ō-TĒ-mē-a)	(excessive) urea and nitrogenous substances in the blood
diuresis . . . . (*dī*-ū-RĒ-sis) (NOTE: the *a* is dropped from dia- because uresis begins with a vowel.)	condition of urine passing through (increased amount of urine)
dysuria. . . . . (dis-Ū-rē-a)	difficult or painful urination
glycosuria . . . . (glī-kō-SŪ-rē-a)	sugar (glucose) in the urine
hematuria . . . . (*hēm*-a-TŪ-rē-a)	blood in the urine
meatal . . . . (mē-Ā-tal)	pertaining to the meatus
nephrologist. . . . . (ne-FROL-o-jist)	a physician who studies and treats diseases of the kidney
nephrology. . . . . (ne-FROL-o-jē)	study of the kidney (a branch of medicine dealing with diseases of the kidney)
nocturia . . . . (nok-TŪ-rē-a)	night urination

Term	Definition
oliguria................ (*ol*-i-GŪ-rē-a)	scanty urine (amount)
polyuria................ (pol-ē-Ū-rē-a)	much (excessive) urine
pyuria................ (pī-Ū-rē-a)	pus in the urine
urinary................ (Ū-rin-*ār*-ē)	pertaining to urine
urologist................ (ū-ROL-o-jist)	a physician who studies and treats (diseases of) the urinary tract
urology................ (ū-ROL-o-jē)	study of the urinary tract (a branch of medicine dealing with diseases of the male and female urinary systems and the male reproductive system)

EXERCISE 32

Practice saying aloud each of the complementary terms built from word parts on pp. 238-239.

 To hear the terms Chapter 6, Chapter Exercises, Pronunciation.

☐ Place a check mark in the box when you have completed this exercise.

EXERCISE 33

Analyze and define the following complementary terms.

1. nocturia __night urination__
2. urologist __A physician who studies and treats urinary tract__
3. oliguria __scanty urine__
4. azotemia __excessive urea and nitrogenious substances in the blood__
5. hematuria __blood in the urine__
6. urology __study of the urinary tract__
7. polyuria __excessive urine__
8. albuminuria __albumin in the urine__
9. anuria __absence of urine__
10. diuresis __condition of urine passing through__
11. pyuria __pus in the urine__
12. urinary __pertaining to urine__
13. glycosuria __sugar in the urine__
14. meatal __pertaining to the meatus__

15. dysuria _difficult or painful urination_
16. nephrology _study of the kidney_
17. nephrologist _a physician who studies and treats the kidney_

EXERCISE 34

Build the complementary terms for the following definitions by using the word parts you have learned.

1. night urination

    noctur / _-ur1a_
    WR   /   S

2. scanty urine

    WR   /   S

3. pus in the urine

    WR   /   S

4. physician who studies and treats (diseases of) the urinary tract

    WR / CV /   S

5. much (excessive) urine

    P   /   S(WR)

6. (excessive) urea and nitrogenous substances in the blood

    WR   /   S

7. pertaining to urine

    WR   /   S

8. blood in the urine

    WR   /   S(WR)

9. study of the urinary tract

    WR / CV /   S

10. condition of urine passing through (increased amount of urine)

    P / WR /   S

11. absence of urine

    P   /   S(WR)

12. sugar in the urine

    WR   /   S(WR)

13. difficult or painful urination

    P   /   S(WR)

14. albumin in the urine

    WR   /   S(WR)

15. pertaining to the meatus

    WR   /   S

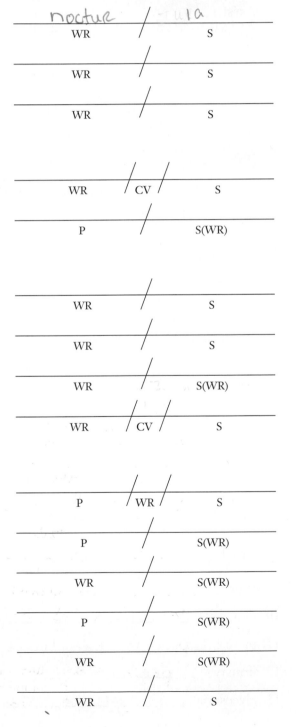

16. study of the kidney

_____ / ___ / ___
WR   CV   S

17. physician who studies and
treats (diseases of) the kidney

_____ / ___ / ___
WR   CV   S

EXERCISE 35

Spell each of the complementary terms built from word parts on pp. 238-239 by having someone dictate them to you.

 To hear and spell the terms select Chapter 6, Chapter Exercises, Spelling. You may type the terms on the screen or write them below in the spaces provided.

☐ Place a check mark in the box if you have completed this exercise using your CD-ROM.

1. _____ 10. _____

2. _____ 11. _____

3. _____ 12. _____

4. _____ 13. _____

5. _____ 14. _____

6. _____ 15. _____

7. _____ 16. _____

8. _____ 17. _____

9. _____

Complementary Terms

Not Built from Word Parts

In some of the following terms, you may recognize word parts you have already learned; however, the full meaning of the terms cannot be discerned by the definition of their word parts.

Term	Definition
catheter (cath) .... (KATH-e-ter)	flexible, tubelike device, such as a urinary catheter, for withdrawing or instilling fluids
distended .... (dis-TEN-ded)	stretched out (a bladder is distended when filled with urine)
diuretic .... (dī-ū-RET-ik)	agent that increases the formation and excretion of urine
enuresis .... (en-ū-RĒ-sis)	involuntary urination
hemodialysis (HD) .... (hē-mō-dī-AL-i-sis)	procedure for removing impurities from the blood because of an inability of the kidneys to do so (Figure 6-16)

 CATHETER
is derived from the Greek **katheter,** meaning a **thing let down.** A catheter lets down the urine from the bladder.

ENURESIS
Nocturnal enuresis, or bedwetting, has been described in early literature and continues to be a problem affecting 15% to 20% of school-aged children. There is no one cause for bed wetting.
Diurnal enuresis is daytime wetting, which may be caused by a small bladder. Various treatments are used to treat diurnal enuresis. Children generally outgrow daytime wetting.

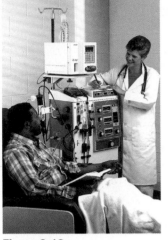

Figure 6-16
Hemodialysis.

MICTURATE
is derived from the Latin **mictus,** meaning **a making of water.** The noun form of micturate is **micturition.** Note the spelling of each. **Micturition** is often misspelled as **micturation.**

URODYNAMIC STUDIES
examines the process of voiding and tests bladder tone, capacity, and pressure along with urine flow and perineal muscle function. **Prostatic cancer,** prostatic hypertrophy, and urethral stricture will diminish urine flow rate.

Complementary Terms—*cont'd*
Not Built from Word Parts

Term	Definition
incontinence (in-KON-ti-nens)	inability to control bladder and/or bowels
micturate (MIK-tū-rāt)	to urinate or void
peritoneal dialysis (pār-i-tō-NĒ-al) (dī-AL-i-sis)	procedure for removing toxic wastes when the kidney is unable to do so; the peritoneal cavity is used as the receptacle for the fluid used in the dialysis (Figure 6-17)
stricture (STRIK-chūr)	abnormal narrowing, such as a urethral stricture
urinal (Ū-rin-al)	receptacle for urine
urinary catheterization (Ū-rin-ār-ē) (kath-e-ter-i-ZĀ-shun)	passage of a catheter into the urinary bladder to withdraw urine (Exercise Figure J)
urodynamics (ū-rō-dī-NAM-iks)	pertaining to the force and flow of urine within the urinary tract
void (voyd)	to empty or evacuate waste material, especially urine

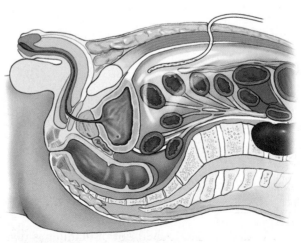

Figure 6-17
Peritoneal dialysis. A sterile dialyzing fluid is instilled into the peritoneal cavity by gravity and dwells there for a period of time ordered by the physician. The fluid, containing the nitrogenous wastes and excess water that a healthy kidney normally removes, is drained from the cavity.

EXERCISE FIGURE J

Fill in the blanks to complete labeling of the diagram.

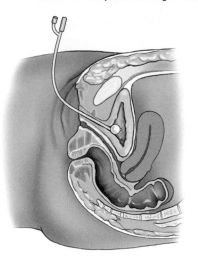

_____ / _____ catheterization. A catheter has been inserted through the urethra and
urine / pertaining to
urine has been drained. The balloon on the end of the catheter has been inflated to hold the catheter in
the bladder for a period of time. This type of catheter is called a *retention catheter*.

EXERCISE 36

Practice saying aloud each of the complementary terms not built from word parts on
pp. 241-242.

 To hear the terms select Chapter 6, Chapter Exercises, Pronunciation.

☐ Place a check mark in the box when you have completed this exercise.

EXERCISE 37

Fill in the blanks with the correct terms.

1. A receptacle for urine is a(n) __urinal__.

2. The procedure for removing impurities from the blood because of the inability of the kidneys to do so is called __hemodidysis__.

3. A __distended__ bladder is stretched out.

4. A flexible, tubelike device for withdrawing or instilling fluids is a(n)
   __Catheter__.

5. The inability to control the bladder and/or bowels is called
   __incontince__.

6. The passage of a catheter into the urinary bladder to withdraw urine is a(n)
   __urinary__ __catheterization__

7. To remove toxic wastes caused by kidney insufficiency by placing dialyzing
   fluid in the peritoneal cavity is called __peritoneal__
   __dialysis__.

8. To void is to _____ _____ _____.

9. An abnormal narrowing is a(n) _____.

10. An agent that increases the formation and excretion of urine is called a(n) _____.

11. Involuntary urination is called _____.

12. _____is another word for void, or urinate.

13. _____is the name given to the force and flow of urine.

EXERCISE 38

Match the terms in the first column with their correct definitions in the second column.

_____ 1. catheter

_____ 2. urinary catheterization

_____ 3. distended

_____ 4. diuretic

_____ 5. hemodialysis

_____ 6. incontinence

_____ 7. void

a. increases the formation and excretion of urine

b. overdevelopment of the kidney

c. inability to control the bladder and/or bowels

d. process for removing impurities from the blood when the kidneys are unable to do so

e. flexible, tubelike device for withdrawing or instilling fluids

f. stretched out

g. passage of a tubelike device into the urinary bladder to remove urine

h. to evacuate or empty waste material, especially urine

EXERCISE 39

Match the terms in the first column with their correct definitions in the second column.

_____ 1. micturate, or urinate

_____ 2. peritoneal dialysis

_____ 3. stricture

_____ 4. urinal

_____ 5. enuresis

_____ 6. urodynamics

a. to void liquid waste

b. receptacle for urine

c. force and flow of urine within the urinary tract

d. absence of urine

e. use of peritoneal cavity to hold dialyzing fluid in the removal of toxic wastes

f. involuntary urination

g. narrowing

EXERCISE 40

Spell each of the complementary terms not built from word parts on pp. 241-242 by having someone dictate them to you.

 To hear and spell the terms select Chapter 6, Chapter Exercises, Spelling. You may type the terms on the screen or write them below in the space provided.

☐ Place a check mark in the box if you have completed this exercise using your CD-ROM.

1. _____   8. _____

2. _____   9. _____

3. _____   10. _____

4. _____   11. _____

5. _____   12. _____

6. _____   13. _____

7. _____

Refer to Appendix E for pharmacology terms related to the urinary system.

Abbreviations

BUN	blood urea nitrogen
cath	catheterization, catheter
ESWL	extracorporeal shock wave lithotripsy
HD	hemodialysis
IVP	intravenous pyelogram
IVU	intravenous urogram
SG	specific gravity
UA	urinalysis
UTI	urinary tract infection
VCUG	voiding cystourethrogram

Refer to Appendix D for a complete list of abbreviations.

EXERCISE 41

1. When imaging is used to diagnose obstructive uropathy, a KUB is usually performed first. An **IVU** _____ _____, also called **IVP** _____ _____, is usually best for confirming or excluding obstruction and determining its level and cause. For further examination a **VCUG** _____ _____ may be performed to evaluate the posterior urethra and check for vesicoureteral reflux.

2. **SG** _____ _____ is one of many tests performed on the urine specimen during a **UA** _____. It measures the concentration of particles, including water and electrolytes in the urine.

3. **BUN** _____ _____ _____ is a laboratory test done on a blood sample to determine kidney function.

4. The number, size, and type of stones are important in determining if **ESWL** _____ _____ _____ _____ is the best method for treating renal calculi.

5. Bladder **cath** _____ carries the risk of **UTI** _____ _____ _____; therefore it is sometimes preferable to use other methods for obtaining urine specimens and managing incontinence.

6. Peritoneal dialysis, **HD** _____, and renal transplant are known as renal replacement therapies.

PRACTICAL APPLICATION

EXERCISE **42** *Interact with Medical Documents*

A. Complete the discharge summary report by writing the medical terms in the blanks. Use the list of definitions with the corresponding numbers.

University Hospital and Medical Center
4700 North Main Street • Wellness, Arizona 54321 • (987) 555-3210

PATIENT NAME: Bruno Oliver
DATE OF BIRTH: 07/30/19XX

CASE NUMBER: 83658-URI
DATE OF ADMISSION: 09/20/20XX
DATE OF DISCHARGE: 09/27/20XX

DISCHARGE SUMMARY

Bruno Oliver is a 32-year-old white man, appearing his stated age, who was admitted to the hospital after presenting himself to the emergency department on 09/20/XX in acute distress. He complained of intermittent pain in the right posterior lumbar area, radiating to the right flank. He has a family history of 1. _____ and has been treated for this condition two other times in the past 10 years.

This patient was admitted to the 2. _____ Unit and was administered intravenous morphine sulfate for pain control. VITAL SIGNS: Low-grade temperature of 99.4. Initial blood pressure was 146/92.

The white blood count, hemoglobin, and hematocrit were normal. The urinalysis showed microscopic 3. _____ .

A 4. _____ revealed 5. _____ in the region of the right renal pelvis. A 6. _____ with a right retrograde 7. _____ confirmed the presence of the three stones in the right kidney. Minimal ureteral obstruction was present.

A percutaneous 8. _____ was completed with no complications. A ureteral stent was inserted as was an indwelling Foley 9. _____ . Drainage from the right kidney was pale yellow in 48 hours. The Foley catheter was removed 3 days postoperatively.

At discharge, the patient is voiding without difficulty. The stones were sent to the laboratory for analysis. The report indicated that they were calcium oxalate.

The patient is to follow up with his urologist in a week to have his ureteral stent removed.

Betsy Begay, MD

BB/mcm

---

1. condition of stones in the kidney
2. study of the urinary tract
3. blood in the urine
4. radiographic image of the abdomen
5. stones
6. visual examination of the bladder
7. radiographic image of the urinary tract
8. incision through the kidney into the renal pelvis to remove a stone
9. flexible, tubelike device

EXERCISE **42** *Interact with Medical Documents—cont'd*

B. Read the operative report and answer the questions following it.

OPERATIVE REPORT

Patient Name: John Allen
Preoperative Diagnosis: Urinary tract obstruction

Date of Operation: May 21, 20XX
Postoperative Diagnosis: Ureterolithiasis

Surgery Performed: Ureteroscopy with calculus extraction

Indications: The patient, a 31-year-old previously healthy man, presented with complaints of flank pain, oliguria, nausea, and chills. The patient denied gross hematuria. A spiral CT scan revealed presence of a ureteral stone.

Procedure: The patient was placed in the dorsal lithotomy position. The area was draped and prepared in the standard manner. Thirty mL of topical anesthesia (1% Lidocaine) was administered, and a penile clamp was applied to ensure retention. The ureteroscope was inserted, with access to the middle third of the ureter gained by passing a guidewire under fluoroscopic control. The guidewire was advanced beyond the stone, and the calculus was delivered through the ureter, engaged in a retrieval basket, and removed. The patient tolerated the procedure well and left the operating room in good condition.

Melvin Peterson, MD, Urologist

---

1. The patient presented with a complaint of
   a. difficult or painful urination.
   b. excessive urine.
   c. scanty urine.
   d. pus in the urine.

2. The presence of a ureteral stone was revealed by
   a. radiographic imaging.
   b. magnetic resonance imaging.
   c. ultrasound.
   d. computed tomography.

3. T F   More than one stone was removed from the ureter.

4. Ureteroscope and ureteral are terms not included in the chapter. Using your knowledge of the meaning of word parts, define these terms.

   a. ureteral _____

   b. ureteroscope _____

EXERCISE **43** *Interpret Medical Terms*

To test your understanding of the terms introduced in this chapter, circle the words that correctly complete the sentences. The italicized words refer to the correct answer.

1. The patient was admitted with a *drooping kidney*, or (**nephromegaly, nephrohypertrophy, nephroptosis**).

2. The patient's radiographic image showed a *stone in the ureter*, or a condition known as (**ureterocele, ureterolithiasis, ureterostenosis**).

3. Because of Mrs. McLean's admission to the intensive care unit with pneumonia and her compromised immune system, her physicians were alert to signs of *pathogenic organisms entering the bloodstream*, or (**fulguration, urodynamics, sepsis**).

4. The physician first suspected diabetes when told of the *excessive amounts of urine* voided, or (**oliguria, polyuria, dysuria**).

5. The physician told the patient with the drooping kidney that it was necessary to *secure the kidney in place* by performing a (**nephropexy, nephrolysis, nephrotripsy**).

6. The patient had a *sudden stoppage of urine formation*, or (**urinary suppression, urinary retention, azoturia**).

7. The patient was scheduled for a *radiographic image of the urinary bladder*, or a (**cystoscopy, cystogram, cystography**).

8. The patient's mother informed the doctor of her son's *involuntary urination*, or (**diuresis, dysuria, enuresis**).

9. The patient was admitted to the hospital for *kidney and ureteral infection*, or (**polycystic kidney disease, urinary retention, urinary tract infection**).

10. *UA* is the abbreviation for (**urine, urinary, urinalysis**).

EXERCISE **44**   *Read Medical Terms in Use*

Practice pronunciation of the terms by reading the following medical document. Use the pronunciation key following the medical terms to assist you in saying the word.

 To hear these terms select Chapter 6, Chapter Exercises, Read Medical Terms in Use.

A 76-year-old woman consulted with her primary care physician because of **hematuria** (*hēm*-a-TŪ-rē-a) and **dysuria** (dis-Ū-rē-a). She was referred to a **urologist** (ū-ROL-o-jist). **Urinalysis** (ū-rin-AL-is-is) disclosed 1+ albumin and mild **pyuria** (pī-Ū-rē-a) in addition to the hematuria. A spiral CT scan was obtained. Mild **nephrolithiasis** (*nef*-rō-lith-Ī-a-sis) was observed but no **hydronephrosis** (*hī*-drō-ne-FRŌ-sis). Finally a **cystoscopy** (sis-TOS-ko-pē) was performed, which showed mild **cystitis** (sis-TĪ-tis). A **urinary tract infection** (Ū-rin-*ār*-ē) (trakt) (in-FEK-shun) was diagnosed and the patient responded favorably to antibiotics. The urologist did not advise **lithotripsy** (LITH-ō-trip-sē) for the **renal calculi** (RĒ-nal) (KAL-kū-lī).

EXERCISE **45**   *Comprehend Medical Terms in Use*

Test your comprehension of terms in the previous medical document by circling the correct answer.

1. Symptoms that prompted the patient to seek treatment from the urologist were:
   a. scanty urine and painful urination
   b. painful urination and bloody urine
   c. pus and blood in the urine
   d. sugar and blood in the urine

2. Which of the following was rejected as treatment for kidney stones?
   a. urinalysis
   b. intravenous urogram
   c. cystoscopy
   d. lithotripsy

3. The CT image revealed which of the following was not present in the kidney?
   a. water
   b. blood
   c. stones
   d. tumor

CHAPTER REVIEW

(•))) CHAPTER REVIEW ON CD-ROM

Use the CD-ROM that accompanies this textbook to play and practice what you have learned in this chapter. The Chapter Exercises, Practice Activities, Animations, and Games allow you to hear, see, and interact with the chapter content.

Chapter Exercises

Exercises in this section of your CD-ROM correlate to exercises in your textbook. You may have completed them as you worked through the chapter.
☐ Pronunciation
☐ Spelling
☐ Read Medical Terms in Use

Practice Activities

Practice in study mode, then test your learning in assessment mode. Keep track of your scores from assessment mode if you wish.

                SCORE

☐ Picture It   _____
☐ Define Word Parts   _____
☐ Build Medical Terms _____
☐ Word Shop   _____
☐ Define Medical Terms _____
☐ Use It   _____
☐ Hear It and Type It: _____
    Clinical Vignettes

Animations
☐ Nephrostomy
☐ Renal
    Anatomy
    Function

Games
☐ Name that Word Part
☐ Term Storm
☐ Term Explorer
☐ Termbusters
☐ Medical Millionaire

REVIEW OF WORD PARTS

Can you define and spell the following word parts?

Combining Forms		Suffixes
albumin/o	olig/o	-esis
azot/o	pyel/o	-gram
blast/o	ren/o	-iasis
cyst/o	son/o	-lysis
glomerul/o	tom/o	-megaly
glyc/o	ureter/o	-ptosis
glycos/o	urethr/o	-rrhaphy
hydr/o	ur/o	-tripsy
lith/o	urin/o	-trophy
meat/o	vesic/o	-uria
nephr/o		
noct/i		

REVIEW OF TERMS

Can you build, analyze, define, pronounce, and spell the following terms *built from word parts*?

Diseases and Disorders	Surgical	Diagnostic	Complementary
cystitis	cystectomy	cystogram	albuminuria
cystocele	cystolithotomy	cystography	anuria
cystolith	cystorrhaphy	cystoscope	azotemia
glomerulonephritis	cystostomy	cystoscopy	diuresis
hydronephrosis	cystotomy	intravenous urogram (IVU)	dysuria
nephritis	lithotripsy	meatoscope	glycosuria
nephroblastoma	meatotomy	meatoscopy	hematuria
nephrohypertrophy	nephrectomy	nephrogram	meatal
nephrolithiasis	nephrolysis	nephrography	nephrologist
nephroma	nephropexy	nephroscopy	nephrology
nephromegaly	nephropyelolithotomy	nephrosonography	nocturia
nephroptosis	nephrostomy	nephrotomogram	oliguria
pyelitis	pyelolithotomy	renogram	polyuria
pyelonephritis	pyeloplasty	retrograde urogram	pyuria
uremia	ureterectomy	ureteroscopy	urinary
ureteritis	ureterostomy	urethroscope	urologist
ureterocele	urethroplasty	urinometer	urology
ureterolithiasis	vesicourethral suspension	voiding cystourethrography (VCUG)	
ureterostenosis	vesicotomy		
urethrocystitis			

Can you define, pronounce, and spell the following terms *not built from word parts?*

Diseases and Disorders	**Surgical**	**Diagnostic**	**Complementary**
epispadias	extracorporeal shock	blood urea nitrogen	catheter (cath)
hypospadias	wave lithotripsy	(BUN)	distended
polycystic kidney disease	(ESWL)	creatinine	diuretic
renal calculus (*pl.* calculi)	fulguration	KUB	enuresis
renal hypertension	renal transplant	specific gravity (SG)	hemodialysis (HD)
sepsis		urinalysis (UA)	incontinence
urinary retention			micturate
urinary suppression			peritoneal dialysis
urinary tract infection (UTI)			stricture
			urinal
			urinary catheterization
			urodynamics
			void

ANSWERS

Exercise Figures

Exercise Figure
A. 1. kidney: nephr/o, ren/o
2. meatus: meat/o
3. ureter: ureter/o
4. bladder: cyst/o, vesic/o
5. urethra: urethr/o

Exercise Figure
B. 1. renal pelvis: pyel/o
2. glomerulus: glomerul/o

Exercise Figure
C. cyst/o/lith

Exercise Figure
D. cyst/o/stomy

Exercise Figure
E. lith/o/tripsy

Exercise Figure
F. nephr/o/stomy

Exercise Figure
G. pyel/o/lith/o/tomy

Exercise Figure
H. ur/o/gram

Exercise Figure
I. urin/o/meter

Exercise Figure
J. urin/ary

Exercise 1
1. g
2. d
3. f
4. c
5. a
6. b
7. e

Exercise 2
1. glomerulus
2. sac, bladder
3. kidney
4. renal pelvis
5. ureter
6. bladder, sac
7. urethra
8. kidney
9. meatus

Exercise 3
1. a. nephr/o
   b. ren/o
2. a. cyst/o
   b. vesic/o
3. ureter/o
4. pyel/o
5. glomerul/o
6. urethr/o
7. meat/o

Exercise 4
1. water
2. urea, nitrogen
3. night
4. stone, calculus
5. cut, section
6. albumin
7. urine, urinary tract
8. sound
9. sugar
10. developing cell, germ cell
11. scanty, few
12. urine, urinary tract
13. sugar

Exercise 5
1. a. glyc/o
   b. glycos/o
2. son/o
3. a. urin/o
   b. ur/o
4. hydr/o
5. blast/o
6. tom/o
7. albumin/o
8. noct/i
9. azot/o
10. lith/o
11. olig/o

Exercise 6
1. c
2. i
3. d
4. f
5. g
6. e
7. a
8. b
9. h

Exercise 7
1. suturing, repairing
2. loosening, dissolution, separating
3. condition
4. nourishment, development
5. urine, urination
6. enlargement
7. drooping, sagging, prolapse
8. surgical crushing
9. record, radiographic image

Exercise 8
1. Pronunciation Exercise

Exercise 9
1. WR S
    nephr/oma
    tumor of the kidney
2. WR CV WR
    cyst/o/lith
        CF
    stone in the bladder
3. WR CV WR S
    nephr/o/lith/iasis
        CF
    condition of stone(s) in the kidney
4. WR S
    ur/emia
    condition of urine (urea) in the blood
5. WR CV S
    nephr/o/ptosis
        CF
    drooping kidney
6. WR CV S
    cyst/o/cele
        CF
    protrusion of the bladder
7. WR CV P S
    nephr/o/hyper/trophy
        CF
    excessive development of the kidney
8. WR S
    cyst/itis
    inflammation of the bladder
9. WR S
    pyel/itis
    inflammation of the renal pelvis
10. WR CV S
    ureter/o/cele
        CF
    protrusion of a ureter
11. WR CV WR S
    hydr/o/nephr/osis
        CF
    abnormal condition of water in the
    kidney
12. WR CV S
    nephr/o/megaly
        CF
    enlargement of a kidney
13. WR CV WR S
    ureter/o/lith/iasis
        CF
    condition of stones(s) in the ureters
14. WR CV WR S
    pyel/o/nephr/itis
        CF
    inflammation of the renal pelvis and
    the kidney
15. WR S
    ureter/itis
    inflammation of a ureter
16. WR S
    nephr/itis
    inflammation of a kidney
17. WR CV WR S
    urethr/o/cyst/itis
        CF
    inflammation of the urethra and
    bladder

18. WR CV S
  ureter/o/stenosis
  ⌣ CF
  narrowing of the ureter
19. WR CV WR S
  nephr/o/blast/oma
  ⌣ CF
  kidney tumor containing developing
    cell

Exercise 10
1. nephr/o/megaly
2. cyst/itis
3. nephr/o/hyper/trophy
4. urethr/o/cyst/itis
5. cyst/o/cele
6. hydr/o/nephr/osis
7. cyst/o/lith
8. glomerul/o/nephr/itis
9. nephr/oma
10. nephr/o/ptosis
11. nephr/itis
12. nephr/o/lith/iasis
13. ureter/o/cele
14. pyel/itis
15. ur/emia
16. ureter/o/stenosis
17. pyel/o/nephr/itis
18. ureter/o/lith/iasis
19. nephr/o/blast/oma

Exercise 11
Spelling Exercise, see text p. 220.

Exercise 12
Pronunciation Exercise

Exercise 13
1. renal calculus
2. urinary retention
3. polycystic kidney disease
4. hypospadias
5. renal hypertension
6. urinary suppression
7. epispadias
8. urinary tract infection
9. sepsis

Exercise 14
1. c   6. e
2. f   7. b
3. d   8. g
4. h   9. i
5. a

Exercise 15
Spelling Exercise; see text p. 222.

Exercise 16
Pronunciation Exercise

Exercise 17
1. WR CV S
  vesic/o/tomy
  ⌣ CF
  incison of the bladder
2. WR CV S
  cyst/o/tomy
  ⌣ CF
  incison of the bladder
3. WR   CV S
  nephr/o/stomy
  ⌣ CF
  creation of an artificial opening into
    the kidney
4. WR CV S
  nephr/o/lysis
  ⌣ CF
  separating the kidney
5. WR   S
  cyst/ectomy
  excision of the bladder
6. WR CV WR CV S
  pyel/o/lith/o/tomy
  ⌣ CF ⌣ CF
  incision of the renal pelvis to remove
    a stone
7. WR CV S
  nephr/o/pexy
  ⌣ CF
  surgical fixation of the kidney
8. WR CV WR CV S
  cyst/o/lith/o/tomy
  ⌣ CF ⌣ CF
  incision of the bladder to remove a
    stone
9. WR   S
  nephr/ectomy
  excision of a kidney
10. WR   S
  ureter/ectomy
  excision of a ureter
11. WR CV S
  cyst/o/stomy
  ⌣ CF
  creation of an artificial opening into
    the bladder
12. WR CV S
  pyel/o/plasty
  ⌣ CF
  surgical repair of the renal pelvis
13. WR CV S
  cyst/o/rrhaphy
  ⌣ CF
  suturing of the bladder
14. WR CV S
  meat/o/tomy
  ⌣ CF
  incision of the meatus

15. WR CV S
  lith/o/tripsy
  ⌣ CF
  surgical crushing of a stone
16. WR CV S
  urethr/o/plasty
  ⌣ CF
  surgical repair of the urethra
17. WR CV WR S
  vesic/o/urethr/al suspension
  ⌣ CF
  suspension pertaining to the bladder
    and urethra
18. WR   CV WR CV WR CV S
  nephr/o/pyel/o/lith/o/tomy
  ⌣ CF ⌣ CF ⌣ CF
  incision through the kidney into the
    renal pelvis to remove a stone
19. WR CV S
  ureter/o/stomy
  ⌣ CF
  creation of an artificial opening into
    the ureter

Exercise 18
1. ureter/o/stomy
2. nephr/ectomy
3. pyel/o/lith/o/tomy
4. cyst/o/rrhaphy
5. nephr/o/lysis
6. nephr/o/stomy
7. urethr/o/plasty
8. cyst/ectomy
9. meat/o/tomy
10. a. cyst/o/tomy
    b. vesic/o/tomy
11. pyel/o/plasty
12. ureter/ectomy
13. nephr/o/pexy
14. cyst/o/lith/o/tomy
15. lith/o/tripsy
16. vesic/o/urethr/al suspension
17. cyst/o/stomy
18. nephr/o/pyel/o/lith/o/tomy

Exercise 19
Spelling Exercise; see text p. 227.

Exercise 20
Pronunciation Exercise

Exercise 21
1. renal transplant
2. fulguration
3. extracorporeal shock wave lithotripsy

Exercise 22
1. b   2. a   3. d

Exercise 23
Spelling Exercise; see text p. 230.

Exercise 24
Pronunciation Exercise

Exercise 25
1. WR CV WR CV S
cyst/o/urethr/o/graphy
   CF   CF
radiographic imaging of the bladder
and the urethra
2. WR CV S
meat/o/scope
   CF
instrument used for visual
examination of the meatus
3. WR CV S
cyst/o/graphy
   CF
radiographic imaging of the bladder
4. WR CV S
urethr/o/scope
   CF
instrument used for visual
examination of the urethra
5. WR CV WR CV S
nephr/o/son/o/graphy
   CF   CF
process of recording the kidney with
sound
6. WR CV S
cyst/o/scope
   CF
instrument used for visual
examination of the bladder
7. WR CV WR CV S
nephr/o/tom/o/gram
   CF   CF
sectional radiographic image of the
kidney
8. WR CV S
cyst/o/gram
   CF
radiographic image of the bladder
9. WR CV S
meat/o/scopy
   CF
visual examination of the meatus
10. WR CV S
nephr/o/gram
   CF
radiographic image of the kidney
11. WR CV S
cyst/o/scopy
   CF
visual examination of the bladder

12. WR CV S
nephr/o/graphy
   CF
radiographic imaging of the kidney
13. WR CV S
urin/o/meter
   CF
instrument used to measure (specific
gravity) urine
14. WR CV S
(intravenous) ur/o/gram
            CF
radiographic image of the urinary
tract (with contrast medium
injected intravenously)
15. WR CV S
(retrograde) ur/o/gram
            CF
radiographic image of the urinary
tract
16. WR CV S
ren/o/gram
   CF
(graphic) record of the kidney
17. WR CV S
nephr/o/scopy
   CF
visual examination of the kidney
18. WR CV S
ureter/o/scopy
   CF
visual examination of the ureter

Exercise 26
1. cyst/o/scopy
2. nephr/o/tom/o/gram
3. intravenous ur/o/gram
4. meat/o/scope
5. urethr/o/scope
6. nephr/o/son/o/graphy
7. cyst/o/gram
8. meat/o/scopy
9. cyst/o/scope
10. cyst/o/urethr/o/graphy
11. cyst/o/graphy
12. nephr/o/gram
13. urin/o/meter
14. ren/o/gram
15. nephr/o/graphy
16. ur/o/gram
17. nephr/o/scopy
18. ureter/o/scopy

Exercise 27
Spelling Exercise; see text p. 236.

Exercise 28
Pronunciation Exercise

Exercise 29
1. KUB
2. specific gravity
3. blood urea nitrogen
4. urinalysis
5. creatinine

Exercise 30
1. c.   4. a
2. b   5. f
3. d

Exercise 31
Spelling Exercise; see text p. 238.

Exercise 32
Pronunciation Exercise

Exercise 33
1. WR S
noct/uria
night urination
2. WR CV S
ur/o/logist
   CF
physician who studies and treats
(diseases of) the urinary tract
3. WR S
olig/uria
scanty urine
4. WR S
azot/emia
(excessive) urea and nitrogenous
substances in the blood
5. WR S
hemat/uria
blood in the urine
6. WR CV S
ur/o/logy
   CF
study of the urinary tract
7. P S(WR)
poly/uria
much (excessive) urine
8. WR S
albumin/uria
albumin in the urine
9. P S(WR)
an/uria
absence of urine
10. P WR S
di/ur/esis
condition of urine passing through
(increased excretion of urine)
11. WR S
py/uria
pus in the urine

12. WR   S
    urin/ary
    pertaining to urine
13. WR   S
    glycos/uria
    sugar in the urine
14. WR   S
    meat/al
    pertaining to the meatus
15. P   S(WR)
    dys/uria
    difficult or painful urination
16. WR   CV   S
    nephr/o/logy
         CF
    study of the kidney
17. WR   CV   S
    nephr/o/logist
         CF
    physician who studies and treats
       diseases of the kidney

Exercise 34
1. noct/uria
2. olig/uria
3. py/uria
4. ur/o/logist
5. poly/uria
6. azot/emia
7. urin/ary
8. hemat/uria
9. ur/o/logy
10. di/ur/esis
11. an/uria
12. glycos/uria
13. dys/uria
14. albumin/uria
15. meat/al
16. nephr/o/logy
17. nephr/o/logist

Exercise 35
Spelling Exercise; see text p. 241.

Exercise 36
Pronunciation Exercise

Exercise 37
1. urinal
2. hemodialysis
3. distended
4. catheter
5. incontinence
6. urinary catheterization
7. peritoneal dialysis
8. evacuate waste material
9. stricture
10. diuretic
11. enuresis
12. micturate
13. urodynamics

Exercise 38
1. e   5. d
2. g   6. c
3. f   7. h
4. a

Exercise 39
1. a   4. b
2. e   5. f
3. g   6. c

Exercise 40
Spelling Exercise; see text p. 245.

Exercise 41
1. intravenous urogram; intravenous
   pyelogram; voiding
   cystourethrogram
2. specific gravity; urinalysis
3. blood urea nitrogen

4. extracorporeal shock wave lithotripsy
5. catheterization; urinary tract infection
6. hemodialysis

Exercise 42
A. 1. nephrolithiasis
   2. urology
   3. hematuria
   4. KUB
   5. calculi
   6. cystoscopy
   7. urogram
   8. nephropyelolithotomy
   9. catheter

B. 1. c
   2. d
   3. F, calculus is singular for stone
   4. a. pertaining to the ureter
      b. instrument for visual examina-
         tion of the ureter

Exercise 43
1. nephroptosis
2. ureterolithiasis
3. sepsis
4. polyuria
5. nephropexy
6. urinary suppression
7. cystogram
8. enuresis
9. urinary tract infection
10. urinalysis

Exercise 44
Reading Exercise

Exercise 45
1. b.   2. d   3. a

NOTES

CHAPTER 7

Male
Reproductive
System

OUTLINE

ANATOMY, 260

WORD PARTS, 262
Combining Forms, 262
Suffix, 264

MEDICAL TERMS, 265
Disease and Disorder Terms, 265
    Built from Word Parts, 265
    Not Built from Word Parts, 268
Surgical Terms, 271
    Built from Word Parts, 271
    Not Built from Word Parts, 274
Diagnostic Terms, 278
    Not Built from Word Parts, 278
Complementary Terms, 279
    Built from Word Parts, 279
    Not Built from Word Parts, 281
Abbreviations, 285

PRACTICAL APPLICATION, 287
Interact with Medical Documents, 287
Interpret Medical Terms, 289
Read Medical Terms in Use, 289
Comprehend Medical Terms in Use, 290

CHAPTER REVIEW, 290

TABLE 7-1 PROSTATE CANCER, 270

OBJECTIVES

Upon completion of this chapter you will be able to:

1. Identify organs and structures of the male reproductive system.

2. Define and spell word parts related to the male reproductive system.

3. Define, pronounce, and spell disease and disorder terms related to the male reproductive system.

4. Define, pronounce, and spell surgical terms related to the male reproductive system.

5. Define, pronounce, and spell diagnostic terms related to the male reproductive system.

6. Define, pronounce, and spell complementary terms related to the male reproductive system.

7. Interpret the meaning of abbreviations related to the male reproductive system.

8. Interpret, read, and comprehend medical language in simulated medical statements and documents.

ANATOMY

Function

The function of the male reproductive system is to produce, sustain, and transport sperm, the male reproductive cell, and to secrete the hormone testosterone (Figure 7-1).

Organs of the Male Reproductive System

Term	Definition
testis, or testicle (*pl.* testes, or testicles)	primary male sex organs, paired, oval-shaped, and enclosed in a sac called the *scrotum*. The testes produce spermatozoa (sperm cells) and the hormone testosterone.
sperm (spermatozoon, *pl.* spermatozoa)	the microscopic male germ cell, which, when united with the ovum, produces a zygote (fertilized egg) that with subsequent development becomes an *embryo*
testosterone	the principal male sex hormone. Its chief function is to stimulate the development of the male reproductive organs and secondary sex characteristics such as facial hair.
seminiferous tubules.	approximately 900 coiled tubes within the testes in which spermatogenesis occurs
epididymis.	coiled duct atop each of the testes that provides for storage, transit, and maturation of spermatozoa; continuous with the vas deferens
vas deferens, ductus deferens, or seminal duct	duct carrying the sperm from the epididymis to the urethra. The **spermatic cord** encloses each vas deferens with nerves, lymphatics, arteries, and veins. (The urethra also connects with the urinary bladder and carries urine outside the body. A circular muscle constricts during intercourse to prevent urination.)
seminal vesicles	two main glands located at the base of the bladder that open into the vas deferens. The glands secrete a thick fluid, which forms part of the semen.
prostate gland	encircles the upper end of the urethra. The prostate gland secretes a fluid that aids in the movement of the sperm and ejaculation.

PROSTATE
Is derived from the Greek *pro,* meaning **before,** and **statis,** meaning **standing** or **sitting.** Anatomically it is the gland standing before the bladder.

Term	Definition
scrotum	sac suspended on both sides of and just behind the penis. The testes are enclosed in the scrotum
penis	male organ of urination and copulation (sexual intercourse)
glans penis	enlarged tip on the end of the penis
prepuce	fold of skin covering the glans penis in uncircumcised males (foreskin of the penis)
semen	composed of sperm, seminal fluids, and other secretions
genitalia (genitals)	reproductive organs (male or female)

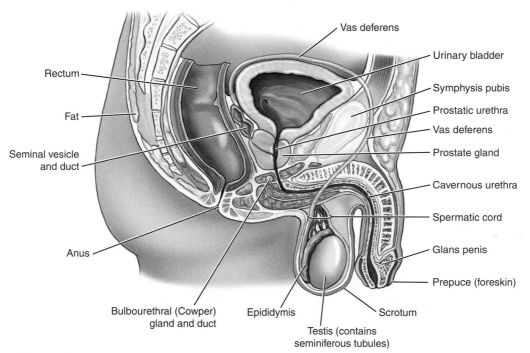

Figure 7-1
Male reproductive organs and associated structures.

EXERCISE 1

Match the anatomic terms in the first column with the correct definitions in the second column.

_____ 1. epididymis

_____ 2. glans penis

_____ 3. penis

_____ 4. prepuce, or foreskin

_____ 5. prostate gland

_____ 6. scrotum

_____ 7. semen

a. sac in which the testes are enclosed

b. structures in testes where the sperm originate

c. duct atop the testis that stores sperm, allows it to mature, and carries it to the vas deferens

d. reproductive organs (male or female)

e. male organ of copulation

_____ 8. seminal vesicles

_____ 9. seminiferous tubules

_____ 10. spermatic cord

_____ 11. testes

_____ 12. vas deferens

_____ 13. genitalia

_____ 14. sperm

_____ 15. testosterone

f. encircles upper end of urethra

g. glands that open into the vas deferens

h. primary male sex organs

i. large tip at end of male organ of copulation

j. the male germ cell

k. fold of skin at tip of penis

l. comprises sperm and secretions

m. male sex hormone

n. encloses the vas deferens with other anatomic structures

o. engorgement of blood

p. duct that carries sperm to the urethra

WORD PARTS

Word parts you need to learn to complete this chapter are listed on the following pages. The exercises at the end of each list help you learn their definitions and spellings.

Combining Forms of the Male Reproductive System

Combining Form	Definition
balan/o	glans penis
epididym/o	epididymis
orchid/o, orchi/o, orch/o, test/o	testis, testicle
prostat/o	prostate gland
vas/o	vessel, duct
vesicul/o	seminal vesicle

EXERCISE 2

Write the definitions of the following combining forms.

1. test/o _____

2. vas/o_____

3. balan/o_____

4. prostat/o _____

5. orch/o _____

6. vesicul/o _____

7. orchi/o_____

8. epididym/o _____

9. orchid/o_____

EXERCISE FIGURE A

Fill in the blanks with combining forms for this diagram of the male reproductive system.

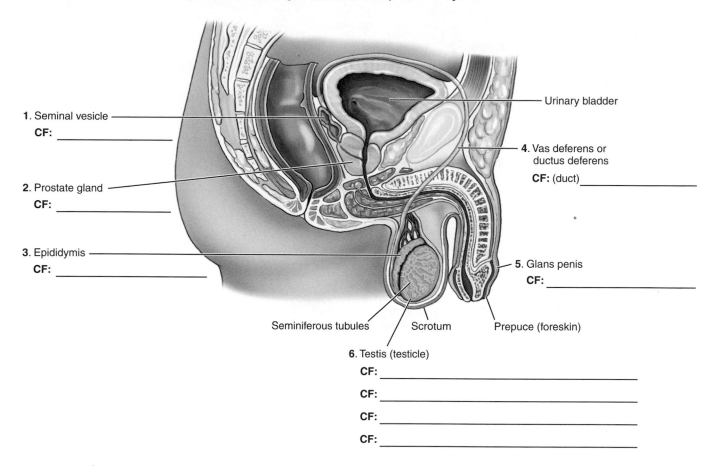

1. Seminal vesicle

    CF: _____

2. Prostate gland

    CF: _____

3. Epididymis

    CF: _____

Urinary bladder

4. Vas deferens or
    ductus deferens

    CF: (duct)_____

5. Glans penis

    CF: _____

Seminiferous tubules   Scrotum   Prepuce (foreskin)

6. Testis (testicle)

    CF: _____

    CF: _____

    CF: _____

    CF: _____

EXERCISE 3

Write the combining form for each of the following terms.

1. vessel, duct   _____

2. prostate
   gland   _____

3. glans
   penis   _____

4. seminal
   vesicle   _____

5. epididymis   _____

6. testicle,
   or testis   a. _____

                  b. _____

                  c. _____

                  d. _____

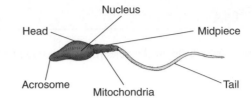

Figure 7-2
Spermatozoon, or sperm. In normal ejaculation there may be as many as 300 to 500 million sperm.

Combining Forms Commonly Used with Male Reproductive System Terms

Combining Form	Definition
andr/o	male
sperm/o, spermat/o	spermatozoon (*pl.* spermatozoa), sperm (Figure 7-2)

EXERCISE 4

Write the definition of the following combining forms.

1. sperm/o _____   3. spermat/o _____

2. andr/o _____

EXERCISE 5

Write the combining form for each of the following.

1. sperm   a. _____   2. male   _____

          b. _____

Suffix

Suffix	Definition
-ism	state of

Refer to Appendix A and Appendix B for alphabetized word parts and their meanings.

EXERCISE 6

Write the definition for the suffix.

1. –ism _____

MEDICAL TERMS

The terms you need to learn to complete this chapter are listed below. The exercises following each list will help you learn the definition and the spelling of each word.

Disease and Disorder Terms

Built from Word Parts

The following terms are built from word parts you have already learned and can be translated literally to find their meanings. Further explanation of terms beyond the definition of their word parts, if needed, is included in parentheses.

Term	Definition
anorchism . . . . (an-OR-kizm)	state of absence of testis (unilateral or bilateral)
balanitis . . . . (*bal*-a-NĪ-tis)	inflammation of the glans penis (Exercise Figure B)
balanorrhea . . . . (*bal*-a-nō-RĒ-a)	discharge from the glans penis
benign prostatic hyperplasia (BPH) . . . . (be-NĪN) (pros-TAT-ik) (*hī*-per-PLĀ-zha)	excessive development pertaining to the prostate gland (nonmalignant enlargement of the prostate gland) (Figure 7-3)
cryptorchidism . . . . (krip-TOR-ki-dizm)	state of hidden testes. (During fetal development, testes are located in the abdominal area near the kidneys. Before birth they move down into the scrotal sac. Failure of the testes to descend from the abdominal cavity into the scrotum before birth results in cryptorchidism, or undescended testicles.) (Exercise Figure C)
epididymitis . . . . (*ep*-i-*did*-i-MĪ-tis)	inflammation of an epididymis
orchiepididymitis . . . . (*or*-kē-ep-i-did-i-MĪ-tis)	inflammation of the testis and epididymis
orchitis, orchiditis, or testitis . . . (or-KĪ-tis) (or-ki-DĪ-tis) (tes-TĪ-tis)	inflammation of the testis or testicle
prostatitis . . . . (pros-ta-TĪ-tis)	inflammation of the prostate gland
prostatocystitis . . . . (pros-*ta*-tō-sis-TĪ-tis)	inflammation of the prostate gland and the bladder
prostatolith . . . . (*pros*-TAT-ō-lith)	stone in the prostate gland
prostatorrhea . . . . (*pros*-ta-tō-RĒ-a)	discharge from the prostate gland
prostatovesiculitis . . . . (*pros*-ta-tō-ves-*ik*-ū-LĪ-tis)	inflammation of the prostate gland and seminal vesicles

EXERCISE FIGURE B

Fill in the blanks with word parts to label the diagram.

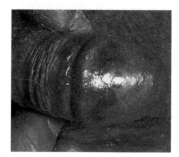

glans penis / inflammation

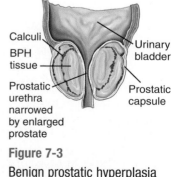

Figure 7-3

Benign prostatic hyperplasia grows inward, causing narrowing of the urethra.

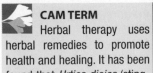

CAM TERM
Herbal therapy uses herbal remedies to promote health and healing. It has been found that *Urtica dioica* (stinging nettles) provides beneficial results in the treatment of symptomatic benign prostatic hyperplasia.

EXERCISE FIGURE C

Fill in the blanks to label the diagram.

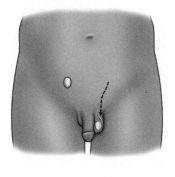

_____ / _____ / _____.
 hidden / testis / state of
The *arrow* shows the path the testis takes in its descent to the scrotal sac before birth.

EXERCISE 7

Practice saying aloud each of the disease and disorder terms built from word parts on p. 265.

 To hear the terms select Chapter 7, Chapter Exercises, Pronunciation.

☐ Place a check mark in the box when you have completed this exercise.

EXERCISE 8

Analyze and define the following disease and disorder terms.

1. prostatolith _____

2. balanitis _____

3. (a) orchitis, (b) orchiditis, or (c) testitis _____

4. prostatovesiculitis _____

5. prostatocystitis _____

6. orchiepididymitis _____

7. prostatorrhea _____

8. epididymitis _____

9. (benign) prostatic hyperplasia _____

10. cryptorchidism _____

11. balanorrhea _____

12. prostatitis _____

13. anorchism _____

EXERCISE 9

Build disease and disorder terms for the following definitions with the word parts you have learned.

1. inflammation of the prostate gland and urinary bladder

   _____ / ___ / _____ / ___
   WR   / CV / WR   / S

2. stone in the prostate gland

   _____ / ___ / _____
   WR   / CV / WR

3. inflammation of the testis   a. _____ / ___
                                      WR   / S

   b. _____ / ___
      WR   / S

   c. _____ / ___
      WR   / S

4. (a nonmalignant) excessive development pertaining to the prostate gland

   benign _____ / ___   _____ / ___
          WR   / S   P   / S(WR)

5. state of hidden testes

   _____ / _____ / ___
   WR   / WR   / S

6. inflammation of the prostate gland and seminal vesicles

   _____ / ___ / _____ / ___
   WR   / CV / WR   / S

7. state of absence of testis

   _____ / _____ / ___
   P   / WR   / S

8. inflammation of the prostate gland

   _____ / ___
   WR   / S

9. inflammation of the testis and the epididymis

   _____ / _____ / ___
   WR   / WR   / S

10. discharge from the glans penis

    _____ / ___ / ___
    WR   / CV / S

11. inflammation of an epididymis

    _____ / ___
    WR   / S

12. inflammation of the glans penis

    _____ / ___
    WR   / S

13. discharge from the prostate gland

    _____ / ___ / ___
    WR   / CV / S

ERECTILE DYSFUNCTION
Oral therapies, such as sildenafil (Viagra), vardenafil (Levitra), and tadalafil (Cialis) are currently first-line treatment for erectile dysfunction and work by relaxing smooth muscle cells and, as such, increasing the flow of blood in the genital area. Second-line treatment includes penile self-injectable drugs and vacuum devices. Surgical implantation of a penile prosthesis is available for men who cannot use or who have not responded to other treatments.

EXERCISE 10

Spell each of the disease and disorder terms built from word parts on p. 265 by having someone dictate them to you.

 To hear and spell the terms select Chapter 7, Chapter Exercises, Spelling. You may type the terms on the screen or write them below in the spaces provided.

☐ Place a check mark in the box if you have completed this exercise using your CD-ROM.

1. _____   9. _____

2. _____   10. _____

3. _____   11. _____

4. _____   12. _____

5. _____   13. _____

6. _____   14. _____

7. _____   15. _____

8. _____

Disease and Disorder Terms

Not Built from Word Parts

In some of the following terms, you may recognize word parts you have already learned; however, the full meaning of the terms cannot be discerned by the definition of their word parts.

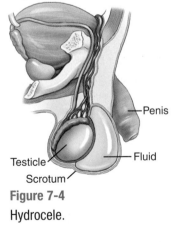

Figure 7-4
Hydrocele.

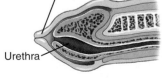

Figure 7-5
Phimosis. Cross section of the penis showing foreskin covering the opening.

Term	Definition
erectile dysfunction (ED) . . . . . (e-REK-tĭl) (dis-FUNK-shun)	the inability of the male to attain or maintain an erection sufficient to perform sexual intercourse (formerly called **impotence**)
hydrocele . . . . (HĪ-drō-sēl)	scrotal swelling caused by a collection of fluid (Figure 7-4)
phimosis . . . . (fi-MŌ-sis)	a tightness of the prepuce (foreskin of the penis) that prevents its retraction over the glans penis; it may be congenital or a result of balanitis. Circumcision is the usual treatment (Figure 7-5).
priapism . . . . (PRĪ-a-pizm)	persistent abnormal erection of the penis accompanied by pain and tenderness
prostate cancer . . . . (PROS-tāt) (KAN-cer)	cancer of the prostate gland (Table 7-1)
testicular carcinoma . . . . (tes-TIK-ū-ler) (*kar*-si-NŌ-ma)	cancer of the testicle

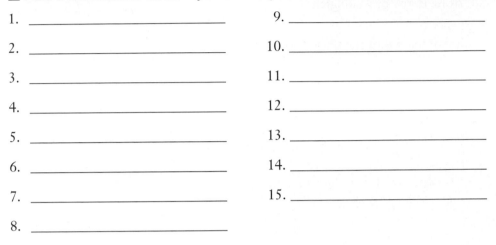

Term	Definition
testicular torsion (tes-TIK-ū-ler) (TOR-shun)	twisting of the spermatic cord causing decreased blood flow to the testis; occurs most often during puberty and often presents with a sudden onset of severe testicular or scrotal pain. Because of lack of blood flow to the testis, it is often considered a surgical emergency.
varicocele (VAR-i-kō-sēl)	enlarged veins of the spermatic cord (Figure 7-6)

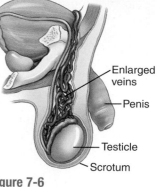

Figure 7-6
Varicocele.

TABLE 7-1

Prostate Cancer

Prostate cancer is the most commonly diagnosed cancer in men and the second most common cause of cancer death among men in the United States. Approximately 95% of all cancers of the prostate are adenocarcinomas arising from epithelial cells.

Diagnostic Procedures
1. Digital rectal examination (DRE)
2. Prostate-specific antigen (PSA)
3. Transrectal ultrasound
4. Transrectal ultrasonically guided biopsy
5. Magnetic resonance imaging with endorectal surface coil

Treatment
Treatment depends on the stage of the prostate cancer, the age of the patient, and choices of treatment by the patient and his physician. Options include the following:
1. **Radical prostatectomy (RP),** which may be performed by retropubic or perineal routes, laparoscopically, or with the use of robotic-assisted devices
2. **Radiation therapy,** which may be performed with an external beam or with radioactive seeds (brachytherapy)
3. **Bilateral orchidectomy** or **hormonal therapy** to reduce the production of testosterone, which fuels the growth of prostate cancer
4. **Chemotherapy,** treating cancer with drugs
5. **Watchful waiting,** with the intent to pursue active therapy on disease progression

Progression of Prostate Cancer

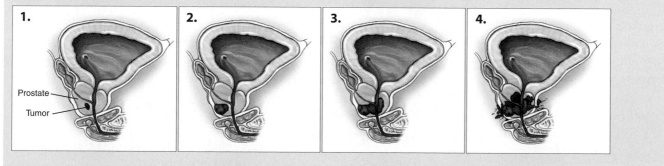

EXERCISE 11

Practice saying aloud each of the disease and disorder terms not built from word parts on pp. 268-269.

 To hear the terms select Chapter 7, Chapter Exercises, Pronunciation.

☐ Place a check mark in the box when you have completed this exercise.

EXERCISE 12

Fill in the blanks with the correct terms.

1. Another way of referring to cancer of the testicle is _____ _____.

2. A tightness of the prepuce is called _____.

3. The condition of having enlarged veins of the spermatic cord is known medically as a(n) _____.

4. A scrotal swelling caused by a collection of fluid is called a(n) _____.

5. Cancer of the prostate gland is called _____ _____.

6. Inability of the man to attain or maintain an erection is called _____ _____.

7. Persistent abnormal erection is called _____.

8. _____ _____ is the twisting of the spermatic cord.

EXERCISE 13

Match the terms in the first column with the correct definitions in the second column.

_____ 1. varicocele

_____ 2. phimosis

_____ 3. testicular carcinoma

_____ 4. erectile dysfunction

_____ 5. hydrocele

_____ 6. prostate cancer

_____ 7. testicular torsion

_____ 8. priapism

a. scrotal swelling caused by a collection of fluid

b. inability to attain or maintain an erection

c. a condition that prevents the retraction of the prepuce

d. enlarged veins of the spermatic cord

e. cancer of the testicle

f. cancer of the prostate gland

g. stone in the prostate gland

h. persistent abnormal erection

i. twisting of the spermatic cord

EXERCISE 14

Spell each of the disease and disorder terms not built from word parts on pp. 268-269 by having someone dictate them to you.

 To hear and spell the terms select Chapter 7, Chapter Exercises, Spelling. You may type the terms on the screen or write them below in the spaces provided.

☐ Place a check mark in the box if you have completed this exercise using your CD-ROM.

1. _____   5. _____

2. _____   6. _____

3. _____   7. _____

4. _____   8. _____

Surgical Terms

Built from Word Parts

The following terms are built from word parts you have already learned and can be translated literally to find their meanings. Further explanation of terms beyond the definitions of their word parts, if needed, is included in parentheses.

Term	Definition
balanoplasty . . . . (BAL-a-nō-*plas*-tē)	surgical repair of the glans penis
epididymectomy . . . . (*ep*-i-*did*-i-MEK-to-mē)	excision of an epididymis
orchidectomy, orchiectomy . . . . (*or*-kid-EK-to-mē) (*or*-kē-EK-to-mē)	excision of the testes (bilateral orchidectomy also is called **castration**)
orchidopexy, orchiopexy . . . . . . (OR-kid-ō-pek-sē) (OR-kē-ō-pek-sē)	surgical fixation of a testicle (performed to bring undescended testicle[s] into the scrotum)
orchidotomy, orchiotomy . . . . . . (*or*-kid-OT-o-mē), (*or*-kē-OT-o-mē)	incision into a testis
orchioplasty . . . . (OR-kē-ō-*plas*-tē)	surgical repair of a testis
prostatectomy . . . . (*pros*-ta-TEK-to-mē)	excision of the prostate gland
prostatocystotomy . . . . (pros-*tat*-ō-sis-TOT-o-mē)	incision into the prostate gland and bladder
prostatolithotomy . . . . (pros-*tat*-ō-li-THOT-o-mē)	incision into the prostate gland to remove a stone
prostatovesiculectomy . . . . (*pros*-tat-ō-ves-*ik*-ū-LEK-to-mē)	excision of the prostate gland and seminal vesicles

Fill in the blanks to label the diagram.

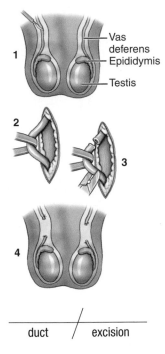

_____ / _____
duct   /   excision

1. incision is made into the covering of the vas
2. vas is exposed
3. segment of vas is excised
4. vas is replaced and skin is sutured

Surgical Terms—cont'd
Built from Word Parts

Term	Definition
vasectomy . . . . (va-SEK-to-mē)	excision of a duct (partial excision of the vas deferens bilaterally, resulting in male sterilization) (Exercise Figure D)
vasovasostomy . . . . (*vas*-ō-vā-SOS-to-mē)	creation of artificial openings between ducts (the severed ends of the vas deferens are reconnected in an attempt to restore fertility in men who have had a vasectomy)
vesiculectomy . . . . (ve-*sik*-ū-LEK-to-mē)	excision of the seminal vesicle(s)

EXERCISE 15

Practice saying aloud each of the surgical terms built from word parts above and on the previous page.

To hear the terms select, Chapter 7, Chapter Exercises, Pronunciation.

☐ Place a check mark in the box when you have completed this exercise.

EXERCISE 16

Analyze and define the following surgical terms.

1. vasectomy _____

2. prostatocystotomy _____

3. orchidotomy, orchiotomy _____

4. epididymectomy _____

5. orchidopexy, orchiopexy _____

6. prostatovesiculectomy _____

7. orchioplasty_____

8. vesiculectomy _____

9. prostatectomy_____

10. balanoplasty _____

11. vasovasostomy_____

12. orchidectomy, orchiectomy_____

13. prostatolithotomy_____

EXERCISE 17

Build surgical terms for the following definitions by using the word parts you have learned.

1. excision of the testis
   a. _____ / _____
        WR   S
   b. _____ / _____
        WR   S

2. surgical repair of the glans penis
   _____ / ____ / _____
     WR   CV   S

3. incision into the prostate gland and bladder
   _____ / ___ / _____ / ___ / _____
     WR   CV   WR   CV   S

4. excision of the seminal vesicle(s)
   _____ / _____
     WR   S

5. incision into the prostate gland to remove a stone
   _____ / ___ / _____ / ___ / _____
     WR   CV   WR   CV   S

6. incision into a testis
   a. _____ / ____ / _____
        WR   CV   S
   b. _____ / ____ / _____
        WR   CV   S

7. excision of the epididymis
   _____ / _____
     WR   S

8. surgical repair of a testis
   _____ / ____ / _____
     WR   CV   S

9. excision of the prostate gland
   _____ / _____
     WR   S

10. excision of a duct (partial excision of the vas deferens)
    _____ / _____
      WR   S

11. excision of the prostate gland and seminal vesicles
    _____ / ___ / _____ / _____
      WR   CV   WR   S

12. surgical fixation of a testicle
    a. _____ / ____ / _____
         WR   CV   S
    b. _____ / ____ / _____
         WR   CV   S

13. creation of artificial openings between the severed ends of the vas deferens

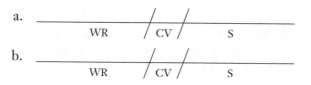
    _____ / ___ / _____ / ___ / _____
      WR   CV   WR   CV   S

EXERCISE 18

Spell each of the surgical terms built from word parts on pp. 271-272 by having someone dictate them to you.

 To hear and spell the terms select Chapter 7, Chapter Exercises, Spelling. You may type the terms on the screen or write them below in the spaces provided.

☐ Place a check mark in the box if you have completed this exercise using your CD-ROM.

1. _____   9. _____

2. _____   10. _____

3. _____   11. _____

4. _____   12. _____

5. _____   13. _____

6. _____   14. _____

7. _____   15. _____

8. _____   16. _____

Surgical Terms

Not Built from Word Parts

In some of the following terms, you may recognize word parts you have already learned; however, the full meaning of the terms cannot be discerned by the definition of their word parts.

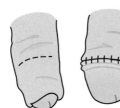

Figure 7-7
Circumcision.

Term	Definition
circumcision . . . . (*ser*-kum-SI-zhun)	surgical removal of the prepuce (foreskin) (Figure 7-7)
hydrocelectomy . . . . (*hī*-drō-sē-LEK-to-mē)	surgical removal of a hydrocele
radical prostatectomy (RP) . . . . (RAD-i-kel) (*pros*-ta-TEK-to-mē)	excision of the prostate gland with its capsule, seminal vesicles, vas deferens, and sometimes pelvic lymph nodes; performed by a retropubic or perineal approach, or laparoscopically; used to treat prostate cancer (Figure 7-8, *B*)
suprapubic prostatectomy . . . . . (sū-pra-PŪ-bik) (*pros*-ta-TEK-to-mē)	excision of the prostate gland through an abdominal incision made above the pubic bone and through an incision in the bladder; used to treat benign prostatic hyperplasia and prostate cancer (Figure 7-8, *A*) (also called **suprapubic transvesical prostatectomy**)

Term	Definition
transurethral incision of the prostate gland (TUIP)......... (trans-ū-RĒ-thral) (in-SIZH-en) (PROS-tāt)	a surgical procedure that widens the urethra by making a few small incisions in the bladder neck and the prostate gland. No prostate tissue is removed. TUIP may be used instead of TURP when the prostate gland is less enlarged.
transurethral microwave thermotherapy (TUMT)......... (trans-ū-RĒ-thral) (MĪ-krō-wāv) (*ther*-mō-THER-a-pē)	a treatment that eliminates excess tissue present in benign prostatic hyperplasia by using heat generated by microwave
transurethral resection of the prostate gland (TURP)......... (trans-ū-RĒ-thral) (rē-SEK-shun) (PROS-tāt)	successive pieces of the prostate gland tissue are resected by using a resectoscope inserted through the urethra. The capsule is left intact; usually performed when the enlarged prostate gland interferes with urination (Figure 7-9).

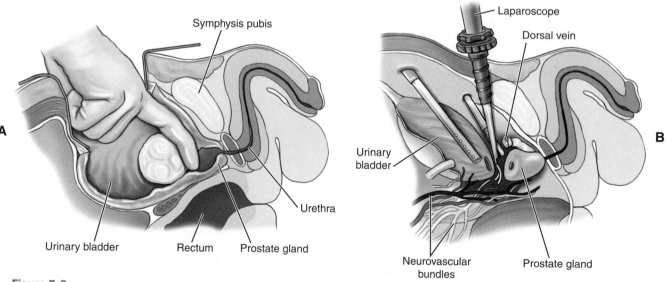

Figure 7-8

A, A large incision surgery. In suprapubic prostatectomy, the surgeon approaches the prostate gland through an incision in the urinary bladder and uses a finger to remove the hyperplastic tissue. A similar incision is used for radical retropubic prostectomy to treat cancer of the prostate. **B,** A small incision surgery. Laparoscopic radical prostatectomy and/or robotic-assisted prostatectomy is a new procedure used to treat early stages of prostate cancer.

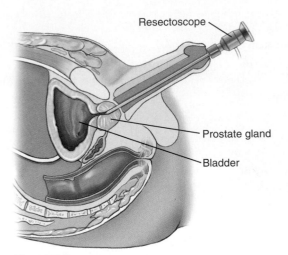

Figure 7-9

Transurethral resection of the prostate gland is used to treat benign prostatic hyperplasia. A resectoscope is inserted through the urethra to the prostate gland. The end of the instrument is equipped to remove pieces of the enlarged prostate gland to relieve bladder outlet obstruction.

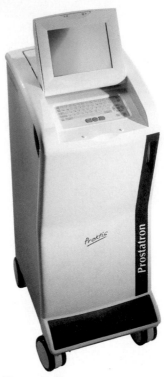

Figure 7-10

Cooled ThermoTherapy device used to treat benign prostatic hyperplasia. Cooled ThermoTherapy delivers precise microwavable energy to heat and destroy prostate tissue while a cooling mechanism protects surrounding tissue.

Surgical Treatments for Benign Prostatic Hyperplasia

Incisional
Transurethral resection of the prostate gland (TURP)
Prostatectomy
Transurethral incision of the prostate gland (TUIP)

Thermotherapy
Transurethral microwave thermotherapy (TUMT)
Cooled ThermoTherapy (Figure 7-10)

Laser
Transurethral laser incision of the prostate gland (TULIP)
Visual laser incision of the prostate gland (VLIP)
Photoselective vaporization of the prostate gland (PVP)

EXERCISE 19

Practice saying aloud each of the surgical terms not built from word parts on pp. 274-275.

 To hear the terms select Chapter 7, Chapter Exercises, Pronunciation.

☐ Place a check mark in the box when you have completed this exercise.

EXERCISE 20

Fill in the blanks with the correct term.

1. The surgery performed to remove the prostate gland through the urinary bladder and an abdominal incision is _____ _____.

2. The surgical procedure performed to remove the prepuce is called a(n) _____.

3. The surgical removal of the prostate gland and surrounding structures, sometimes including pelvic lymph nodes, is called _____ _____.

4. Surgical removal of a hydrocele is _____.

5. _____ _____ _____ is a treatment for benign prostatic hyperplasia that uses heat generated by microwave.

6. A surgical procedure for benign prostatic hyperplasia that widens the urethra by making small incisions is called _____ _____ of the _____ _____.

7. Pieces of prostate gland tissue are removed with a resectoscope during the surgical procedure called _____ _____ of the _____ _____.

EXERCISE 21

Spell each of the surgical terms not built from word parts on pp. 274-275 by having someone dictate them to you.

 To hear and spell the terms select Chapter 7, Chapter Exercises, Spelling. You may type the terms on the screen or write them below in the spaces provided.

☐ Place a check mark in the box if you have completed this exercise using your CD-ROM.

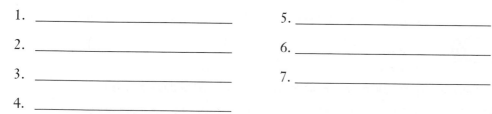

1. _____   5. _____

2. _____   6. _____

3. _____   7. _____

4. _____

Diagnostic Terms
Not Built from Word Parts

In some of the following terms, you may recognize word parts you have already learned; however, the full meaning of the terms cannot be discerned by the definition of their word parts.

Term	Definition
DIAGNOSTIC IMAGING	

transrectal ultrasound . . . .
    (trans-REK-tal)
    (UL-tra-sound)
	an ultrasound procedure used to diagnose prostate cancer. Sound waves are sent and received by a transducer in the form of a probe that is placed into the rectum. The sound waves are transformed into an image of the prostate gland.

LABORATORY	

prostate-specific antigen
 (PSA) . . . .
    (PROS-tāt) (spe-SIF-ik)
    (AN-ti-jen)
	a blood test that measures the level of prostate-specific antigen in the blood. Elevated test results may indicate the presence of prostate cancer or excess prostate tissue, as found in benign prostatic hyperplasia.

OTHER	

digital rectal examination
 (DRE) . . . .
    (DIJ-i-tal) (REK-tal)
    (eg-*zam*-i-NĀ-shun)
	a physical examination in which the physician inserts a finger into the rectum and feels for the size and shape of the prostate gland through the rectal wall. Used to screen for BPH and cancer of the prostate. BPH usually presents as a uniform, nontender enlargement, whereas cancer usually presents as a stony hard nodule.

EXERCISE 22

Practice saying aloud each of the diagnostic terms not built from word parts above.

 To hear the terms select Chapter 7, Chapter Exercises, Pronunciation.

☐ Place a check mark in the box when you have completed this exercise.

EXERCISE 23

Fill in the blanks with the correct terms.

1. A physical examination in which the physician feels for the size and shape of the prostate gland through the rectal wall is called _____ _____ _____.

2. A blood test that, when elevated, may indicate the presence of prostate cancer is called_____ _____.

3. A diagnostic ultrasound procedure used to obtain images of the prostate gland is called _____ _____.

EXERCISE 24

Spell each of the diagnostic terms not built from word parts on p. 278 by having someone dictate them to you.

To hear and spell the terms select Chapter 7, Chapter Exercises, Spelling. You may type the terms on the screen or write them below in the spaces provided.

☐ Place a check mark in the box if you have completed this exercise using your CD-ROM.

1. _____   3. _____

2. _____

Complementary Terms

Built from Word Parts

The following terms are built from word parts you have already learned and can be translated literally to find their meanings. Further explanation of terms beyond the definitions of their word parts, if needed, is included in parentheses.

Term	Definition
andropathy............... (an-DROP-a-thē)	disease of the male (specific to the male, such as testitis)
aspermia.................. (a-SPER-mē-a)	condition of without sperm (or semen or ejaculation)
oligospermia.............. (ol-i-gō-SPER-mē-a)	condition of scanty sperm (in the semen; may contribute to infertility)
spermatolysis............. (sper-ma-TOL-i-sis)	dissolution (destruction) of sperm

AZOOSPERMIA
refers to the lack of live sperm in the semen, whereas aspermia generally means no semen or ejaculation and therefore no sperm. Azoospermia and oligospermia are terms frequently used in relation to male infertility.

EXERCISE 25

Practice saying aloud each of the complementary terms not built from word parts above.

To hear the terms select Chapter 7, Chapter Exercises, Pronunciation.

☐ Place a check mark in the box when you have completed this exercise.

EXERCISE 26

Analyze and define the following complementary terms.

1. oligospermia _____

2. andropathy _____

3. spermatolysis_____

4. aspermia _____

EXERCISE 27

Build the complementary terms for the following definitions by using the word parts you have learned.

1. dissolution (destruction) of sperm

_____ / _____ / _____
  WR   CV   S

2. condition of without spermatozoa (or semen or ejaculate)

_____ / _____ / _____
  P   WR   S

3. disease of the male

_____ / _____ / _____
  WR   CV   S

4. condition of scanty sperm (in the semen)

_____ / ____ / _____ / _____
  WR   CV   WR   S

EXERCISE 28

Spell each of the complementary terms built from word parts on p. 279 by having someone dictate them to you.

 To hear and spell the terms select Chapter 7, Chapter Exercises, Spelling. You may type the terms on the screen or write them below in the spaces provided.

☐ Place a check mark in the box if you have completed this exercise using your CD-ROM.

1. _____   3. _____

2. _____   4. _____

Complementary Terms

Not Built from Word Parts

In some of the following terms, you may recognize word parts you have already learned; however, the full meaning of the terms cannot be discerned by the definition of their word parts.

Term	Definition
acquired immunodeficiency syndrome (AIDS) . . . . (*im*-ū-nō-de-FISH-en-sē) (SIN-drōm)	a disease that affects the body's immune system, transmitted by exchange of body fluid during the sexual act, reuse of contaminated needles, or receiving contaminated blood transfusions (also called **acquired immune deficiency syndrome**)
artificial insemination . . . . (ar-ti-FISH-al) (in-sem-i-NĀ-shun)	introduction of semen into the vagina by artificial means
chlamydia . . . . (kla-MID-ē-a)	a sexually transmitted disease, sometimes referred to as a **silent STD** because many people are not aware they have the disease. Symptoms that occur when the disease becomes serious are painful urination and discharge from the penis in men and genital itching, vaginal discharge, and bleeding between menstrual periods in women. The causative agent is *C. trachomatis.*
coitus . . . . (KŌ-i-tus)	sexual intercourse between male and female (also called **copulation**)
condom . . . . (KON-dum)	cover for the penis worn during coitus to prevent conception and the spread of sexually transmitted disease
ejaculation . . . . (ē-jak-ū-LĀ-shun)	ejection of semen from the male urethra
genital herpes . . . . (JEN-i-tal) (HER-pēz)	sexually transmitted disease caused by *Herpesvirus hominis* type 2 (also called **herpes simplex virus**)
gonads . . . . (GŌ-nads)	male and female sex glands
gonorrhea . . . . (gon-ō-RĒ-a)	contagious, inflammatory sexually transmitted disease caused by a bacterial organism that affects the mucous membranes of the genitourinary system
heterosexual . . . . (*het*-er-ō-SEKS-shū-al)	person who is attracted to a member of the opposite sex
homosexual . . . . (*hō*-mō-SEKS-shū-al)	person who is attracted to a member of the same sex

Complementary Terms—*cont'd*
Not Built from Word Parts

HUMAN PAPILLOMAVIRUS
infection in women is thought
to be a major cause of cervical
cancer.

Term	Definition
human immunodeficiency virus (HIV) (*im*-ū-nō-de-FISH-en-sē)	a type of retrovirus that causes AIDS. HIV infects T-helper cells of the immune system, allowing for opportunistic infections such as candidiasis, *Pneumocystis jiroveci* pneumonia, tuberculosis, and Kaposi sarcoma
human papillomavirus (HPV) (HŪ-man) (*pap*-i-LŌ-ma-*vi*-rus)	a prevalent sexually transmitted disease causing benign or cancerous growths in male and female genitals (also called **venereal warts**)
orgasm (ŌR-gazm)	climax of sexual stimulation
prosthesis (pros-THĒ-sis)	an artificial replacement of an absent body part (a penile prosthesis may be implanted to treat erectile dysfunction if first-line therapies are not effective)
puberty (PŪ-ber-tē)	period when secondary sex characteristics develop and the ability to reproduce sexually begins
sexually transmitted disease (STD) (SEKS-ū-al-ē) (TRANS-mi-ted) (di-ZĒZ)	diseases, such as syphilis, gonorrhea, and genital herpes, transmitted during sexual contact (also called **venereal disease** and **sexually transmitted infection [STI]**)
sterilization (star-i-li-ZĀ-shun)	process that renders an individual unable to produce offspring
syphilis (SIF-i-lis)	chronic infection caused by the bacterium *Treponema pallidum*, which usually is transmitted by sexual contact, may be acquired in utero, or (less often) contracted through direct contact with infected tissue. If untreated, the infection usually progresses through three clinical stages with a latent period. The initial local infection quickly becomes systemic with widespread dissemination of the bacterium.
trichomoniasis (*trik*-ō-mō-NĪ-a-sis)	a sexually transmitted disease caused by a one-cell organism, *Trichomonas*. It infects the genitourinary tract. Men may be asymptomatic or may develop urethritis, an enlarged prostate gland, or epididymitis. Women have vaginal itching, dysuria, and vaginal or urethral discharge.

**LIST OF MALE AND
FEMALE SEXUALLY
TRANSMITTED DISEASES**
acquired immunodeficiency
    syndrome
human immunodeficiency virus
    infections
syphilis
genital herpes
venereal warts (human
    papillomavirus)
gonorrhea
chlamydia
trichomoniasis
cytomegalovirus infections

VENEREAL
is derived from **Venus,**
the goddess of love. In
ancient times it was noted that
the disease was part of the misfortunes of love.

EXERCISE 29

Practice saying aloud each of the complementary terms not built from word parts on pp. 281-282.

 To hear the terms select Chapter 7, Chapter Exercises, Pronunciation.

☐ Place a check mark in the box when you have completed this exercise.

EXERCISE 30

Write the definitions of the following complementary terms.

1. puberty _____

2. orgasm _____

3. gonorrhea _____

4. homosexual _____

5. coitus _____

6. genital herpes _____

7. heterosexual _____

8. syphilis _____

9. ejaculation _____

10. gonads _____

11. sexually transmitted disease _____

12. sterilization _____

13. human papillomavirus _____

14. acquired immunodeficiency syndrome _____

15. trichomoniasis _____

16. artificial insemination _____

17. chlamydia _____

18. condom _____

19. prosthesis _____

20. human immunodeficiency virus _____

EXERCISE 31

Match the terms in the first column with their correct definitions in the second column.

_____ 1. coitus

_____ 2. ejaculation

_____ 3. human papillomavirus

_____ 4. gonads

_____ 5. genital herpes

_____ 6. gonorrhea

_____ 7. heterosexual

_____ 8. orgasm

_____ 9. condom

_____ 10. prosthesis

a. male and female sex glands

b. climax of sexual stimulation

c. one who is attracted to a member of the opposite sex

d. STD caused by _Herpesvirus hominis_ type 2

e. ejection of semen

f. an artificial replacement for an absent body part

g. sexual intercourse between man and woman

h. venereal warts

i. contagious and inflammatory STD

j. cover for the penis worn during coitus

k. one who is attracted to a member of the same sex

EXERCISE 32

Match the terms in the first column with their correct definitions in the second column.

_____ 1. homosexual

_____ 2. STD

_____ 3. sterilization

_____ 4. syphilis

_____ 5. puberty

_____ 6. AIDS

_____ 7. trichomoniasis

_____ 8. artificial insemination

_____ 9. chlamydia

_____ 10. HIV

a. abbreviation for diseases such as syphilis, gonorrhea, and genital herpes

b. a disease that affects the body's immune system

c. a type of retrovirus that causes AIDS

d. a chronic infection that can be transmitted by sexual contact or acquired in utero

e. introduction of semen into the vagina by means other than intercourse

f. one who is attracted to members of the same sex

g. a prevalent STD caused by a bacterium, _C. trachomatis_ (silent STD)

h. process rendering an individual unable to produce offspring

i. an STD caused by a one-cell organism, _Trichomonas_

j. period when the ability to sexually reproduce begins

EXERCISE 33

Spell each of the complementary terms not built from word parts on pp. 281-282 by having someone dictate them to you.

 To hear and spell the terms select Chapter 7, Chapter Exercises, Spelling. You may type the terms on the screen or write them below in the spaces provided.

☐ Place a check mark in the box if you have completed this exercise using your CD-ROM.

1. _____   11. _____

2. _____   12. _____

3. _____   13. _____

4. _____   14. _____

5. _____   15. _____

6. _____   16. _____

7. _____   17. _____

8. _____   18. _____

9. _____   19. _____

10. _____   20. _____

Refer to Appendix E for pharmacology terms related to the male reproductive system.

Abbreviations

AIDS.....................	acquired immunodeficiency syndrome
BPH	benign prostatic hyperplasia
DRE	digital rectal examination
ED	erectile dysfunction
HIV......................	human immunodeficiency virus
HPV	human papillomavirus
PSA	prostate-specific antigen
RP	radical prostatectomy
STD	sexually transmitted disease
TUIP.....................	transurethral incision of the prostate
TUMT.....................	transurethral microwave thermotherapy
TURP	transurethral resection of the prostate

Refer to Appendix D for a complete list of abbreviations.

EXERCISE 34

Write the meaning of the abbreviations in the following sentences.

1. The physician performed a **DRE** _____ _____ _____ on the patient to assist in diagnosing **BPH** _____ _____ _____. Surgical treatments for BPH include prostatectomy, **TURP** _____ _____ of the _____ gland, **TUMT** _____ _____ _____, and **TUIP** _____ _____ of the_____ gland.

2. **AIDS** _____ _____ _____ is an **STD** _____ _____ _____. **HIV** _____ _____ _____ is a type of retrovirus that causes AIDS. **HPV** _____ _____ is an STD that causes female and male venereal warts.

3. **PSA** _____ _____ is a laboratory test used to diagnose cancer of the prostate.

4. **RP** _____ _____ is a surgical procedure to treat prostate cancer.

5. **ED** _____ _____ was formerly referred to as impotence.

PRACTICAL APPLICATION

EXERCISE 35 *Interact with Medical Documents*

A. Complete the emergency department report by writing the medical terms in the blanks. Use the list of definitions with the corresponding numbers.

University Hospital and Medical Center
4700 North Main Street • Wellness, Arizona 54321 • (987) 555-3210

PATIENT NAME: Andrew Nguyen
DATE OF BIRTH: 07/27/19XX

CASE NUMBER: 19504-MRSS
DATE OF ADMISSION: 08/23/20XX

Emergency Department Report

CHIEF COMPLAINT: Severe lower abdominal pain and the inability to void for the past 12 hours.

PRESENT ILLNESS: Andrew Nguyen is a 75-year-old Asian American man who came into the emergency department at 3 AM stating that he was in great pain and could not urinate. He had not been seen by a physician for several years but claimed to be in good health except for "a little high blood pressure." The patient reports urinary frequency, 1. _____ x 2, hesitancy, intermittency, and diminished force and caliber of the urinary stream. He also has postvoid dribbling and the sensation of not having completely emptied the bladder. Earlier today, he had 2. _____ at the end of urination.

MEDICATION ALLERGIES: None

CURRENT MEDICATIONS: Benadryl 25 mg at bedtime.

PHYSICAL EXAM: Temperature, 98.6. Blood pressure, 140/90. Pulse, 98. Respirations, 24. Palpation of the abdomen shows a suprapubic mass approximately three fingerbreadths below the umbilicus, dull to percussion and slightly tender.

IMPRESSION: 3. _____ bladder distention caused by urinary outlet obstruction, probably from 4. _____
_____ _____.

PLAN:
Indwelling Foley catheter for relief of urinary obstruction.
5. _____ consult.

Eleanor Adams, MD

EA/mcm

---

1. night urination
2. blood in the urine
3. pertaining to urine

4. nonmalignant excessive development pertaining to the prostate gland (enlargement of the prostate gland)
5. study of the urinary tract

EXERCISE **35**   *Interact with Medical Documents—cont'd*

B. Read the letter reviewing a patient's progress and answer the questions following it.

Michigan Oncology Group
44976 East Lincoln
Detroit, MI 97654

January 23, 20XX

Kathryn S. Marcus, MD
Internal Medicine Services
2301 North Brinkley
Detroit, MI 97654

RE: Brindley, John F.
DOB: 08/24/1941

Dear Dr. Marcus:

It is now three years since he had brachytherapy using radioactive seeds for his T2a, Gleason 5 prostate cancer. He continues voiding uncomfortably with nocturia and a prostate obstructive score of 3.

His weight is stable at 209 pounds and blood pressure is 122/82. He has no adenopathy. DRE reveals a smooth prostate with no nodules and no suspicious areas. There is a slight asymmetry with greater prominence on the right side. The PSA remains 0.1 as of August 20, 20XX.

He is doing well and is likely cured of his cancer. He continues to experience some erectile dysfunction. I would like to continue seeing him on a yearly basis with a repeat PSA. He will continue seeing you as needed.

_____

Joseph P. Potter, MD

JPP/bko

---

1. In addition to uncomfortable urination, the patient's symptoms include:
   a. pus in the urine
   b. excessive urine
   c. night urination
   d. blood in the urine

2. Brachytherapy using radioactive seeds were used to treat:
   a. benign prostatic hyperplasia
   b. prostate cancer
   c. erectile dysfunction

3. Which diagnostic test revealed "a smooth prostate"?
   a. transrectal ultrasound
   b. prostate-specific antigen
   c. digital rectal examination

4. Three years after treatment, the patient:
   a. appears to be cancer free
   b. shows disease progression
   c. has been recommended for a radical prostatectomy

EXERCISE 36 *Interpret Medical Terms*

To test your understanding of the terms introduced in this chapter, circle the words that correctly complete the sentences. The italicized words refer to the correct answer.

1. A *discharge from the glans penis* is referred to medically as (**balanitis, balanorrhea, balanorrhaphy**).

2. The surgical procedure circumcision is the removal of the *foreskin*, or (**glans penis, testes, prepuce**).

3. *A person who is attracted to a member of the opposite sex* is (**heterosexual, homosexual**).

4. The patient had a diagnosis of (**oligospermia, phimosis, impotence**), or *a narrowing of the opening of the prepuce*.

5. The *operation for the surgical fixation of the testicle* is (**orchidopexy, orchidotomy, orchioplasty**).

6. An *artificial replacement* or (**condom, prosthesis, artificial insemination**) may be used to correct erectile dysfunction when first-line therapies are not effective.

7. The following is a treatment for benign prostatic hyperplasia using heat (**transurethral prostatectomy, suprapubic prostatectomy, transurethral microwave thermotherapy**).

EXERCISE 37 *Read Medical Terms in Use*

Practice pronunciation of the terms by reading the following medical document. Use the pronunciation key following the medical term to assist you in saying the word.

 To hear these terms select Chapter 7, Chapter Exercises, Read Medical Terms in Use.

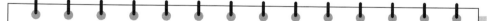

A 62-year-old man was found to have an elevated **prostate-specific antigen** (PROS-tāt) (spe-SIF-ik) (AN-ti-jen) test during a routine physical examination. At the age of 42 years he underwent a **vasectomy** (va-SEK-to-mē). The patient denies having nocturia or any significant change in his urinary stream. **Digital rectal examination** (DIJ-i-tal) (REK-tal) (eg-*zam*-i-NĀ-shun) revealed a mildly enlarged prostate gland with a 1.0 cm nodule of the right lobe. The urologist performed a **transrectal ultrasound** (trans-REK-tal) (UL-tra-sound) and biopsy. A diagnosis of adenocarcinoma of the prostate was made. The patient elected to undergo a **suprapubic prostatectomy** (sū-pra-PŪ-bik) (*pros*-ta-TEK-to-mē). Urinary incontinence complicated his postoperative course but this lasted for only 3 months. No **erectile dysfunction** (e-REK-tīl) (dis-FUNK-shun) was reported. His prognosis for full recovery should be excellent.

EXERCISE **38** *Comprehend Medical Terms in Use*

Test your comprehension of the terms in the previous medical document by circling the correct answer.

1. Before being diagnosed with cancer of the prostate the patient had surgery for:
   a. sterilization
   b. excision of the seminal vesicle
   c. removal of the prepuce
   d. repair of the glans penis

2. The patient chose which of the following types of treatment for prostate cancer?
   a. radiation
   b. chemotherapy
   c. surgery
   d. hormonal therapy

3. After surgery the patient:
   a. had absence of sperm
   b. had persistent abnormal erection
   c. had a narrowing of the opening of the prepuce of the glans penis
   d. was able to have an erection

4. Using word parts you have already learned, write the definition of terms used in this document from previous chapters.
   a. urin/ary _____
   b. ur/o/logist _____
   c. bi/opsy _____
   d. dia/gnosis _____
   e. aden/o/carcinoma _____

CHAPTER REVIEW

CHAPTER REVIEW ON CD-ROM

Use the CD-ROM that accompanies this textbook to play and practice what you have learned in this chapter. The Chapter Exercises, Practice Activities, Animations, and Games allow you to hear, see, and interact with the chapter content.

Chapter Exercises

Exercises in this section of your CD-ROM correlate to exercises in your textbook. You may have completed them as you worked through the chapter.
☐ Pronunciation
☐ Spelling
☐ Read Medical Terms in Use

Practice Activities

Practice in study mode, then test your learning in assessment mode. Keep track of your scores from assessment mode if you wish.

SCORE
☐ Picture It _____
☐ Define Word Parts _____
☐ Build Medical Terms _____
☐ Word Shop _____
☐ Define Medical Terms _____
☐ Use It _____
☐ Hear It and Type It: _____
   Clinical Vignettes

Animations
☐ Sperm Production
☐ Testicular Torsion

Games
☐ Name that Word Part
☐ Term Storm
☐ Term Explorer
☐ Termbusters
☐ Medical Millionaire

REVIEW OF WORD PARTS

Can you define and spell the following word parts?

Combining Forms		Suffix
andr/o	prostat/o	-ism
balan/o	sperm/o	
epididym/o	spermat/o	
orch/o	test/o	
orchi/o	vas/o	
orchid/o	vesicul/o	

REVIEW OF TERMS

Can you build, analyze, define, pronounce, and spell the following terms *built from word parts?*

Diseases and Disorders	Surgical	Complementary
anorchism	balanoplasty	andropathy
balanitis	epididymectomy	aspermia
balanorrhea	orchidectomy, orchiectomy	oligospermia
benign prostatic hyperplasia (BPH)	orchidopexy, orchiopexy	spermatolysis
cryptorchidism	orchidotomy, orchiotomy	
epididymitis	orchioplasty	
orchiepididymitis	prostatectomy	
orchitis, orchiditis, or testitis	prostatocystotomy	
prostatitis	prostatolithotomy	
prostatocystitis	prostatovesiculectomy	
prostatolith	vasectomy	
prostatorrhea	vasovasostomy	
prostatovesiculitis	vesiculectomy	

Can you define, pronounce, and spell the following terms *not built from word parts?*

Diseases and Disorders	Surgical	Diagnostic	Complementary
erectile dysfunction (ED)	circumcision	digital rectal examination (DRE)	acquired immunodeficiency syndrome (AIDS)
hydrocele	hydrocelectomy		artificial insemination
phimosis	radical prostatectomy (RP)	prostate-specific antigen (PSA)	chlamydia
priapism	suprapubic prostatectomy	transrectal ultrasound	coitus
prostate cancer	transurethral incision of the prostate gland (TUIP)		condom
testicular carcinoma			ejaculation
testicular torsion	transurethral microwave thermotherapy (TUMT)		genital herpes
varicocele			gonads
	transurethral resection of the prostate gland (TURP)		gonorrhea
			heterosexual
			homosexual
			human immunodeficiency virus (HIV)
			human papillomavirus (HPV)
			orgasm
			prosthesis
			puberty
			sexually transmitted disease (STD)
			sterilization
			syphilis
			trichomoniasis

ANSWERS

Exercise Figures

Exercise Figure

A. 1. seminal vesicle: vesicul/o
2. prostate gland: prostat/o
3. epididymis: epididym/o
4. vas deferens or ductus deferens: vas/o
5. glans penis: balan/o
6. testis: orchid/o, orchi/o, orch/o, test/o

Exercise Figure

B. balan/itis

Exercise Figure

C. crypt/orchid/ism

Exercise Figure

D. vas/ectomy

Exercise 1
1. c
2. i
3. e
4. k
5. f
6. a
7. l
8. g
9. b
10. n
11. h
12. p
13. d
14. j
15. m

Exercise 2
1. testis, testicle
2. vessel, duct
3. glans penis
4. prostate gland
5. testis, testicle
6. seminal vesicle
7. testis, testicle
8. epididymis
9. testis, testicle

Exercise 3
1. vas/o
2. prostat/o
3. balan/o
4. vesicul/o
5. epididym/o
6. a. orchid/o
   b. orchi/o
   c. orch/o
   d. test/o

Exercise 4
1. sperm
2. male
3. sperm

Exercise 5
1. a. sperm/o
   b. spermat/o
2. andr/o

Exercise 6
1. state of

Exercise 7
Pronunciation Exercise

Exercise 8
1. WR CV WR
   prostat/o/lith
   CF
   stone in the prostate gland
2. WR S
   balan/itis
   inflammation of the glans penis
3. a. WR S
   orch/itis
   b. WR S
   orchid/itis
   c. WR S
   test/itis
   inflammation of the testis
4. WR CV WR S
   prostat/o/vesicul/itis
   CF
   inflammation of the prostate gland and seminal vesicles
5. WR CV WR S
   prostat/o/cyst/itis
   CF
   inflammation of the prostate gland and bladder
6. WR WR S
   orchi/epididym/itis
   inflammation of the testis and epididymis
7. WR CV S
   prostat/o/rrhea
   CF
   discharge from the prostate gland
8. WR S
   epididym/itis
   inflammation of an epididymis
9. WR S P S(WR)
   (benign) prostat/ic hyper/plasia
   (nonmalignant) excessive development pertaining to the prostate gland
10. WR WR S
    crypt/orchid/ism
    state of hidden testis
11. WR CV S
    balan/o/rrhea
    CF
    discharge from the glans penis
12. WR S
    prostat/itis
    inflammation of prostate gland
13. P WR S
    an/orch/ism
    state of absence of testis

Exercise 9
1. prostat/o/cyst/itis
2. prostat/o/lith
3. a. orchid/itis
   b. orch/itis
   c. test/itis
4. (benign) prostat/ic hyper/plasia
5. crypt/orchid/ism
6. prostat/o/vesicul/itis
7. an/orch/ism
8. prostat/itis
9. orchi/epididym/itis
10. balan/o/rrhea
11. epididym/itis
12. balan/itis
13. prostat/o/rrhea

Exercise 10
Spelling Exercise; see text p. 269.

Exercise 11
Pronunciation Exercise

Exercise 12
1. testicular carcinoma
2. phimosis
3. varicocele
4. hydrocele
5. prostate cancer
6. erectile dysfunction
7. priapism
8. testicular torsion

Exercise 13
1. d
2. c
3. e
4. b
5. a
6. f
7. i
8. h

Exercise 14
Spelling Exercise; see text p. 271.

Exercise 15
Pronunciation Exercise

Exercise 16
1. WR   S
   vas/ectomy
   excision of a duct
2. WR   CV WR CV   S
   prostat/o/cyst/o/tomy
           CF   CF
   incision into the prostate gland and
   bladder
3. a.   WR CV   S
      orchid/o/tomy
             CF
   b.   WR CV S
      orchi/o/tomy
            CF
      incision into a testis
4. WR   S
   epididym/ectomy
   excision of an epididymis
5. a.   WR CV   S
      orchid/o/pexy
             CF
   b.   WR CV S
      orchi/o/pexy
            CF
      surgical fixation of a testicle
6. WR   CV WR   S
   prostat/o/vesicul/ectomy
           CF
   excision of the prostate gland and
   seminal vesicles
7. WR   CV   S
   orchid/o/plasty
          CF
   surgical repair of a testis
8. WR   S
   vesicul/ectomy
   excision of the seminal vesicle(s)
9. WR   S
   prostat/ectomy
   excision of the prostate gland
10. WR CV   S
    balan/o/plasty
           CF
    surgical repair of the glans penis
11. WR CV WR CV S
    vas/o/vas/o/stomy
        CF   CF
    creation of artificial openings
    between ducts
12. a.   WR   S
      orchid/ectomy
   b.   WR   S
      orchi/ectomy
      excision of the testis

13. WR   CV WR CV S
    prostat/o/lith/o/tomy
            CF   CF
    incision into prostate gland to
    remove a stone

Exercise 17
1. a. orchid/ectomy
   b. orchi/ectomy
2. balan/o/plasty
3. prostat/o/cyst/o/tomy
4. vesicul/ectomy
5. prostat/o/lith/o/tomy
6. a. orchid/o/tomy
   b. orchi/o/tomy
7. epididym/ectomy
8. orchi/o/plasty
9. prostat/ectomy
10. vas/ectomy
11. prostat/o/vesicul/ectomy
12. a. orchid/o/pexy
    b. orchi/o/pexy
13. vas/o/vas/o/stomy

Exercise 18
Spelling Exercise; see text p. 274.

Exercise 19
Pronunciation Exercise

Exercise 20
1. suprapubic prostatectomy
2. circumcision
3. radical prostatectomy
4. hydrocelectomy
5. transurethral microwave
   thermotherapy
6. transurethral incision (of the) prostate
   gland
7. transurethral resection (of the)
   prostate gland

Exercise 21
Spelling Exercise; see text p. 277.

Exercise 22
Pronunciation Exercise

Exercise 23
1. digital rectal examination
2 prostate-specific antigen
3. transrectal ultrasound

Exercise 24
Spelling Exercise; see text p. 279.

Exercise 25
Pronunciation Exercise

Exercise 26
1. WR   CV WR S
   olig/o/sperm/ia
         CF
   condition of scanty sperm
2. WR CV S
   andr/o/pathy
         CF
   disease of the male
3. WR   CV S
   spermat/o/lysis
           CF
   dissolution of sperm
4. P   WR   S
   a/sperm/ia
         CF
   condition of without sperm

Exercise 27
1. spermat/o/lysis
2. a/sperm/ia
3. andr/o/pathy
4. olig/o/sperm/ia

Exercise 28
Spelling Exercise; see text p. 280.

Exercise 29
Pronunciation Exercise

Exercise 30
1. period when secondary sex characteristics develop and the ability to sexually reproduce begins
2. climax of sexual stimulation
3. contagious, inflammatory sexually
   transmitted disease
4. person who is attracted to a member
   of the same sex
5. sexual intercourse between male and
   female
6. sexually transmitted disease caused by
   the *herpesvirus hominis* type 2
7. person who is attracted to a member
   of the oppostite sex
8. chronic infection caused by bacterium that can be transmitted by sexual contact, acquired in utero, or by
   contact with infected tissue
9. ejection of semen from the male
   urethra
10. male and female sex glands
11. a disease transmitted during sexual
    contact
12. process rendering an individual un-
    able to produce offspring
13. an STD causing growths on the male
    and female genitalia

14. a disease transmitted by exchange of body fluids during the sexual act, reuse of contaminated needles, or contaminated blood transfusions
15. STD caused by a one-cell organism, *Trichomonas;* it affects the genitourinary system
16. introduction of semen into the vagina by artificial means
17. STD caused by bacterium, *C. trachomatis*
18. a cover for the penis worn during coitus
19. an artificial replacement of an absent body part
20. a type of retrovirus that causes AIDS

Exercise 31

1. g	6. i
2. e	7. c
3. h	8. b
4. a	9. j
5. d	10. f

Exercise 32

1. f	6. b
2. a	7. i
3. h	8. e
4. d	9. g
5. j	10. c

Exercise 33
Spelling Exercise; see text p. 285.

Exercise 34
1. digital rectal examination; benign prostatic hyperplasia; transurethral resection (of the) prostate; transurethral microwave thermotherapy; transurethral incision (of the) prostate
2. acquired immunodeficieny syndrome; sexually transmitted disease; human immunodeficiency virus; human papillomavirus
3. prostate-specific antigen
4. radical prostatectomy

Exercise 35

A. 1. nocturia
2. hematuria
3. urinary
4. benign prostatic hyperplasia
5. urology

B. 1. c
2. b
3. c
4. a

Exercise 36
1. balanorrhea
2. prepuce
3. heterosexual
4. phimosis
5. orchidopexy
6. prosthesis
7. transurethral microwave thermotherapy

Exercise 37
Reading Exercise

Exercise 38
1. a
2. c
3. d
4. a. pertaining to urine
   b. a physician who studies and treats diseases of the urinary tract
   c. view of life
   d. state of complete knowledge
   e. cancerous tumor of glandular tissue

NOTES

CHAPTER 8

Female Reproductive System

OUTLINE

ANATOMY, 298

WORD PARTS, 301
Combining Forms, 301
Prefix and Suffixes, 304

MEDICAL TERMS, 305
Disease and Disorder Terms, 305
    Built from Word Parts, 305
    Not Built from Word Parts, 310
Surgical Terms, 314
    Built from Word Parts, 314
    Not Built from Word Parts, 319
Diagnostic Terms, 325
    Built from Word Parts, 325
    Not Built from Word Parts, 330
Complementary Terms, 333
    Built from Word Parts, 333
    Not Built from Word Parts, 335
Abbreviations, 337

PRACTICAL APPLICATION, 338
Interact with Medical Documents, 338
Interpret Medical Terms, 340
Read Medical Terms in Use, 341
Comprehend Medical Terms in Use, 342

CHAPTER REVIEW, 342

TABLE 8-1 TYPES OF HYSTERECTOMIES, 315

TABLE 8-2 TYPES OF SURGERIES PERFORMED TO TREAT MALIGNANT BREAST TUMORS, 315

TABLE 8-3 ENDOSCOPIC SURGERY, 328

OBJECTIVES

Upon completion of this chapter you will be able to:

1. Identify organs and structures of the female reproductive system.

2. Define and spell word parts related to the female reproductive system.

3. Define, pronounce, and spell disease and disorder terms related to the female reproductive system.

4. Define, pronounce, and spell surgical terms related to the female reproductive system.

5. Define, pronounce, and spell diagnostic terms related to the female reproductive system.

6. Define, pronounce, and spell complementary terms related to the female reproductive system.

7. Interpret the meaning of abbreviations related to the female reproductive system.

8. Interpret, read, and comprehend medical language in simulated medical statements and documents.

ANATOMY

Function

The female reproductive system produces the female egg cells and hormones and also provides for conception and pregnancy (Figure 8-1).

Internal Organs of the Female Reproductive System

THE GRAAFIAN FOLLICLE
is named for Dutch anatomist Reinier de *Graaf,* who discovered the sac in 1672.

THE FALLOPIAN TUBE
was named in honor of Gabriele Fallopius because he described it in his works. Fallopius also gave the *vagina* and the *placenta* their names.

Term	Definition
ovaries	pair of almond-shaped organs located in the pelvic cavity. Egg cells are formed and stored in the ovaries.
ovum (*pl.* ova)	female egg cell
graafian follicles	100,000 microscopic sacs that make up a large portion of the ovaries. Each follicle contains an immature ovum. Normally one graafian follicle develops to maturity monthly between puberty and menopause. It moves to the surface of the ovary and releases the ovum, which passes into the uterine tube.
uterine, or fallopian, tubes	pair of 5-inch (12-cm) tubes, attached to the uterus, that provide a passageway for the ovum to move from the ovary to the uterus
fimbria (*pl.* fimbriae)	finger-like projection at the free end of the uterine tube
uterus	pear-sized and pear-shaped muscular organ that lies in the pelvic cavity, except during pregnancy when it enlarges and extends up into the abdominal cavity. Its functions are menstruation, pregnancy, and labor.
endometrium	inner lining of the uterus
myometrium	muscular middle layer of the uterus
perimetrium	outer thin layer that covers the surface of the uterus
corpus, or body	large central portion of the uterus
fundus	rounded upper portion of the uterus
cervix (Cx)	narrow lower portion of the uterus
vagina	a 3-inch (7-8 cm) tube that connects the uterus to the outside of the body
hymen	fold of membrane found near the opening of the vagina
rectouterine pouch	pouch between the posterior wall of the uterus and the anterior wall of the rectum (also called **Douglas cul-de-sac**)

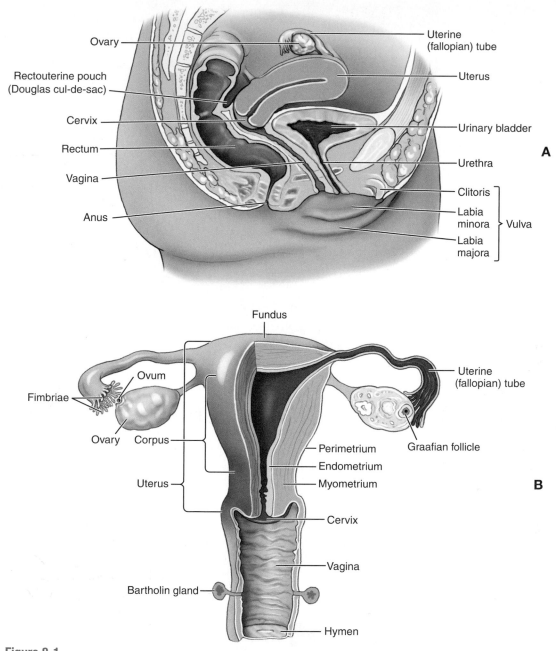

Figure 8-1
Female reproductive organs. **A,** Sagittal view. **B,** Frontal view.

Glands of the Female Reproductive System

Term	Definition
Bartholin glands	pair of mucus-producing glands located on each side of the vagina and just above the vaginal opening
mammary glands, or breasts . . .	milk-producing glands of the female. Each breast consists of 15 to 20 divisions, or lobes (Figure 8-2).
mammary papilla	breast nipple
areola	pigmented area around the breast nipple

BARTHOLIN GLANDS
were described by Caspar Bartholin, a Danish anatomist, in 1675.

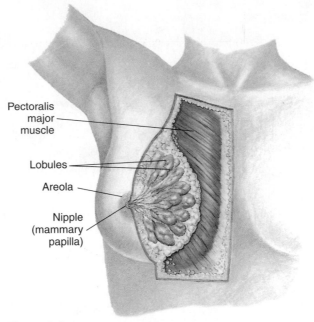

Pectoralis major muscle

Lobules

Areola

Nipple (mammary papilla)

Figure 8-2
Female breast.

External Female Reproductive Structures

Term	Definition
vulva, or external genitals	two pairs of lips (labia major and labia minora) that surround the vagina
clitoris	highly erogenous erectile body located anterior to the urethra
perineum	pelvic floor in both the male and female. In females it usually refers to the area between the vaginal opening and the anus.

EXERCISE  1

Match the definitions in the first column with the anatomic terms in the second column.

_C_ 1. organs in which egg cells are formed

_F_ 2. lower portion of the uterus

_G_ 3. lining of the uterus

_B_ 4. upper portion of the uterus

_D_ 5. pelvic floor

_E_ 6. ends of uterine tubes

_H_ 7. large central portion of the uterus

_A_ 8. layer that covers the uterus

_I_ 9. muscle layer of the uterus

a. perimetrium

b. fundus

c. ovaries

d. perineum

e. fimbriae

f. cervix

g. endometrium

h. corpus

i. myometrium

j. ovum

EXERCISE 2

Match the definitions in the first column with the anatomic terms in the second column.

_B_ 1. connects the uterus to the outside
of the body

_C_ 2. mucus-producing glands located
on each side of the vagina

_D_ 3. breast

_K_ 4. female egg cells

_E_ 5. external genitals

_F_ 6. passageway for ovum

_G_ 7. pigmented area around the nipple

_L_ 8. microscopic sacs in the ovaries

_I_ 9. muscular organ

_J_ 10. nipples

_H_ 11. rectouterine pouch

a. ovary

b. vagina

c. Bartholin glands

d. mammary gland

e. vulva

f. uterine tube

g. areola

h. Douglas cul-de-sac

i. uterus

j. mammary papillae

k. ova

l. graafian follicles

WORD PARTS

Word parts you need to learn to complete this chapter are listed on the following pages. The exercises at the end of each list will help you learn their definitions and spellings.

Combining Forms of the Female Reproductive System

Combining Form	Definition
arche/o	first, beginning
cervic/o, trachel/o. . . . . (NOTE: *trachel/o* also means *neck, necklike*.)	cervix
colp/o, vagin/o	vagina
culd/o	cul-de-sac
episi/o, vulv/o	vulva
gynec/o, gyn/o	woman
hymen/o	hymen
hyster/o, metr/o, metr/i, uter/o . . . . (NOTE: the combining vowel *i* or *o* may be used with metr/.)	uterus
mamm/o, mast/o	breast

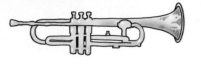

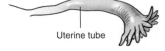

Uterine tube

Figure 8-3

Salpinx is derived from the Greek term for trumpet. The term was used for the uterine tubes because of their trumpet-like shape.

Combining Forms of the Female Reproductive System—*cont'd*

Combining Form	Definition
men/o	menstruation
oophor/o	ovary
perine/o	perineum
salping/o	uterine tube (fallopian tube) (Figure 8-3)

EXERCISE FIGURE A

Fill in the blanks with combining forms in this diagram of the frontal view of the female reproductive system.

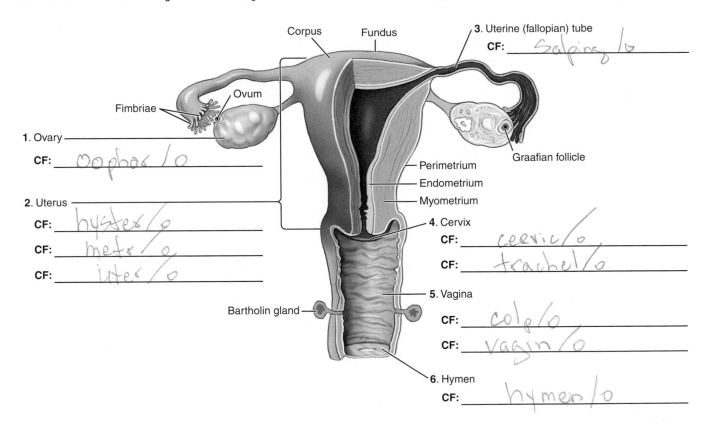

Corpus   Fundus

3. Uterine (fallopian) tube
CF: _Salping/o_

Ovum

Fimbriae

1. Ovary
CF: _Oophor/o_

Graafian follicle

Perimetrium
Endometrium
Myometrium

2. Uterus
CF: _hyster/o_
CF: _metr/o_
CF: _uter/o_

4. Cervix
CF: _cervic/o_
CF: _trachel/o_

5. Vagina
CF: _colp/o_
CF: _vagin/o_

Bartholin gland

6. Hymen
CF: _hymen/o_

EXERCISE FIGURE B

Fill in the blanks with combining forms in this diagram showing the external reproductive organs.

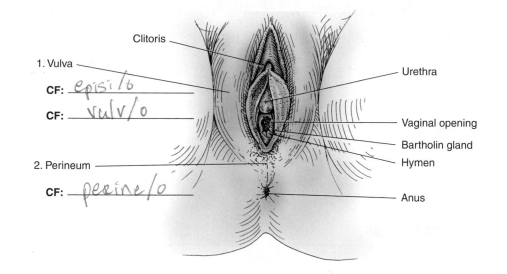

Clitoris

1. Vulva

CF: _episi/o_

CF: _vulv/o_

Urethra

Vaginal opening

Bartholin gland

Hymen

2. Perineum

CF: _perine/o_

Anus

EXERCISE 3

Write the definitions of the following combining forms.

1. vagin/o _vagina_
2. oophor/o _ovary_
3. metr/o, metr/i _uterus_
4. uter/o _uterus_
5. hymen/o _hymen_
6. hyster/o _uterus_
7. men/o _menstruation_
8. episi/o _vulva_
9. cervic/o _cervix_
10. colp/o _vagina_

11. gynec/o _woman_
12. mamm/o _breast_
13. perine/o _perineum_
14. salping/o _uterine tube_
15. vulv/o _vulva_
16. mast/o _breast_
17. arche/o _first, beginning_
18. culd/o _cul-de-sac_
19. gyn/o _woman_
20. trachel/o _cervix_

EXERCISE 4

Write the combining form for each of the following terms.

1. vulva a. _episi/o_
         b. _vulv/o_

2. breast a. _mamm/o_
          b. _mast/o_

3. menstruation _men/o_

4. ovary _oophor/o_

5. uterine tube _salping/o_

6. perineum _perine/o_

7. vagina
   a. _colp/o_
   b. _vagin/o_

8. uterus
   a. _hyster/o_
   b. _metr/o_
   c. _metr/i_

9. woman
   a. _gynec/o_
   b. _gyn/o_

10. hymen _hymen/o_

11. cul-de-sac _culd/o_

12. cervix
   a. _cervic/o_
   b. _trachel/o_

13. first, beginning _arche/o_

Prefix and Suffixes

> **ATRESIA**
> literally means **no perforation or hole.** It is composed of the Greek words **a,** meaning **without,** and **tresis,** meaning **perforation.** The term may be used alone, as in "atresia of the vagina," or combined with other word parts, as in "gynatresia," meaning closure of a part of the female genital tract, usually the vagina.

Prefix	Definition
peri-	surrounding (outer)

Suffixes	Definition
-atresia	absence of a normal body opening; occlusion; closure
-ial	pertaining to
-salpinx	uterine tube (fallopian tube) (Figure 8-3)

(NOTE: for learning purposes *salpinx* and *atresia* are presented as suffixes.)

EXERCISE 5

Write the prefix or suffix for each of the following.

1. uterine tube _salpinx_

2. pertaining to _ial_

3. surrounding _peri_

4. absence of a normal body opening _atresia_

EXERCISE 6

Write the definitions of the following prefix and suffixes.

1. –salpinx _uterine tube_

2. peri- _surrounding_

3. –ial _pertaining to_

4. –atresia _absence of a normal body opening_

Refer to Appendix A and Appendix B for alphabetized word parts and their meanings.

MEDICAL TERMS

The terms you need to learn to complete this chapter are listed on the following pages. The exercises following each list will help you learn the definition and spelling of each word.

Disease and Disorder Terms

Built from Word Parts

The following terms are built from word parts you have already learned and can be translated literally to find their meanings. Further explanation of terms beyond the definition of their word parts, if needed, is included in parentheses.

Term	Definition
amenorrhea . . . . (a-*men*-ō-RĒ-a)	absence of menstrual discharge
Bartholin adenitis . . . . (BAR-tō-lin) (*ad*-e-NĪ-tis)	inflammation of a Bartholin gland (also called **bartholinitis**)
cervicitis. . . . . (ser-vi-SĪ-tis)	inflammation of the cervix (see Figure 8-7)
colpitis, vaginitis. . . . . (kol-PĪ-tis), (vaj-i-NĪ-tis)	inflammation of the vagina (see Figure 8-7)
dysmenorrhea. . . . . (dis-*men*-ō-RĒ-a)	painful menstrual discharge
endocervicitis. . . . . (en-dō-*ser*-vi-SĪ-tis)	inflammation of the inner (lining) of the cervix
endometritis . . . . (en-dō-mē-TRĪ-tis)	inflammation of the inner (lining) of the uterus (endometrium) (see Figure 8-7)
hematosalpinx . . . . (*hem*-a-tō-SAL-pinks)	blood in the uterine tube
hydrosalpinx. . . . . (hī-drō-SAL-pinks)	water in the uterine tube (see Exercise Figure H)
hysteratresia. . . . . (his-ter-a-TRĒ-zha)	closure of the uterus (uterine cavity)
mastitis. . . . . (*mas*-TĪ-tis)	inflammation of the breast
menometrorrhagia . . . . (men-ō-*met*-rō-RĀ-jea)	rapid flow of blood from the uterus at menstruation (and between menstrual cycles; increased amount) (see Figure 8-7)
menorrhagia. . . . . (men-ō-RĀ-jea)	rapid flow of blood at menstruation (increased amount)
metrorrhagia. . . . . (mē-trō-RĀ-jea)	rapid flow of blood from the uterus (between menstrual cycles)
myometritis . . . . (*mī*-o-me-TRĪ-tis)	inflammation of the uterine muscle (myometrium)

Disease and Disorder Terms—cont'd

Built from Word Parts

Term	Definition
oligomenorrhea . . . . (*ol*-i-gō-*men*-ō-RĒ-a)	scanty menstrual flow (less often)
oophoritis . . . . (ō-of-o-RĪ-tis)	inflammation of the ovary
perimetritis . . . . (*per*-i-me-TRĪ-tis)	inflammation surrounding the uterus (peri- metrium)
pyosalpinx . . . . (pī-ō-SAL-pinks)	pus in the uterine tube
salpingitis . . . . (*sal*-pin-JĪ-tis)	inflammation of the uterine tube (Exercise Figure C and Figure 8-7)
salpingocele . . . . (sal-PING-gō-sēl)	hernia of the uterine tube
vulvovaginitis . . . . (*vul*-vō-vaj-i-NĪ-tis)	inflammation of the vulva and vagina

EXERCISE FIGURE C

Fill in the blanks with combining forms to label the diagram.

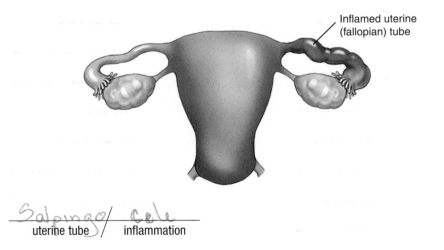

Inflamed uterine
(fallopian) tube

Salpingo / cele
uterine tube / inflammation

EXERCISE 7

Practice saying aloud each of the disease and disorder terms built from word parts on
p. 305 and above.

To hear the terms select Chapter 8, Chapter Exercises, Pronunciation.

☐ Place a check mark in the box when you have completed this exercise.

EXERCISE 8

Analyze and define the following disease and disorder terms.

1. colpitis _____

2. cervicitis _____

3. hydrosalpinx _____

4. hematosalpinx _____

5. metrorrhagia _____

6. oophoritis _____

7. (Bartholin) adenitis _____

8. vulvovaginitis _____

9. salpingocele _Inflammation of uterine tube_

10. menometrorrhagia _____

11. amenorrhea _____

12. dysmenorrhea _____

13. mastitis _____

14. perimetritis _____

15. myometritis _____

16. endometritis _____

17. endocervicitis _____

18. pyosalpinx _____

19. hysteratresia _____

20. salpingitis _____

21. vaginitis _____

22. menorrhagia _____

23. oligomenorrhea _____

EXERCISE 9

Build disease and disorder terms for the following definitions with the word parts you have learned.

1. inflammation of the breast

   _____ / _____
   WR   S

2. rapid flow of blood from the uterus (between menstrual cycles)

   _____ / _____ / _____
   WR   CV   S

3. inflammation of the uterine tube

   _____ / _____
   WR   S

4. inflammation of the vulva and vagina

   _____ / _____ / _____ / _____
   WR   CV   WR   S

5. absence of menstrual discharge

   _____ / _____ / _____ / _____
   P   WR   CV   S

6. inflammation of the cervix

   _____ / _____
   WR   S

7. inflammation of (Bartholin) gland   Bartholin _____ / _____
                                                  WR   S

8. water in the uterine tube

   _____ / _____ / _____
   WR   CV   S

9. painful menstrual discharge

   _____ / _____ / _____ / _____
   P   WR   CV   S

10. blood in the uterine tube

    _____ / _____ / _____
    WR   CV   S

11. inflammation of the vagina   a. _____ / _____
                                     WR   S

                                  b. _____ / _____
                                     WR   S

12. rapid flow of blood from the uterus at menstruation (and between menstrual cycles)

    _____ / _____ / _____ / _____ / _____
    WR   CV   WR   CV   S

13. inflammation of the ovary

    _____ / _____
    WR   S

14. hernia of the uterine tube

    _____ / _____ / _____
    WR   CV   S

15. inflammation surrounding the uterus (outer layer)

    _____ / _____ / _____
    P   WR   S

16. inflammation of the inner
    (lining) of the uterus

    _____ / _____ / _____
    P   WR   S

17. inflammation of the inner
    (lining) of the cervix

    _____ / _____ / _____
    P   WR   S

18. inflammation of the
    uterine muscle

    _____ / CV / _____ / _____
    WR   WR   S

19. pus in the uterine tube

    _____ / CV / _____
    WR   S

20. closure of the uterus
    (uterine cavity)

    _____ / _____
    WR   S

21. scanty menstrual flow
    (less often)

    _____ / CV / _____ / CV / _____
    WR   WR   S

22. rapid flow of blood at
    menstruation (increased
    amount)

    _____ / CV / _____
    WR   S

EXERCISE **10**

Spell each of the disease and disorder terms built from word parts on pp. 305-306 by
having someone dictate them to you.

 To hear and spell the terms select Chapter 8, Chapter Exercises, Spelling. You may
type the terms on the screen or write them below in the spaces provided.

☐ Place a check mark in the box if you have completed this exercise using your CD-ROM.

1. _____   13. _____

2. _____   14. _____

3. _____   15. _____

4. _____   16. _____

5. _____   17. _____

6. _____   18. _____

7. _____   19. _____

8. _____   20. _____

9. _____   21. _____

10. _____   22. _____

11. _____   23. _____

12. _____

Disease and Disorder Terms

Not Built from Word Parts

In some of the following terms, you may recognize word parts you have already learned; however, the full meaning of the terms cannot be discerned by the definition of their word parts.

Term	Definition
adenomyosis . . . . (ad-e-nō-mī-Ō-sis)	growth of endometrium into the muscular portion of the uterus
breast cancer . . . . (brest) (KAN-cer)	malignant tumor of the breast (Figure 8-4)
cervical cancer . . . . (SER-vi-kal) (KAN-cer)	malignant tumor of the cervix, which progresses from cellular dysplasia to carcinoma. Its cause is linked to human papillomavirus infection.
endometrial cancer . . . . (en-dō-MĒ-trē-al) (KAN-cer)	malignant tumor of the endometrium (also called **uterine cancer**)
endometriosis . . . . (*en*-dō-*mē*-trē-Ō-sis)	abnormal condition in which endometrial tissue grows outside of the uterus in various areas in the pelvic cavity, including ovaries, uterine tubes, intestines, and uterus (Figure 8-5)
fibrocystic breast disease . . . . . (fī-brō-SIS-tik) (di-ZĒZ)	a disorder characterized by one or more benign cysts in the breast

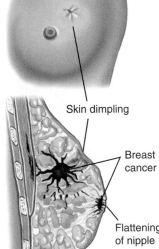

Figure 8-4

Clinical signs of breast cancer.

Skin dimpling

Breast cancer

Flattening of nipple

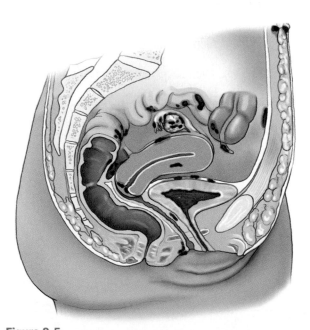

Figure 8-5

Endometriosis. Spots indicate common sites of endometrial deposits.

Term	Definition
fibroid tumor . . . . (FĪ-broyd) (TŪ-mor)	benign fibroid tumor of the uterine muscle (also called **myoma of the uterus** or **leiomyoma**) (Figure 8-6)
ovarian cancer . . . . (ō-VAR-ē-an) (KAN-cer)	malignant tumor of the ovary
pelvic inflammatory disease (PID) . . . . (PEL-vik) (in-FLAM-a-tor-ē) (di-ZĒZ)	inflammation of the female pelvic organs that can be caused by many different pathogens. If untreated, the infection may spread upward from the vagina, involving the uterus, uterine tubes, ovaries, and other pelvic organs. An ascending infection may result in infertility and, in acute cases, fatal septicemia (Figure 8-7).
prolapsed uterus . . . . (PRŌ-lapsd) (Ū-ter-us)	downward displacement of the uterus into the vagina (also called **hysteroptosis**) (Exercise Figure D)
toxic shock syndrome (TSS) . . . (TOX-ik) (shok) (SIN-drōm)	a severe illness characterized by high fever, rash, vomiting, diarrhea, and myalgia, followed by hypotension and, in severe cases, shock and death; usually affects menstruating women using tampons; caused by *Staphylococcus aureus* and *Streptococcus pyogenes*.
vesicovaginal fistula . . . . (ves-i-kō-VAJ-i-nal) (FIS-tū-la)	abnormal opening between the bladder and the vagina (Exercise Figure E)

CAM TERM
Massage therapy is the manual manipulation of soft tissue, incorporating stroking, kneading, and percussion motions. Benefits of massage therapy during breast cancer treatment include increased dopamine levels, lymphocytes, and natural killer cells and a decrease in depression and anger.

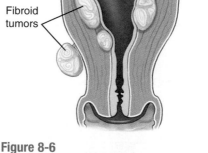

Figure 8-6
Fibroid tumors (also called myomas or leiomyomas).

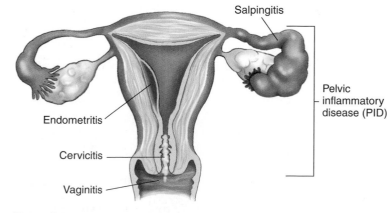

Figure 8-7
Ascending infection of the female reproductive system as seen in pelvic inflammatory disease.

EXERCISE FIGURE **D**

Fill in the blanks to label the diagram.

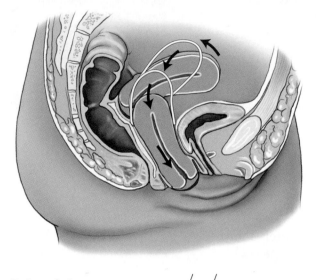

Prolapsed uterus or _____ / _____ / _____
                       uterus / cv / prolapse

EXERCISE FIGURE **E**

Fill in the blanks to label the diagram.

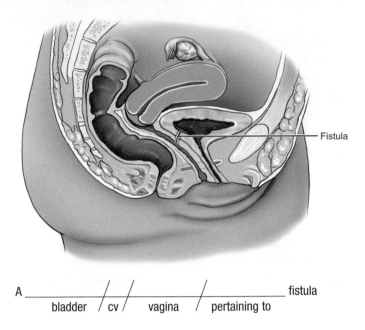

— Fistula

A _____ / ___ / _____ / _____ fistula
   bladder / cv / vagina / pertaining to

EXERCISE **11**

Practice saying aloud each of the disease and disorder terms not built from word parts on pp. 310-311.

 To hear the terms, select Chapter 8, Chapter Exercises, Pronunciation.

☐ Place a check mark in the box when you have completed this exercise.

EXERCISE **12**

Fill in the blanks with the correct definitions.

1. prolapsed uterus _____

2. pelvic inflammatory disease_____

3. vesicovaginal fistula _____

4. fibroid tumor _____

5. endometriosis _____

6. adenomyosis _____

7. toxic shock syndrome_____

8. fibrocystic breast disease _____

9. ovarian cancer_____

10. breast cancer_____

11. cervical cancer _____

12. endometrial cancer_____

EXERCISE 13

Write the term for each of the following.

1. abnormal opening between the bladder and the vagina _____
   _____

2. benign tumor of the uterine muscle _____ _____

3. inflammation of the female pelvic organs _____
   _____ _____

4. downward displacement of the uterus into the vagina
   _____ _____

5. endometrial tissue in the pelvic cavity _____

6. growth of endometrium into the muscular portion of the uterus
   _____

7. affects menstruating women using tampons _____
   _____ _____

8. one or more benign cysts in the breast _____
   _____ _____

9. a malignant tumor of the breast _____ _____

10. also called uterine cancer _____ _____

11. malignant tumor of the ovaries _____ _____

12. malignant tumor of the cervix _____ _____

EXERCISE 14

Spell each of the disease and disorder terms not built from word parts on pp. 310-311 by having someone dictate them to you.

 To hear and spell the terms select Chapter 8, Chapter Exercises, Spelling. You may type the terms on the screen or write them below in the spaces provided.

☐ Place a check mark in the box if you have completed this exercise using your CD-ROM.

1. _____   7. _____

2. _____   8. _____

3. _____   9. _____

4. _____   10. _____

5. _____   11. _____

6. _____   12. _____

Surgical Terms
Built from Word Parts

The following terms are built from word parts you have already learned and can be translated literally to find their meanings. Further explanation of terms beyond the definitions of their word parts, if needed, is included in parentheses.

Term	Definition
cervicectomy (*ser*-vi-SEK-to-mē)	excision of the cervix
colpoperineorrhaphy (*kol*-pō-*per*-i-nē-OR-a-fē)	suture of the vagina and perineum (performed to mend perineal vaginal tears)
colpoplasty (KOL-pō-*plas*-tē)	surgical repair of the vagina
colporrhaphy (*kol*-POR-a-fē)	suture of the vagina (wall of the vagina)
episioperineoplasty (e-*piz*-ē-ō-*per*-i-NĒ-o-plas-tē)	surgical repair of the vulva and perineum
episiorrhaphy (e-*piz*-ē-OR-a-fē)	suture of (a tear in) the vulva
hymenectomy (*hī*-men-EK-to-mē)	excision of the hymen
hymenotomy (*hī*-men-OT-o-mē)	incision of the hymen
hysterectomy (*his*-te-REK-to-mē)	excision of the uterus (Table 8-1) (Exercise Figure F)
hysteropexy (HIS-ter-ō-*pek*-sē)	surgical fixation of the uterus
hysterosalpingo-oophorectomy (*his*-ter-ō-sal-*ping*-gō-Ō-*of*-o-REK-to-mē)	excision of the uterus, uterine tubes, and ovaries (Exercise Figure F)
mammoplasty (MAM-ō-*plas*-tē)	surgical repair of the breast (performed to enlarge or reduce in size, to lift, or to reconstruct after removal of a tumor)
mastectomy (mas-TEK-to-mē)	surgical removal of a breast (Table 8-2)
oophorectomy (ō-of-o-REK-to-mē)	excision of an ovary

Term	Definition
perineorrhaphy (*per*-i-nē-OR-a-fē)	suture of (a tear in) the perineum
salpingectomy (*sal*-pin-JEK-to-mē)	excision of a uterine tube
salpingo-oophorectomy (sal-ping-gō-ō-*of*-o-REK-to-mē)	excision of the uterine tube and ovary (Exercise Figure F)
salpingostomy (*sal*-ping-GOS-to-mē)	creation of an artificial opening in a uterine tube (performed to restore patency)
trachelectomy (*trā*-ke-LEK-to-mē)	excision of the cervix
trachelorrhaphy (trā-ke-LOR-a-fē)	suture of the cervix
vulvectomy (vul-VEK-to-mē)	excision of the vulva

TABLE 8-1

Types of Hysterectomies

Subtotal hysterectomy	Excision of the uterus, excluding cervix; rarely performed
Total hysterectomy	Excision of the uterus (abdominal, vaginal, or laparoscopic)
Panhysterectomy	Excision of the uterus, ovaries, and uterine tubes (abdominal)
Radical hysterectomy	Excision of the uterus, ovaries, uterine tubes; lymph nodes, upper portion of the vagina, and the surrounding tissues (abdominal)
Laparoscopic-assisted vaginal hysterectomy	Vaginal excision of the uterus with the use of the laparoscope to view the abdominopelvic cavity. Laparoscopic instruments are used to sever the ligaments that hold the uterus in place.

TABLE 8-2

Types of Surgeries Performed to Treat Malignant Breast Tumors

Radical mastectomy	Removal of breast tissue, nipple, underlying muscle, and lymph nodes; also called *Halsted mastectomy* (seldom used)
Modified radical mastectomy	Removal of breast tissue, nipple, and lymph nodes
Simple mastectomy	Removal of breast tissue and usually the nipple; referred to as a *total mastectomy*
Subcutaneous mastectomy	Removal of breast tissue, preserving the overlying skin, nipple, and areola, so that the breast may be reconstructed
Lumpectomy	Removal of the cancerous lesion only; also called *tylectomy*

EXERCISE FIGURE F

Fill in the blanks to label the diagram.

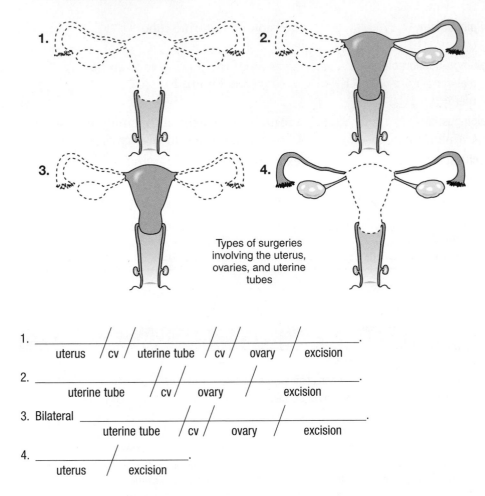

Types of surgeries involving the uterus, ovaries, and uterine tubes

1. _____ / cv / _____ / cv / _____ / _____ .
       uterus   cv   uterine tube   cv   ovary   excision

2. _____ / cv / _____ / _____ .
       uterine tube   cv   ovary   excision

3. Bilateral _____ / cv / _____ / _____ .
       uterine tube   cv   ovary   excision

4. _____ / _____ .
       uterus   excision

EXERCISE 15

Practice saying aloud each of the surgical terms built from word parts on pp. 314-315.

 To hear the terms select Chapter 8, Chapter Exercises, Pronunciation.

☐ Place a check mark in the box when you have completed this exercise.

EXERCISE 16

Analyze and define the following surgical terms.

1. colporrhaphy_____

2. colpoplasty _____

3. episiorrhaphy _____

4. hymenotomy_____

5. hysteropexy _____

6. vulvectomy _____

7. perineorrhaphy _____

8. salpingostomy _____

9. salpingo-oophorectomy _____

10. oophorectomy _____

11. mastectomy _____

12. salpingectomy _____

13. cervicectomy _____

14. colpoperineorrhaphy _____

15. episioperineoplasty _____

16. hymenectomy _____

17. hysterosalpingo-oophorectomy _____

18. hysterectomy _____

19. mammoplasty _____

20. trachelorrhaphy _____

21. trachelectomy _____

EXERCISE 17

Build surgical terms for the following definitions by using the word parts you have learned.

1. suture of the vagina

　　_____ / _____ / _____
　　WR　　　　 CV　　　　S

2. excision of the cervix

　　_____ / _____
　　WR　　　　　　S

3. suture of the vulva

　　_____ / _____ / _____
　　WR　　　　 CV　　　　S

4. surgical repair of the vulva and perineum

　　_____ / ____ / _____ / ____ / _____
　　WR　　 CV　　WR　　 CV　　 S

5. surgical repair of the vagina

　　_____ / _____ / _____
　　WR　　　　 CV　　　　S

6. suture of the vagina and perineum

　　_____ / ____ / _____ / ____ / _____
　　WR　　 CV　　WR　　 CV　　 S

7. excision of the uterus, ovaries, and uterine tubes

　　_____ / ____ / _____ / ____ / _____ / ____
　　WR　　 CV　　WR　　 CV　　 WR　　 S

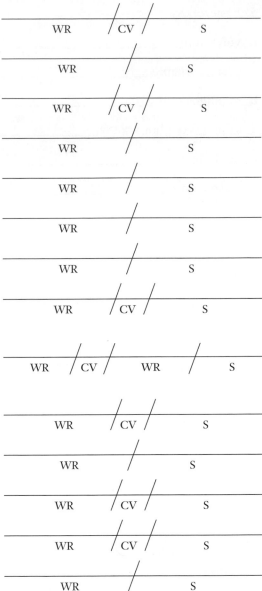

8. surgical fixation of the uterus _____ / ___ / _____
    WR   CV   S

9. excision of the hymen _____ / _____
    WR   S

10. incision of the hymen _____ / ___ / _____
    WR   CV   S

11. excision of the uterus _____ / _____
    WR   S

12. excision of the ovary _____ / _____
    WR   S

13. surgical removal of a breast _____ / _____
    WR   S

14. excision of a uterine tube _____ / _____
    WR   S

15. suture of the perineum _____ / ___ / _____
    WR   CV   S

16. excision of the uterine
    tube and ovary _____ / ___ / _____ / _____
    WR   CV   WR   S

17. creation of an artificial
    opening in the uterine tube _____ / ___ / _____
    WR   CV   S

18. excision of the vulva _____ / _____
    WR   S

19. surgical repair of the breast _____ / ___ / _____
    WR   CV   S

20. suture of the cervix _____ / ___ / _____
    WR   CV   S

21. excision of the cervix _____ / _____
    WR   S

EXERCISE 18

Spell each of the surgical terms built from word parts on pp. 314-315 by having someone
dictate them to you.

 To hear and spell the terms select Chapter 8, Chapter Exercises, Spelling. You may
type the terms on the screen or write them below in the spaces provided.

☐ Place a check mark in the box if you have completed this exercise using your CD-ROM.

1. _____   6. _____

2. _____   7. _____

3. _____   8. _____

4. _____   9. _____

5. _____   10. _____

11._____   17._____

12._____   18._____

13._____   19._____

14._____   20._____

15._____   21._____

16._____

Surgical Terms

Not Built from Word Parts

In some of the following terms, you may recognize word parts you have already learned; however, the full meaning of the terms cannot be discerned by the definition of their word parts.

Term	Definition
anterior and posterior colporrhaphy (A&P repair) . . . . (kol-POR-a-fē)	when a weakened vaginal wall results in a cystocele (protrusion of the bladder against the anterior wall of the vagina) and a rectocele (protrusion of the rectum against the posterior wall of the vagina), an A&P repair corrects the condition (Exercise Figure G)
conization. . . . . (*kon*-i-ZĀ-shun)	the surgical removal of a cone-shaped area of the cervix; used in the treatment for noninvasive cervical cancer (also called **cone biopsy**)
dilation and curettage (D&C) . . (dī-LA-shun) (kū-re-TAHZH)	dilation (widening) of the cervix and scraping of the endometrium with an instrument called a *curette*. It is performed to diagnose disease, to correct bleeding, and to empty uterine contents (Figure 8-8).
endometrial ablation. . . . . (en-dō-MĒ-trē-al) (ab-LĀ-shun)	a procedure to destroy or remove the endometrium by use of laser or thermal energy; used to treat abnormal uterine bleeding (Figure 8-9)
laparoscopy or laparoscopic surgery . . . . (*lap*-a-ROS-ko-pē) (*lap*-a-rō-SKOP-ik)	visual examination of the abdominal cavity, accomplished by inserting a laparoscope through a tiny incision near the umbilicus. It is used for surgical procedures such as tubal sterilization (closure of the uterine tubes), hysterectomy, oophorectomy, or biopsy of the ovaries. It may also be used to diagnose endometriosis (Figure 8-10).
myomectomy . . . . (mī-ō-MEK-to-mē)	excision of a fibroid tumor (myoma) from the uterus

DILATION OR DILATATION
are both used in the presentation of dilation and curettage. Dilation is the more common usage and is used in this text.

ABLATION
is from the Latin **ablatum,** meaning **to carry away.** In surgery **ablation** means **removal** or **excision,** especially by cutting with laser or electrical energy.

Surgical Terms—cont'd
Not Built from Word Parts

Term	Definition
sentinel lymph node biopsy . . . (SEN-tin-el) (limf) (nōd) (BĪ-op-sē)	an injection of blue dye and/or radioactive isotope is used to identify the sentinel lymph node(s), the first in the axillary chain and most likely to contain metastases of breast cancer. The nodes are removed and microscopically examined. If negative, no more nodes are removed (Figure 8-11).
stereotactic breast biopsy . . . . (ster-ē-ō-TAK-tik) (brest) (BĪ-op-sē)	a technique that combines mammography and computer-assisted biopsy to obtain tissue from a breast lesion (Figure 8-12)
tubal ligation. . . . . (lī-GĀ-shun)	closure of the uterine tubes for sterilization by cutting, tying, or cauterizing (also called **tubal sterilization** and "**tying of tubes**") (Figure 8-11)
uterine artery embolization (UAE). . . . . (ū-ter-in) (AR-ter-ē) (*em*-be-li-ZĀ-shun)	minimally invasive procedure used to treat fibroids of the uterus by blocking arteries that supply blood to the fibroids. First, an arteriogram is used to identify the vessels. Once identified, tiny gelatin beads, about the size of grains of sand, are inserted into the vessels to create a blockage. The blockage stops the blood supply to the fibroids causing them to shrink.

UTERINE ARTERY EMBOLIZATION (UAE) provides an alternative to hysterectomy as a treatment for fibroid tumors. A hysterectomy is a major surgery involving general anesthesia and has considerably more recovery time. UAE is performed with local anesthesia and is often done on an outpatient basis.

EXERCISE FIGURE G

Fill in the blanks to complete the labeling of the diagrams.

Anterior and posterior _____ / ___ / _____ corrects the conditions of:
  vagina / cv / suturing

1. _____
   bladder / cv / protrusion

2. Rectocele

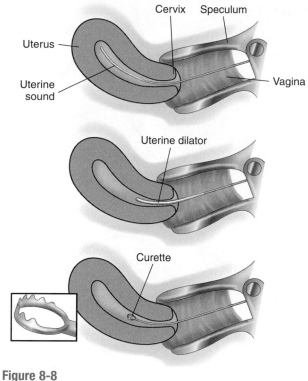

Figure 8-8
Dilation and curettage.

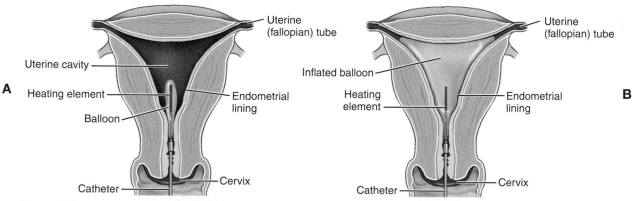

Figure 8-9
Endometrial ablation. **A,** The balloon catheter (deflated) is inserted through the cervix into the uterine cavity. **B,** The balloon is inflated with a solution of 5% dextrose and water and heated to 87°C for 8 minutes, ablating the endometrial lining.

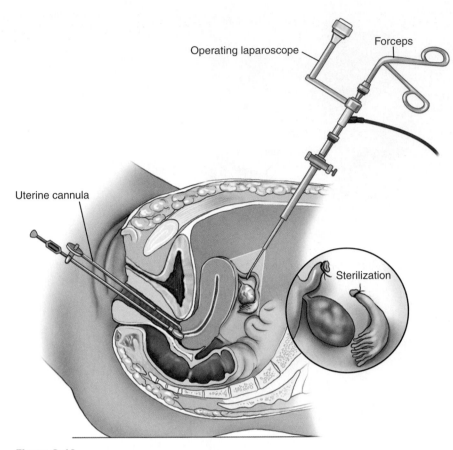

Figure 8-10
Laparoscopic tubal sterilization.

SENTINEL LYMPH NODE BIOPSY

was first developed for patients with melanoma. It is now used to determine metastasis of breast cancer to the lymph nodes. Previously, surgeons would remove 10 to 20 lymph nodes to determine the spread of cancer, often causing lymphedema, which can lead to painful and permanent swelling of the arm. With sentinel lymph node biopsy, if negative, additional lymph nodes are not removed.

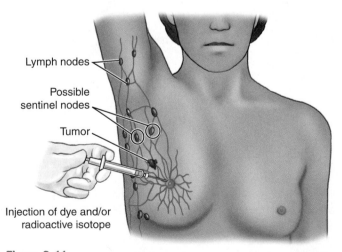

Figure 8-11
Preparation for sentinel lymph node biopsy. The process of identifying the sentinel node(s) is performed in the nuclear medicine department of radiology. The biopsy is performed in surgery.

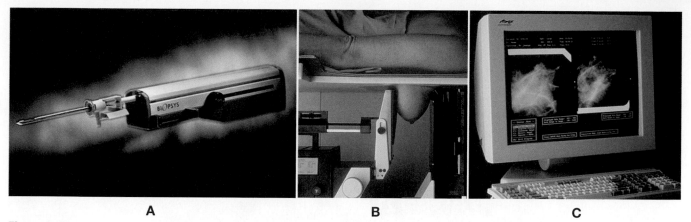

A   **B**   **C**

Figure 8-12
Stereotactic breast biopsy is the least invasive method of obtaining tissue to determine if a nonpalpable breast lesion is benign or malignant. Benefits include less pain and scarring, a shorter recovery time, and less expense than conventional surgery. The patient is placed prone on a special table with the breast suspended through an opening. The breast is placed in a mammography machine under the table. A digital mammogram is produced on a computer monitor to identify the exact location of the lesion. The biopsy instrument is guided by a radiologist or surgeon. Tissue obtained from the lesion is examined microscopically. **A,** The mammotome is used to obtain the specimen for biopsy. **B,** The patient is positioned for stereotactic breast biopsy. **C,** The mammogram appears digitally and is used to determine the placement of the biopsy needle.

EXERCISE 19

Practice saying aloud each of the surgical terms not built from word parts on pp. 319-320.

To hear the terms select Chapter 8, Chapter Exercises, Pronunciation.

☐ Place a check mark in the box when you have completed this exercise.

EXERCISE 20

Fill in the blanks with the correct term.

1. A procedure used for sterilization of the woman is _____
   _____.

2. The surgery used to repair a cystocele and rectocele is a(n) _____
   and _____ _____.

3. D&C is the abbreviation for _____ and _____.

4. _____ _____ _____ is a technique
   used to obtain tissue from a breast lesion.

5. Excision of a fibroid tumor from the uterus is called _____.

6. A procedure to destroy endometrium by laser or thermal energy is called
   _____ _____.

7. A procedure used to treat uterine fibroids by blocking the blood supply is
   called _____ _____ _____.

8. Surgical removal of a cone-shaped area of the cervix is called

_____.

9. A procedure to identify metastasis of breast cancer in the axillary lymph nodes for biopsy is called _____ _____

_____ _____.

10. A surgical procedure performed through a tiny incision near the umbilicus is called _____ or _____ _____.

EXERCISE 21

Match the surgical procedures in the first column with the corresponding organs in the second column. You may use the answers in the second column more than once.

_____ 1. dilation and curettage

_____ 2. laparoscopic surgery for sterilization

_____ 3. tubal ligation

_____ 4. anterior and posterior colporrhaphy repair

_____ 5. myomectomy

_____ 6. stereotactic breast biopsy

_____ 7. conization

_____ 8. endometrial ablation

_____ 9. sentinel lymph node biopsy

_____ 10. uterine artery embolization

a. uterine tubes

b. vagina

c. uterus

d. ovaries

e. vulva

f. mammary glands

g. lymph nodes

EXERCISE 22

Spell each of the surgical terms not built from word parts on pp. 319-320 by having someone dictate them to you.

 To hear and spell the terms select Chapter 8, Chapter Exercises, Spelling. You may type the terms on the screen or write them below in the spaces provided.

☐ Place a check mark in the box if you have completed this exercise using your CD-ROM.

1. _____

2. _____

3. _____

4. _____

5. _____

6. _____

7. _____

8. _____

9. _____

10. _____

Diagnostic Terms

Built from Word Parts

The following terms are built from word parts you have already learned and can be translated literally to find their meanings. Further explanation of terms beyond the definitions of their word parts, if needed, is included in parentheses.

Term	Definition
DIAGNOSTIC IMAGING	
hysterosalpingogram . . . . (*his*-ter-ō-*sal*-PING-gō-gram)	radiographic image of the uterus and uterine tubes (after an injection of a contrast agent) (Exercise Figure H)
mammogram . . . . (MAM-ō-gram)	radiographic image of the breast (Figure 8-13)
mammography . . . . (ma-MOG-ra-fē)	radiographic imaging of the breast (also called **digital mammography** when images are obtained using computed radiography or direct digital radiography) (Figure 8-13)
sonohysterography (SHG) . . . . . (son-ō-*his*-ter-OG-ra-fē)	process of recording the uterus by use of sound (an ultrasound procedure)
ENDOSCOPY	
colposcope . . . . (KOL-pō-skōp)	instrument used for visual examination of the vagina (and cervix)
colposcopy . . . . (kol-POS-ko-pē)	visual examination (with a magnified view) of the vagina (and cervix)
culdoscope . . . . (KUL-dō-skōp)	instrument used for visual examination of Douglas cul-de-sac (rectouterine pouch)
culdoscopy . . . . (kul-DOS-ko-pē)	visual examination of Douglas cul-de-sac (rectouterine pouch) (Exercise Figure I)
hysteroscope . . . . (HIS-ter-ō-skōp)	instrument used for visual examination of the uterus (uterine cavity)
hysteroscopy . . . . (*his*-ter-OS-ko-pē)	visual examination of the uterus (uterine cavity)
OTHER	
culdocentesis . . . . (*kul*-dō-sen-TĒ-sis)	surgical puncture to remove fluid from Douglas cul-de-sac (rectouterine pouch) (Exercise Figure I)

SONOHYSTEROGRAPHY
is a technique for evaluating the uterine cavity. Saline solution is injected into the uterine cavity, followed by transvaginal sonography. It is used preoperatively to assess polyps, myomas, and adhesions.

ENDOSCOPY
dates back to the time of Hippocrates (460-375 BC), who mentions using a speculum to look into a rectum to see where it was affected. By the end of the nineteenth century, **cystoscopy, proctoscopy, laryngoscopy,** and **esophagoscopy** were well established. Use of the **endoscope** for surgery was not widely practiced in the United States until the 1970s when gynecologists started performing **laparoscopic tubal sterilization.** The first ectopic pregnancy was removed by laparoscopic surgery in 1973, the first **laparoscopic appendectomy** occurred in 1983, and the first laparoscopic **cholecystectomy** in 1989. See Table 8-3 for a list of endoscopic surgeries.

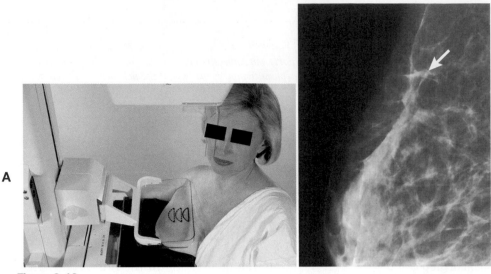

A

B

Figure 8-13
A, Mammography. **B,** Mammogram. *Arrow* points to lesion confirmed by biopsy to be infiltrating ductal carcinoma.

EXERCISE FIGURE H

Fill in the blanks to complete the labeling of the diagram.

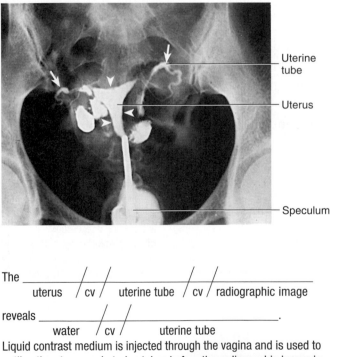

Uterine tube

Uterus

Speculum

The _____/_____/_____
    uterus / cv / uterine tube / cv / radiographic image

reveals _____/_____/_____.
      water / cv /   uterine tube

Liquid contrast medium is injected through the vagina and is used to outline the uterus and uterine tubes before the radiographic image is made. This procedure usually is performed to determine whether obstructions exist in the uterine tubes causing sterility.

EXERCISE FIGURE **I**

Fill in the blanks to complete the labeling of the diagram.

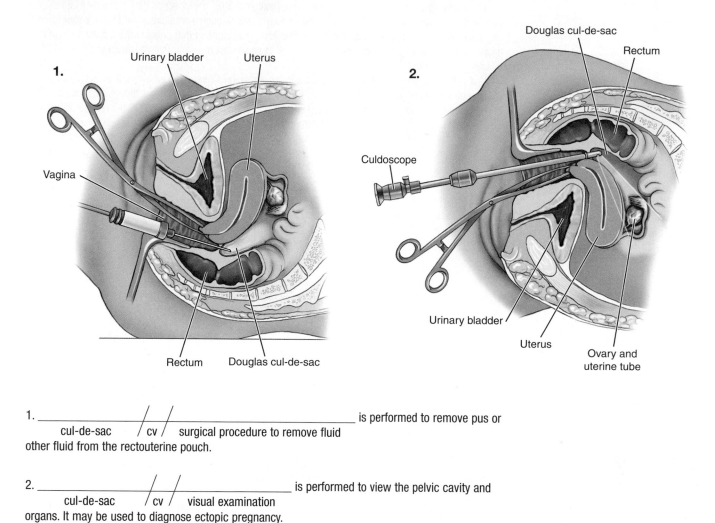

1.
Urinary bladder   Uterus
Vagina
Rectum   Douglas cul-de-sac

2.
Douglas cul-de-sac
Rectum
Culdoscope
Urinary bladder
Uterus
Ovary and uterine tube

1. _____ is performed to remove pus or
   cul-de-sac   / cv /   surgical procedure to remove fluid
other fluid from the rectouterine pouch.

2. _____ is performed to view the pelvic cavity and
   cul-de-sac   / cv /   visual examination
organs. It may be used to diagnose ectopic pregnancy.

TABLE 8-3

Endoscopic Surgery

Endoscopic surgery includes the use of a slender, flexible fiberoptic endoscope that is inserted into a natural body cavity, such as the mouth, or other body areas through a small incision. Three or four other tiny incisions may be made to accommodate visualization equipment that projects the patient's internal organs and structures onto a television screen and to accommodate other instruments and devices needed to complete the surgery.

Because the surgeon performs endoscopic surgery, sometimes referred to as *videoscopic surgery,* by viewing a video monitor, the surgeon must master a new set of skills. Although it is thought that endoscopic surgery will not replace large-incision surgery, its use is in demand because of the reduced trauma and medical cost to the patient. Continued advances in technology will improve and expand its use.

Operative setup for laparoscopic hysterectomy.

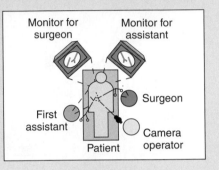

Types of Endoscopic Surgery

Instrument	Procedure	Type of Surgery
arthroscope	arthroscopy or arthroscopic surgery	biopsy ligament repair meniscus repair synovectomy
colonoscope	colonoscopy	polypectomy
hysteroscope	hysteroscopy	myomectomy polypectomy
laparoscope	laparoscopy or laparoscopic surgery	adhesiolysis appendectomy bariatric surgery cholecystectomy herniorrhaphy hysterectomy myomectomy oophorectomy ovarian biopsy ovarian cystectomy prostatectomy splenectomy tubal ligation
thoracoscope	thoracoscopy	biopsy wedge resection of the lung

EXERCISE 23

Practice saying aloud each of the diagnostic terms built from word parts on p. 325.

 To hear the terms select Chapter 8, Chapter Exercises, Pronunciation.

☐ Place a check mark in the box when you have completed this exercise.

EXERCISE 24

Analyze and define the following diagnostic terms.

1. colposcopy _____

2. mammogram _____

3. colposcope _____

4. hysteroscopy _____

5. hysterosalpingogram _____

6. culdoscope _____

7. culdoscopy _____

8. culdocentesis _____

9. mammography _____

10. hysteroscope _____

11. sonohysterography _____

EXERCISE 25

Build diagnostic terms that correspond to the following definitions by using the word parts you have learned.

1. radiographic image of the uterus and uterine tubes

_____ / ____ / _____ / ____ / ____
WR   / CV /   WR   / CV /   S

2. visual examination of the vagina (and cervix)

_____ / ____ / _____
WR   / CV /   S

3. instrument used for visual examination of the vagina (and cervix)

_____ / ____ / _____
WR   / CV /   S

4. visual examination of the uterus

_____ / ____ / _____
WR   / CV /   S

5. radiographic image of the breast

_____ / ____ / _____
WR   / CV /   S

6. instrument used for visual examination of Douglas cul-de-sac

_____ / ____ / _____
WR   / CV /   S

7. visual examination of Douglas cul-de-sac

_____ / ____ / _____
WR   / CV /   S

8. surgical puncture to remove
fluid from Douglas cul-de-sac   _____ / ___ / ___
                                        WR   CV   S

9. instrument used for visual
examination of the uterus   _____ / ___ / ___
                                   WR   CV   S

10. radiographic imaging
of the breast   _____ / ___ / ___
                       WR   CV   S

11. process of recording
the uterus with sound   ___ / ___ / ___ / ___ / ___
                          WR   CV   WR   CV   S

EXERCISE 26

Spell each of the diagnostic terms built from word parts on p. 325 by having someone dictate them to you.

 To hear and spell the terms select Chapter 8, Chapter Exercises, Spelling. You may type the terms on the screen or write them below in the spaces provided.

☐ Place a check mark in the box if you have completed this exercise using your CD-ROM.

1. _____   7. _____

2. _____   8. _____

3. _____   9. _____

4. _____   10. _____

5. _____   11. _____

6. _____

Diagnostic Terms

Not Built from Word Parts

In some of the following terms, you may recognize word parts you have already learned; however, the full meaning of the terms cannot be discerned by the definition of their word parts.

Term	Definition
DIAGNOSTIC IMAGING	
transvaginal sonography (TVS) . . . . (trans-VAJ-i-nal) (so-NOG-ra-fē)	an ultrasound procedure that uses a transducer placed in the vagina to obtain images of the ovaries, uterus, cervix, uterine tubes, and surrounding structures; used to diagnose masses such as ovarian cysts or tumors, to monitor pregnancy, and to evaluate ovulation for the treatment of infertility (Figure 8-14)

Term	Definition
LABORATORY	
CA-125 (cancer antigen-125 tumor marker)	a blood test used in the detection of ovarian cancer. It is also used to monitor treatment and to determine the extent of the disease.
Pap smear	a cytological study of cervical and vaginal secretions used to determine the presence of abnormal or cancerous cells; most commonly used to detect cancers of the cervix (also called **Papanicolaou** [*pap*-a-NIK-*kō*-la-oo] **smear** and **Pap test** (Figure 8-15)

PAP SMEAR
is named after Dr. George N. Papanicolaou (1883–1962), a Greek physician practicing in the United States, who developed the cell smear method for the diagnosis of cancer in 1943. The test may be used for tissue specimen from any organ but is most commonly used on cervical and vaginal secretions. The Pap smear is 95% accurate in detecting cervical carcinoma. In 1966 a liquid-based screening system was approved by the Food and Drug Administration as an alternative for the conventional Pap smear. This system improves detection of squamous intraepithelial lesions.

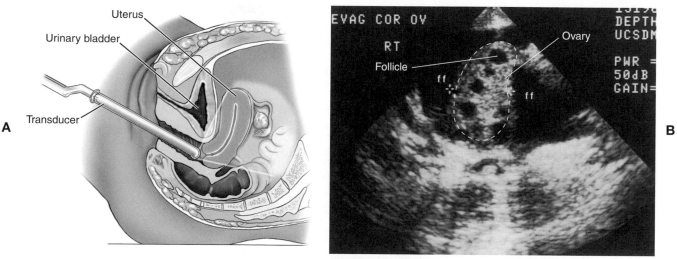

A

B

Figure 8-14

Transvaginal sonography. **A,** Transducer placed in the vagina. **B,** Transvaginal sagittal image of the right ovary with multiple follicles, showing free fluid surrounding the ovary.

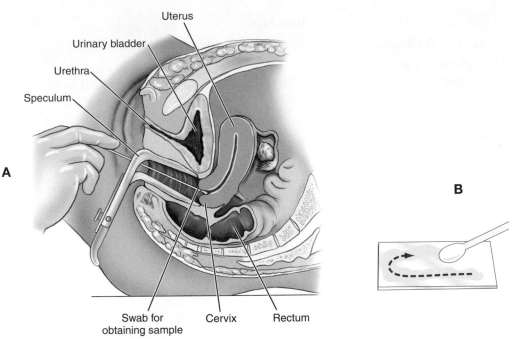

Figure 8-15

Pap smear. **A,** Obtaining the specimen. **B,** Transferring the specimen to a glass slide, where it will be stained and studied under a microscope in the laboratory.

EXERCISE 27

Practice saying aloud each of the diagnostic terms not built from word parts on pp. 330-331.

 To hear the terms select Chapter 8, Chapter Exercises, Pronunciation.

☐ Place a check mark in the box when you have completed this exercise.

EXERCISE 28

Fill in the blanks with the correct definition.

1. Pap smear _____

2. transvaginal sonography _____

3. CA-125 _____

EXERCISE 29

Write the term for each of the following.

1. study of cervical and vaginal secretions _____ _____

2. blood test used to detect ovarian cancer _____

3. obtains images of the ovaries, uterus, cervix, uterine tubes, and surrounding structures _____ _____

EXERCISE 30

Spell each of the disease and disorder terms not built from word parts on pp. 330-331 by
having someone dictate them to you.

 To hear and spell the terms select Chapter 8, Chapter Exercises, Spelling. You may
type the terms on the screen or write them below in the spaces provided.

☐ Place a check mark in the box if you have completed this exercise using your CD-ROM.

1. _____   3. _____

2. _____

Complementary Terms

Built from Word Parts

*The following terms are built from word parts you have already learned and can be translated
literally to find their meanings. Further explanation of terms beyond the definition of their word
parts, if needed, is included in parentheses.*

Term	Definition
gynecologist . . . . (gīn-ek-OL-o-jist)	a physician who studies and treats diseases of women (female reproductive system)
gynecology (GYN) . . . . (gīn-ek-OL-o-jē)	study of women (a branch of medicine deal- ing with diseases of the female reproduc- tive system)
gynopathic . . . . (gīn-ō-PATH-ik)	pertaining to diseases of women
leukorrhea . . . . (lū-kō-RĒ-a)	white discharge (from the vagina)
mastalgia . . . . (mas-TAL-ja)	pain in the breast
mastoptosis . . . . (mas-top-TŌ-sis)	sagging breast
menarche . . . . (me-NAR-kē)	beginning of menstruation (usually occurring between the ages of 11 and 16)
vaginal . . . . (VAJ-i-nal)	pertaining to the vagina
vulvovaginal . . . . (vul-vō-VAJ-i-nal)	pertaining to the vulva and vagina

EXERCISE 31

Practice saying aloud each of the complementary terms built from word parts above.

 To hear the terms select Chapter 8, Chapter Exercises, Pronunciation.

☐ Place a check mark in the box when you have completed this exercise.

EXERCISE 32

Analyze and define the following complementary terms.

1. gynecologist _____

2. gynecology _____

3. vulvovaginal _____

4. mastalgia _____

5. menarche _____

6. leukorrhea _____

7. gynopathic _____

8. mastoptosis _____

9. vaginal _____

EXERCISE 33

Build complementary terms that correspond to the following definitions by using the word parts you have learned.

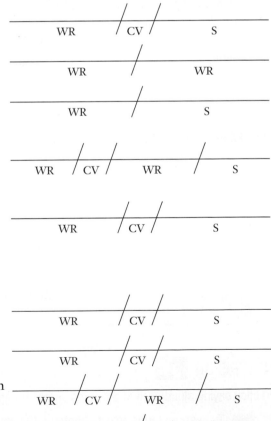

1. white discharge (from the vagina)

    WR / CV /   S

2. beginning of menstruation

    WR /   WR

3. pain in the breast

    WR /   S

4. pertaining to the vulva and vagina

    WR / CV /   WR /   S

5. a physician who studies and treats (diseases of) women

    WR / CV /   S

6. study of women (branch of medicine dealing with diseases of the female reproductive system)

    WR / CV /   S

7. sagging breast

    WR / CV /   S

8. pertaining to diseases of women

    WR / CV /   WR /   S

9. pertaining to the vagina

    WR /   S

EXERCISE 34

Spell each of the complementary terms built from word parts on p. 333 by having someone dictate them to you.

 To hear and spell the terms select Chapter 8, Chapter Exercises, Spelling. You may type the terms on the screen or write them below in the spaces provided.

☐ Place a check mark in the box if you have completed this exercise using your CD-ROM.

1. _____   6. _____

2. _____   7. _____

3. _____   8. _____

4. _____   9. _____

5. _____

Complementary Terms

Not Built from Word Parts

In some of the following terms, you may recognize word parts you have already learned; however, the full meaning of the terms cannot be discerned by the definition of their word parts.

Term	Definition
dyspareunia . . . . (*dis*-pa-RŪ-nē-a)	difficult or painful intercourse
fistula . . . . (FIS-tū-la)	abnormal passageway between two organs or between an internal organ and the body surface
hormone replacement therapy (HRT)	replacement of hormones to treat symptoms associated with menopause (also called **estrogen replacement therapy [ERT]**)
menopause . . . . (MEN-o-pawz)	cessation of menstruation, usually around the ages of 48 to 53 years
premenstrual syndrome (PMS) . . . . (prē-MEN-stroo-al) (SIN-drom)	a syndrome involving physical and emotional symptoms occurring in the 10 days before menstruation. Symptoms include nervous tension, irritability, mastalgia, edema, and headache. Its cause is not fully understood.
speculum . . . . (SPEK-ū-lum)	instrument for opening a body cavity to allow visual inspection (Figure 8-16)

Figure 8-16
Vaginal speculum.

EXERCISE 35

Practice saying aloud each of the complementary terms not built from word parts on p. 335.

 To hear the terms select Chapter 8, Chapter Exercises, Pronunciation.

☐ Place a check mark in the box when you have completed this exercise.

EXERCISE 36

Write the definitions of the following terms.

1. menopause _____

2. dyspareunia _____

3. fistula _____

4. premenstrual syndrome _____

5. speculum _____

6. hormone replacement therapy _____

EXERCISE 37

Write the term for each of the following.

1. abnormal passageway _____

2. painful intercourse _____

3. cessation of menstruation _____

4. syndrome involving physical
   and emotional symptoms _____ _____

5. instrument for opening a body cavity _____

6. replacement of hormones to treat symptoms associated with
   menopause _____ _____ _____

EXERCISE 38

Spell each of the complementary terms not built from word parts on p. 335 by having someone dictate them to you.

 To hear and spell the terms select Chapter 8, Chapter Exercises, Spelling. You may type the terms on the screen or write them below in the spaces provided.

☐ Place a check mark in the box if you have completed this exercise using your CD-ROM.

1. _____   4. _____

2. _____   5. _____

3. _____   6. _____

Refer to Appendix E for pharmacology terms related to the female reproductive system.

Abbreviations

A&P repair	anterior and posterior colporrhaphy
Cx	cervix
D&C.	dilation and curettage
FBD.	fibrocystic breast disease
GYN.	gynecology
HRT.	hormone replacement therapy
PID	pelvic inflammatory disease
PMS	premenstrual syndrome
SHG.	sonohysterography
TAH/BSO	total abdominal hysterectomy/bilateral salpingo-oophorectomy
TSS.	toxic shock syndrome
TVH.	total vaginal hysterectomy
TVS.	transvaginal sonography
UAE.	uterine artery embolization

Refer to Appendix D for a complete list of abbreviations.

EXERCISE 39

Write the meaning for each of the abbreviations in the following sentences.

1. To repair a cystocele and rectocele the patient is scheduled in surgery for an **A&P repair** _____ & _____ _____ .

2. Following a **TAH/BSO** _____ _____ _____ and _____ _____ the gynecologist ordered **HRT** _____ _____ _____ for the patient.

3. **SHG** _____ and **TVS** _____ _____ are diagnostic ultrasound procedures used to assist in diagnosing diseases and disorders of the female reproductive organs.

4. When performing a **TVH** _____ _____ _____ the surgeon removes the uterus through the vagina without a surgical incision into the abdomen.

5. **D&C** _____ & _____ is the dilation of the **Cx** _____ and scraping of the endometrium.

6. **FBD** _____ _____ _____ is the most common breast problem of women in their 20s.

7. A female patient with probable **PID** _____ _____ _____ was referred to the **GYN** _____ clinic for evaluation and care.

8. The medical management of **PMS** _____ _____ emphasizes the relief of symptoms.

9. **UAE** _____ _____ _____ offers a minimally invasive treatment option for some women with symptomatic fibroid tumors.

PRACTICAL APPLICATION

EXERCISE 40   *Interact with Medical Documents*

A. Complete the progress note by writing the medical terms in the blanks. Use the list of definitions with the corresponding numbers on the next page.

University Hospital and Medical Center
4700 North Main Street • Wellness, Arizona 54321 • (987) 555-3210

PATIENT NAME: Sandra Garcia   **CASE NUMBER:** 05632-FRS
DATE OF BIRTH: 11/01/19XX   **DATE:** 11/14/20XX

PROGRESS NOTE

Sandra Garcia is a 48-year-old Puerto Rican woman here for follow-up after a suspicious mass in the left breast was discovered during routine 1. _____.

Family history is positive for 2. _____ in a maternal aunt.

Past medical history includes 3. _____ for 4. _____ and 5. _____. She has been on 6. _____ since age 46 years.

The patient consented to a 7. _____ _____ _____.

Pathology report is as follows:

GROSS DESCRIPTION: Received labeled "breast biopsy" is an ovoid mass of predominantly adipose breast tissue measuring 4.5 × 3.0 × 1.3 cm. Sectioning reveals a focal area of suspicious 8. _____. Frozen section reveals fat 9. _____ and evidence of malignancy in an area measuring 0.25 cm in the center of the specimen. The surgeon is so informed.

MICROSCOPIC DESCRIPTION: Microscopic examination of the frozen section specimen confirms the presence of fat necrosis. There is focal duct epithelial 10. _____ exhibiting a papillomatous pattern. A well-differentiated adenocarcinoma was found in this area. Occasional breast parenchymal fragments are also identified and show fibrocystic changes. These are predominantly nonproliferative, although in slide D, a small radial scar containing ducts showing proliferative fibrocystic changes with significant atypia and adjacent sclerosing adenosis is identified.

DIAGNOSIS: Left breast biopsy:
1. Papillary ductal carcinoma, well differentiated.
2. Radial scar.
3. Nonproliferative and proliferative fibrocystic changes with significant atypia.
4. Focal sclerosing adenosis.

_____
Marcus Weldon, MD

MW/mcm

1. radiographic imaging of the breast
2. cancerous tumor
3. excision of the uterus
4. growth of endometrium into the muscular portion of the uterus
5. abnormal condition in which endometrial tissue occurs in various areas of the pelvic cavity
6. abbreviation for replacement of hormones to treat menopause
7. combines mammography and computer-assisted biopsy to obtain tissue from a breast lesion
8. abnormal hard spot
9. abnormal condition of death (dead tissue because of disease)
10. excessive development (of cells)

B. Read the chart note and answer the questions following it.

47820 CARLSON, SARA R.   _ □ X

File Patient Navigate Custom Fields Help

| Patient Chart | Lab | Rad | Notes | Documents | Rx | Scheduling | Images | Billing |

Name: **CARLSON, SARA R.**   MR#: **47820**   Sex: **F**
DOB: **2/15/19XX**

CHART NOTE

ENCOUNTER DATE: 11/13/20XX

HISTORY: This 37-year-old gravida 2 para 2 African American woman was referred by her primary care provider. She complains of fullness in the pelvic region and menometrorrhagia. She admits to frequency and urgency of urination. Also, she complains of fatigue. The patient's last menstrual period was two weeks ago. Her mother was treated for ovarian cancer.

PHYSICAL EXAMINATION: Upon bimanual pelvic examination, an ill-defined mass was palpable on left lateral portion of the uterus.

DIAGNOSTIC STUDIES: Pap smear results showed normal cytology. CA-125 results were normal. Transvaginal sonography confirmed the presence of a pedunculated fibroid tumor. The uterine tubes and ovaries were normal.

IMPRESSION: Fibroid tumor.

RECOMMENDATION: We discussed the benefits of having a vaginal hysterectomy with bilateral salpingo-oophorectomy in view of her mother's history of ovarian cancer. The patient declined this approach because of the desire to have another child. A laparoscopic myomectomy is therefore recommended.

Electronically signed by: Patrick Fuller, MD 11/14/20XX 3:34 PM

PF/dlb

| Start | Log On/Off | Print | Edit |

---

1. The patient's symptoms include:
   a. absence of menstrual discharge
   b. scanty menstrual flow
   c. increased amount of menstrual flow during menses and bleeding between periods
   d. painful menstruation

2. The CA-125 diagnostic study was used to detect the presence of:
   a. ovarian cancer
   b. cervical cancer
   c. endometrial cancer
   d. endometriosis

3. The recommended procedure, a myomectomy, will entail the surgical excision of:
   a. a breast
   b. the uterus
   c. ovarian cancer
   d. a fibroid tumor

EXERCISE **41** *Interpret Medical Terms*

To test your understanding of the terms introduced in this chapter, circle the words that correctly complete the sentences. The italicized words refer to the correct answer.

1. The patient was diagnosed as having *painful menstruation*, or (**oligomenorrhea, dysmenorrhea, amenorrhea**).

2. *Inflammation of the inner lining of the uterus* is (**endocervicitis, endometritis, endometriosis**).

3. The patient is scheduled in surgery for a *salpingectomy*, which is the excision of the (**uterine tube, ovary, uterus**).

4. An *episiorrhaphy* is a (**suture of the vulva, discharge from the vulva, rapid discharge from the vulva**).

5. A *surgical procedure to reduce breast size* is called reduction (**mammogram, mammography, mammoplasty**).

6. A *hysterosalpingo-oophorectomy* is the excision of the (**uterus, uterine tubes, and ovaries; uterus, ovaries, and cervix; uterus, uterine tubes, and vagina**).

7. *Blood in the uterine tube* is called (**hematosalpinx, hydrosalpinx, pyosalpinx**).

8. *Endometrial tissue occurring in various areas of the pelvic cavity* is called (**adenomyosis, endometriosis, hysteratresia**).

9. The doctor requested a (**hysteroscope, colposcope, speculum**) *to open the vagina for visual examination.*

10. A severe illness *that may affect menstruating women after using tampons is* (**TVS, TSS, TVH**).

EXERCISE 42 Read Medical Terms in Use

Practice pronunciation of the terms by reading the following information on cancers of the female reproductive system. Use the pronunciation key following the medical terms to assist you in saying the words.

To hear these terms select Chapter 8, Chapter Exercises, Read Medical Terms in Use.

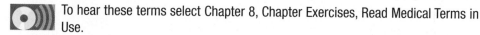

CANCERS OF THE FEMALE REPRODUCTIVE SYSTEM

Breast Cancer

The breast is the second most common site of cancer in women. More than 80% of **breast cancer** (brest) (KAN-cer) is infiltrating ductal cancer (IDC), which originates in the mammary ducts. The rate of growth depends on hormonal influences. As long as the cancer remains in the duct, it is considered noninvasive and is called *ductal carcinoma in situ (DCIS)*.

Mammography (ma-MOG-ra-fē) is the most common method used for diagnosing cancer of the breast. Confirmation is done with a biopsy obtained by conventional surgery or **stereotactic breast biopsy** (ster-ē-ō-TAK-tik) (brest) (BĪ-op-sē). Treatment may include lumpectomy, **mastectomy** (mas-TEK-to-mē), chemotherapy, radiation therapy, and hormonal therapy.

Cervical Cancer

In many regions of the world **cervical cancer** (SER-vi-kal) (KAN-cer) is the leading cause of death in women. Cervical cancer resembles a sexually transmitted disease, a feature that distinguishes it from other cancers. Abnormal **vaginal** (VAJ-i-nal) bleeding is the most common symptom. **Pap smear** followed by **colposcopy** (kol-POS-ko-pē) biopsy is used to diagnose this disease. Surgical treatment options are **conization** (*kon*-i-ZĀ-shun), cryosurgery, laser ablation, and **hysterectomy** (*his*-te-REK-to-mē). Chemotherapy and radiation therapy may also be used. **Trachelectomy** (*trā*-ke-LEK-to-mē) may be performed in patients with small primary tumors who may wish to bear children in the future. A vaccine for human papillomavirus is now available and can be used for the prevention of cervical cancer.

Endometrial Cancer

Currently 75% of women diagnosed with **endometrial cancer** (en-dō-MĒ-trē-al) (KAN-cer) are postmenopausal. Inappropriate bleeding is the only warning sign; hence early diagnosis is common. Pelvic examination, Pap smear, and endometrial sampling are used to diagnose this disease. Treatment is **hysterosalpingo-oophorectomy** (*his*-ter-ō-sal-*ping*-gō-ō-*of*o-REK-to-mē), which may be followed by chemotherapy and radiation therapy. **Laparoscopic** (lap-a-RŌ-skop-ik)-assisted **vaginal hysterectomy** (VAJ-i-nal) (his-te-REK-to-mē) may also be used.

Ovarian Cancer

Ovarian cancer (ō-VAR-ē-an) (KAN-cer) is the sixth most common form of cancer in women. Early symptoms are often absent or associated with other problems; thus early diagnosis is uncommon. Early symptoms include abdominal discomfort and bloating; later stages include abdominal or pelvic pain and urinary or menstrual irregularities. **CA-125** and **transvaginal sonography** (trans-VAJ-i-nal) (so-NOG-ra-fē) are used in diagnosing this disease. Treatment is total abdominal **hysterectomy** (his-te-REK-to-mē) and bilateral **salpingo-oophorectomy** (sal-ping-gō-ō-*of*o-REK-to-mē) and removal of as much additional involved tissue as possible.

Chemotherapy is usually prescribed, followed a year later by a second-look **laparoscopy** (*lap*-a-ROS-ko-pē) to determine the presence or absence of the tumor.

EXERCISE 43 *Comprehend Medical Terms in Use*

Test your comprehension of the terms in the previous box by circling the correct answer.

1. Which of the following diagnostic tests would the physician use to diagnose ovarian cancer?
   a. colposcopy biopsy
   b. transvaginal sonography
   c. Pap smear
   d. mammography

2. T   F   Surgery is a treatment option for breast, cervical, endometrial, and ovarian cancer.

3. T   F   Excision of the uterus, uterine tubes, and ovaries is an accepted surgical treatment for both endometrial and ovarian cancer.

4. An instrument for visualization of the vagina is used to obtain a biopsy to confirm the diagnosis of cancer of the:
   a. ovary
   b. breast
   c. uterine tube
   d. cervix

CHAPTER REVIEW

CHAPTER REVIEW ON CD-ROM

Use the CD-ROM that accompanies this textbook to play and practice what you have learned in this chapter. The Chapter Exercises, Practice Activities, Animations, and Games allow you to hear, see, and interact with the chapter content.

Chapter Exercises

Exercises in this section of your CD-ROM correlate to exercises in your textbook. You may have completed them as you worked through the chapter.
☐ Pronunciation
☐ Spelling
☐ Read Medical Terms in Use

Practice Activities

Practice in study mode, then test your learning in assessment mode. Keep track of your scores from assessment mode if you wish.

                                          SCORE
☐ Picture It   _____
☐ Define Word Parts   _____
☐ Build Medical Terms   _____
☐ Word Shop   _____
☐ Define Medical Terms   _____
☐ Use It   _____
☐ Hear It and Type It: _____
   Clinical Vignettes

Animations
☐ Pelvic Inflammatory Disease

Games
☐ Name that Word Part
☐ Term Storm
☐ Term Explorer
☐ Termbusters
☐ Medical Millionaire

REVIEW OF WORD PARTS

Can you define and spell the following word parts?

Combining Forms		**Prefix**	**Suffixes**
arche/o	men/o	peri-	-atresia
cervic/o	metr/i		-ial
colp/o	metr/o		-salpinx
culd/o	oophor/o		
episi/o	perine/o		
gyn/o	salping/o		
gynec/o	trachel/o		
hymen/o	uter/o		
hyster/o	vagin/o		
mamm/o	vulv/o		
mast/o			

REVIEW OF TERMS

Can you build, analyze, define, pronounce, and spell the following terms *built from word parts?*

Diseases and Disorders	**Surgical**	**Diagnostic**	**Complementary**
amenorrhea	cervicectomy	colposcope	gynecologist
Bartholin adenitis	colpoperineorrhaphy	colposcopy	gynecology (GYN)
cervicitis	colpoplasty	culdocentesis	gynopathic
colpitis	colporrhaphy	culdoscope	leukorrhea
dysmenorrhea	episioperineoplasty	culdoscopy	mastalgia
endocervicitis	episiorrhaphy	hysterosalpingogram	mastoptosis
endometritis	hymenectomy	hysteroscope	menarche
hematosalpinx	hymenotomy	hysteroscopy	vaginal
hydrosalpinx	hysterectomy	mammogram	vulvovaginal
hysteratresia	hysteropexy	mammography	
mastitis	hysterosalpingo-	sonohysterography (SHG)	
menometrorrhagia	oophorectomy		
menorrhagia	mammoplasty		
metrorrhagia	mastectomy		
myometritis	oophorectomy		
oligomenorrhea	perineorrhaphy		
oophoritis	salpingectomy		
perimetritis	salpingo-oophorectomy		
pyosalpinx	salpingostomy		
salpingitis	trachelectomy		
salpingocele	trachelorrhaphy		
vaginitis	vulvectomy		
vulvovaginitis			

Can you define, pronounce, and spell the following terms *not built from word parts?*

Diseases and Disorders	**Surgical**	**Diagnostic**	**Complementary**
adenomyosis	anterior and posterior colpor-rhaphy (A&P repair)	CA-125	dyspareunia
breast cancer		Pap smear	fistula
cervical cancer	conization	transvaginal sonography (TVS)	hormone replacement therapy (HRT)
endometrial cancer	dilation and curettage (D&C)		
endometriosis	endometrial ablation		menopause
fibrocystic breast disease (FBD)	laparoscopy		premenstrual syndrome (PMS)
fibroid tumor	myomectomy		speculum
ovarian cancer	sentinel lymph node biopsy		
pelvic inflammatory disease (PID)	stereotactic breast biopsy		
	tubal ligation		
prolapsed uterus	uterine artery embolization (UAE)		
toxic shock syndrome (TSS)			
vesicovaginal fistula			

ANSWERS

Exercise Figures

Exercise Figure

A. 1. ovary: oophor/o
   2. uterus: hyster/o, metr/o (metr/i), uter/o
   3. uterine, or fallopian, tube: salping/o
   4. cervix: cervic/o, trachel/o
   5. vagina: colp/o, vagin/o
   6. hymen: hymen/o

Exercise Figure

B. 1. vulva: episi/o, vulv/o
   2. perineum: perine/o

Exercise Figure

C. salping/itis

Exercise Figure

D. hyster/o/ptosis

Exercise Figure

E. vesic/o/vagin/al

Exercise Figure

F. 1. hyster/o/salping/o/-oophor/ectomy
   2. salping /o/-oophor/ectomy
   3. salping/o/-oophor/ectomy
   4. hyster/ectomy

Exercise Figure

G. colp/o/rrhaphy, cyst/o/cele

Exercise Figure

H. hyster/o/salping/o/gram, hydr/o/salpinx

Exercise Figure

I. 1. culd/o/centesis
   2. culd/o/scopy

Exercise 1

1. c	6. e
2. f	7. h
3. g	8. a
4. b	9. i
5. d	

Exercise 2

1. b	7. g
2. c	8. l
3. d	9. i
4. k	10. j
5. e	11. h
6. f	

Exercise 3

1. vagina
2. ovary
3. uterus
4. uterus
5. hymen
6. uterus
7. menstruation
8. vulva
9. cervix
10. vagina
11. woman
12. breast
13. perineum
14. uterine tube
15. vulva
16. breast
17. first, beginning
18. cul-de-sac
19. woman
20. cervix

Exercise 4

1. a. episi/o
   b. vulv/o
2. a. mamm/o
   b. mast/o
3. men/o
4. oophor/o
5. salping/o
6. perine/o
7. a. vagin/o
   b. colp/o
8. a. uter/o
   b. metr/i, metr/o
   c. hyster/o
9. a. gynec/o
   b. gyn/o
10. hymen/o
11. culd/o
12. a. cervic/o
    b. trachel/o
13. arche/o

Exercise 5

1. -salpinx
2. -ial
3. peri-
4. -atresia

Exercise 6

1. uterine tube
2. surrounding
3. pertaining to
4. absence of a normal body opening, occlusion, closure

Exercise 7

Pronunciation Exercise

Exercise 8

1. WR   S
   colp/itis
   inflammation of the vagina
2. WR   S
   cervic/itis
   inflammation of the cervix
3. WR CV   S
   hydr/o/salpinx
   ⌣
   CF
   water in the uterine tube
4. WR CV   S
   hemat/o/salpinx
   ⌣
   CF
   blood in the uterine tube
5. WR CV   S
   metr/o/rrhagia
   ⌣
   CF
   rapid flow of blood from the uterus (between menstrual cycles)
6. WR   S
   oophor/itis
   inflammation of the ovary
7.   WR   S
   (Bartholin) aden/itis
   inflammation of (Bartholin) gland
8. WR CV WR   S
   vulv/o/vagin/itis
   ⌣
   CF
   inflammation of the vulva and vagina
9. WR   CV S
   salping/o/cele
   ⌣
   CF
   hernia of the uterine tube
10. WR CV WR CV   S
    men/o/metr/o/rrhagia
    ⌣   ⌣
    CF   CF
    rapid flow of blood from the uterus at menstruation (and between menstrual cycles)
11. P WR CV S
    a/men/o/rrhea
    ⌣
    CF
    absence of menstrual discharge
12. P   WR CV S
    dys/men/o/rrhea
    ⌣
    CF
    painful menstrual discharge
13. WR   S
    mast/itis
    inflammation of the breast

14. P WR S
    peri/metr/itis
    inflammation surrounding the uterus
    (outer layer)
15. WR CV WR S
    my/o/metr/itis
      CF
    inflammation of the uterine muscle
16. P WR S
    endo/metr/itis
    inflammation of the inner (lining) of
    the uterus
17. P WR S
    endo/cervic/itis
    inflammation of the inner (lining) of
    the cervix
18. WR CV S
    py/o/salpinx
      CF
    pus in the uterine tube
19. WR S
    hyster/atresia
    closure of the uterus (uterine cavity)
20. WR S
    salping/itis
    inflammation of the uterine tube
21. WR S
    vagin/itis
    inflammation of the vagina
22. WR CV S
    men/o/rrhagia
      CF
    rapid flow of blood at menstruation
    (increased amount)
23. WR CV WR CV S
    olig/o/men/o/rrhea
      CF   CF
    scanty menstrual flow (less often)

Exercise 9
1. mast/itis
2. metr/o/rrhagia
3. salping/itis
4. vulv/o/vagin/itis
5. a/men/o/rrhea
6. cervic/itis
7. (Bartholin) aden/itis
8. hydr/o/salpinx
9. dys/men/o/rrhea
10. hemat/o/salpinx
11. a. colp/itis
    b. vagin/itis
12. men/o/metr/o/rrhagia
13. oophor/itis
14. salping/o/cele
15. peri/metr/itis
16. endo/metr/itis
17. endo/cervic/itis
18. my/o/metr/itis
19. py/o/salpinx
20. hyster/atresia

21. olig/o/men/o/rrhea
22. men/o/rrhagia

Exercise 10
Spelling Exercise; see text p. 309.

Exercise 11
Pronunciation Exercise

Exercise 12
1. downward placement of the uterus
   into the vagina
2. inflammation of the female pelvic
   organs
3. abnormal opening between the bladder and vagina
4. benign fibroid tumor of the uterine
   muscle
5. abnormal condition in which endometrial tissue grows in various areas
   of the pelvic cavity
6. growth of endometrium into the
   muscular portion of the uterus
7. a severe illness characterized by high
   fever, vomiting, diarrhea, and myalgia
8. a disorder characterized by one or
   more benign cysts
9. malignant tumor of the ovary
10. malignant tumor of the breast
11. malignant tumor of the cervix
12. malignant tumor of the endometrium

Exercise 13
1. vesicovaginal fistula
2. fibroid tumor
3. pelvic inflammatory disease
4. prolapsed uterus
5. endometriosis
6. adenomyosis
7. toxic shock syndrome
8. fibrocystic breast disease
9. breast cancer
10. endometrial cancer
11. ovarian cancer
12. cervical cancer

Exercise 14
Spelling Exercise; see text p. 313.

Exercise 15
Pronunciation Exercise

Exercise 16
1. WR CV S
   colp/o/rrhaphy
      CF
   suture of the vagina
2. WR CV S
   colp/o/plasty
      CF
   surgical repair of the vagina

3. WR CV S
   episi/o/rrhaphy
      CF
   suture of the vulva (tear)
4. WR CV S
   hymen/o/tomy
      CF
   incision of the hymen
5. WR CV S
   hyster/o/pexy
      CF
   surgical fixation of the uterus
6. WR S
   vulv/ectomy
   excision of the vulva
7. WR CV S
   perine/o/rrhaphy
      CF
   suture of the perineum (tear)
8. WR CV S
   salping/o/stomy
      CF
   creation of an artificial opening in the
   uterine tube
9. WR CV WR S
   salping/o/-oophor/ectomy
         CF
   excision of the uterine tube and ovary
10. WR S
    oophor/ectomy
    excision of an ovary
11. WR S
    mast/ectomy
    surgical removal of a breast
12. WR S
    salping/ectomy
    excision of a uterine tube
13. WR S
    cervic/ectomy
    excision of the cervix
14. WR CV WR CV S
    colp/o/perine/o/rrhaphy
      CF   CF
    suture of the vagina and perineum
15. WR CV WR CV S
    episi/o/perine/o/plasty
      CF   CF
    surgical repair of the vulva and
    perineum
16. WR S
    hymen/ectomy
    excision of the hymen
17. WR CV WR CV WR S
    hyster/o/salping/o/-oophor/ectomy
       CF   CF
    excision of the uterus, uterine tubes,
    and ovaries

18. WR   S
    hyster/ectomy
    excision of the uterus
19. WR   CV   S
    mamm/o/plasty
         CF
    surgical repair of the breast
20. WR   CV   S
    trachel/o/rrhaphy
           CF
    suture of the cervix
21. WR   S
    trachel/ectomy
    excision of the cervix

Exercise 17
1. colp/o/rrhaphy
2. cervic/ectomy
3. episi/o/rrhaphy
4. episi/o/perine/o/plasty
5. colp/o/plasty
6. colp/o/perine/o/rrhaphy
7. hyster/o/salping/o/-oophor/ectomy
8. hyster/o/pexy
9. hymen/ectomy
10. hymen/o/tomy
11. hyster/ectomy
12. oophor/ectomy
13. mast/ectomy
14. salping/ectomy
15. perine/o/rrhaphy
16. salping/o/-oophor/ectomy
17. salping/o/stomy
18. vulv/ectomy
19. mamm/o/plasty
20. trachel/o/rrhaphy
21. trachel/ectomy

Exercise 18
Spelling Exercise; see text p. 318.

Exercise 19
Pronunciation Exercise

Exercise 20
1. tubal ligation
2. anterior and posterior colporrhaphy
3. dilation and curettage
4. stereotactic breast biopsy
5. myomectomy
6. endometrial ablation
7. uterine artery embolization
8. conization
9. sentinel lymph node biopsy
10. laparoscopy or laparoscopic surgery

Exercise 21
1. c   6. f
2. a   7. c
3. a   8. c
4. b   9. g
5. c   10. c

Exercise 22
Spelling Exercise; see text p. 324.

Exercise 23
Pronunciation Exercise

Exercise 24
1. WR   CV   S
   colp/o/scopy
        CF
   visual examination of the vagina
2. WR   CV   S
   mamm/o/gram
         CF
   radiographic image of the breast
3. WR   CV   S
   colp/o/scope
        CF
   instrument used for visual
      examination of the vagina
4. WR   CV   S
   hyster/o/scopy
          CF
   visual examination of the uterus
5. WR   CV   WR   CV   S
   hyster/o/salping/o/gram
         CF   CF
   radiographic image of the uterus and
      uterine tubes
6. WR   CV   S
   culd/o/scope
        CF
   instrument used for visual examina-
      tion of the Douglas cul-de-sac
7. WR   CV   S
   culd/o/scopy
        CF
   visual examination of the Douglas
      cul-de-sac
8. WR   CV   S
   culd/o/centesis
        CF
   surgical puncture to remove fluid
      from the Douglas cul-de-sac
9. WR   CV   S
   mamm/o/graphy
         CF
   radiographic imaging of the breast

10. WR   CV   S
    hyster/o/scope
           CF
    instrument used for visual
       examination of the uterus
11. WR   CV   WR   CV   S
    son/o/hyster/o/graphy
        CF   CF
    process of recording the uterus with
       sound

Exercise 25
1. hyster/o/salping/o/gram
2. colp/o/scopy
3. colp/o/scope
4. hyster/o/scopy
5. mamm/o/gram
6. culd/o/scope
7. culd/o/scopy
8. culd/o/centesis
9. hyster/o/scope
10. mamm/o/graphy
11. son/o/hyster/o/graphy

Exercise 26
Spelling Exercise; see text p. 330.

Exercise 27
Pronunciation Exercise

Exercise 28
1. cytological study of cervical and vaginal secretions used to determine the
   presence of abnormal or cancerous
   cells
2. an ultrasound procedure that obtains
   images of the ovaries, uterus, cervix,
   and uterine tubes
3. a blood test used to detect and monitor treatment of ovarian cancer

Exercise 29
1. Pap smear
2. CA-125
3. transvaginal sonography

Exercise 30
Spelling Exercise; see text p. 333.

Exercise 31
Pronunciation Exercise

Exercise 32
1. WR   CV   S
   gynec/o/logist
         CF
   a physician who studies and treats
      (diseases of) women

2. WR CV S
   gynec/o/logy
       CF
   study of women (branch of medicine
      dealing with diseases of the female
      reproductive system)
3. WR CV WR S
   vulv/o/vagin/al
       CF
   pertaining to the vulva and vagina
4. WR S
   mast/algia
   pain in the breast
5. WR WR
   men/arche
   beginning of menstruation
6. WR CV S
   leuk/o/rrhea
       CF
   white discharge (from the vagina)
7. WR CV WR S
   gyn/o/path/ic
       CF
   pertaining to diseases of women
8. WR CV S
   mast/o/ptosis
       CF
   sagging breast
9. WR S
   vagin/al
   pertaining to the vagina

Exercise 33
1. leuk/o/rrhea
2. men/arche
3. mast/algia
4. vulv/o/vagin/al
5. gynec/o/logist
6. gynec/o/logy
7. mast/o/ptosis
8. gyn/o/path/ic
9. vagin/al

Exercise 34
Spelling Exercise; see text p. 335.

Exercise 35
Pronunciation Exercise

Exercise 36
1. cessation of menstruation
2. difficult or painful intercourse
3. abnormal passageway between two organs or between an internal organ and
   the body surface
4. a syndrome involving physical and
   emotional symptoms occurring during
   the 10 days before menstruation
5. instrument for opening a body cavity
   to allow for visual inspection
6. replacement of hormones to treat
   symptoms associated with menopause

Exercise 37
1. fistula
2. dyspareunia
3. menopause
4. premenstrual syndrome
5. speculum
6. hormone replacement therapy

Exercise 38
Spelling Exercise; see text p. 336.

Exercise 39
1. anterior; posterior colporrhaphy
2. total abdominal hysterectomy and
   bilateral salpingo-oophorectomy;
   hormone replacement therapy
3. sonohysterogram and transvaginal
   sonography
4. total vaginal hysterectomy
5. dilation and curettage; cervix
6. fibrocystic breast disease
7. pelvic inflammatory disease;
   gynecology
8. premenstrual syndrome
9. uterine artery embolization

Exercise 40
A. 1. mammography
   2. carcinoma
   3. hysterectomy
   4. adenomyosis
   5. endometriosis
   6. HRT
   7. stereotactic breast biopsy
   8. induration
   9. necrosis
   10. hyperplasia

Exercise 40
B. 1. c
   2. a
   3. d

Exercise 41
1. dysmenorrhea
2. endometritis
3. uterine tube
4. suture of the vulva
5. mammoplasty
6. uterus, uterine tubes, and ovaries
7. hematosalpinx
8. endometriosis
9. speculum
10. TSS

Exercise 42
Reading Exercise

Exercise 43
1. b
2. *T*
3. *T*
4. d

CHAPTER 9

Obstetrics and Neonatology

OUTLINE

ANATOMY, 352

WORD PARTS, 354
Combining Forms, 354
Prefixes, 357
Suffixes, 358

MEDICAL TERMS, 359
Obstetric Disease and Disorder Terms, 359
    Built from Word Parts, 359
    Not Built from Word Parts, 361
Neonatology Disease and Disorder Terms, 364
    Built from Word Parts, 364
    Not Built from Word Parts, 366
Obstetric Surgical Terms, 368
    Built from Word Parts, 368
Obstetric Diagnostic Terms, 369
    Built from Word Parts, 369
Obstetric and Neonatal Complementary Terms, 372
    Built from Word Parts, 372
    Not Built from Word Parts, 378
Abbreviations, 383

PRACTICAL APPLICATION, 384
Interact with Medical Documents, 384
Interpret Medical Terms, 385
Read Medical Terms in Use, 386
Comprehend Medical Terms in Use, 386

CHAPTER REVIEW, 387

OBJECTIVES

Upon completion of this chapter you will be able to:

1. Identify organs and structures relating to pregnancy.

2. Define and spell word parts related to obstetrics and neonatology.

3. Define, pronounce, and spell disease and disorder terms related to obstetrics and neonatology.

4. Define, pronounce, and spell surgical and diagnostic terms related to obstetrics.

5. Define, pronounce, and spell complementary terms related to obstetrics and neonatology.

6. Interpret the meaning of abbreviations related to obstetrics and neonatology.

7. Interpret, read, and comprehend medical language in simulated medical statements and documents.

ANATOMY

Obstetrics is the branch of medicine that deals with childbirth and the care of the mother before, during, and after birth. **Neonatology** is the branch of medicine that deals with the diagnosis and treatment of disorders of the newborn.

Terms Relating to Pregnancy

Term	Definition
gamete	mature germ cell, either sperm (male) or ovum (female)
ovulation	expulsion of a mature ovum from an ovary (Figure 9-1)
conception, or fertilization	beginning of pregnancy, when the sperm enters the ovum. Fertilization normally occurs in the uterine tubes (Figure 9-1).
zygote	cell formed by the union of the sperm and the ovum
embryo	unborn offspring in the stage of development from implantation of the zygote to the end of the second month of pregnancy. This period is characterized by rapid growth of the embryo.
fetus	unborn offspring from the beginning of the third month of pregnancy until birth (Figure 9-2)
gestation, pregnancy	development of a new individual from conception to birth
gestation period	duration of pregnancy; approximately 9 months (38-42 weeks), which can be divided into three equal periods of time called *trimesters*
implantation	embedding of the zygote in the uterine lining. The process normally begins about 7 days after fertilization and continues for several days (Figure 9-1).
placenta, or afterbirth	a structure that grows on the wall of the uterus during pregnancy and allows for nourishment of the unborn child (Figure 9-1)
amniotic, or amnionic, sac	membranous bag that surrounds the fetus before delivery (also called **bag of water**) (Figure 9-1)
chorion	outermost layer of the fetal membrane
amnion	innermost layer of the fetal membrane
amniotic, or amnionic, fluid	fluid within the amniotic sac, which surrounds the fetus

SKIN CHANGES THAT OCCUR THROUGHOUT PREGNANCY
- **striae gravidarum:** "stretch marks" occurring on the abdomen, breast, buttocks, and thighs from weakening of elastic tissues
- **linea nigra:** dark medial line extending from the pubis upward
- **chloasma:** hyperpigmentation of blotchy brown macules usually evenly distributed over the cheeks and forehead

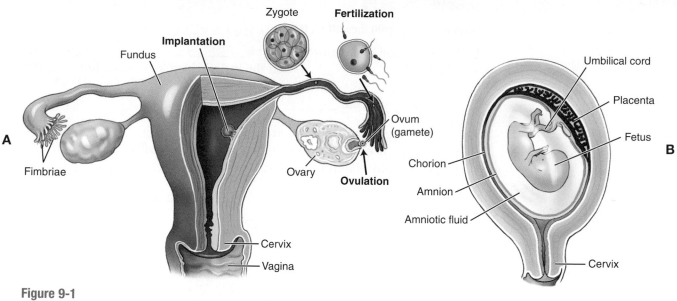

Figure 9-1
A, Ovulation, fertilization, and implantation. **B,** Development of the fetus.

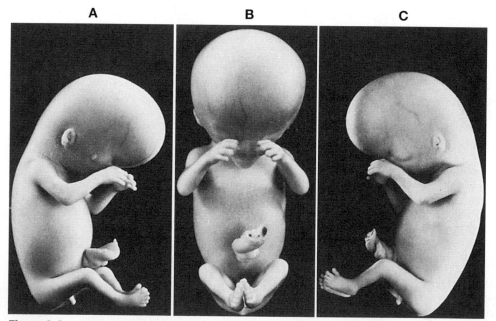

Figure 9-2
Human male fetus at 68 days (1.85 inches, 47 mm). **A,** Right. **B,** front. **C,** left.

Fill in the blanks with the correct terms.

1. The expulsion of a mature ovum, or _____, from an ovary is called _____. When the male gamete enters the female gamete, _____ occurs, and a(n) _____ is formed. This marks the beginning of the _____ period.

2. Once the zygote is implanted, it becomes a(n) _____ until the end of the second month of gestation. The unborn offspring from the beginning of the third month until birth is called a(n) _____.

3. The fetus is surrounded by a(n) _____ sac, which has an outermost layer, called the _____, and an innermost layer, called the _____. This sac contains the _____ fluid that surrounds the fetus.

WORD PARTS

Combining Forms of Obstetrics and Neonatology

Word parts you need to learn to complete this chapter are listed on the following pages. The exercises at the end of each list will help you learn their definitions and spelling.

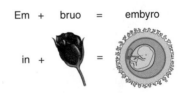

Em + bruo = embyro

in + =

Figure 9-3
Embryo comes from the Greek *em,* meaning *in,* plus *bruo,* meaning to *bud* or *shoot.*

PUERPER
is made up of two Latin word roots: **puer,** meaning **child,** and per, meaning **through.**

Combining Form	Definition
amni/o, amnion/o	amnion, amniotic fluid
chori/o	chorion
embry/o	embryo, to be full (Figure 9-3)
fet/o, fet/i	fetus, unborn child
(NOTE: both *i* and *o* may be used as combining vowels with fet.)	
gravid/o	pregnancy
lact/o.	milk
nat/o.	birth
omphal/o.	umbilicus, navel
par/o, part/o	bear, give birth to, labor, childbirth
puerper/o	childbirth

EXERCISE FIGURE A

Fill in the blanks with combining forms in this diagram of fetal development.

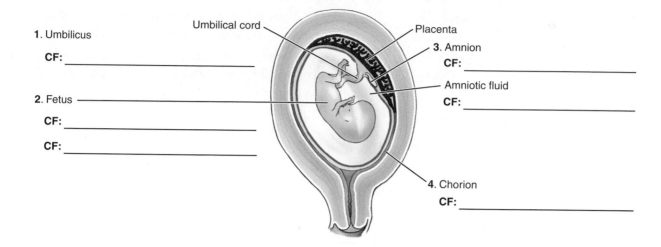

1. Umbilicus

   CF: _____

2. Fetus —————————————

   CF: _____

   CF: _____

Umbilical cord

Placenta

3. Amnion

   CF: _____

Amniotic fluid

   CF: _____

4. Chorion

   CF: _____

EXERCISE 2

Write the definitions of the following combining forms.

1. fet/o, fet/i _____

2. lact/o _____

3. par/o, part/o _____

4. omphal/o_____

5. amni/o, amnion/o_____

6. puerper/o _____

7. gravid/o_____

8. nat/o _____

9. chori/o_____

10. embry/o_____

EXERCISE 3

Write the combining form for each of the following terms.

1. milk   _____

2. fetus   a. _____

          b. _____

3. chorion   _____

4. amnion,
   amniotic
   fluid   a. _____

          b. _____

5. childbirth _____

6. bear, give
   birth to,
   labor,
   childbirth a. _____

          b. _____

7. pregnancy _____

8. embryo   _____

9. birth   _____

10. umbilicus,
    navel   _____

Combining Forms Commonly Used in Obstetrics and Neonatology

Combining Form	Definition
cephal/o	head
esophag/o	esophagus (tube leading from the throat to the stomach) (see Figure 11-1)
pelv/o, pelv/i .... (NOTE: both *i* and *o* may be used as the combining vowel with pelv.)	pelvic bone, pelvis (see Chapter 14 Exercise Figure A and Exercise Figure B)
prim/i .... (NOTE: the combining vowel is *i*.)	first
pseud/o.................	false
pylor/o	pylorus (pyloric sphincter) (see Figure 11-2)
terat/o...................	malformations

TERAT/O
is translated literally as monster; however, in terms containing terat/o relating to obstetrics, terat/o refers to malformations or abnormal development.

EXERCISE 4

Write the definition of the following combining forms.

1. prim/i_____   5. pseud/o _____

2. pylor/o _____   6. pelv/o, pelv/i _____

3. cephal/o _____   7. terat/o _____

4. esophag/o _____

EXERCISE 5

Write the combining form for each of the following.

1. head   _____   5. first   _____

2. pylorus   _____   6. malformations _____

3. false   _____   7. pelvic
                                               bone,
4. esophagus   _____   pelvis   a. _____

                                                         b. _____

Prefixes

Prefix	Definition
ante-, pre-	before
micro-	small
multi-	many
nulli-	none
post-	after

EXERCISE 6

Write the definitions of the following prefixes.

1. post-_____

2. multi-_____

3. nulli- _____

4. micro- _____

5. ante-_____

6. pre- _____

EXERCISE 7

Write the prefix for each of the following definitions.

1. none _____

2. small _____

3. many _____

4. before   a. _____

      b. _____

5. after _____

Suffixes

-RRHEXIS
is the last of the four **-rrh** suffixes to be learned. The other three introduced in earlier chapters are **-rrhea** (flow or discharge), **-rrhagia** (rapid flow [of blood]), and **-rrhaphy** (suturing, repair).

Suffix	Definition
-amnios	amnion, amniotic fluid
-cyesis	pregnancy
-e	noun suffix, no meaning
-is	noun suffix, no meaning
-partum	childbirth, labor
-rrhexis	rupture
-tocia	birth, labor
-um	noun suffix, no meaning
-us	noun suffix, no meaning

 The noun suffix **-a** covered in Chapter 4 also has no meaning.

Refer to Appendix A and Appendix B for alphabetized word parts and their meanings.

EXERCISE 8

Write the definitions of the following suffixes.

1. -rrhexis _____

2. -tocia _____

3. -cyesis _____

4. -partum _____

5. -amnios _____

EXERCISE 9

Write the suffix for each of the following definitions.

1. birth, labor _____

2. rupture _____

3. childbirth, labor _____

4. pregnancy _____

5. amnion, amniotic fluid _____

EXERCISE 10

Write the noun suffixes introduced in this chapter that have no meaning.

1. _____

2. _____

3. _____

4. _____

MEDICAL TERMS

The terms you need to learn to complete this chapter are listed next. The exercises following each list will help you learn the definition and the spelling of each word.

Obstetric Disease and Disorder Terms

Built from Word Parts

The following terms are built from word parts you have already learned and can be translated literally to find their meanings. Further explanation of terms beyond the definition of their word parts, if needed, is included in parentheses.

Term	Definition
amnionitis.............. (*am*-nē-ō-NĪ-tis)	inflammation of the amnion
chorioamnionitis........... (*kor*-ē-ō-*am*-nē-ō-NĪ-tis)	inflammation of the chorion and amnion
choriocarcinoma........... (*kor*-ē-ō-*kar*-si-NŌ-ma)	cancerous tumor of the chorion
dystocia .... (dis-TŌ-sha)	difficult labor
hysterorrhexis............. (*his*-ter-ō-REK-sis)	rupture of the uterus
oligohydramnios........... (*ol*-i-gō-hī-DRAM-nē-os)	scanty amnion water (less than the normal amount of amniotic fluid; 500 ml or less)
polyhydramnios .... (*pol*-ē-hī-DRAM-nē-os)	much amnion water (more than the normal amount of amniotic fluid; 2000 ml or more) (also called **hydramnios**)

EXERCISE 11

Practice saying aloud each of the obstetric disease and disorder terms built from word parts on p. 359.

 To hear the terms select Chapter 9, Chapter Exercises, Pronunciation.

☐ Place a check mark in the box when you have completed this exercise.

EXERCISE 12

Analyze and define the following disease and disorder terms.

1. chorioamnionitis_____

2. choriocarcinoma_____

3. dystocia _____

4. amnionitis _____

5. hysterorrhexis _____

6. oligohydramnios_____

7. polyhydramnios _____

EXERCISE 13

Build disease and disorder terms for the following definitions by using the word parts you have learned.

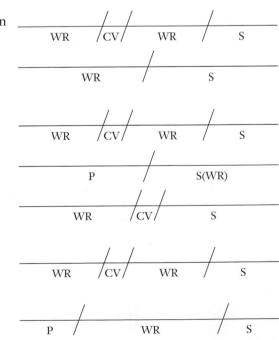

1. cancerous tumor of the chorion

       WR   /CV/   WR   /   S

2. inflammation of the amnion

            WR   /   S

3. inflammation of the chorion and amnion

       WR   /CV/   WR   /   S

4. difficult labor

            P   /   S(WR)

5. rupture of the uterus

            WR   /CV/   S

6. scanty amnion water (less than normal amniotic fluid)

       WR   /CV/   WR   /   S

7. much amnion water (more than normal amniotic fluid)

            P   /   WR   /   S

EXERCISE 14

Spell each of the obstetric disease and disorder terms built from word parts on p. 359 by having someone dictate them to you.

 To hear and spell the terms select Chapter 9, Chapter Exercises, Spelling. You may type the terms on the screen or write them below in the spaces provided.

☐ Place a check mark in the box if you have completed this exercise using your CD-ROM.

1. _____   5. _____

2. _____   6. _____

3. _____   7. _____

4. _____

Obstetric Disease and Disorder Terms

Not Built from Word Parts

In some of the following terms you may recognize word parts you have already learned; however, the full meaning of the terms cannot be discerned by the definition of their word parts.

Term	Definition
abortion . . . . (a-BOR-shun)	termination of pregnancy by the expulsion from the uterus of an embryo before fetal viability, usually before 20 weeks of gestation
abruptio placentae . . . . (ab-RUP-shē-ō) (pla-SEN-tē)	premature separation of the placenta from the uterine wall (Figure 9-5, *A*)
eclampsia . . . . (e-KLAMP-sē-a)	severe complication and progression of preeclampsia characterized by convulsion and coma (see *preeclampsia* on the next page). Eclampsia is a potentially life-threatening disorder.
ectopic pregnancy . . . . (ek-TOP-ik) (PREG-nan-sē)	pregnancy occurring outside the uterus, commonly in the uterine tubes (Figure 9-4)
placenta previa . . . . (pla-SEN-ta) (PRĒ-vē-a)	abnormally low implantation of the placenta on the uterine wall. (Dilation of the cervix can cause separation of the placenta from the uterine wall, resulting in bleeding. With severe hemorrhage, a cesarean section may be necessary to save the mother's life.) (Figure 9-5, *B*)

TYPES OF ABORTION

Spontaneous abortion is the termination of pregnancy that occurs naturally. It is commonly referred to as *miscarriage*.

Induced abortion is the intentional termination of pregnancy by surgical or medical intervention.

Therapeutic abortion is an induced abortion performed because of health risks to the mother or for fetal disease.

Elective abortion is an induced abortion performed at the request of the woman.

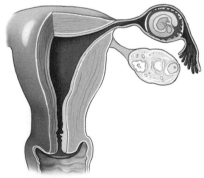

Figure 9-4
Ectopic pregnancy.

Obstetric Disease and Disorder Terms—*cont'd*

Not Built from Word Parts

Term	Definition
preeclampsia . . . . (prē-ē-KLAMP-sē-a)	abnormal condition encountered during pregnancy or shortly after delivery characterized by high blood pressure, edema, and proteinuria, but with no convulsions or coma. The cause is unknown; if not successfully treated the condition will progress to eclampsia. Eclampsia is the third most common cause of maternal death in the United States after hemorrhage and infection.

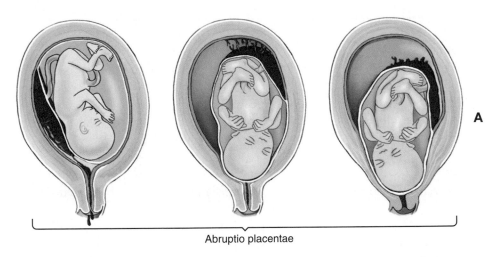

Abruptio placentae

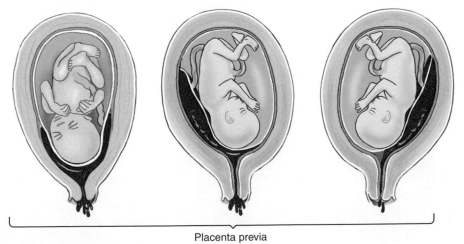

Placenta previa

Figure 9-5
A, Various stages of abruptio placentae. **B,** Placenta previa.

EXERCISE 15

Practice saying aloud each of the obstetric disease and disorder terms not built from word parts on pp. 361-362.

 To hear the terms select Chapter 9, Chapter Exercises, Pronunciation.

☐ Place a check mark in the box when you have completed this exercise.

EXERCISE 16

Write the definitions of the following terms.

1. abruptio placentae _____

2. abortion _____

3. placenta previa _____

4. eclampsia _____

5. ectopic pregnancy _____

6. preeclampsia _____

EXERCISE 17

Write the term for each of the following definitions.

1. premature separation of the placenta from the uterine wall _____

2. severe complication and progression of preeclampsia _____

3. termination of pregnancy by the expulsion from the uterus of an embryo _____

4. pregnancy occurring outside the uterus _____

5. abnormally low implantation of the placenta on the uterine wall _____

6. characterized by high blood pressure, edema, and proteinuria, but with no convulsions or coma _____

EXERCISE 18

Spell each of the obstetric disease and disorder terms not built from word parts on
pp. 361-362 by having someone dictate them to you.

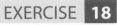 To hear and spell the terms select Chapter 9, Chapter Exercises, Spelling. You may
type the terms on the screen or write them below in the spaces provided.

☐ Place a check mark in the box if you have completed this exercise using your CD-ROM.

1. _____   4. _____

2. _____   5. _____

3. _____   6. _____

Neonatology Disease and Disorder Terms

Built from Word Parts

*The following terms are built from word parts you have already learned and can be translated
literally to find their meanings. Further explanation of terms beyond the definition of their word
parts, if needed, is included in parentheses.*

Term	Definition
microcephalus . . . . (*mī*-krō-SEF-a-lus)	(fetus with a very) small head
omphalitis . . . . (*om*-fa-LĪ-tis)	inflammation of the umbilicus
omphalocele . . . . (OM-fal-ō-*sēl*)	herniation at the umbilicus (a part of the intestine protrudes through the abdominal wall at birth) (Exercise Figure B)
pyloric stenosis . . . . (pī-LOR-ik) (ste-NŌ-sis)	narrowing pertaining to the pyloric sphincter. (Congenital pyloric stenosis occurs in 1 of every 200 newborns.)
tracheoesophageal fistula . . . . (*trā*-kē-ō-ē-SOF-a-*jē*-al) (FIS-tū-la)	abnormal passageway pertaining to the esophagus and the trachea (between the esophagus and trachea)

EXERCISE 19

Practice saying aloud each of the neonatology disease and disorder terms built from word
parts above.

 To hear the terms select Chapter 9, Chapter Exercises, Pronunciation.

☐ Place a check mark in the box when you have completed this exercise.

EXERCISE FIGURE B

Fill in the blanks to label the diagram.

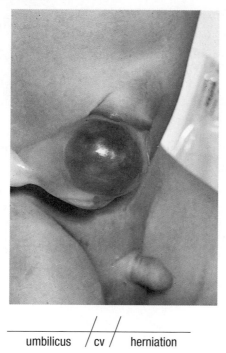

_____ / cv / _____
 umbilicus   herniation

EXERCISE 20

Analyze and define the following disease and disorder terms.

1. pyloric (stenosis) _____

2. omphalocele _____

3. omphalitis _____

4. microcephalus _____

5. tracheoesophageal (fistula) _____

EXERCISE 21

Build disease and disorder terms for the following definitions by using the word parts you have learned.

1. hernia at the umbilicus

2. (fetus with a very) small head

3. (narrowing) pertaining to the pyloric sphincter

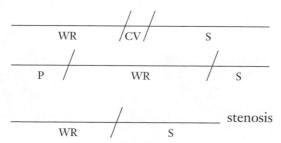

4. abnormal passageway pertaining to the esophagus and the trachea (between the esophagus and trachea)

_____ / ___ / _____ / ___ fistula
WR   /CV/   WR   / S

5. inflammation of the umbilicus   _____

WR   /   S

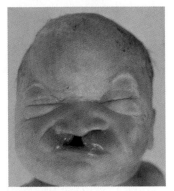

Figure 9-6
Cleft lip and palate.

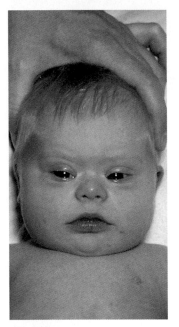

Figure 9-7
Down syndrome.

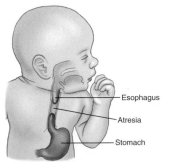

Figure 9-8
Esophageal atresia.

EXERCISE 22

Spell each of the neonatology disease and disorder terms built from word parts on p. 364 by having someone dictate them to you.

 To hear and spell the terms select Chapter 9, Chapter Exercises, Spelling. You may type the terms on the screen or write them below in the spaces provided.

☐ Place a check mark in the box if you have completed this exercise using your CD-ROM.

1. _____   4. _____

2. _____   5. _____

3. _____

Neonatology Disease and Disorder Terms

Not Built from Word Parts

In some of the following terms you may recognize word parts you have already learned; however, the full meaning of the terms cannot be discerned by the definition of their word parts.

Term	Definition
cleft lip and palate . . . . (kleft) (lip) (PAL-at)	congenital split of the lip and roof of the mouth (*cleft* indicates a fissure) (Figure 9-6)
Down syndrome . . . . (down) (SIN-drōme)	congenital condition characterized by varying degrees of mental retardation and multiple defects (formerly called **mongolism**) (Figure 9-7)
erythroblastosis fetalis . . . . (e-rith-rō-blas-TŌ-sis) (fē-TAL-is)	condition of the newborn characterized by hemolysis of the erythrocytes. The condition is usually caused by incompatibility of the infant's and mother's blood, occurring when the mother's blood is Rh negative and the infant's blood is Rh positive.
esophageal atresia . . . . (ē-sof-a-JĒ-al) (a-TRĒ-zha)	congenital absence of part of the esophagus. Food cannot pass from the baby's mouth to the stomach (Figure 9-8).

Term	Definition
fetal alcohol syndrome....... (FĒ-tal) (AL-kō-hol) (SIN-drōm)	a condition caused by excessive alcohol consumption by the mother during pregnancy. Various birth defects may present, including central nervous system dysfunction and malformations of the skull and face.
gastroschisis .... (gas-TROS-ki-sis)	a congenital fissure of the abdominal wall not at the umbilicus. Enterocele, protrusion of the intestine, is usually present (Figure 9-9).
respiratory distress syndrome (RDS).................... (RES-pi-ra-tōr-ē) (di-STRESS) (SIN-drōm)	a respiratory complication in the newborn, especially in premature infants. In premature infants RDS is caused by normal immaturity of the respiratory system resulting in compromised respiration (formerly called **hyaline membrane disease**).
spina bifida............... (SPĪ-na) (BIF-i-da)	congenital defect in the vertebral column caused by the failure of the vertebral arch to close. If the meninges protrude through the opening the condition is called *meningocele*. Protrusion of both the meninges and spinal cord is called *meningomyelocele*. Both terms are covered in Chapter 15 (Figure 9-10).

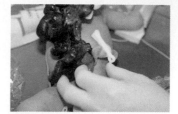

Figure 9-9
Gastroschisis.

CAM TERM
Acupressure is the ancient practice of applying finger pressure to specific acupoints on the body to preserve and restore health. Studies have demonstrated that acupressure on specific acupoints reduces labor pain and shortens length of delivery time.

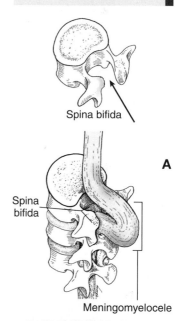

Spina bifida

A

Spina bifida

Meningomyelocele

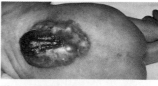

B

Figure 9-10
A, Drawings of spina bifida and meningomyelocele. **B,** Photograph of meningomyelocele.

EXERCISE 23

Practice saying aloud each of the neonatology disease and disorder terms not built from word parts found on pp. 366-367.

 To hear the terms select Chapter 9, Chapter Exercises, Pronunciation.

☐ Place a check mark in the box when you have completed this exercise.

EXERCISE 24

Match the terms in the first column with their correct definitions in the second column.

_____ 1. Down syndrome
_____ 2. cleft lip and palate
_____ 3. spina bifida
_____ 4. erythroblastosis fetalis
_____ 5. fetal alcohol syndrome
_____ 6. respiratory distress syndrome
_____ 7. esophageal atresia
_____ 8. gastroschisis

a. defect of the vertebral column
b. respiratory complication
c. split of the lip and roof of the mouth
d. caused by incompatibility of the infant's and the mother's blood
e. congenital fissure of the abdominal wall
f. congenital condition characterized by mental retardation
g. congenital absence of part of the esophagus
h. causes various birth defects, including central nervous system dysfunction

EXERCISE 25

Spell each of the neonatal disease and disorder terms not built from word parts on pp. 366-367 by having someone dictate them to you.

To hear and spell the terms select Chapter 9, Chapter Exercises, Spelling. You may type the terms on the screen or write them below in the spaces provided.

☐ Place a check mark in the box if you have completed this exercise using your CD-ROM.

1. _____   5. _____

2. _____   6. _____

3. _____   7. _____

4. _____   8. _____

Obstetric Surgical Terms

Built from Word Parts

The following terms are built from word parts you have already learned and can be translated literally to find their meanings. Further explanation of terms beyond the definition of their word parts, if needed, is included in parentheses.

Term	Definition
amniotomy . . . . (*am*-nē-OT-o-mē)	incision into the amnion (rupture of the fetal membrane to induce labor)
episiotomy . . . . (e-*piz*-ē-OT-o-mē)	incision of the vulva (perineum), sometimes performed during delivery (also called **perineotomy**) (Figure 9-11)

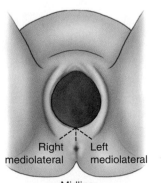

Right mediolateral   Left mediolateral

Midline

Figure 9-11
Episiotomies.

Obstetric Diagnostic Terms

Built from Word Parts

Term	Definition
DIAGNOSTIC IMAGING	
pelvic sonography .... (PEL-vik) (so-NOG-ra-fē)	pertaining to the pelvis, process of recording sound (pelvic ultrasound is used to evaluate the fetus and pregnancy) (Figure 9-12)
OTHER	
amniocentesis .... (*am*-nē-ō-sen-TĒ-sis)	surgical puncture to aspirate amniotic fluid (the needle is inserted through the abdominal and uterine walls, using ultrasound to guide the needle). The fluid is used for the assessment of fetal health and maturity to aid in diagnosing fetal abnormalities (Figure 9-13).
amnioscope .... (AM-nē-ō-skōp)	instrument used for visual examination of the amniotic fluid (and the fetus)
amnioscopy .... (*am*-nē-OS-ko-pē)	visual examination of amniotic fluid (and the fetus)

Pelvic sonography, also called **pelvic ultrasonography, pelvic ultrasound,** or **obstetric ultrasonography,** is used extensively to evaluate the fetus and the pregnancy. It is noninvasive, harmless, and especially suited for this evaluation because the presence of amniotic fluid enhances sound. Some specific uses for pelvic sonography are:

1. to diagnose an abnormal pregnancy early
2. to determine the age of the fetus
3. to measure fetal growth and rate
4. to determine fetal position

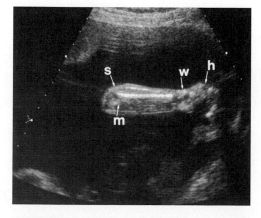

Figure 9-12

An ultrasound image showing the forearm of a fetus. The skinline *(s)*, muscle *(m)*, wrist *(w)*, and hand *(h)* are in view. The first ultrasound examination was used in obstetrics in 1958.

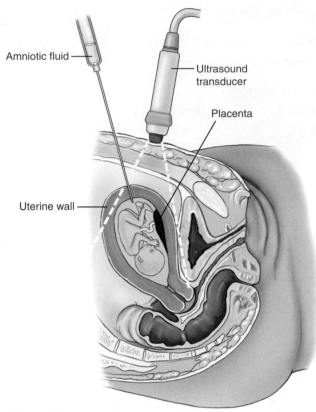

Amniotic fluid

Ultrasound transducer

Placenta

Uterine wall

Figure 9-13
Amniocentesis. Ultrasound is used to guide the needle through the abdominal and uterine walls.

EXERCISE 26

Practice saying aloud each of the obstetric surgical and diagnostic terms built from word parts on pp. 368-369.

To hear the terms select Chapter 9, Chapter Exercises, Pronunciation.

☐ Place a check mark in the box when you have completed this exercise.

EXERCISE 27

Analyze and define the following obstetric surgical and diagnostic terms.

1. episiotomy_____

2. amniotomy _____

3. amnioscope _____

4. pelvic sonography_____

5. amniocentesis _____

6. amnioscopy_____

EXERCISE 28

Build obstetric surgical and diagnostic terms for the following definitions by using the word parts you have learned.

1. incision into the amnion

                WR   /CV/   S

2. incision of the vulva

                WR   /CV/   S

3. visual examination of the amniotic fluid (and fetus)

                WR   /CV/   S

4. surgical puncture to aspirate amniotic fluid

                WR   /CV/   S

5. instrument used for visual examination of the amniotic fluid (and fetus)

                WR   /CV/   S

6. pertaining to the pelvis, process of recording sound

                WR   /   S

                WR   /CV/   S

EXERCISE 29

Spell each of the obstetric surgical and diagnostic terms built from word parts on pp. 368-369 by having someone dictate them to you.

 To hear and spell the terms select Chapter 9, Chapter Exercises, Spelling. You may type the terms on the screen or write them below in the spaces provided.

☐ Place a check mark in the box if you have completed this exercise using your CD-ROM.

1. _____

2. _____

3. _____

4. _____

5. _____

6. _____

Obstetric and Neonatal Complementary Terms

Built from Word Parts

The following terms are built from word parts you have already learned and can be translated literally to find their meanings. Further explanation of terms beyond the definition of their word parts, if needed, is included in parentheses.

Term	Definition
amniochorial (*am*-nē-ō-KOR-ē-al)	pertaining to the amnion and chorion
amniorrhea (*am*-nē-ō-RĒ-a)	discharge (escape) of amniotic fluid
amniorrhexis (*am*-nē-ō-REK-sis)	rupture of the amnion
antepartum (*an*-tē-PAR-tum)	before childbirth (reference to the mother)
embryogenic (*em*-brē-ō-JEN-ik)	producing an embryo
embryoid (EM-brē-oyd)	resembling an embryo
fetal (FĒ-tal)	pertaining to the fetus
gravida (GRAV-i-da)	pregnant (woman)
gravidopuerperal (*grav*-i-dō-pū-ER-per-al)	pertaining to pregnancy and childbirth (from delivery until reproductive organs return to normal)
intrapartum (*in*-tra-PAR-tum)	within (during) labor and childbirth
lactic (LAK-tik)	pertaining to milk
lactogenic (*lak*-tō-JEN-ik)	producing milk (by stimulation)
lactorrhea (*lak*-tō-RĒ-a)	(spontaneous) discharge of milk
multigravida (mul-ti-GRAV-i-da)	many pregnancies (a woman who has been pregnant two or more times)
multipara (multip) (mul-TIP-a-ra)	many births (a woman who has given birth to two or more viable offspring)
natal (NĀ-tal)	pertaining to birth
neonate (NĒ-ō-nāt)	new birth (an infant from birth to 4 weeks of age) (synonymous with **newborn [NB]**) (Exercise Figure C)
neonatologist (nē-ō-nā-TOL-o-jist)	physician who studies and treats disorders of the newborn

Term	Definition
neonatology . . . . (nē-ō-nā-TOL-o-jē)	study of the newborn (branch of medicine that deals with diagnosis and treatment of disorders in newborns)
nulligravida . . . . (nul-li-GRAV-i-da)	no pregnancies (a woman who has never been pregnant)
nullipara . . . . (nu-LIP-a-ra)	no births (a woman who has not given birth to a viable offspring)
para . . . . (PAR-a)	birth (a woman who has given birth to a viable offspring)
postnatal . . . . (pōst-NĀ-tal)	pertaining to after birth (reference to the newborn)
postpartum . . . . (pōst-PAR-tum)	after childbirth (reference to the mother)
prenatal . . . . (prē-NĀ-tal)	pertaining to before birth (reference to the newborn)
primigravida . . . . (prī-mi-GRAV-i-da)	first pregnancy (a woman in her first pregnancy)
primipara (primip) . . . . (prī-MIP-a-ra)	first birth (a woman who has given birth to one viable offspring)
pseudocyesis . . . . (sū-dō-sī-Ē-sis)	false pregnancy
puerpera . . . . (pū-ER-per-a)	childbirth (a woman who has just given birth)
puerperal . . . . (pū-ER-per-al)	pertaining to (immediately after) childbirth
teratogen . . . . (TER-a-tō-jen)	any agent producing malformations (in the developing embryo). Teratogens include chemical agents such as drugs, alcohol, viruses, x-rays, and environmental factors such as age or health of the mother.
teratogenic . . . . (ter-a-tō-JEN-ik)	producing malformations (in the developing embryo)
teratology . . . . (ter-a-TOL-o-jē)	study of malformations (usually in regard to malformations caused by teratogens on the developing embryo)

EXERCISE FIGURE C

Fill in the blanks to label the diagram.

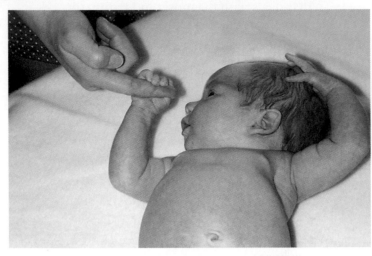

_____ / _____ / __e___
  new   / birth /

Terms Relating to Mother and Newborn

	Before Birth	After Birth
Mother	antepartum	postpartum
Newborn	prenatal	postnatal

Comparing Terms with gravid/o and par/o

gravid/o—pregnant	**par/o—birth**
nulli/gravid/a—no pregnancies	nulli/par/a—no births
primi/gravid/a—first pregnancy	primi/par/a—first birth
multi/gravid/a—many pregnancies	multi/par/a—many births

EXERCISE 30

Practice saying aloud each of the complementary terms built from word parts on pp. 372-373.

 To hear the terms select Chapter 9, Chapter Exercises, Pronunciation.

☐ Place a check mark in the box when you have completed this exercise.

EXERCISE 31

Analyze and define the following obstetric and neonatal complementary terms.

1. puerpera _____

2. amniorrhexis _____

3. antepartum _____

4. pseudocyesis _____

5. prenatal _____

6. lactic _____

7. lactorrhea _____

8. amniorrhea _____

9. multipara _____

10. embryogenic _____

11. embryoid _____

12. fetal _____

13. gravida _____

14. amniochorial _____

15. multigravida _____

16. lactogenic _____

17. natal _____

18. gravidopuerperal _____

19. neonatology _____

20. nullipara _____

21. para _____

22. primigravida _____

23. postpartum _____

24. neonate _____

25. primipara _____

26. puerperal _____

27. nulligravida _____

28. intrapartum _____

29. teratogen _____

30. postnatal _____

31. teratology _____

32. neonatologist _____

33. teratogenic _____

EXERCISE 32

Build the complementary terms for the following definitions by using the word parts you have learned.

1. pertaining to the amnion and chorion

_____ / ___ / _____ / ___
WR　　 CV　　 WR　　　 S

2. before childbirth (reference to the mother)

_____ / _____ / ___
P　　　 WR　　　 S

3. producing an embryo

_____ / ___ / ___
WR　　 CV　　 S

4. pertaining to the fetus

_____ / ___
WR　　　 S

5. pertaining to before birth (reference to the newborn)

_____ / _____ / ___
P　　　 WR　　　 S

6. pertaining to milk

_____ / ___
WR　　　 S

7. (spontaneous) discharge of milk

_____ / ___ / ___
WR　　 CV　　 S

8. discharge (escape) of amniotic fluid

_____ / ___ / ___
WR　　 CV　　 S

9. false pregnancy

_____ / ___ / ___
WR　　 CV　　 S

10. (stimulating) the production of milk

_____ / ___ / ___
WR　　 CV　　 S

11. rupture of the amnion

_____ / ___ / ___
WR　　 CV　　 S

12. resembling an embryo

_____ / ___
WR　　　 S

13. pregnant (woman)

_____ / ___
WR　　　 S

14. pertaining to pregnancy and childbirth

_____ / ___ / _____ / ___
WR　　 CV　　 WR　　　 S

15. many births

_____ / _____ / ___
P　　　 WR　　　 S

16. pertaining to birth

_____ / ___
WR　　　 S

17. new birth (an infant from birth to 4 weeks of age)

_____ / _____ / ___
P　　　 WR　　　 S

18. study of the newborn

___P___ / ___WR___ /CV/ S

19. no births

___P___ / ___WR___ / S

20. birth

___WR___ / S

21. first pregnancy

___WR___ /CV/ ___WR___ / S

22. after childbirth (reference to the mother)

___P___ / ___WR___ / S

23. first birth

___WR___ /CV/ ___WR___ / S

24. many pregnancies

___P___ / ___WR___ / S

25. pertaining to (immediately after) childbirth

___WR___ / S

26. no pregnancies

___P___ / ___WR___ / S

27. any agent producing malformations

___WR___ /CV/ S

28. childbirth

___WR___ / S

29. within (during) labor and childbirth

___P___ / ___WR___ / S

30. producing malformations

___WR___ /CV/ S

31. physician who studies and treats disorders of the newborn

___P___ / ___WR___ /CV/ S

32. pertaining to after birth (reference to the newborn)

___P___ / ___WR___ / S

33. study of malformations

___WR___ /CV/ S

EXERCISE 33

Spell each of the complementary terms built from word parts on pp. 372-373 by having someone dictate them to you.

To hear and spell the terms select Chapter 9, Chapter Exercises, Spelling. You may type the terms on the screen or write them below in the spaces provided.

☐ Place a check mark in the box if you have completed this exercise using your CD-ROM.

1. _____ 18. _____

2. _____ 19. _____

3. _____ 20. _____

4. _____ 21. _____

5. _____ 22. _____

6. _____ 23. _____

7. _____ 24. _____

8. _____ 25. _____

9. _____ 26. _____

10. _____ 27. _____

11. _____ 28. _____

12. _____ 29. _____

13. _____ 30. _____

14. _____ 31. _____

15. _____ 32. _____

16. _____ 33. _____

17. _____

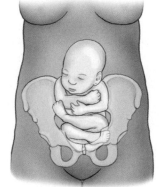

Breech presentation

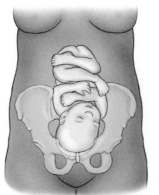

Cephalic presentation

Figure 9-14

A, Breech presentation.
B, Cephalic presentation.

Obstetric and Neonatal Complementary Terms

Not Built from Word Parts

In some of the following terms you may recognize word parts you have already learned; however, the full meaning of the terms cannot be discerned by the definition of their word parts.

Term	Definition
breech presentation . . . . (brēch)	parturition (act of giving birth) in which the buttocks, feet, or knees emerge first (Figure 9-14, *A*)
cephalic presentation . . . . (se-FAL-ik)	parturition (act of giving birth) in which any part of the head emerges first. It is the most common presentation (Figure 9-14, *B*).

Term	Definition
cesarean section (CS, C-section) (se-ZĀR-ē-an)	the birth of a baby through an incision in the mother's abdomen and uterus (may also be spelled **caesarean**)
colostrum (k-LOS-trem)	thin, milky fluid secreted by the breast during pregnancy and during the first days after birth before lactation begins
congenital anomaly (kon-JEN-i-tal) (a-NOM-a-lē)	abnormality present at birth
in vitro fertilization (IVF) (in-VĒ-trō) (*fer*-ti-li-ZĀ-shun)	a method of fertilizing human ova outside the body and placing the zygote into the uterus; used when infertility is present (Figure 9-15)
lactation (lak-TĀ-shun)	the secretion of milk
lochia (LŌ-kē-a)	vaginal discharge after childbirth
meconium (me-KŌ-nē-um)	first stool of the newborn (greenish black)
midwife (MID-wīf)	an individual who practices midwifery
midwifery (MID-wif-rē)	the practice of assisting in childbirth
obstetrician (*ob*-ste-TRISH-an)	physician who specializes in obstetrics
obstetrics (OB) (ob-STET-riks)	medical specialty dealing with pregnancy, childbirth, and puerperium
parturition (*par*-tū-RISH-un)	act of giving birth
premature infant	infant born before completing 37 weeks of gestation (also called **preterm infant**)
puerperium (pū-er-PĒ-rē-um)	period from delivery until the reproductive organs return to normal (approximately 6 weeks)
quickening (KWIK-en-ing)	the first feeling of movement of the fetus in utero by the pregnant woman. It usually occurs between 16 and 20 weeks of gestation.
stillborn (STIL-born)	born dead

CESAREAN SECTION (C-SECTION)

The origin of this term has no relation to the birth of Julius Caesar, as is commonly believed. One suggested etymology is that from 715 to 672 BC it was Roman law that the operation be performed on dying women in the last few months of pregnancy in the hope of saving the child. At that time the operation was called a *caeso matris utero*, which means **the cutting of the mother's uterus.**

MIDWIFERY

Midwives who practice midwifery supervise pregnancy, labor, delivery, and puerperium. They assist with delivery independently, care for the newborn, and obtain medical assistance as necessary. A midwife may or may not be a registered nurse. Education, certification, and licensure vary by state and country.

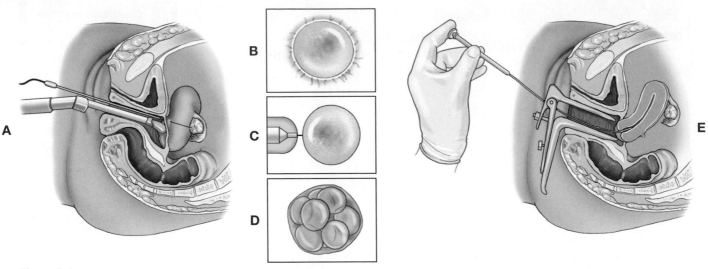

Figure 9-15
In vitro fertilization (IVF). After ovarian stimulation ova are retrieved from the ovary by ultrasound-guided transvaginal needle aspiration **(A)**. The ova are fertilized outside the body in a dish with spermatozoa obtained from semen **(B)**. A technique using a single sperm called intracytoplasmic sperm injection may also be used **(C)**. After 48 hours the fertilized ova (zygotes) **(D)** are injected into the uterus for implantation **(E)**. The first pregnancy after in vitro fertilization was reported more than 3 decades ago. Since then **assisted reproductive technology (ART)** has achieved hundreds of thousands of pregnancies worldwide. One in 80 to 100 births in the United States is a result of IVF.

EXERCISE 34

Practice saying aloud each of the complementary terms not built from word parts on pp. 378-379.

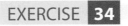 To hear the terms select Chapter 9, Chapter Exercises, Pronunciation.

☐ Place a check mark in the box when you have completed this exercise.

EXERCISE 35

Match the definitions in the first column with the correct terms in the second column.

_____ 1. vaginal discharge		a. lochia
_____ 2. medical specialty		b. obstetrician
_____ 3. abnormality present at birth		c. premature infant
		d. meconium
_____ 4. period after delivery		e. obstetrics
_____ 5. giving birth		f. parturition

_____ 6. physician specializing
in obstetrics

_____ 7. buttocks, feet, or knees first

_____ 8. first stool

_____ 9. born before completing
37 weeks of gestation

_____ 10. birth through an abdominal
and uterine incision

f. parturition

g. puerperium

h. cesarean section

i. congenital anomaly

j. breech presentation

EXERCISE 36

Match the definitions in the first column with the correct terms in the second column.

_____ 1. assisting in childbirth

_____ 2. onc who assists in childbirth

_____ 3. secretion of milk

_____ 4. head first

_____ 5. born dead

_____ 6. movement of the fetus

_____ 7. secreted before lactation

_____ 8. used when infertility is present

a. quickening

b. lactation

c. cephalic presentation

d. colostrum

e. midwife

f. stillborn

g. in vitro fertilization

h. midwifery

EXERCISE 37

Write the definitions of the following terms.

1. meconium _____

2. obstetrics _____

3. premature infant _____

4. lochia _____

5. puerperium _____

6. parturition _____

7. obstetrician _____

8. congenital anomaly _____

9. breech presentation _____

10. cesarean section _____

11. quickening _____

12. lactation _____

13. cephalic presentation _____

14. colostrum _____

15. midwife _____

16. stillborn _____

17. midwifery _____

18. in vitro fertilization _____

EXERCISE 38

Spell each of the complementary terms not bult from word parts on pp. 378-379 by having someone dictate them to you.

 To hear and spell the terms select Chapter 9, Chapter Exercises, Spelling. You may type the terms on the screen or write them below in the spaces provided.

☐ Place a check mark in the box if you have completed this exercise using your CD-ROM.

1. _____   10. _____

2. _____   11. _____

3. _____   12. _____

4. _____   13. _____

5. _____   14. _____

6. _____   15. _____

7. _____   16. _____

8. _____   17. _____

9. _____   18. _____

Abbreviations

CS, C-section	cesarean section
DOB.	date of birth
EDD.	expected (estimated) date of delivery
FAS	fetal alcohol syndrome
IVF.	in vitro fertilization
LMP.	last menstrual period
LNMP	last normal menstrual period
multip	multipara
NB.	newborn
OB.	obstetrics
primip	primipara
RDS.	respiratory distress syndrome

Refer to Appendix D for a complete list of abbreviations.

Refer to Appendix E for pharmacology terms related to obstetrics and neonatology.

EXERCISE 39

Write the definition of the following abbreviations.

1. OB _____

2. EDD _____ _____ of _____

3. LMP _____ _____ _____

4. DOB _____ _____ _____

5. NB _____

6. multip _____

7. C/S, C-section _____ _____

8. LNMP _____ _____ _____ _____

9. RDS _____ _____ _____

10. primip _____

11. FAS _____ _____ _____

12. IVF _____ _____ _____

LAMAZE
is a method of psychophysical preparation for childbirth started in the 1950s by a French obstetrician, Fernand Lamaze. The method requires classes and practice before and coaching during labor and delivery.

PRACTICAL APPLICATION

EXERCISE **40** *Interact with Medical Documents*

A. Complete the progress note by writing the medical terms in the blanks. Use the list of definitions with the corresponding numbers.

University Hospital and Medical Center

4700 North Main Street • Wellness, Arizona 54321 • (987) 555-3210

PATIENT NAME: Gloria Cisneros   **CASE NUMBER:** 17432-OBN

DATE OF BIRTH: 08/26/19XX   **DATE:** 09/23/20XX

PROGRESS NOTE

HISTORY: Gloria Cisneros is a 24-year-old married Latina 1. _____ 3, 2. _____ 2 who is here today with her husband. Her 3. _____ is 1 week from today. She has received 4. _____ care here at the Medical Center Obstetrics Clinic since her second month of pregnancy. This 5. _____ has been uncomplicated with no spotting, albuminuria, hypertension, edema, or glycosuria. Patient has attended Lamaze classes with her husband.

PHYSICAL EXAM: Her breasts are large. She has gained 2 pounds since her last visit and she has gained 25 pounds throughout her pregnancy. Her current weight is 164 pounds. Her cervix is 1 cm dilated. Routine 6. _____ _____ reveals a single 7. _____ and indicates adequate pelvis for normal size delivery. 8. _____ presentation is cephalic.

PLAN: Patient will return to clinic once a week until delivery.

_____
Heather Strom, MD

HS/mcm

---

1. pregnant (woman)
2. birth
3. abbreviation for expected delivery date
4. pertaining to before birth (reference to the newborn)
5. development of a new individual from conception to birth
6. pertaining to the pelvis, process of recording sound
7. unborn offspring from second month of pregnancy
8. pertaining to the fetus

B. Read the following radiology report and answer the questions following it.

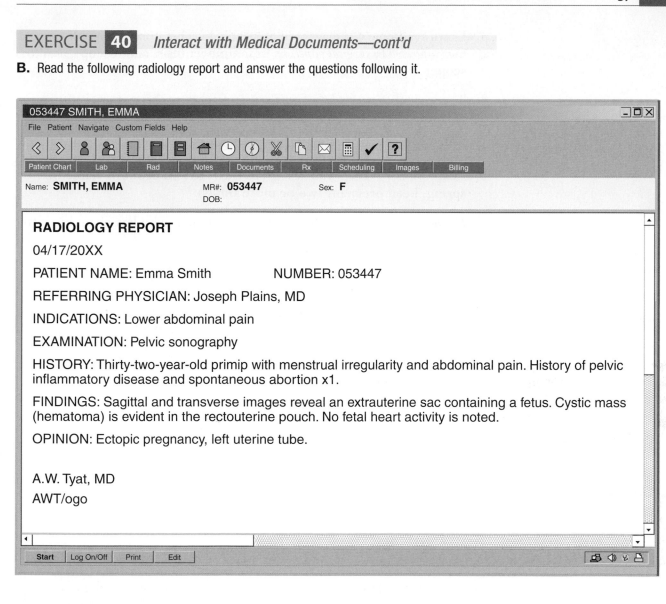

053447 SMITH, EMMA

File   Patient   Navigate   Custom Fields   Help

Patient Chart | Lab | Rad | Notes | Documents | Rx | Scheduling | Images | Billing

Name: **SMITH, EMMA**   MR#: **053447**   Sex: **F**
                              DOB:

RADIOLOGY REPORT

04/17/20XX

PATIENT NAME: Emma Smith   NUMBER: 053447

REFERRING PHYSICIAN: Joseph Plains, MD

INDICATIONS: Lower abdominal pain

EXAMINATION: Pelvic sonography

HISTORY: Thirty-two-year-old primip with menstrual irregularity and abdominal pain. History of pelvic inflammatory disease and spontaneous abortion x1.

FINDINGS: Sagittal and transverse images reveal an extrauterine sac containing a fetus. Cystic mass (hematoma) is evident in the rectouterine pouch. No fetal heart activity is noted.

OPINION: Ectopic pregnancy, left uterine tube.

A.W. Tyat, MD
AWT/ogo

Start | Log On/Off | Print | Edit

1. The patient has:
   a. been pregnant two or more times
   b. given birth to two or more viable offspring
   c. borne one viable offspring
   d. never been pregnant

2. T F   The patient has experienced one abortion
3. T F   Radiographic images were used to determine the findings.

To test your understanding of the terms introduced in this chapter, circle the words that correctly complete the sentences. The italicized words refer to the correct answer.

1. The premature infant was diagnosed as having *respiratory distress syndrome*, a disease of the (**umbilicus, erythrocytes, lungs**).

2. Because of inadequate uterine contractions, the patient was experiencing *difficult labor*, or (**dysphasia, dystocia, dysuria**).

3. Down syndrome was diagnosed prenatally by laboratory analysis of *amniotic fluid aspirated by surgical puncture*, or (**amniocentesis, amnioscopy, amnioscope**).

4. The word that means *before childbirth* (reference to the mother) is (**intrapartum, antepartum, postpartum**).

5. *Nulligravida* is a woman who (**has never been pregnant, has not given birth**).

6. *Multipara* is a woman who has (**given birth to two or more viable offspring, been pregnant two or more times**).

7. *Primigravida* is a woman (**in her first pregnancy, who has given birth to one child**).

8. The word that means the *act of giving birth* is (**parturition, puerperium, gravidopuerperal**).

9. *Rupture of the uterus* is called (**hysterorrhaphy, hysterorrhexis, hysteroptosis**).

10. Fetal alcohol syndrome is *producing malformations* or (**quickening, colostrum, teratogenic**) in nature.

EXERCISE **42** *Read Medical Terms in Use*

Practice pronunciation of the terms by reading the following medical document. Use the pronunciation key following the medical term to assist you in saying the words.

 To hear these terms select Chapter 9, Chapter Exercises, Read Medical Terms in Use.

Jane Anne is a 34-year-old **gravida** (GRAV-i-da) 2 **para** (PAR-a) 1 woman. Her LMP was April 20, 20XX. The EDD is January 2, 20XX. The **obstetrician** (ob-ste-TRISH-an) prescribed folic acid to prevent **spina bifida** (SPĪ-na) (BIF-i-da). The patient's first pregnancy was complicated by **preeclampsia** (prē-ē-KLAMP-sē-a) and a **breech** (brēch) **presentation,** which required a **cesarean section** (se-ZĀR-ē-an) (SEK-shun). **Pelvic sonography** (PEL-vik) (so-NOG-ra-fē) showed a single female fetus with normal development. She went on to deliver a healthy baby 3 days before her expected delivery date.

EXERCISE **43** *Comprehend Medical Terms in Use*

Test your comprehension of terms in the above medical document by circling the correct answer.

1. T F Jane Anne has been pregnant twice and has given birth once.

2. The obstetrician prescribed folic acid to prevent congenital:
   a. split of the lip and roof of the mouth
   b. mental retardation
   c. absence of part of the esophagus
   d. defect of the vertebral column

3. During her first pregnancy the patient had:
   a. abnormally low implantation of the placenta on the uterine wall
   b. high blood pressure, edema, and proteinuria
   c. premature separation of the placenta from the uterine wall
   d. convulsions and coma

4. T F The fetal presentation of the patient's first pregnancy was cephalic.

CHAPTER REVIEW

◉))) CHAPTER REVIEW ON CD-ROM

Use the CD-ROM that accompanies this textbook to play and practice what you have learned in this chapter. The Chapter Exercises, Practice Activities, Animations, and Games allow you to hear, see, and interact with the chapter content.

Chapter Exercises	Practice Activities	Animations	Games
Exercises in this section of your CD-ROM correlate to exercises in your textbook. You may have completed them as you worked through the chapter.	Practice in study mode, then test your learning in assessment mode. Keep track of your scores from assessment mode if you wish.	☐ Ectopic Pregnancy	☐ Name that Word Part
			☐ Term Storm
			☐ Term Explorer
			☐ Termbusters
			☐ Medical Millionaire

Chapter Exercises	Practice Activities	SCORE
☐ Pronunciation	☐ Picture It	
☐ Spelling	☐ Define Word Parts	_____
☐ Read Medical Terms in Use	☐ Build Medical Terms	_____
	☐ Word Shop	_____
	☐ Define Medical Terms	_____
	☐ Use It	_____
	☐ Hear It and Type It: Clinical Vignettes	_____

REVIEW OF WORD PARTS

Can you define and spell the following word parts?

Combining Forms		Prefixes	Suffixes
amni/o	lact/o	ante-	-amnios
amnion/o	nat/o	micro-	-cyesis
cephal/o	omphal/o	multi-	-e
chori/o	par/o	nulli-	-is
embry/o	part/o	post-	-partum
esophag/o	pelv/o	pre-	-rrhexis
fet/i	pelv/i		-tocia
fet/o	prim/i		-um
gravid/o	pseud/o		-us
	puerper/o		
	pylor/o		
	terat/o		

REVIEW OF TERMS

Can you build, analyze, define, pronounce, and spell the following terms *built from word parts?*

Diseases and Disorders (Obstetrics)	Diseases and Disorders (Neonatology)	Surgical (Obstetrics)	Diagnostic (Obstetrics)	Complementary (Obstetrics and Neonatology)	
amnionitis	microcephalus	amniotomy	amniocentesis	amniochorial	multigravida
chorioamnionitis	omphalitis	episiotomy	amnioscope	amniorrhea	multipara (multip)
choriocarcinoma	omphalocele		amnioscopy	amniorrhexis	natal
dystocia	pyloric stenosis		pelvic	antepartum	neonate
hysterorrhexis	tracheoesophageal		sonography	embryogenic	neonatologist
oligohydramnios	fistula			embryoid	neonatology
polyhydramnios				fetal	nulligravida
				gravida	nullipara
				gravidopuerperal	para
				intrapartum	postnatal
				lactic	postpartum
				lactogenic	prenatal
				lactorrhea	primigravida
					primipara (primip)
					pseudocyesis
					puerpera
					puerperal
					teratogen
					teratogenic
					teratology

Can you define, pronounce, and spell the following terms *not built from word parts?*

Diseases and Disorders (Obstetrics)	Diseases and Disorders (Neonatology)	Complementary (Obstetrics and Neonatology)
abortion	cleft lip and palate	breech presentation
abruptio placentae	Down syndrome	cephalic presentation
eclampsia	erythroblastosis fetalis	cesarean section (CS, C-section)
ectopic pregnancy	esophageal atresia	colostrum
placenta previa	fetal alcohol syndrome (FAS)	congenital anomaly
preeclampsia	gastroschisis	in vitro fertilization (IVF)
	respiratory distress syndrome (RDS)	lactation
	spina bifida	lochia
		meconium
		midwife
		midwifery
		obstetrician
		obstetrics (OB)
		parturition
		premature infant
		puerperium
		quickening
		stillborn

ANSWERS

Exercise Figures

Exercise Figure
A. 1. umbilicus: omphal/o
2. fetus: fet/o, fet/i
3. amnion, amniotic fluid: amni/o, amnion/o
4. chorion: chori/o

Exercise Figure
B. omphal/o/cele

Exercise Figure
C. neo/nat/e

Exercise 1
1. gamete; ovulation; fertilization; zygote; gestation
2. embryo; fetus
3. amniotic; chorion; amnion; amniotic

Exercise 2
1. fetus, unborn child
2. milk
3. bear, give birth to, labor, childbirth
4. umbilicus, navel
5. amnion, amniotic fluid
6. childbirth
7. pregnancy
8. birth
9. chorion
10. embryo, to be full

Exercise 3
1. lact/o
2. a. fet/o, b. fet/i
3. chori/o
4. a. amni/o, b. amnion/o
5. puerper/o
6. a. par/o, b. part/o
7. gravid/o
8. embry/o
9. nat/o
10. omphal/o

Exercise 4
1. first
2. pylorus
3. head
4. esophagus
5. false
6. pelvic bone, pelvis
7. malformations

Exercise 5
1. cephal/o
2. pylor/o
3. pseud/o

4. esophag/o
5. prim/i
6. terat/o
7. a. pelv/i, b. pelv/o

Exercise 6
1. after   4. small
2. many   5. before
3. none   6. before

Exercise 7
1. nulli-   4. a. ante-
2. micro-   b. pre-
3. multi-   5. post-

Exercise 8
1. rupture
2. birth, labor
3. pregnancy
4. childbirth, labor
5. amnion, amniotic fluid

Exercise 9
1. -tocia   4. -cyesis
2. -rrhexis   5. -amnios
3. -partum

Exercise 10
1. -e   3. -us
2. -is   4. -um
Answers may be in any order.

Exercise 11
Pronunciation Exercise

Exercise 12
1. WR CV WR   S
   chori/o/amnion/itis
        CF
   inflammation of the chorion and amnion
2. WR CV WR   S
   chori/o/carcin/oma
        CF
   cancerous tumor of the chorion
3. P   S(WR)
   dys/tocia
   difficult labor
4. WR   S
   amnion/itis
   inflammation of the amnion
5. WR CV S
   hyster/o/rrhexis
        CF
   rupture of the uterus

6. WR CV WR   S
   olig/o/hydr/amnios
        CF
   scanty amnion water (less than the normal amount of amniotic fluid)
7. P   WR   S
   poly/hydr/amnios
   much amnion water (more than the normal amount of amniotic fluid)

Exercise 13
1. chori/o/carcin/oma
2. amnion/itis
3. chori/o/amnion/itis
4. dys/tocia
5. hyster/o/rrhexis
6. olig/o/hydr/amnios
7. poly/hydr/amnios

Exercise 14
Spelling Exercise; see text p. 361.

Exercise 15
Pronunciation Exercise

Exercise 16
1. premature separation of the placenta from the uterine wall
2. termination of pregnancy by the expulsion from the uterus of an embryo
3. abnormally low implantation of the placenta on the uterine wall
4. severe complication and progression of preeclampsia
5. pregnancy occurring outside the uterus
6. abnormal condition, encountered during pregnancy or shortly after delivery, of high blood pressure, edema, and proteinuria

Exercise 17
1. abruptio placentae
2. eclampsia
3. abortion
4. ectopic pregnancy
5. placenta previa
6. preeclampsia

Exercise 18
Spelling Exercise; see text p. 364.

Exercise 19
Pronunciation Exercise

Exercise 20
1. WR S
   pylor/ic (stenosis)
   narrowing pertaining to the pyloric
     sphincter
2. WR   CV S
   omphal/o/cele
        CF
   hernia at the umbilicus
3. WR   S
   omphal/itis
   inflammation of the umbilicus
4. P   WR   S
   micro/cephal/us
   (fetus with a very) small head
5. WR CV WR   S
   trache/o/esophag/eal (fistula)
        CF
   abnormal passageway (between)
     pertaining to the esophagus
       and the trachea

Exercise 21
1. omphal/o/cele
2. micro/cephal/us
3. pylor/ic (stenosis)
4. trache/o/esophag/eal (fistula)
5. omphal/itis

Exercise 22
Spelling Exercise; see text p. 366.

Exercise 23
Pronunciation Exercise

Exercise 24
1. f   5. h
2. c   6. b
3. a   7. g
4. d   8. e

Exercise 25
Spelling Exercise; see text p. 368.

Exercise 26
Pronunciation Exercise

Exercise 27
1. WR CV S
   episi/o/tomy
        CF
   incision of the vulva (perineum)
2. WR CV S
   amni/o/tomy
        CF
   incision into the amnion (rupture of
     the fetal membrane to induce labor)

3. WR CV S
   amni/o/scope
        CF
   instrument for visual examination of
     amniotic fluid (and fetus)
4. WR S WR CV S
   pelv/ic son/o/graphy
              CF
   pertaining to the pelvis, process of
     recording sound
5. WR CV   S
   amni/o/centesis
        CF
   surgical puncture to aspirate amniotic
     fluid
6. WR CV S
   amni/o/scopy
        CF
   visual examination of amniotic fluid
     (and fetus)

Exercise 28
1. amni/o/tomy
2. episi/o/tomy
3. amni/o/scopy
4. amni/o/centesis
5. amni/o/scope
6. pelv/ic son/o/graphy

Exercise 29
Spelling Exercise; see text p. 371.

Exercise 30
Pronunciation Exercise

Exercise 31
1. WR   S
   puerper/a
   childbirth
2. WR CV S
   amni/o/rrhexis
        CF
   rupture of the amnion
3. P   WR S
   ante/part/um
   before childbirth
4. WR CV S
   pseud/o/cyesis
        CF
   false pregnancy
5. P WR S
   pre/nat/al
   pertaining to before birth
6. WR S
   lact/ic
   pertaining to milk

7. WR CV S
   lact/o/rrhea
        CF
   (spontaneous) discharge of milk
8. WR CV S
   amni/o/rrhea
        CF
   discharge (escape) of amniotic fluid
9. P   WR S
   multi/par/a
   many births
10. WR CV S
    embry/o/genic
        CF
    producing an embryo
11. WR   S
    embry/oid
    resembling an embryo
12. WR S
    fet/al
    pertaining to the fetus
13. WR S
    gravid/a
    pregnant (woman)
14. WR CV WR S
    amni/o/chori/al
        CF
    pertaining to the amnion and chorion
15. P   WR S
    multi/gravid/a
    many pregnancies
16. WR CV S
    lact/o/genic
        CF
    producing milk (by stimulation)
17. WR S
    nat/al
    pertaining to birth
18. WR CV WR   S
    gravid/o/puerper/al
           CF
    pertaining to pregnancy and
      childbirth
19. P WR CV S
    neo/nat/o/logy
           CF
    study of the newborn
20. P   WR S
    nulli/par/a
    no births
21. WR S
    par/a
    birth
22. WR CV WR S
    prim/i/gravid/a
           CF
    first pregnancy

23. P WR S
    post/part/um
    after childbirth
24. P WR S
    neo/nat/e
    new birth (an infant from birth to
    4 weeks of age, synonymous with
    newborn)
25. WR CV WR S
    prim/i/par/a
      CF
    first birth
26. WR S
    puerper/al
    pertaining to (immediately after)
    childbirth
27. P WR S
    nulli/gravid/a
    no pregnancies
28. P WR S
    intra/part/um
    within (during) labor and childbirth
29. WR CV S
    terat/o/gen
      CF
    any agent producing malformations
    (in the developing embryo)
30. P WR S
    post/nat/al
    pertaining to after birth
31. WR CV S
    terat/o/logy
      CF
    study of malformations (in the
    developing embryo)
32. P WR CV S
    neo/nat/o/logist
        CF
    physician who studies and treats
    disorders of the newborn
33. WR CV S
    terat/o/genic
      CF
    producing malformations

Exercise 32
1. amni/o/chori/al
2. ante/part/um
3. embry/o/genic
4. fet/al
5. pre/nat/al
6. lact/ic
7. lact/o/rrhea
8. amni/o/rrhea
9. pseud/o/cyesis
10. lact/o/genic
11. amni/o/rrhexis
12. embry/oid
13. gravid/a

14. gravid/o/puerper/al
15. multi/par/a
16. nat/al
17. neo/nat/e
18. neo/nat/o/logy
19. nulli/par/a
20. par/a
21. prim/i/gravid/a
22. post/part/um
23. prim/i/par/a
24. multi/gravid/a
25. puerper/al
26. nulli/gravid/a
27. terat/o/gen
28. puerper/a
29. intra/part/um
30. terat/o/genic
31. neo/nat/o/logist
32. post/nat/al
33. terat/o/logy

Exercise 33
Spelling Exercise; see text p. 378.

Exercise 34
Pronunciation Exercise

Exercise 35
1. a	6. b
2. e	7. j
3. i	8. d
4. g	9. c
5. f	10. h

Exercise 36
1. h	5. f
2. e	6. a
3. b	7. d
4. c	8. g

Exercise 37
1. first stool of the newborn
2. medical specialty dealing with pregnancy, childbirth, and puerperium
3. infant born before completing 37 weeks of gestation
4. vaginal discharge after childbirth
5. period after delivery until the reproductive organs return to normal
6. act of giving birth
7. physician who specializes in obstetrics
8. abnormality present at birth
9. parturition in which the buttocks, feet, or knees emerge first
10. birth of a baby through an incision in the mother's abdomen and uterus
11. first feeling of movement of the fetus in utero by the pregnant woman
12. secretion of milk
13. parturition in which any part of the head emerges first

14. fluid secreted by the breast during pregnancy and after birth until lactation begins
15. an individual who practices midwifery
16. born dead
17. the practice of assisting in childbirth
18. a method of fertilizing human ova outside the body

Exercise 38
Spelling Exercise; see text p. 382.

Exercise 39
1. obstetrics
2. expected (estimated) date of delivery
3. last menstrual period
4. date of birth
5. newborn
6. multipara
7. cesarean section
8. last normal menstrual period
9. respiratory distress syndrome
10. primapara
11. fetal alcohol syndrome
12. in vitro fertilization

Exercise 40
A.
1. gravida	5. gestation
2. para	6. pelvic sonography
3. EDD	7. fetus
4. prenatal	8. fetal

B.
1. c
2. *T*
3. *F*, sonography was used

Exercise 41
1. lungs
2. dystocia
3. amniocentesis
4. antepartum
5. has never been pregnant
6. given birth to two or more viable offspring
7. in her first pregnancy
8. parturition
9. hysterorrhexis
10. teratogenic

Exercise 42
Reading Exercise

Exercise 43
1. *T*
2. d
3. b
4. *F*, the fetal presentation was breech.

CHAPTER 10

Cardiovascular, Immune, and Lymphatic Systems and Blood

OUTLINE

ANATOMY, 394

WORD PARTS, 403
Combining Forms, 403
Prefix, 406
Suffixes, 406

MEDICAL TERMS, 408
Disease and Disorder Terms, 408
    Built from Word Parts, 408
    Not Built from Word Parts, 413
Surgical Terms, 422
    Built from Word Parts, 422
    Not Built from Word Parts, 425
Diagnostic Terms, 431
    Built from Word Parts, 431
    Not Built from Word Parts, 436
Complementary Terms, 444
    Built from Word Parts, 444
    Not Built from Word Parts, 448, 452
Abbreviations, 455

PRACTICAL APPLICATION, 458
Interact with Medical Documents, 458
Interpret Medical Terms, 460
Read Medical Terms in Use, 461
Comprehend Medical Terms in Use, 461

CHAPTER REVIEW, 462

TABLE 10-1 TYPES OF ANGIOGRAPHY, 432

TABLE 10-2 UNDERSTANDING A LIPID PROFILE, 440

OBJECTIVES

Upon completion of this chapter you will be able to:

1. Identify the organs and structures of the cardiovascular and lymphatic systems and blood and the function of the immune system.

2. Define and spell word parts related to the cardiovascular and lymphatic systems and blood.

3. Define, pronounce, and spell disease and disorder terms related to the cardiovascular and lymphatic systems and blood.

4. Define, pronounce, and spell surgical terms related to the cardiovascular and lymphatic systems and blood.

5. Define, pronounce, and spell diagnostic terms related to the cardiovascular system and blood.

6. Define, pronounce, and spell complementary terms related to the cardiovascular and immune systems and blood.

7. Interpret the meaning of abbreviations presented in the chapter.

8. Interpret, read, and comprehend medical language in simulated medical statements and documents.

ANATOMY

At first glance this may seem like an overabundance of material to cover in one chapter. It is a lot of material, but as you will see the systems have interactive functions, and learning the terms for these systems at the same time will be beneficial.

The functions are interactive in many ways. The lymphatic and immune systems support each other by providing an immune response to invading microorganisms and foreign substances. The lymphatic system and blood share macrophages and lymphocytes. Lymph is drained into large veins of the cardiovascular system, and the cardiovascular system is responsible for circulating blood throughout the body.

Cardiovascular System

Function

The cardiovascular system pumps and transports blood throughout the body. It consists of the heart and a closed network of blood vessels composed of arteries, capillaries, and veins. The heart pumps blood containing oxygen and nutrients to body tissues through the arteries. The exchange of gases, nutrients, and waste between the blood and body tissue takes place in the capillaries. The blood carrying carbon dioxide and waste is carried from the tissues through veins to organs of excretion.

Structures of the Cardiovascular System

Term	Definition
heart	muscular cone-shaped organ the size of a fist, located behind the sternum (breast bone) and between the lungs. The pumping action of the heart circulates blood throughout the body. The heart consists of two upper chambers, the *right atrium* and the *left atrium* (*pl.* atria), and two lower chambers, the *right ventricle* and the *left ventricle* (*pl.* ventricles). The atria receive blood returning from the body through the veins. The ventricles pump blood through the arteries from the heart back to the body tissue. The atrial septum separates the atria and the ventricular septum separates the ventricles. The tricuspid and mitral valves are referred to as the atrioventricular (AV) valves (Figure 10-1). Valves of the heart keep the blood flowing in one direction.
tricuspid valve	located between the right atrium and right ventricle
mitral valve	located between the left atrium and left ventricle

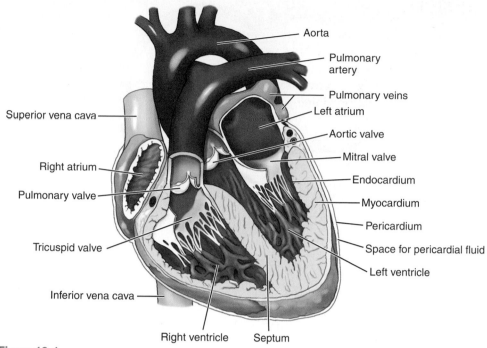

Figure 10-1
Interior of the heart.

Term	Definition
semilunar valves	pulmonary and aortic valves located between the right ventricle and the pulmonary artery and between the left ventricle and the aorta
pericardium	two-layer sac consisting of an external fibrous and an internal serous layer. The serous layer secretes a fluid that facilitates movement of the heart. This layer also covers the heart and is called the epicardium.
three layers of the heart	
epicardium	covers the heart
myocardium	middle, thick, muscular layer
endocardium	inner lining of the heart
blood vessels	tubelike structures that carry blood throughout the body (Figure 10-2)
arteries	blood vessels that carry blood away from the heart. All arteries, with the exception of the pulmonary artery, carry oxygen and other nutrients from the heart to the body cells. The *pulmonary artery*, in contrast, carries carbon dioxide and other waste products from the heart to the lungs.

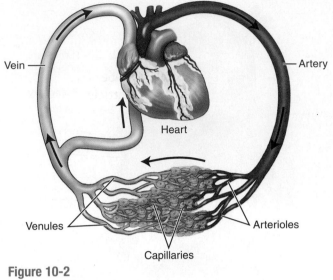

Figure 10-2
Types of blood vessels.

Structures of the Cardiovascular System—*cont'd*

Term	Definition
arterioles	smallest arteries
aorta	largest artery in the body, originating at the left ventricle and descending through the thorax and abdomen
veins	blood vessels that carry blood back to the heart. All veins, with the exception of the pulmonary veins, carry blood containing carbon dioxide and other waste products. The pulmonary veins carry oxygenated blood from the lungs to the heart.
venules	smallest veins
venae cavae	largest veins in the body. The *inferior vena cava* carries blood to the heart from body parts below the diaphragm, and the *superior vena cava* returns the blood to the heart from the upper part of the body.
capillaries	microscopic blood vessels that connect arterioles with venules. Materials are passed between the blood and tissue through the capillary walls.

EXERCISE 1

Match the anatomic terms for the cardiovascular system in the first column with the correct definitions in the second column.

_____ 1. aorta

_____ 2. arteries

_____ 3. arterioles

_____ 4. atria

_____ 5. mitral valve

_____ 6. capillaries

_____ 7. endocardium

_____ 8. serous pericardium

_____ 9. heart

_____ 10. atrioventricular valves

a. lies between the left atrium and left ventricle

b. pumps blood throughout the body

c. smallest arteries

d. inner lining of the heart

e. largest artery in the body

f. connect arterioles with venules

g. blood vessels that carry blood away from the heart

h. layer of the pericardial sac that lies closest to the myocardium

i. upper chambers of the heart

j. tricuspid and mitral valves

EXERCISE 2

Match the anatomic terms for the cardiovascular system in the first column with the correct definitions in the second column.

_____ 1. myocardium

_____ 2. parietal pericardium

_____ 3. pericardium

_____ 4. semilunar valves

_____ 5. atrial septum

_____ 6. tricuspid valve

_____ 7. veins

_____ 8. ventricles

_____ 9. venules

_____ 10. vena cava

a. carries blood back to the heart

b. two-layer sac

c. smallest veins

d. lines the pericardial sac

e. lower chambers of the heart

f. largest vein in the body

g. allows the double layer of the covering of the heart to move without friction

h. located between the right ventricle and the pulmonary artery and between the left ventricle and the aorta

i. carries oxygenated blood away from the heart

j. located between the right atrium and the right ventricle

k. muscular layer of the heart

l. separates the atria

Blood

Function

The primary function of blood is to maintain internal balance in the body. Activities of the blood include **transportation** of nutrients, waste, oxygen, carbon dioxide, and hormones; **protection** provided by certain cells that protect the body against microorganisms; and **regulation** by controlling body temperature and maintaining fluid and electrolyte balance.

Composition of Blood

Term	Definition
blood..................	composed of *plasma* and *formed elements*, such as erythrocytes, leukocytes, and thrombocytes (platelets) (Figure 10-3)
plasma	clear, straw-colored, liquid portion of blood in which cells are suspended. Plasma is approximately 90% water and comprises approximately 55% of the total blood volume.
cells (formed elements)	
erythrocytes...........	red blood cells that carry oxygen. Erythrocytes develop in bone marrow.
leukocytes	white blood cells that combat infection and respond to inflammation. There are five types of white blood cells (Figure 10-4).
platelets (thrombocytes).........	one of the formed elements in the blood that is responsible for aiding in the clotting process
serum................	clear, watery fluid portion of the blood that remains after a clot has formed

Neutrophil

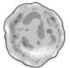

Eosinophil

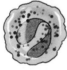

Basophil

Lymphocyte

Monocyte

Figure 10-4

Types of leukocytes. Each leukocyte plays a different role in providing immune responses to pathogens, foreign agents, allergies, and abnormal body cells.

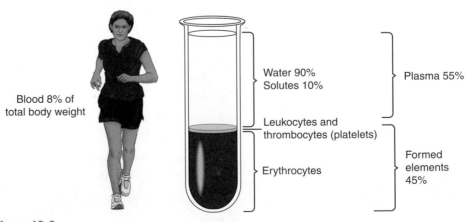

Blood 8% of total body weight

Water 90%
Solutes 10%

Plasma 55%

Leukocytes and thrombocytes (platelets)

Erythrocytes

Formed elements 45%

Figure 10-3

Composition of blood.

Lymphatic System

Function

Three functions of the lymphatic system are to return excessive tissue fluid to the blood, absorb fats and fat-soluble vitamins from the small intestine and transport them to the blood, and provide defense against infection.

The lymphatic system functions through a network of vessels, ducts, nodes, and organs. The collected interstitial fluid called lymph travels away from body tissue toward the heart and is drained into the cardiovascular system through ducts in the upper chest. Breathing and muscle action help propel lymph through the vessels (Figure 10-5).

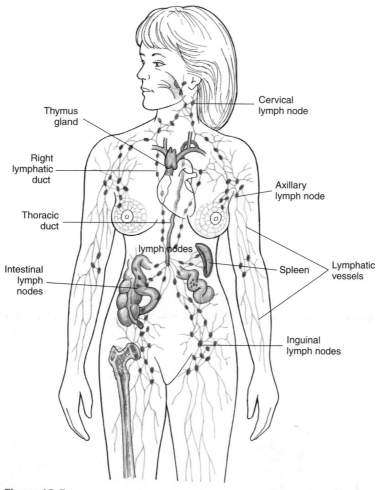

Figure 10-5
Lymphatic system.

Structures of the Lymphatic System

Term	Definition
lymph	transparent, colorless, tissue fluid that, on entering the lymphatic system, is called lymph. Lymph contains lymphocytes and monocytes and flows in a one-way direction to the heart. Lymph is similar to blood plasma.
lymphatic vessels	similar to veins, lymphatic vessels transport lymph from body tissues to the chest, where it enters the cardiovascular system. The vessels begin as capillaries spread throughout the body then merge into larger tubes that eventually become ducts in the chest. They provide a one-way flow for lymph gathered from the tissues to ducts in the chest, where lymph enters through veins into the circulatory system.
lymph nodes	small, spherical bodies composed of lymphoid tissue. They may be singular or grouped together along the path of the lymph vessels. The nodes filter lymph to keep substances such as bacteria and other foreign agents from entering the blood. They also produce lymphocytes.
spleen	located in the left side of the abdominal cavity between the stomach and the diaphragm. In adulthood, the spleen is the largest lymphatic organ in the body. Blood, rather than lymph, flows through the spleen. Blood is cleansed of microorganisms in the spleen. The spleen stores blood and destroys worn out red blood cells.
thymus gland	one of the primary lymphatic organs, it is located anterior to the ascending aorta and posterior to the sternum between the lungs. It plays an important role in the development of the body's immune system, particularly from infancy to puberty. Around puberty the thymus gland atrophies so that most of the gland is connective tissue.

Fill in the blanks with anatomic terms for blood and the lymphatic systems.

The function of the blood is to maintain internal balance in the body. The liquid portion of blood is called (1) _Plasma_, in which (2) _erythrocytes_, (3) _leukocytes_, and (4) _platelets_ are suspended. (5) _platelets_ aid in clotting blood; (6) _Serum_ is the clear liquid that remains after a clot is formed. The lymphatic system provides defense against infection. The lymphatic system is composed of the fluid (7) _lymph_; small spherical bodies (8) _lymph nodes_; vessels for transporting lymph, the (9) _Spleen_, which is the largest lymphatic organ; and the (10) _thymus_ gland.

Immune System

Function

The immune system protects the body against pathogens (bacteria, fungi, and viruses), foreign agents that cause allergic reactions (e.g., peanuts) or toxins (e.g., insect bites), and abnormal body cells (e.g., cancer). However, it does not have its own organs and structures. Its function depends on organs and structures of other body systems, including the spleen, liver, intestinal tract, lymph nodes, and bone marrow.

The immune system has three lines of defense; the first is the prevention of foreign substances from entering the body. Unbroken skin and mucous membranes act as mechanical barriers. Ear wax and saliva act as chemical barriers.

If the first line of defense is penetrated by microorganisms, a second line of defense continues to battle disease. Second-line defenses include inflammation and fever plus phagocytosis, a process in which some of the white blood cells destroy the invading microorganisms. Also activated are protective proteins such as interferons, which fight viruses, and natural killer (NK) cells, which are effective against microorganisms and cancer cells (Figure 10-6).

Specific immunity, the third line of defense, provides protection against specific pathogens, such as the polio virus, by forming specific antibodies to fight against the infectious agent.

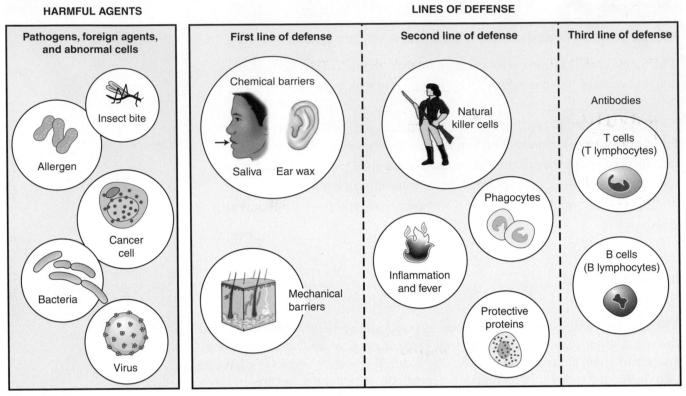

HARMFUL AGENTS   **LINES OF DEFENSE**

Figure 10-6
Three lines of defense provided by the immune system to protect the body against pathogens, foreign agents, and cancer.

EXERCISE   4

Complete the following exercise for the immune system.

1. The function of the immune system is to _Peotect the body against pathogens, foreign agents and abnormal cells_ .

2. List five organs and structures from other body systems used by the immune system to carry out its function.

   a. _Spleen_

   b. _liver_

   c. _intestinal tract_

   d. _lymph nodes_

   e. _bone marrow_

3. The three lines of defense used by the immune system are:

   a. _Prevention of foreign substances from entering_ body

   b. _Unbroken skin and mucс membranes act as barriecs_ mechinal

   c. _Ear wax and Saliva act as chemical barrien_

WORD PARTS

Word parts you need to learn to complete this chapter are listed on the following pages. The exercises at the end of each list willl help you learn their definitions and spellings.

Combining Forms of the Cardiovascular and Lymphatic Systems and Blood

Combining Form	Definition
angi/o	vessel (usually refers to blood vessel)
aort/o	aorta
arteri/o	artery
atri/o	atrium
cardi/o	heart
lymphaden/o	lymph node
lymph/o	lymph, lymph tissue
myel/o	bone marrow
(NOTE: myel/o also means *spinal cord;* see Chapter 15)	
phleb/o, ven/o	vein
plasm/o	plasma
splen/o	spleen
(NOTE: only one *e* in the word root for spleen)	
thym/o	thymus gland
valv/o, valvul/o	valve
ventricul/o	ventricle

VITAL AIR
It was believed in ancient times that arteries carried air. Vital air, or **pneuma,** did not allow blood in the arteries. A cut in an artery allowed vital air to escape and blood to replace it. The Greek **arteria,** meaning **windpipe,** was given for this reason.

VENTRICLE
is derived from the Latin **venter,** meaning **little belly.** It was first applied to the belly and then to the stomach. Later it was extended to mean any small cavity in an organ or body.

EXERCISE FIGURE A

Fill in the blanks with combining forms in this diagram of a cutaway section of the heart.

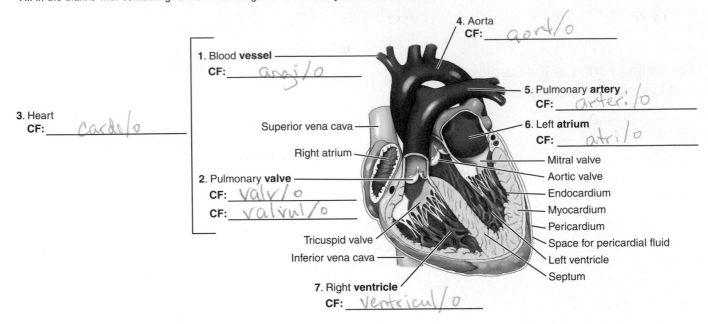

4. Aorta
CF: _aort/o_

1. Blood **vessel**
CF: _angi/o_

3. Heart
CF: _cardi/o_

Superior vena cava

Right atrium

2. Pulmonary **valve**
CF: _valv/o_
CF: _valvul/o_

Tricuspid valve

Inferior vena cava

5. Pulmonary **artery**
CF: _arteri/o_

6. Left **atrium**
CF: _atri/o_

Mitral valve
Aortic valve
Endocardium
Myocardium
Pericardium
Space for pericardial fluid
Left ventricle
Septum

7. Right **ventricle**
CF: _ventricul/o_

EXERCISE 5

Write the definitions of the following combining forms.

1. cardi/o _heart_
2. atri/o _atrium_
3. plasm/o _plasma_
4. angi/o _vessel_
5. ven/o _vein_
6. aort/o _aorta_
7. valv/o _valve_
8. splen/o _spleen_

9. thym/o _thymus gland_
10. phleb/o _vein_
11. ventricul/o _ventricle_
12. arteri/o _artery_
13. valvul/o _valve_
14. lymph/o _lymph_
15. lymphaden/o _lymph node_
16. myel/o _bone marrow_

EXERCISE 6

Write the combining form for each of the following terms.

1. artery _arteri/o_

2. vein
   a. _ven/o_
   b. _phleb/o_

3. heart _cardio_

4. atrium _atri/o_

5. ventricle _ventricul/o_

6. lymph, lymph tissue _lymph/o_

7. aorta _lymph/o_

8. vessel (usually blood vessel) _angi/o_

9. valve
   a. _valv/o_
   b. _valvul/o_

10. spleen _splen/o_

11. plasma _plasm/o_

12. thymus gland _thym/o_

13. lymph node _lymphaden/o_

14. bone marrow _myel/o_

Combining Forms Commonly Used with the Cardiovascular and Lymphatic Systems and Blood Terms

Combining Form	Definition
ather/o	yellowish, fatty plaque
ech/o...................	sound
electr/o.................	electricity, electrical activity
isch/o	deficiency, blockage
therm/o.................	heat
thromb/o................	clot

EXERCISE 7

Write the definition of the following combining forms.

1. ech/o _sound_

2. thromb/o _clot_

3. isch/o _deficiency_

4. therm/o _heat_

5. ather/o _yellowish, fatty plaque_

6. electr/o _electricity, electrical activity_

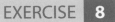

EXERCISE 8

Write the combining form for each of the following.

1. clot _thromb/o_   5. heat _therm/o_

2. sound _ech/o_   6. electricity,
                                        electrical
3. deficiency,   activity _electr/o_
   blockage _isch/o_

4. yellowish,
   fatty plaque _ather/o_

Prefix

Prefix	Definition
brady-	slow

Suffixes

COMPARING -GRAPH, -GRAPHY, AND -GRAM
-graph is the instrument used to record, i.e., the machine, as in **telegraph** or **electrocardiograph** and also means record, as in **radiograph.**
-graphy is the process of recording, the act of setting down or registering a record, as in **photography** or **electroencephalography.**
-gram is the record (picture, radiographic image, or tracing), as in **telegram** or **electrocardiogram.**

Suffix	Definition
-ac	pertaining to
-apheresis	removal
-graph	instrument used to record; record
-odynia	pain
-penia	abnormal reduction in number
-poiesis	formation
-sclerosis	hardening

Refer to Appendix A and Appendix B for alphabetical lists of word parts and their meanings.

EXERCISE 9

Write the definitions of the following prefix and suffixes.

1. brady- _____slow_____

2. -graph _____instrument used to record_____

3. -penia _____abnormal reduction in number_____

4. -sclerosis _____hardening_____

5. -odynia _____pain_____

6. -apheresis _____removal_____

7. -poiesis _____formation_____

8. -ac _____pertaining to_____

EXERCISE 10

Write the suffix or prefix for each of the following.

1. formation _____-poiesis_____

2. pertaining to _____-ac_____

3. hardening _____-sclerosis_____

4. instrument used to record; record _____-graph_____

5. abnormal reduction in number _____-penia_____

6. pain _____-odynia_____

7. slow _____brady-_____

8. removal _____-apheresis_____

MEDICAL TERMS

The terms you need to learn to complete this chapter are listed below. The exercises following each list will help you learn the definition and the spelling of each word.

Disease and Disorder Terms

Built from Word Parts

The following terms are built from word parts you have already learned and can be translated literally to find their meanings. Further explanation of terms beyond the definition of their word parts, if needed, is included in parentheses.

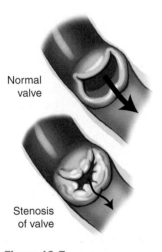

Normal
valve

Stenosis
of valve

Figure 10-7
Aortic stenosis.

EXERCISE FIGURE B

Fill in the blanks to label the diagram.

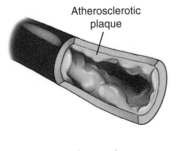

Atherosclerotic
plaque

___fatty___ / ___cv___ / ___hardening___
plaque

Term	Definition
CARDIOVASCULAR SYSTEM	
angioma .... (an-jē-Ō-ma)	tumor composed of blood vessels
angiostenosis .... (an-jē-ō-ste-NŌ-sis)	narrowing of a blood vessel
aortic stenosis .... (ā-OR-tik) (ste-NŌ-sis)	narrowing pertaining to aorta (narrowing of the aortic valve) (Figure 10-7)
arteriosclerosis............. (ar-*tēr*-ē-ō-skle-RŌ-sis)	hardening of the arteries
atherosclerosis............. (*ath*-er-ō-skle-RŌ-sis)	hardening of fatty plaque (deposited on the arterial wall) (Exercise Figure B)
bradycardia............... (brad-ē-KAR-dē-a) (NOTE: the *i* in cardi/o has been dropped)	condition of a slow heart (rate less than 60 beats per minute)
cardiodynia............... (*kar*-dē-ō-DIN-ē-a) (NOTE: the *o* is attached to -odynia and not a combining vowel)	pain in the heart
cardiomegaly .... (*kar*-dē-ō-MEG-a-lē)	enlargement of the heart
cardiomyopathy .... (kar-dē-ō-mī-OP-a-thē)	disease of the heart muscle
cardiovalvulitis .... (kar-dē-ō-val-vū-LĪ-tis)	inflammation of the valves of the heart (also referred to as **valvulitis**)
endocarditis .... (*en*-dō-kar-DĪ-tis)	inflammation of the inner (lining) of the heart (particularly heart valves)
ischemia.................. (is-KĒ-mē-a)	deficiency of blood (flow)
myocarditis............... (*mī*-ō-kar-DĪ-tis)	inflammation of the muscle of the heart

Term	Definition
pericarditis .... (per-i-kar-DĪ-tis)	inflammation of the sac surrounding the heart (see Figure 10-12)
phlebitis .... (fle-BĪ-tis)	inflammation of a vein
polyarteritis .... (pol-ē-ar-te-RĪ-tis) (NOTE: the *i* in arteri/o has been dropped)	inflammation of many (sites in the) arteries
tachycardia............... (*tak*-i-KAR-dē-a) (NOTE: the *i* in cardi/o has been dropped)	abnormal state of rapid heart (rate of more than 100 beats per min)
thrombophlebitis .... (*throm*-bō-fle-BĪ-tis)	inflammation of a vein associated with a clot

BLOOD

hematoma .... (*hē*-ma-TŌ-ma)	tumor of blood (collection of blood resulting from a broken blood vessel)
multiple myeloma........... (mi-e-LŌ-ma)	tumors of the bone marrow
pancytopenia .... (pan-sī-tō-PĒ-nē-a)	abnormal reduction of all (blood) cells
thrombosis .... (throm-BŌ-sis)	abnormal condition of a (blood) clot
thrombus .... (THROM-bus)	(blood) clot (attached to the interior wall of an artery or vein)

LYMPHATIC SYSTEM

lymphadenitis............. (*lim*-fad-e-NĪ-tis)	inflammation of the lymph nodes
lymphadenopathy........... (lim-*fad*-e-NOP-a-thē)	disease of the lymph nodes (characterized by abnormal enlargement of the lymph nodes associated with an infection or malignancy)
lymphoma................. (lim-FŌ-ma)	tumor of lymphatic tissue (malignant)
splenomegaly .... (*splē*-nō-MEG-a-lē)	enlargement of the spleen
thymoma.................. (thī-MŌ-ma)	tumor of the thymus gland

CAM TERM
Meditation is a mental practice focusing attention on a single activity such as breathing, an image, or a sound to calm and still the mind. Research has demonstrated the efficacy of meditation to improve blood pressure and cardiac autonomic nervous system tone.

Multiple myeloma in the United States comprises approximately 10% of all blood malignancies. It most often occurs between 65 and 70 years of age. Most patients are asymptomatic until the disease is advanced. Symptoms and signs are varied and may include bone pain and fractures, infections, weight loss, anemia, and fatigue. Treatments include chemotherapy and stem cell transplantation. Multiple myeloma is seldom cured.

EMBOLUS, THROMBUS
An *embolus* circulates in the bloodstream until it becomes lodged in a vessel, whereas a **thrombus** is attached to the interior wall of a vessel. When a **thrombus** breaks away and circulates in the bloodstream, it becomes known as an *embolus*.

EXERCISE 11

Practice saying aloud each of the disease and disorder terms built from word parts on pp. 408-409.

 To hear the terms select Chapter 10, Chapter Exercises, Pronunciation.

☐ Place a check mark in the box when you have completed this exercise.

EXERCISE 12

Analyze and define the following terms.

1. endocarditis_____

2. bradycardia _____

3. cardiomegaly_____

4. arteriosclerosis _____

5. cardiovalvulitis _____

6. (multiple) myeloma _____

7. tachycardia _____

8. angiostenosis _____

9. thrombus _____

10. ischemia _____

11. pericarditis _____

12. cardiodynia _____

13. aortic stenosis _____

14. thrombosis _____

15. atherosclerosis _____

16. myocarditis _____

17. angioma_____

18. thymoma _____

19. lymphoma _____

20. lymphadenitis _____

21. splenomegaly _____

22. hematoma _____

23. polyarteritis _____

24. cardiomyopathy _____

25. lymphadenopathy _____

26. thrombophlebitis _____

27. phlebitis _____

28. pancytopenia _____

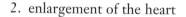

EXERCISE 13

Build disease and disorder terms for the following definitions by using the word parts you have learned.

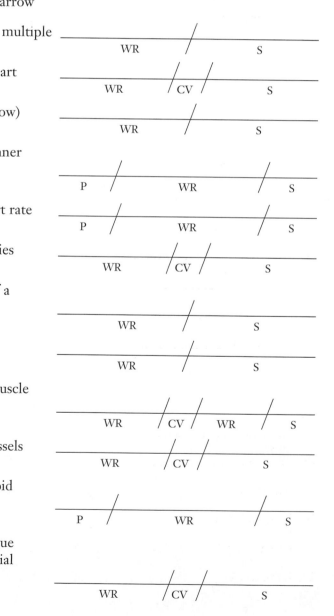

1. tumors of the bone marrow

    multiple _____/_____
             WR   /   S

2. enlargement of the heart
    _____/___/_____
    WR   / CV /   S

3. deficiency of blood (flow)
    _____/_____
    WR   /   S

4. inflammation of the inner
   (layer) of the heart
    ___/_____/___
    P /   WR   / S

5. condition of slow heart rate
    ___/_____/___
    P /   WR   / S

6. hardening of the arteries
    _____/___/_____
    WR   / CV /   S

7. abnormal condition of a
   (blood) clot
    _____/_____
    WR   /   S

8. pain in the heart
    _____/_____
    WR   /   S

9. inflammation of the muscle
   of the heart
    _____/___/_____/___
    WR   / CV / WR / S

10. narrowing of blood vessels
    _____/___/_____
    WR   / CV /   S

11. abnormal state of a rapid
    heart rate
    ___/_____/___
    P /   WR   / S

12. hardening of fatty plaque
    (deposited on the arterial
    wall)
    _____/___/_____
    WR   / CV /   S

13. tumor composed of blood
    vessels

    _____ / _____
    WR   S

14. inflammation of the valves
    of the heart

    _____ / ____ / _____ / _____
    WR   CV   WR   S

15. pertaining to the aorta
    (narrowing)

    _____ / _____ stenosis
    WR   S

16. inflammation of the sac
    surrounding the heart

    _____ / _____ / _____
    P   WR   S

17. tumor of lymphatic tissue

    _____ / _____
    WR   S

18. tumor of the thymus gland

    _____ / _____
    WR   S

19. enlargement of the spleen

    _____ / ____ / _____
    WR   CV   S

20. tumor (mass) of blood

    _____ / _____
    WR   S

21. inflammation of lymph nodes

    _____ / _____
    WR   S

22. disease of the heart muscle

    ____ / ____ / _____ / ____ / ___
    WR   CV   WR   CV   S

23. inflammation of many
    (sites in the) arteries

    _____ / _____ / _____
    P   WR   S

24. disease of the lymph nodes

    _____ / ____ / _____
    WR   CV   S

25. inflammation of a vein
    associated with a clot

    _____ / ____ / _____ / _____
    WR   CV   WR   S

26. inflammation of a vein

    _____ / _____
    WR   S

27. (blood) clot

    _____ / _____
    WR   S

28. abnormal reduction of
    all (blood) cells

    _____ / _____ / ____ / _____
    P   WR   CV   S

EXERCISE 14

Spell each of the disease and disorder terms built from word parts on pp. 408-409 by having someone dictate them to you.

 To hear and spell the terms select Chapter 10, Chapter Exercises, Spelling. You may type the terms on the screen or write them below in the spaces provided.

☐ Place a check mark in the box if you have completed this exercise using your CD-ROM.

1. _____   15. _____

2. _____   16. _____

3. _____   17. _____

4. _____   18. _____

5. _____   19. _____

6. _____   20. _____

7. _____   21. _____

8. _____   22. _____

9. _____   23. _____

10. _____   24. _____

11. _____   25. _____

12. _____   26. _____

13. _____   27. _____

14. _____   28. _____

Disease and Disorder Terms

Not Built from Word Parts

In some of the following terms, you may recognize word parts you have already learned; however, the full meaning of the terms cannot be discerned by the definition of their word parts.

Term	Definition
CARDIOVASCULAR SYSTEM	
acute coronary syndrome (ACS) (a-KŪT) (KOR-o-nar-ē) (SIN-drōme)	sudden symptoms of insufficient blood supply to the heart indicating **unstable angina** or **acute myocardial infarction**
aneurysm (AN-ū-rizm)	ballooning of a weakened portion of an arterial wall (Figure 10-8)
angina pectoris (an-JĪ-na) (PEK-to-ris)	chest pain, which may radiate to the left arm and jaw, that occurs when there is an insufficient supply of blood to the heart muscle

ACUTE CORONARY SYNDROME (ACS) is an umbrella term used when a patient seeks care at an emergency care facility for symptoms of **acute angina** or **myocardial infarction not yet diagnosed.** Treatment includes rapid assessment to determine the diagnosis and treatment of symptoms to possibly minimize heart damage.

 ANGINA PECTORIS was believed by the ancients to be a disorder of the breast. The Latin *angere*, meaning *to throttle*, was used to represent the sudden pain and was added to *pectus*, meaning **breast.**

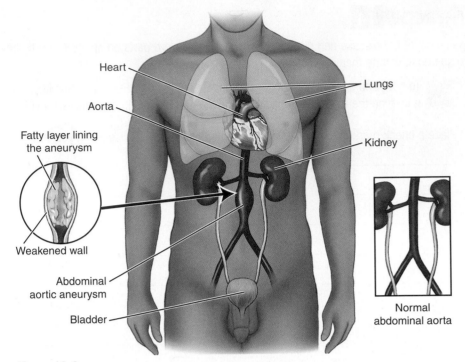

Figure 10-8

Abdominal aortic aneurysm. An abdominal aortic aneurysm (AAA) located in the abdominal area of the aorta, the main blood vessel that transports blood away from the heart. Surgery is the primary treatment for this most common site of aortic aneurysm. Because the success rate of surgery is much lower once the aneurysm has ruptured, more emphasis is being placed on diagnosis. AAAs sometimes can be detected by physical examination but are more frequently detected by abdominal ultrasound. A newer procedure called endovascular stent-graft, which uses laparoscopy to place an endovascular stent-graft into the area of the aneurysm, is now an option for treatment.

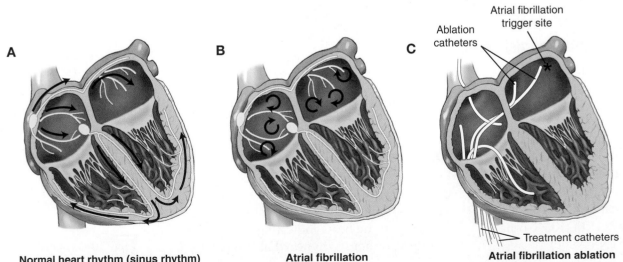

Figure 10-9

Atrial fibrillation. **A,** Normal heart rhythm. **B,** Atrial fibrillation showing chaotic, rapid electrical impulses. **C,** Atrial fibrillation ablation, which destroys the abnormal cells that trigger atrial fibrillation. Ablation is used to treat atrial fibrillation if drug therapy is not effective.

Disease and Disorder Terms—*cont'd*
Not Built from Word Parts

Term	Definition

CARDIOVASCULAR SYSTEM, CONT'D

arrhythmia . . . .
(ā-RITH-mē-a)

any disturbance or abnormality in the heart's normal rhythmic pattern

atrial fibrillation (AFib) . . . .
(Ā-trē-al) (fi-bri-LĀ-shun)

a cardiac arrhythmia characterized by chaotic, rapid electrical impulses in the atria. The atria quiver instead of contracting, causing irregular ventricular response and the ejection of a reduced amount of blood. The blood that remains in the atria becomes static, increasing the risk of clot formation, which may lead to a stroke. Two types of AFib are **paroxysmal atrial fibrillation (PAF),** which is intermittent, and **chronic atrial fibrillation,** which is sustained (Figure 10-9).

cardiac arrest . . . .
(KAR-dē-ak) (a-REST)

sudden cessation of cardiac output and effective circulation, which requires cardiopulmonary resuscitation (CPR)

cardiac tamponade . . . .
(KAR-dē-ak)
(tam-po-NĀD)

acute compression of the heart caused by fluid accumulation in the pericardial cavity

coarctation of the aorta . . . .
(kō-ark-TĀ-shun)

congenital cardiac condition characterized by a narrowing of the aorta (Figure 10-10)

congenital heart disease . . . . . .
(kon-JEN-i-tal)
(hart) (di-ZĒZ)

heart abnormality present at birth

congestive heart failure
(CHF) . . . .
(kon-JES-tiv) (hart)
(fāl-ūr)

inability of the heart to pump enough blood through the body to supply the tissues and organs with nutrients and oxygen

coronary artery
disease (CAD) . . . .
(KOR-o-nar-ē)
(AR-te-rē) (di-ZĒZ)

a condition that reduces the flow of blood through the coronary arteries to the myocardium, denying the myocardial tissue of sufficient oxygen and nutrients to function fully; most often caused by coronary atherosclerosis (also called **heart failure** [HF])

coronary occlusion . . . .
(KOR-o-nar-ē)
(o-KLŪ-zhun)

obstruction of an artery of the heart, usually from atherosclerosis. Coronary occlusion can lead to acute myocardial infarction.

deep vein thrombosis (DVT) . . . .
(dēp) (vān) (throm-BŌ-sis)

condition of thrombus in a deep vein of the body. Most often occurs in the lower extremities. A clot can break off and travel to the lungs, causing a pulmonary embolism.

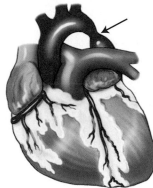

Figure 10-10
Coarctation of the aorta.

CORONARY
is derived from the Latin **coronalis,** meaning **crown** or **wreath.** It describes the arteries encircling the heart.

Disease and Disorder Terms—*cont'd*

Not Built from Word Parts

Term	Definition
CARDIOVASCULAR SYSTEM, CONT'D	
hypertensive heart disease (HHD).............. (*hī*-per-TEN-siv) (hart) (di-ZĒZ)	disorder of the heart brought about by persistent high blood pressure
intermittent claudication ...... (*in*-ter-MIT-nt) (klaw-di-KĀ-shun)	pain and discomfort in calf muscles while walking; a condition seen in occlusive artery disease.
mitral valve stenosis .... (MĪ-tral) (ste-NŌ-sis)	a narrowing of the mitral valve from scarring, usually caused by episodes of rheumatic fever
myocardial infarction (MI) ..... (mī-ō-KAR-dē-al) (in-FARK-shun)	death (necrosis) of a portion of the myocardium caused by lack of oxygen resulting from an interrupted blood supply (also called **heart attack**)
peripheral arterial disease (PAD) .... (pe-RIF-er-al) (ar-TER-ē-al) (di-ZĒZ)	disease of the arteries, other than those of the heart and brain, that affects blood circulation, such as atherosclerosis and Raynaud disease. The most common symptom of peripheral atherosclerosis is intermittent claudication.
rheumatic heart disease....... (rū-MAT-ik) (hart) (di-ZĒZ)	damage to the heart muscle or heart valves caused by one or more episodes of **rheumatic fever**
varicose veins.............. (VAR-i-kōs) (vānz)	distended or tortuous veins usually found in the lower extremities (Figure 10-11)

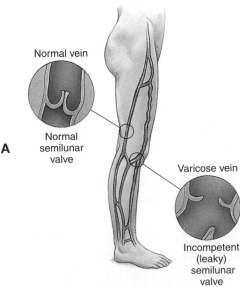
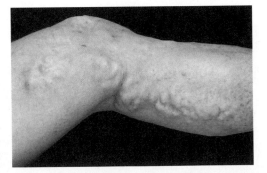

Normal vein

Normal semilunar valve

A

Varicose vein

Incompetent (leaky) semilunar valve

B

Figure 10-11

A, Normal and varicose veins. **B,** Appearance of varicose veins.

Varicose Veins and Current Treatment

Varicose veins usually occur in the superficial veins of the legs, which return approximately 15% of the blood back to the heart. One-way valves in the veins help move the blood upward. When these valves fail, or the veins lose their elasticity, the blood flows backward, pools, and forms varicose veins. Approximately 80 million Americans, mostly women, have varicose veins or small, shallow spider veins. Causes are heredity, obesity, pregnancy, illness, or injury. Ligation and stripping was previously considered the primary surgical procedure for treatment.

Current Treatment

Endovenous laser ablation—Closure of varicose veins by application of heat within the vein.

Ambulatory phlebectomy—Tiny punctures are made in the skin through which the varicose veins are pulled out. Local anesthetic is used, and the procedure is minimally invasive.

Sclerotherapy—Sclerotherapy takes less than an hour and requires no anesthesia. A solution is injected into the varicose vein and destroys it over several months. Sclerotherapy isn't effective on varicose veins that extend into the groin area.

Laser or intense pulsed light—This noninvasive technique is used to remove spider veins. The light causes the veins to shrink and collapse.

Common Types of Anemia

- **Acute blood loss anemia**—reduction in hemoglobin and hematocrit as a result of hemorrhage
- **Iron-deficiency anemia**—insufficient amount of iron in the body to produce hemoglobin; frequently caused by chronic blood loss
- **Pernicious anemia**—ineffective production of red blood cells from vitamin B_{12} deficiency
- **Hemolytic anemia**—reduced life of red blood cells (e.g., sickle cell anemia)
- **Anemia of chronic inflammation**—ineffective red blood cell production from chronic disease
- **Aplastic anemia**—resulting from bone marrow failure

HODGKIN DISEASE was first described in 1832 by Thomas Hodgkin, a pathologist at Guy's Hospital in London. In 1865 the name *Hodgkin's disease* was given to the condition by another English physician, Sir Samuel Wilks.

Term	Definition
BLOOD	
anemia (a-NĒ-mē-a)	reduction in the amount of hemoglobin in the red blood cells. Anemia may be caused by blood loss or decrease in the production or increase in the destruction of red blood cells.
embolus (*pl.* emboli) (EM-bō-lus) (EM-bo-lī)	blood clot or foreign material, such as air or fat, that enters the bloodstream and moves until it lodges at another point in the circulation
hemophilia (hē-mō-FIL-ē-a)	inherited bleeding disease most commonly caused by a deficiency of the coagulation factor VIII
leukemia (lū-KĒ-mē-a)	malignant disease characterized by excessive increase in abnormal white blood cells formed in the bone marrow
LYMPHATIC SYSTEM	
Hodgkin disease (HOJ-kin) (di-ZĒZ)	malignant disorder of the lymphatic tissue characterized by progressive enlargement of the lymph nodes, usually beginning in the cervical nodes
infectious mononucleosis (in-FEK-shus) (*mon*-ō-nū-klē-Ō-sis)	an acute infection caused by the Epstein-Barr virus characterized by swollen lymph nodes, sore throat, fatigue, and fever. The disease affects mostly young people and is usually transmitted by saliva.

EXERCISE 15

Practice saying aloud each of the disease and disorder terms not built from word parts on pp. 413-417.

 To hear the terms select Chapter 10, Chapter Exercises, Pronunciation.

☐ Place a check mark in the box when you have completed this exercise.

EXERCISE 16

Fill in the blanks with the correct terms.

1. A congenital cardiac condition characterized by a narrowing of the aorta is called _____ of the aorta.

2. A blood clot or foreign material that enters the bloodstream and moves until it lodges at another point in the circulation is called a(n) _____.

3. Sudden cessation of cardiac output and effective circulation is referred to as a(n) _____ _____.

4. _____ heart disease is the name given to a heart abnormality present at birth.

5. Veins that are distended or tortuous are called _____ _____.

6. Obstruction of an artery of the heart, usually from atherosclerosis, is called a(n) _____ _____.

7. _____ is the name given to the ballooning of a weakened portion of an artery wall.

8. _____ disease is the name given to a malignant disorder of lymphatic tissue characterized by enlarged lymph nodes.

9. _____ _____ _____ is a condition most often caused by atherosclerosis.

10. _____ _____ is a cardiac condition characterized by chest pain caused by an insufficient blood supply to the cardiac muscle.

11. Death of a portion of myocardial muscle caused by lack of oxygen resulting from an interrupted blood supply is called a(n) _____ _____.

12. _____ _____ is a cardiac arrhythmia.

13. Any disturbance or abnormality in the heart's normal rhythmic pattern is called a(n) _____.

14. A disorder of the heart brought about by a persistently high blood pressure is called _____ heart disease.

15. _____ _____ _____ is the inability of the heart to pump enough blood through the body to supply tissues and organs.

16. _____ _____ _____ is a disease of the arteries that affects blood circulation.

17. _____ is an inherited bleeding disease most commonly caused by a deficiency of the coagulation factor VIII.

18. _____ is a malignant disease in which the number of abnormal white blood cells formed in the bone marrow is excessively increased.

19. A reduction in the amount of hemoglobin in the red blood cells results in a condition known as _____.

20. _____ _____ is an infection caused by the Epstein-Barr virus.

21. _____ _____ is a condition in which a patient has pain and discomfort in calf muscles while walking.

22. Acute compression of the heart caused by fluid accumulation in the pericardial cavity is known as _____ _____.

23. Episodes of rheumatic fever can cause _____ _____ _____ and _____ _____ _____.

24. _____ _____ _____ usually occurs in the deep veins of the lower extremities.

25. _____ _____ _____ is insufficient blood supply to the heart, indicating unstable angina or myocardial infarction.

EXERCISE 17

Match the terms in the first column with the correct definitions in the second column.

_____ 1. anemia

_____ 2. aneurysm

_____ 3. angina pectoris

_____ 4. arrhythmia

_____ 5. cardiac arrest

_____ 6. cardiac tamponade

_____ 7. coarctation of the aorta

_____ 8. congenital heart disease

_____ 9. congestive heart failure

_____ 10. coronary occlusion

_____ 11. intermittent claudication

_____ 12. deep vein thrombosis

_____ 13. coronary artery disease

_____ 14. peripheral arterial disease

a. sudden cessation of cardiac output and effective circulation

b. obstruction of an artery of the heart, usually from atherosclerosis

c. ballooning of a weak portion of an arterial wall

d. reduction of the amount of hemoglobin in the blood

e. any disturbance or abnormality in the heart's normal rhythmic pattern

f. chest pain occurring because of insufficient blood supply to the heart muscle

g. inability of the heart to pump enough blood through the body to supply tissues or organs

h. pain in calf muscles while walking

i. congenital cardiac condition with narrowing of the aorta

j. acute compression of the heart caused by fluid in the pericardial cavity

k. heart abnormality present at birth

l. clot in a deep vein

m. disease of the arteries, such as atherosclerosis, that affects blood circulation

n. a condition that reduces the flow of blood through the coronary arteries

EXERCISE 18

Match the terms in the first column with the correct definitions in the second column.

_____ 1. embolus

_____ 2. atrial fibrillation

_____ 3. hemophilia

_____ 4. infectious mononucleosis

_____ 5. Hodgkin disease

_____ 6. hypertensive heart disease

_____ 7. leukemia

_____ 8. myocardial infarction

_____ 9. mitral valve stenosis

_____ 10. acute coronary syndrome

_____ 11. varicose veins

_____ 12. rheumatic heart disease

a. inherited bleeding disease most commonly caused by a deficiency of the coagulation factor VIII

b. heart disorder brought on by persistent high blood pressure

c. distended or tortuous veins

d. excessive increase of abnormal white blood cells formed in the bone marrow

e. characterized by chaotic, rapid electrical impulses of the atria

f. caused by episodes of rheumatic fever

g. symptoms indicating unstable angina or myocardial infarction

h. a disease that affects mostly young people; characterized by swollen lymph glands

i. blood clot or foreign material that enters the bloodstream and moves until it lodges at another point

j. malignant disorder of lymphatic tissue with enlargement of lymph nodes

k. death of a portion of myocardium caused by lack of oxygen resulting from an interrupted blood supply

l. narrowing of the valve between the left atrium and left ventricle

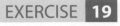

EXERCISE

Spell each of the disease and disorder terms not built from word parts on pp. 413-417 by having someone dictate them to you.

To hear and spell the terms select Chapter 10, Chapter Exercises, Spelling. You may type the terms on the screen or write them below in the spaces provided.

☐ Place a check mark in the box if you have completed this exercise using your CD-ROM.

1. _____   14. _____

2. _____   15. _____

3. _____   16. _____

4. _____   17. _____

5. _____   18. _____

6. _____   19. _____

7. _____   20. _____

8. _____   21. _____

9. _____   22. _____

10. _____   23. _____

11. _____   24. _____

12. _____   25. _____

13. _____   26. _____

PERCUTANEOUS CORONARY INTERVENTION (PCI) includes a range of procedures, such as **coronary angioplasty** and **percutaneous transluminal coronary angioplasty** used to treat coronary artery disease. The procedure is usually performed by an invasive cardiologist.

EXERCISE FIGURE C

Fill in the blanks to label the diagram.

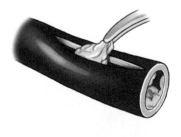

within / artery / excision

Surgical Terms

Built from Word Parts

The following terms are built from word parts you have already learned and can be translated literally to find their meanings. Further explanation of terms beyond the definition of their word parts, if needed, is included in parentheses.

Term	Definition
CARDIOVASCULAR SYSTEM	
angioplasty . . . . (AN-jē-ō-*plas*-tē)	surgical repair of a blood vessel
atherectomy . . . . (ath-er-EK-to-mē)	excision of fatty plaque (from a blocked artery using a specialized catheter and a rotary cutter)
endarterectomy . . . . (*end*-ar-ter-EK-to-mē) (NOTE: the *o* from *endo-* is dropped for easier pronunciation)	excision within the artery (excision of plaque from the arterial wall). This procedure is usually named for the artery to be cleaned out, such as carotid endarterectomy, which means removal of plaque from the wall of the carotid artery (Exercise Figure C).

Term	Definition
pericardiocentesis .... (*per*-i-kar-dē-ō-sen-TĒ-sis)	surgical puncture to aspirate fluid from the outer layer (pericardial sac) (used to treat cardiac tamponade) (Figure 10-12)
phlebectomy............... (fle-BEK-to-mē)	excision of a vein
phlebotomy................. (fle-BOT-o-mē)	incision into a vein (to remove blood or to give blood or intravenous fluids) (also called **venipuncture**)
valvuloplasty............... (VAL-vū-lō-*plas*-tē)	surgical repair of a valve (cardiac or venous)

LYMPHATIC SYSTEM

splenectomy............... (splē-NEK-to-mē)	excision of the spleen
splenopexy................. (SPLĒ-nō-*peks*-ē)	surgical fixation of the spleen
thymectomy .... (thī-MEK-to-mē)	excision of the thymus gland

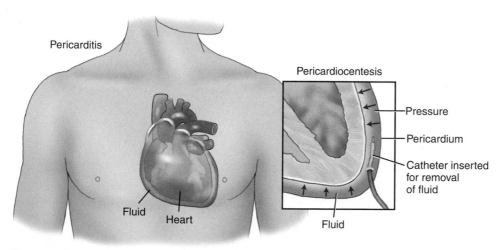

Pericarditis

Pericardiocentesis

Pressure

Pericardium

Catheter inserted for removal of fluid

Fluid   Heart

Fluid

Figure 10-12
Pericarditis may produce excess fluid in the pericardium. If the fluid seriously affects the heart's ability to pump blood, pericardiocentesis may be performed to remove the fluid.

EXERCISE 20

Practice saying aloud each of the surgical terms built from word parts on pp. 422-423.

 To hear the terms select Chapter 10, Chapter Exercises, Pronunciation.

☐ Place a check mark in the box when you have completed this exercise.

EXERCISE **21**

Analyze and define the following surgical terms.

1. pericardiocentesis _____

2. thymectomy _____

3. angioplasty _____

4. splenopexy _____

5. valvuloplasty _____

6. endarterectomy _____

7. phlebotomy _____

8. splenectomy _____

9. phlebectomy _____

10. atherectomy _____

EXERCISE **22**

Build surgical terms for the following definitions by using the word parts you have learned.

1. excision within the artery

   _____ / _____ / _____
   P   WR   S

2. surgical fixation of the spleen

   _____ / ____ / _____
   WR   CV   S

3. surgical repair of a valve

   _____ / ____ / _____
   WR   CV   S

4. incision into a vein

   _____ / ____ / _____
   WR   CV   S

5. excision of the thymus gland

   _____ / _____
   WR   S

6. surgical puncture to aspirate
   fluid from the outer layer
   of the heart

   _____ / _____ / ____ / _____
   P   WR   CV   S

7. surgical repair of a blood
   vessel

   _____ / ____ / _____
   WR   CV   S

8. excision of the spleen

   _____ / _____
   WR   S

9. excision of a vein

   _____ / _____
   WR   S

10. excision of fatty plaque

   _____ / _____
   WR   S

EXERCISE 23

Spell each of the surgical terms built from word parts on pp. 422-423 by having someone dictate them to you.

 To hear and spell the terms select Chapter 10, Chapter Exercises, Spelling. You may type the terms on the screen or write them below in the spaces provided.

☐ Place a check mark in the box if you have completed this exercise using your CD-ROM.

1. _____   6. _____

2. _____   7. _____

3. _____   8. _____

4. _____   9. _____

5. _____   10. _____

Surgical Terms

Not Built from Word Parts

In some of the following terms, you may recognize word parts you have already learned; however, the full meaning of the terms cannot be discerned by the definition of their word parts.

Term	Definition
CARDIOVASCULAR SYSTEM	
aneurysmectomy . . . . (*an*-ū-riz-MEK-to-mē)	surgical excision of an aneurysm
atrial fibrillation ablation . . . . . . (Ā-tre-al) (fi-bri-LĀ-shun) (ab-LĀ-shun)	a procedure in which abnormal cells that trigger atrial fibrillation are destroyed by using radiofrequency energy (see Figure 10-7)
cardiac pacemaker . . . . (KAR-dē-ak) (PĀS-mā-kr)	battery-powered apparatus implanted under the skin with leads placed on the heart (Figure 10-13, *A*) or in the chamber of the heart (Figure 10-13, *B*)
coronary artery bypass graft (CABG) . . . . (KOR-o-nar-ē) (AR-te-rē) (BĪ-pas) (graft)	surgical technique to bring a new blood supply to heart muscle by detouring around blocked arteries (Figure 10-14)
coronary stent . . . . (KOR-o-nar-ē) (stent)	a supportive scaffold device implanted in the coronary artery; used to prevent closure of the artery after angioplasty or atherectomy (Figure 10-15)
embolectomy . . . . (*em*-bo-LEK-to-mē)	surgical removal of an embolus or clot (usually with a balloon catheter, inflating the balloon beyond the clot, then pulling the balloon back to the incision and bringing the clot with it)

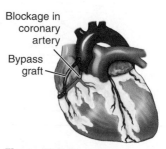

Blockage in coronary artery

Bypass graft

Figure 10-14
Coronary artery bypass graft.

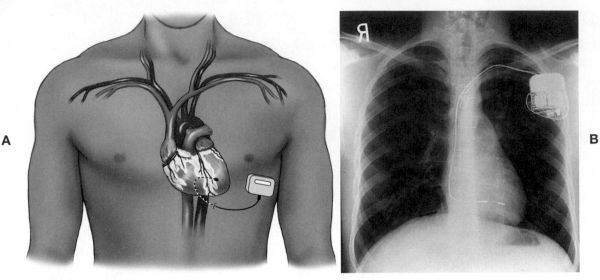

Figure 10-13

A, Cardiac pacemaker. The leads are implanted surgically on the epicardium through a thoracotomy. **B,** Chest radiograph of a patient with a cardiac pacemaker in which leads are implanted transvenously under fluoroscopic guidance. A pacemaker is used to treat irreversible complete heart block, which is caused by failure of the sinus node impulse to reach the ventricles.

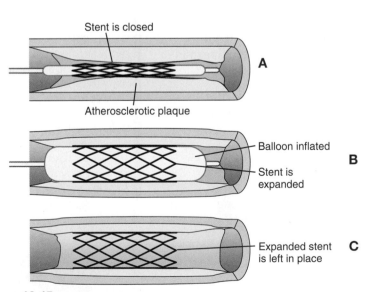

Stent is closed

Atherosclerotic plaque

A

Balloon inflated

Stent is expanded

B

Expanded stent is left in place

C

Figure 10-15

Coronary stent. **A,** Stent at the site of plaque formation. **B,** Inflated balloon and expanded stent. **C,** Implanted stent with balloon removed.

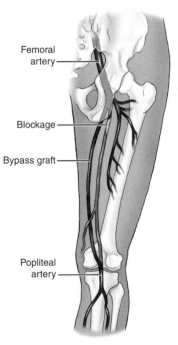

Femoral artery

Blockage

Bypass graft

Popliteal artery

Figure 10-16

Femoropopliteal bypass.

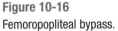

Surgical Terms—*cont'd*

Not Built from Word Parts

Term	Definition
CARDIOVASCULAR SYSTEM, CONT'D	
femoropopliteal bypass . . . . (*fem*-o-rō-pop-LIT-ē-al) (BĪ-pass)	surgery to establish an alternate route from femoral artery to popliteal artery to bypass an obstruction (Figure 10-16)
implantable cardiac defibrillator (ICD) . . . . (im-PLANT-a-bl) (KAR-dē-ak) (dē-FIB-ri-lā-tor)	a device implanted in the body that continuously monitors the heart rhythm. If life-threatening arrhythmias occur, the device delivers an electric shock to convert the arrhythmia back to a normal rhythm (Figure 10-17).
intracoronary thrombolytic therapy . . . . (in-tra-KOR-o-nar-ē) (*throm*-bō-LIT-ik) (THER-a-pē)	an injection of an intravenous medication to dissolve blood clots in coronary (blood) vessels
percutaneous transluminal coronary angioplasty (PTCA) . . . (*per*-kū-TĀ-nē-us) (trans-LŪ-min-al) (KOR-o-nar-ē) (AN-jē-ō-*plas*-tē)	procedure in which a balloon is passed through a blood vessel into a coronary artery to the area where plaque is formed. Inflation of the balloon compresses the plaque against the vessel wall, expanding the inner diameter of the blood vessel, which allows the blood to circulate more freely (also called **balloon angioplasty**) (Figure 10-18).

Thrombolytic Therapy for Acute Myocardial Infarction

Intracoronary thrombolytic therapy is the administration of a medication that breaks blood clots apart (thrombolysis) before they become hardened. It is sometimes used in emergency departments (for acute myocardial infarction) and is administered immediately after the diagnosis is made. The drugs, such as streptokinase, tPA (alteplase), or recombinant tissue plasminogen activator (rtPA) (reteplase), are administered intravenously. Emergency percutaneous transluminal coronary angioplasty (PTCA) appears to be more effective than thrombolytic therapy for acute myocardial infarction. However, thrombolytic therapy can be administered in an emergency department when PTCA is not readily available.

CARDIAC RESYNCHRONIZATION THERAPY (CRT),

also called biventricular pacing, is the use of an implantable device, alone or in combination with an ICD, that provides simultaneous pacing of both ventricles of the heart. CRT is used in the treatment of severe congestive heart failure. (see Figure 10-17)

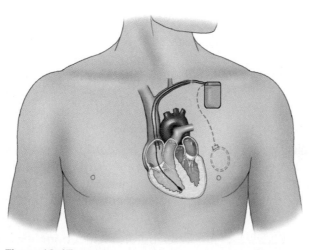

Figure 10-17
An implantable cardiac defibrillator.

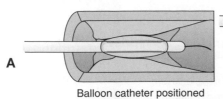
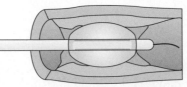
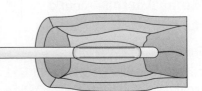

A, Balloon catheter positioned in stenotic area

Inflated balloon presses plaque against arterial wall expanding the size of vessel opening

Balloon is deflated and blood flow reestablished

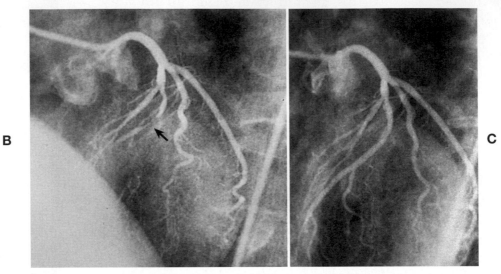

B

C

Figure 10-18

Percutaneous transluminal coronary angioplasty. **A,** Balloon dilation. **B,** Coronary arteriogram before PTCA. The *arrow* indicates the stenotic area, estimated at 95% minimum blood flow distal to the lesion. **C,** Coronary arteriogram after PTCA in the same patient. Blood flow is estimated to be 100%.

BONE MARROW
is a spongy tissue found in the hollow part of the larger bones of the body. It is made up of both a solid and liquid portion. Stem cells within the bone marrow turn into platelets, red blood cells, and white blood cells. **Bone marrow aspiration** and **bone marrow biopsy** are both used to obtain specimens for study. Each provides complementary information about the condition of blood cells. Bone marrow aspiration is performed first if both are being performed on the patient. Information from both procedures is used for staging, monitoring, and diagnosing diseases and conditions of the blood such as anemia, leukemia, lymphoma, and multiple myeloma.

Surgical Terms—*cont'd*
Not Built from Word Parts

Term	Definition
BLOOD	
bone marrow aspiration . . . . (bōn) (MAR-ō) (as-pi-RĀ-shun)	a syringe is used to aspirate a sample of the liquid portion of the bone marrow, usually from the ilium, for study; used to diagnose, stage, and monitor disease and condition of the blood cells (Figure 10-19)
bone marrow biopsy . . . . (bōn) (MAR-ō) (BĪ-op-sē)	a needle puncture to obtain a sample of bone marrow, usually from the ilium, for study; used to diagnose, stage, and monitor disease and condition of the blood cells
bone marrow transplant . . . . (bōn) (MAR-ō) (TRANS-plant)	infusion of normal bone marrow cells from a donor with matching cells and tissue to a recipient with a certain type of leukemia or anemia

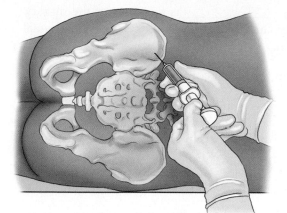
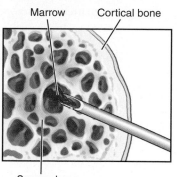

Figure 10-19
Bone marrow aspiration. Study of the bone marrow can be used to identify the presence of leukemia or other malignancies or to determine the cause of anemia.

EXERCISE 24

Practice saying aloud each of the surgical terms not built from word parts on pp. 425-428.

To hear the terms select Chapter 10, Chapter Exercises, Pronunciation.

☐ Place a check mark in the box when you have completed this exercise.

EXERCISE 25

1. The procedure used to treat atrial fibrillation using radio frequency energy is called atrial fibrillation _____.

2. The procedure in which a balloon is passed through a blood vessel into a coronary artery (where plaque is formed) to compress plaque against the vessel wall when the balloon is inflated is called _____

   _____ _____ _____.

3. To regulate the heart rate, the physician may insert a(n) _____

   _____ with leads on or in the patient's heart.

4. Bone marrow aspiration and biopsy are used to diagnose, stage, and monitor disease and conditions of the _____ _____.

5. The surgery performed to detour blood around a blocked artery so that a new blood supply can be given to heart muscles is called _____

   _____ _____ _____.

6. The surgical excision of an aneurysm is called a(n) _____ .

7. A(n) _____ _____ is the name of the surgery performed to establish an alternate route from femoral artery to popliteal artery to bypass an obstruction.

8. An injection of a medication in a blocked coronary vessel to dissolve blood clots is called _____ _____ therapy.

9. _____ _____ _____ is a procedure to transfuse bone marrow cells to a recipient from a donor with matching tissue and cells.

10. _____ is the surgical removal of an embolus, or clot.

11. A supportive scaffold device used to prevent closure of a coronary artery is called a(n) _____ _____.

12. _____ _____ _____ is used to treat life-threatening arrhythmias.

EXERCISE 26

Match the terms in the first column with their correct definitions in the second column.

_____ 1. aneurysmectomy

_____ 2. coronary artery bypass graft

_____ 3. femoropopliteal bypass

_____ 4. bone marrow aspiration

_____ 5. cardiac pacemaker

_____ 6. atrial fibrillation ablation

_____ 7. percutaneous transluminal coronary angioplasty

_____ 8. bone marrow biopsy

_____ 9. bone marrow transplant

_____ 10. intracoronary thrombolytic therapy

_____ 11. embolectomy

_____ 12. coronary stent

_____ 13. implantable cardiac defibrillator

a. compressing plaque against a blood vessel wall by inflating a balloon passed through the blood vessel

b. use of medication to dissolve blood clots in a blocked coronary vessel

c. used to obtain a sample of bone marrow

d. apparatus implanted under the skin to regulate the heartbeat

e. a procedure using radio frequency energy

f. monitors and corrects heart rhythms

g. supportive scaffold device implanted in an artery

h. excision of a weakened, ballooning blood vessel wall

i. normal bone marrow cells infused from a donor with matching tissues and cells into a recipient with leukemia

j. surgical removal of an embolus

k. surgical procedure to establish an alternate route from the femoral artery to the popliteal artery to bypass an obstruction

l. aspiration of a sample of the liquid portion of bone marrow

m. diverts blood past a blocked artery in the heart

Spell each of the surgical terms not built from word parts on pp. 425-428 by having someone dictate them to you.

 To hear and spell the terms select Chapter 10, Chapter Exercises, Spelling. You may type the terms on the screen or write them below in the spaces provided.

☐ Place a check mark in the box if you have completed this exercise using your CD-ROM.

1. _____   8. _____

2. _____   9. _____

3. _____   10. _____

4. _____   11. _____

5. _____   12. _____

6. _____   13. _____

7. _____

Diagnostic Terms

Built from Word Parts

The following terms are bult from word parts you have already learned and can be translated literally to find their meanings. Further explanation of terms beyond the definition of their word parts, if needed, is included in parentheses.

Term	Definition
CARDIOVASCULAR SYSTEM	
Diagnostic Imaging	
angiography . . . . (an-jē-OG-ra-fē)	radiographic imaging of blood vessels (the procedure is named for the vessel to be studied, e.g., *femoral angiography* or *coronary angiography*) (Table 10-1)
angioscope . . . . (AN-jē-ō-skōp)	instrument used for visual examination of a blood vessel
angioscopy . . . . (an-jē-OS-ko-pē)	visual examination of a blood vessel
aortogram . . . . (ā-OR-to-gram)	radiographic image of the aorta (after an injection of contrast media)
arteriogram . . . . (ar-TER-ē-ō-gram)	radiographic image of an artery (after an injection of contrast media) (Figure 10-20)
venogram . . . . (VĒ-nō-gram)	radiographic image of a vein (after an injection of contrast media) (Figure 10-21)
venography . . . . (vē-NOG-ra-fē)	radiographic imaging of a vein (after an injection of contrast media)

TABLE 10-1

Types of Angiography

Coronary Artery Visualization

Coronary angiography, commonly called cardiac catheterization, is an **invasive procedure** in which a catheter is inserted into the coronary vessels, dye is injected, and images are recorded. It is considered the best technique for determining the percentage of blockage in the coronary arteries.

Coronary computed tomography angiography (CCTA) also called a *heart scan* is a noninvasive procedure used to assist in the diagnosis of coronary artery disease. Two types of scanners used are:

• **multislice spiral CT scanner (MSCT)** is capable of scanning multiple images during each gantry rotation. The scanner can produce images of a beating heart and detailed cross-sectional images of the arteries. The first 4-slice scanner was first used in the 1990s and is now a 64-slice scanner.

• **electronic beam CT scanner (EBCT)** uses an electron beam to create three-dimensional images of the heart. EBCT, developed in the early 1980s is faster than MSCT and produces an accurate **coronary artery calcification (CAC)** score, also called coronary calcium score **(CCS),** which is predictive of the presence of coronary artery stenosis as a result of the build up of plaque on the arterial wall; may be used as a screening test for CAD.

Other Vascular Visualization

Magnetic resonance angiography (MRA) is a **noninvasive procedure** that does not require catheterization or the injection of dye and uses specialized MR imaging to study vascular structures of the body. MRA may be chosen over CTA because there is no exposure to ionizing radiation and contrast media.

Computed tomography angiography (CTA) is a **noninvasive procedure** that uses a high-resolution CT system to study vascular structures of the body after the injection of intravenous contrast media.

Digital subtraction angiography is a procedure in which an image is taken and stored in the computer, then contrast medium is injected. A second image is taken and stored in the computer. The computer compares the two images and subtracts the first image from the second, removing structures not being studied. DSA enables better visualization of the arteries than regular angiography (Figure 10-22).

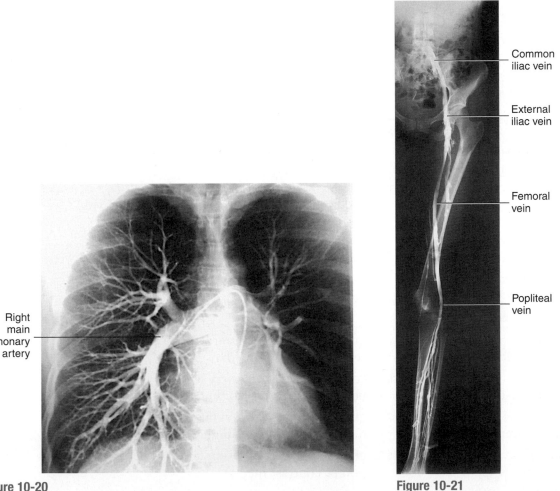

Figure 10-20
Arteriogram showing the right main pulmonary artery. This procedure (arteriography) is performed after injection of contrast material.

Figure 10-21
Normal venogram, lower left limb.

Diagnostic Terms—*cont'd*

Built from Word Parts

Term	Definition
Cardiovascular Procedures	
echocardiogram (ECHO) . . . . (ek-ō-KAR-dē-ō-gram)	record of the heart (structure and motion) using sound (used to detect valvular disease and evaluate heart function)
electrocardiogram (ECG, EKG) . . . . (ē-*lek*-trō-KAR- dē-ō-gram)	record of the electrical activity of the heart (Exercise Figure D)
electrocardiograph . . . . (ē-*lek*-trō-KAR-dē-ō-graf)	instrument used to record the electrical activity of the heart
electrocardiography . . . . (ē-*lek*-trō-*kar*- dē-OG-ra-fē)	process of recording the electrical activity of the heart

EXERCISE FIGURE D

Fill in the blanks to complete labeling of the diagram.

Lead II

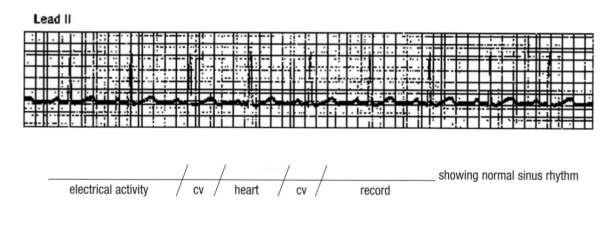

_____ / cv / heart / cv / _____ showing normal sinus rhythm
electrical activity   cv   heart   cv   record

EXERCISE 28

Practice saying aloud each of the diagnostic terms built from word parts on pp. 431-433.

 To hear the terms select Chapter 10, Chapter Exercises, Pronunciation.

☐ Place a check mark in the box when you have completed this exercise.

EXERCISE 29

Analyze and define the following diagnostic terms.

1. electrocardiograph _____

2. venogram _____

3. angiography _____

4. echocardiogram _____

5. aortogram _____

6. electrocardiogram _____

7. arteriogram _____

8. electrocardiography _____

9. angioscopy _____

10. venography _____

11. angioscope _____

EXERCISE 30

Build diagnostic terms that correspond to the following definitions by using the word parts you have learned.

1. instrument used to record
   the electrical activity of
   the heart

   _____ / ___ / _____ / ___ / ___
   WR   CV   WR   CV   S

2. radiographic image of an
   artery (after an injection
   of contrast media)

   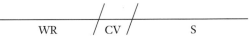
   WR   CV   S

3. radiographic image
   of a vein (after an injection
   of contrast media)

   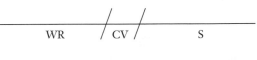
   WR   CV   S

4. radiographic imaging
   of a blood vessel

   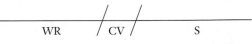
   WR   CV   S

5. record of the electrical
   activity of the heart

   _____ / ___ / _____ / ___ / ___
   WR   CV   WR   CV   S

6. record of the heart
(structure and motion)
by using sound

   _____ / _____ / _____ / _____ / _____
   WR   CV   WR   CV   S

7. radiographic image of
the aorta (after an injection
of contrast media)

   _____ / _____ / _____
   WR   CV   S

8. process of recording the
electrical activity of the
heart

   _____ / _____ / _____ / _____ / _____
   WR   CV   WR   CV   S

9. visual examination
of a blood vessel

   _____ / _____ / _____
   WR   CV   S

10. radiographic imaging
of a vein

   _____ / _____ / _____
   WR   CV   S

11. instrument used for visual
examination of a blood vessel

   _____ / _____ / _____
   WR   CV   S

EXERCISE 31

Spell each of the diagnostic terms built from word parts on pp. 431-433 by having someone dictate them to you.

To hear and spell the terms select Chapter 10, Chapter Exercises, Spelling. You may type the terms on the screen or write them below in the spaces provided.

☐ Place a check mark in the box if you have completed this exercise using your CD-ROM.

1. _____   7. _____

2. _____   8. _____

3. _____   9. _____

4. _____   10. _____

5. _____   11. _____

6. _____

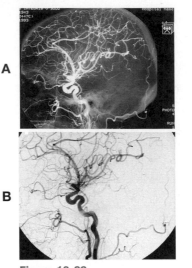

Figure 10-22
Digital subtraction angiography (DSA). **A,** Lateral digital **nonsubtracted** carotid artery. **B,** Lateral digital **subtracted** carotid artery. By removing undesired images, the image of the carotid artery is of high quality.

CHEMICAL STRESS TESTING
is the **use of drugs to simulate the stress of physical exercise** in the body. It is used to study patients who are unable to exercise.

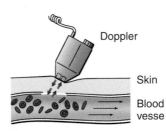

Figure 10-23
Doppler ultrasound showing the red blood cells reflecting sound.

Diagnostic Terms

Not Built from Word Parts

In some of the following terms, you may recognize word parts you have already learned; however, the full meaning of the terms cannot be discerned by the definition of their word parts.

Term	Definition
CARDIOVASCULAR SYSTEM	
Diagnostic Imaging	
digital subtraction angiography (DSA) (DIJ-i-tal) (sub-TRAK-shun) (an-jē-OG-ra-fē)	a process of digital radiographic imaging of the blood vessels that "subtracts" or removes structures not being studied (Figure 10-22 and Table 10-1)
Doppler ultrasound (DOP-ler) (UL-tra-sound)	a study that uses sound for detection of blood flow within the vessels; used to assess intermittent claudication, deep vein thrombosis, and other blood flow abnormalities (Figure 10-23)
exercise stress test (EK-ser-sīz) (stres) (test)	a study that evaluates cardiac function during physical stress by riding a bike or walking on a treadmill. Electrocardiography, echocardiography, and nuclear medicine scanning are three types of tests performed to measure cardiac function while exercising. Echocardiography is fast becoming the preferred choice of testing over electrocardiography.
single-photon emission computed tomography (SPECT) (SING-el-fō-ton) (ē-MISH-on) (com-PŪ-td) (tō-MOG-ra-fē)	a nuclear medicine scan that visualizes the heart from several different angles. A tracer substance such as sestamibi or thallium is injected intravenously. The SPECT scanner creates images from the tracer absorbed by the body tissues. It is used to assess damage to cardiac tissue (Figure 10-24).

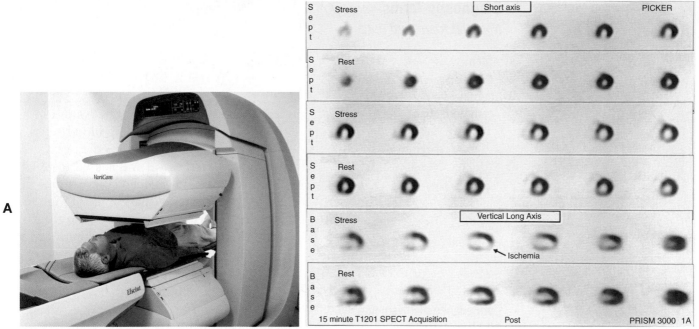

Figure 10-24

A, Single-photon emission computed tomography (SPECT) camera system. **B,** Thallium-201 myocardial perfusion scan comparing stress and redistribution (resting) images in various planes of the heart (short axis and long axis). A perfusion defect is identified in the stress images but not seen in the redistribution (rest) images. This finding is indicative of ischemia.

Term	Definition
thallium test .... (THĀL-ē-um) (test)	a nuclear medicine test used to diagnose coronary artery disease and assess revascularization after coronary artery bypass surgery. Thallium, a radioactive isotope, is injected into the body intravenously; a radiation detector is placed over the heart and images are recorded. Thallium is taken up by the normal myocardial cells, but not in ischemia or infarction. These areas are identified as "cold" spots on the images produced. Thallium testing can be performed when the patient is at rest or it can be part of a stress test.
transesophageal echocardiogram **(TEE)** .... (trans-e-sof-a-JĒ-al) (ek-ō-KAR-dē-ō-gram)	an ultrasound test that examines cardiac function and structure by using an ultrasound probe placed in the esophagus, which provides views of the heart structures

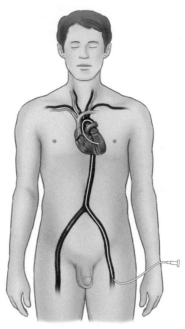

Figure 10-25
Cardiac catherization.

Sphygmomanometer

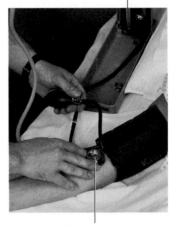

Stethoscope

Figure 10-26
Measurement of blood pressure.

STETHOSCOPE
is a term derived from the Greek **stethos**, meaning **chest**, and **scopeo**, meaning **to view** or **examine**. It means **to see** what is in the body by listening to the body sounds. The stethoscope was first called a **baton** or **cylinder**.

Diagnostic Terms—*cont'd*
Not Built from Word Parts

Term	Definition
Cardiovascular Studies	
cardiac catheterization (KAR-dē-ak) (*kath*-e-ter-i-ZĀ-shun)	an examination to determine the condition of the heart and surrounding blood vessels. A catheter is passed into the heart through a blood vessel and is used to record pressures and inject a contrast medium, enabling the visualization of the coronary arteries, great vessels, and the heart chambers; used most frequently to evaluate chest pain and coronary artery disease (also called **coronary angiography**) (Figure 10-25).
impedance plethysmography (IPG) (im-PĒD-ans) (pleth-iz-MOG-rā-fē)	measures venous flow of the extremities with a plethysmograph to detect clots by measuring changes in blood volume and resistance (impedance) in the vein; used to detect deep vein thrombosis
Other	
auscultation (*aws*-kul-TĀ-shun)	hearing sounds within the body through a stethoscope
blood pressure (BP)	pressure exerted by the blood against the blood vessel walls. A blood pressure measurement written as systolic pressure (120) and diastolic pressure (80) is commonly recorded as 120/80 (Figure 10-26).
percussion (per-KUSH-un)	tapping of a body surface with the fingers to determine the density of the part beneath (Figure 10-27)
pulse (puls)	the number of times per minute the heartbeat is felt on the arterial wall. The pulse rate is most commonly felt over the radial artery; however, the pulsations can be felt over a number of sites, including the femoral and carotid arteries.
sphygmomanometer (*sfig*-mō-ma-NOM-e-ter)	device used for measuring blood pressure (see Figure 10-26)
stethoscope (STETH-ō-scōp)	an instrument used to hear internal body sounds; used for performing auscultation and blood pressure measurement (see Figure 10-26)

Term	Definition

Laboratory

C-reactive protein (CRP) . . . .
(rē-AK-tiv) (prō-TĒN))

a blood test to measure the amount of C-reactive protein in the blood, which, when elevated, indicates inflammation in the body. It is sometimes used in assessing the risk of cardiovascular disease.

creatine phosphokinase (CPK) . .
(KRĒ-a-tin)
(fos-fō-KĪ-nās)

a blood test used to measure the level of creatine phosphokinase, an enzyme of heart and skeletal muscle released into the blood after muscle injury or necrosis. The test is useful in evaluating patients with acute myocardial infarction.

homocysteine . . . .
(hō-mō-SIS-tēn)

a blood test used to measure the amount of homocysteine in the blood. Homocysteine is an amino acid that, if elevated, may indicate an increased risk of cardiovascular disease.

lipid profile . . . .
(LIP-id) (PRŌ-fīl)

a blood test used to measure the amount of lipids in a sample of blood. This test is used to evaluate the risk of developing cardiovascular disease and to monitor therapy of existing disease. Results provide levels of total cholesterol, high-density lipoprotein (HDL), low-density lipoprotein (LDL), very-low-density lipoprotein (VLDL), and triglycerides (Box 10-3).

troponin . . . .
(TRŌ-pō-nin)

a blood test that measures troponin, a heart muscle enzyme. Troponins are released into the blood approximately 3 hours after necrosis of the heart muscle and may remain elevated from 7 to 10 days. The test is useful in the diagnosis of a myocardial infarction.

BLOOD

Laboratory

coagulation time . . . .
(kō-ag-ū-LĀ-shun)

blood test to determine the time it takes for blood to form a clot

complete blood count (CBC)
and differential count (Diff) . . . .

basic blood screening that measures hemoglobin, hematocrit, red blood cell number and morphology (size and shape), leukocyte count, and white blood cell differential (types of white blood cells) and platelet count. The test is automated, thus done easily and rapidly, and provides a tremendous amount of information about the blood.

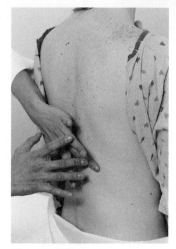

Figure 10-27
Percussion techniques.

A BIOMARKER
is a naturally occurring substance of certain body cells that can be measured in the blood and used to aid in the diagnosis of various disorders. Troponin, creatinine phosphokinase, homocystine, and C-reactive protein are biomarkers, and elevated levels are used in diagnosing various disorders occurring in the body.

Diagnostic Terms—cont'd
Not Built from Word Parts

Term	Definition
hematocrit (HCT)............ (hē-MAT-o-crit)	a blood test to measure the volume and number of red blood cells. It is used in the diagnosis and evaluation of anemic patients.
hemoglobin (Hgb)........... (HĒ-mō-glō-bin)	blood test used to determine the concentration of oxygen-carrying components (hemoglobin) in red blood cells
prothrombin time (PT) .... (prō-THROM-bin)	blood test used to determine certain coagulation activity defects and to monitor anticoagulation therapy for patients taking Coumadin, an oral anticoagulant medication. (Activated partial thromboplastin time [PTT] is used to monitor anticoagulation therapy for patients taking heparin, an intravenous anticoagulant medication.)

PT/INR stands for prothrombin time/international normalized ratio. Most institutions now, on the recommendation of the World Health Organization, report both absolute numbers and INR numbers, which provide uniform PT results to physicians worldwide.

TABLE 10-2
Understanding a Lipid Profile

Terms

Cholesterol—a compound important in the production of sex hormones, steroids, cell membranes, and bile acids. Cholesterol is produced by the body and contained in foods such as animal fats. Cholesterol is transported by lipoproteins.

   High-density lipoprotein (HDL)—a type of lipoprotein that removes cholesterol from the tissues and transports it to the liver to be excreted in the bile. Elevated levels of HDL are considered protective against development of atherosclerosis, which may lead to coronary artery disease. HDL is often referred to as the "good" cholesterol.

   Low-density lipoprotein (LDL)—a tye of lipoprotein that transports cholesterol to the tissue and deposits it on the walls of the arteries. High levels of LDL are associated with the presence of atherosclerosis, which may lead to coronary artery disease. LDL is often referred to as the "bad" cholesterol.

Total cholesterol—the total amount of cholesterol contained in the HDL and LDL.

Triglycerides (TGs)—a form of fat in the blood. Triglycerides are synthesized in the liver and used to store energy. Test results are used to assess the risk of coronary artery disease.

   Very-low-density lipoprotein (VLDL)—a type of lipoprotein that transports most of the triglycerides in the blood. Elevated levels of VLDL, to a lesser degree than LDL, indicate a risk for developing coronary artery disease.

Example of Lipid Profile Lab Report

Tests	Results	Flag	Normal Range
Cholesterol, total	188 mg/dL		100-199 mg/dL
Triglycerides	287 mg/dL	High	0-149 mg/dL
HDL cholesterol	50 mg/dL		40-59 mg/dL
VLDL cholesterol calc	57 mg/dL	High	5-40 mg/dL
LDL cholesterol calc	81 mg/dL		0-99 mg/dL

EXERCISE 32

Practice saying aloud each of the diagnostic terms not built from word parts on pp. 436-440.

To hear the terms select Chapter 10, Chapter Exercises, Pronunciation.

☐ Place a check mark in the box when you have completed this exercise.

EXERCISE 33

Fill in the blanks with the correct terms.

1. A device for measuring blood pressure is called a(n) _____.

2. _____ _____ is a blood test that determines the time it takes for blood to form a clot.

3. _____ _____ _____ and _____ _____ are the names of basic blood-screening tests.

4. A study that uses sound for detection of blood flow within blood vessels is called _____ _____.

5. A(n) _____ is an instrument used to hear internal body sounds.

6. Pressure exerted by blood against the blood vessel walls is called _____ _____.

7. A blood test used to determine certain coagulation activity defects and to monitor oral anticoagulation therapy is called _____ _____.

8. _____ _____ is a procedure in which a catheter is introduced into the heart to record pressures and enable the visualization of the heart chambers.

9. A blood test used to determine the oxygen-carrying component in the red blood cells is called _____.

10. _____ _____ measures venous flow of the extremities.

11. A nuclear medicine test used to diagnose coronary artery disease is _____ _____.

12. _____ _____ is a test in which an ultrasound probe provides views of the heart structures from the esophagus.

13. A nuclear medicine test that visualizes the heart from different angles is called a(n) _____ _____ _____ _____.

14. _____ _____ _____ evaluates cardiac function during physical stress.

15. A process of radiographic imaging of blood vessels that removes structures not being studied is called _____ _____ _____.

16. Hearing sounds within the body through a stethoscope is called _____.

17. A blood test to measure an enzyme of the heart released into the bloodstream after muscle injury is called _____ _____.

18. An elevated _____ _____ indicates inflammation in the body.

19. _____ is the number of times the heartbeat is felt on the arterial wall.

20. _____ is an amino acid that if elevated, indicates an increased risk of cardiovascular disease.

21. _____ is a heart muscle enzyme released into the bloodstream approximately 3 hours after heart muscle necrosis.

22. _____ _____ is the name of the blood test that measures the amount of lipids in the blood.

23. Tapping of the body surface with fingers to determine density is called _____.

24. A test of the red blood cells used in the diagnosis and evaluation of anemic patients is called _____.

EXERCISE 34

Match the terms in the first column with their correct definition in the second column.

_____ 1. cardiac catheterization

_____ 2. stethoscope

_____ 3. complete blood count and differential count

_____ 4. coagulation time

_____ 5. hemoglobin

_____ 6. Doppler ultrasound

_____ 7. prothrombin time

_____ 8. sphygmomanometer

_____ 9. single-photon emission computed tomography

_____ 10. digital subtraction angiography

a. device used for measuring blood pressure

b. digital radiographic imaging of blood vessels

c. test to determine certain coagulation activity defects

d. passage of a catheter into the heart to evaluate coronary artery disease

e. visualizes the heart from several different angles

f. used to assess revascularization after CABG

g. oxygen-carrying component of the red blood cell

h. basic blood-screening test

i. an ultrasound test that provides views of the heart from the esophagus

_____ 11. thallium test

_____ 12. transesophageal echocardiogram

j. study in which sound is used to determine the flow of blood within the vessels

k. test to determine the number of red blood cells

l. used to perform auscultation and blood pressure measurement

m. determines the time it takes for blood to form a clot

EXERCISE 35

Match the terms in the first column with the correct definitions in the second column.

_____ 1. exercise stress test

_____ 2. impedance plethysmography

_____ 3. percussion

_____ 4. C-reactive protein

_____ 5. auscultation

_____ 6. blood pressure

_____ 7. creatine phosphokinase

_____ 8. hematocrit

_____ 9. homocysteine

_____ 10. pulse

_____ 11. lipid profile

_____ 12. troponin

a. measures the volume and number of red blood cells

b. determines density

c. blood test to determine inflammation or risk of cardiovascular disease

d. measures cardiac function during physical stress

e. measures the level of an enzyme released into the blood after muscle injury

f. hearing sounds through a stethoscope

g. measures blood flow of the extremities

h. pressure exerted by blood against the blood vessel walls

i. measures the amount of an amino acid in the blood

j. measured most often over the radial artery

k. results provide levels of cholesterol, HDL, LDL, VLDL, and triglycerides

l. measures an enzyme released within hours after damage to the heart muscle

EXERCISE 36

Spell each of the diagnostic terms not built from word parts on pp. 436-440 by having someone dictate them to you.

 To hear and spell the terms select Chapter 10, Chapter Exercises, Spelling. You may type the terms on the screen or write them below in the spaces provided.

☐ Place a check mark in the box if you have completed this exercise using your CD-ROM.

1. _____   3. _____

2. _____   4. _____

5. _____   15. _____

6. _____   16. _____

7. _____   17. _____

8. _____   18. _____

9. _____   19. _____

10. _____   20. _____

11. _____   21. _____

12. _____   22. _____

13. _____   23. _____

14. _____   24. _____

Complementary Terms
Built from Word Parts

The following terms are built from word parts you have already learned and can be translated literally to find their meanings. Further explanation of terms beyond the definition of their word parts, if needed, is included in parentheses.

Term	Definition
CARDIOVASCULAR SYSTEM	
atrioventricular (AV) . . . . (ā-trē-ō-ven-TRIK-ū-ler)	pertaining to the atrium and ventricle
cardiac . . . . (KAR-dē-ak)	pertaining to the heart
cardiogenic . . . . (*kar*-dē-ō-JEN-ik)	originating in the heart
cardiologist . . . . (*kar*-dē-OL-o-jist)	physician who studies and treats diseases of the heart
cardiology . . . . (*kar*-dē-OL-o-jē)	study of the heart (a branch of medicine that deals with diseases of the heart and blood vessels)
hypothermia . . . . (*hī*-pō-THER-mē-a)	condition of (body) temperature that is below (normal sometimes induced for various surgical procedures, such as bypass surgery)
intravenous (IV) . . . . (in-tra-VĒ-nus)	pertaining to within the vein
phlebologist . . . . (fle-BOL-o-jist)	physician who studies and treats diseases of the veins
phlebology . . . . (fle-BOL-o-jē)	study of veins (a branch of medicine that deals with diseases of the veins)

AN ELECTROPHYSIOLOGIST is a cardiologist who specializes in the diagnosis and treatment of patients with arrhythmias.

Term	Definition
BLOOD	
hematologist............... (hē-ma-TOL-o-jist)	physician who studies and treats diseases of the blood
hematology................ (hē-ma-TOL-o-jē)	study of the blood (a branch of medicine that deals with diseases of the blood)
hematopoiesis .... (hē-ma-tō-poy-Ē-sis)	formation of blood (cells)
hemolysis................. (hē-MOL-i-sis)	dissolution of (red) blood (cells)
hemostasis................. (hē-mō-STĀ-sis)	stoppage of bleeding
myelopoiesis............... (mī-e-lō-poy-Ē-sis)	formation of bone marrow
plasmapheresis .... (plaz-ma-fe-RĒ-sis)	removal of plasma (from withdrawn blood)
thrombolysis............... (throm-BOL-i-sis)	dissolution of a clot

EXERCISE 37

Practice saying aloud each of the complementary terms built from word parts on pp. 444-445.

To hear the terms select Chapter 10, Chapter Exercises, Pronunciation.

☐ Place a check mark in the box when you have completed this exercise.

EXERCISE 38

Analyze and define the following complementary terms.

1. hypothermia _____

2. hematopoiesis _____

3. cardiology _____

4. cardiologist _____

5. hemolysis _____

6. hematologist _____

7. cardiac _____

8. hematology _____

9. plasmapheresis _____

10. hemostasis _____

11. cardiogenic _____

12. myelopoiesis _____

13. thrombolysis _____

14. atrioventricular _____

15. intravenous _____

16. phlebologist _____

17. phlebology _____

EXERCISE 39

Build the complementary terms for the following definitions by using the word parts you have learned.

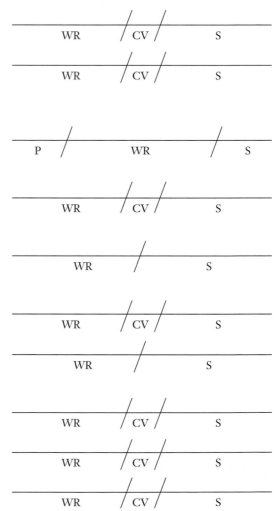

1. study of the heart

    _____ / ___ / _____
    WR   CV   S

2. formation of blood (cells)

    _____ / ___ / _____
    WR   CV   S

3. condition of (body) temperature that is below (normal)

    ___ / _____ / _____
    P   WR   S

4. dissolution of (red) blood (cells)

    _____ / ___ / _____
    WR   CV   S

5. removal of plasma (from withdrawn blood)

    _____ / _____
    WR   S

6. physician who studies and treats diseases of the blood

    _____ / ___ / _____
    WR   CV   S

7. pertaining to the heart

    _____ / _____
    WR   S

8. physician who studies and treats diseases of the heart

    _____ / ___ / _____
    WR   CV   S

9. study of the blood

    _____ / ___ / _____
    WR   CV   S

10. stoppage of bleeding

    _____ / ___ / _____
    WR   CV   S

11. formation of bone marrow   _____
    WR   / CV /   S

12. originating in the heart   _____
    WR   / CV /   S

13. dissolution of a clot   _____
    WR   / CV /   S

14. pertaining to the
    atrium and ventricle   _____
    WR / CV /   WR   /   S

15. pertaining to within
    the vein   _____
    P /   WR   /   S

16. study of veins   _____
    WR   / CV /   S

17. physician who studies
    and treats diseases of
    the vein   _____
    WR   / CV /   S

EXERCISE 40

Spell each of the complementary terms built from word parts on pp. 444-445 by having someone dictate them to you.

To hear and spell the terms select Chapter 10, Chapter Exercises, Spelling. You may type the terms on the screen or write them below in the spaces provided.

☐ Place a check mark in the box if you have completed this exercise using your CD-ROM.

1. _____   10. _____

2. _____   11. _____

3. _____   12. _____

4. _____   13. _____

5. _____   14. _____

6. _____   15. _____

7. _____   16. _____

8. _____   17. _____

9. _____

Complementary Terms
Not Built from Word Parts

In some of the following terms, you may recognize word parts you have already learned; however, the full meaning of the terms cannot be discerned by the definition of their word parts.

Term	Definition
CARDIOVASCULAR SYSTEM	
cardiopulmonary resuscitation (CPR)...................... (*kar*-dē-ō-PUL-mo-nar-ē) (rē-*sus*-i-TĀ-shun)	emergency procedure consisting of artificial ventilation and external cardiac massage
defibrillation............... (dē-fib-ri-LĀ-shun)	application of an electric shock to the myocardium through the chest wall to restore normal cardiac rhythm (Figure 10-28)
diastole.................... (dī-AS-tō-lē)	phase in the cardiac cycle in which the ventricles relax between contractions (diastolic is the lower number of a blood pressure reading)
extracorporeal .... (*ek*-stra-kōr-POR-ē-al)	occurring outside the body. During open-heart surgery extracorporeal circulation occurs when blood is diverted outside the body to a heart-lung machine.
extravasation .... (ek-strav-a-SĀ-shun)	escape of blood from the blood vessel into the tissue
fibrillation................. (fi-bri-LĀ-shun)	rapid, quivering, noncoordinated contractions of the atria and ventricles
heart murmur.............. (MER-mer)	a short-duration humming sound of cardiac or vascular origin
hypercholesterolemia......... (*hī*-per-k-*les*-ter-ol-Ē-mē-a)	excessive amount of cholesterol in the blood; associated with heightened risk of cardiovascular disease
hyperlipidemia .... (*hī*-per-lip-i-DĒ-mē-a)	excessive amount of fats (triglycerides and cholesterol) in the blood
hypertension................ (*hī*-per-TEN-shun)	blood pressure that is above normal (greater than 140/90)
hypertriglyceridemia.......... (*hī*-per-trī-*glis*-er-rī-DĒ-mē-a)	excessive amount of triglycerides in the blood; associated with an increased risk of cardiovascular disease
hypotension .... (*hī*-pō-TEN-shun)	blood pressure that is below normal (less than 90/60)
lipids..................... (LIP-ids)	fats and fatlike substances that serve as a source of fuel in the body and are an important constituent of cell structure
lumen .... (LŪ-men)	space within a tubular part or organ, such as the space within a blood vessel

Term	Definition
CARDIOVASCULAR SYSTEM, CONT'D	
occlude...... (o-KLŪD)	to close tightly, to block
systole...... (SIS-tō-lē)	phase in the cardiac cycle in which the ventricles contract (systolic is the upper number of a blood pressure reading)
vasoconstrictor...... (*vās*-ō-kon-STRIK-tor)	agent or nerve that narrows the blood vessels
vasodilator...... (*vās*-ō-DĪ-lā-tor)	agent or nerve that enlarges the blood vessels
venipuncture...... (VEN-i-*punk*-chur)	puncture of a vein to remove blood, instill a medication, or start an intravenous infusion
BLOOD	
anticoagulant...... (*an*-tī-kō-AG-ū-lant)	agent that slows the clotting process
dyscrasia...... (dis-KRĀ-zha)	abnormal or pathologic condition of the blood
hemorrhage...... (HEM-o-rij)	rapid loss of blood, as in bleeding

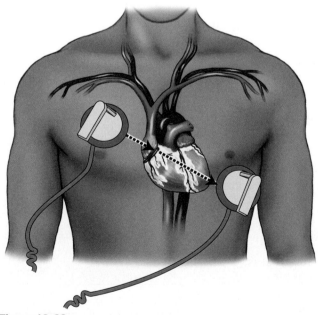

Figure 10-28
Placement of defibrillator paddles on the chest.

EXERCISE 41

Practice saying aloud each of the complementary terms not built from word parts on pp. 448-449.

 To hear the terms select Chapter 10, Chapter Exercises, Pronunciation.

☐ Place a check mark in the box when you have completed this exercise.

EXERCISE 42

Write the term for each of the following definitions.

1. agent that narrows the
   blood vessels   _____

2. space within a tubelike
   structure   _____

3. emergency procedure
   consisting of artificial
   ventilation and external
   cardiac massage   _____   _____

4. phase in the cardiac cycle
   in which the ventricles relax   _____

5. noncoordinated contractions
   of the atria and ventricles   _____

6. blood pressure that is below
   normal   _____

7. escape of blood from the
   blood vessel into the tissue   _____

8. puncture of a vein to remove
   blood   _____

9. phase in the cardiac cycle in
   which the ventricles contract   _____

10. agent that enlarges the
    blood vessels   _____

11. blood pressure that is
    above normal   _____

12. to close tightly   _____

13. excessive amount of
    triglycerides in the blood   _____

14. excessive amount of fat
    in the blood   _____

15. rapid flow of blood   _____

16. agent that slows the
    clotting process   _____

17. excessive amount of
    cholesterol in the blood   _____

18. pathologic condition
    of the blood   _____

19. a humming sound of cardiac
    or vascular origin   _____   _____

20. occurring outside the body   _____

21. fat and fat substances   _____

22. used to restore normal
    cardiac rhythm   _____

EXERCISE 43

Write the definitions of the following terms.

1. lumen_____

2. extravasation _____

3. hypercholesterolemia_____

4. venipuncture_____

5. vasodilator _____

6. hypertension_____

7. cardiopulmonary resuscitation _____

8. systole _____

9. hypotension _____

10. vasoconstrictor _____

11. diastole _____

12. fibrillation _____

13. occlude _____

14. hyperlipidemia _____

15. hypertriglyceridemia _____

16. dyscrasia _____

17. hemorrhage_____

18. anticoagulant _____

19. extracorporeal _____

20. heart murmur _____

21. lipid _____

22. defibrillation _____

EXERCISE **44**

Spell each of the complementary terms not built from word parts on pp. 448-449 by having someone dictate them to you.

 To hear and spell the terms select Chapter 10, Chapter Exercises, Spelling. You may type the terms on the screen or write them below in the spaces provided.

☐ Place a check mark in the box if you have completed this exercise using your CD-ROM.

1._____	12._____
2._____	13._____
3._____	14._____
4._____	15._____
5._____	16._____
6._____	17._____
7._____	18._____
8._____	19._____
9._____	20._____
10._____	21._____
11._____	22._____

IMMUNE SYSTEM

Complementary Terms

Not Built From Word Parts

Term	Definition
allergen. . . . . (AL-er-jen)	an environmental substance capable of producing an immediate hypersensitivity in the body (allergy). Common allergens are house dust, pollen, animal dander, and various foods.
allergist. . . . . (AL-er-jist)	a physician who studies and treats allergic conditions

Term	Definition
anaphylaxis................ (*an*-a-fe-LAK-sis)	an exaggerated, life-threatening reaction to a previously encountered antigen such as bee venom, peanuts, or latex. Symptoms range from mild, with patients experiencing hives or sneezing, to severe symptoms such as drop in blood pressure and blockage of the airway, which can lead to death within minutes (also called **anaphylactic shock**).
antibiotic................. (*an*-tī-bī-OT-ik)	a drug that targets microorganisms to kill or halt growth or replication
antibodies................ (AN-ti-bod-ēz)	a substance produced by lymphocytes that inactivates or destroys antigens (also called **immunoglobulins**)
antigen................... (AN-ti-jen)	a substance that triggers an immune response when introduced into the body. Examples of antigens are transplant tissue, toxins, and infectious organisms.
autoimmune disease........ (aw-tō-i-MŪN) (di-ZĒZ)	a disease caused by the body's inability to distinguish its own cells from foreign bodies, thus producing antibodies that attack its own tissue. **Rheumatoid arthritis** and **systemic lupus erythematosus** are examples of autoimmune diseases.
immune.................. (i-MŪN)	being resistant to specific invading pathogens
immunodeficiency.......... (*im*-ū-nō-de-FISH-en-sē)	deficient immune response caused by the immune system dysfunction brought on by disease (HIV infection) or immunosuppressive drugs (prednisone)
immunologist.............. (im-ū-NOL-o-jist)	a physician who studies and treats immune system disorders
immunology............... (im-ū-NOL-o-jē)	the branch of medicine dealing with immune system disorders
infection.................. (in-FEK-shun)	the invasion of pathogens in body tissue. An infection may remain localized if the body's defense mechanisms are effective. If the infection persists it may become acute, subacute, or chronic. A systemic infection occurs when the pathogen causing a local infection gains access to the vascular or lymphatic system and becomes disseminated throughout the body.
phagocytosis.............. (fā-gō-sī-TŌ-sis)	a process in which some of the white blood cells destroy the invading microorganism and old cells

IMMUNITY

occurs in three ways:

- **natural immunity** between mother and child before birth and after birth through breast milk
- **active immunity** by the body producing antibodies in response to an infectious disease such as tuberculosis
- **artificial immunity** by receiving vaccinations to produce antibodies. Artificial immunity is used for many common diseases such as measles and mumps. Vaccines new to the market in 2006 were for rotavirus, which causes severe diarrhea in children; human papillomavirus, which is linked to cervical cancer; and a vaccine to prevent shingles in the elderly.

Complementary Terms—*cont'd*
Not Built From Word Parts

Term	Definition
vaccine . . . . (vak-SĒN)	a suspension of inactivated microorganisms administered by injection, mouth, or nasal spray to prevent infectious diseases by inducing immunity

EXERCISE 45

Practice saying aloud each of the complementary terms not built from word parts on pp. 453-454.

 To hear the terms select Chapter 10, Chapter Exercises, Pronunciation.

☐ Place a check mark in the box when you have completed this exercise.

EXERCISE 46

Match the immune system terms in the first column with the phrases in the second column.

_____ 1. allergen

_____ 2. antibiotic

_____ 3. autoimmune disease

_____ 4. immunologist

_____ 5. antigen

_____ 6. immune

_____ 7. allergist

_____ 8. antibodies

_____ 9. immunodeficiency

_____ 10. phagocytosis

_____ 11. vaccine

_____ 12. infection

_____ 13. immunology

_____ 14. anaphylaxis

a. deficient immune response

b. a branch of medicine

c. administered by injection or orally to prevent infectious diseases

d. inactivates or destroys antigens

e. house dust, pollen, animal dander

f. transplant tissue, toxin, infectious organisms

g. treats allergic conditions

h. white blood cells destroy invading microorganisms

i. an invasion of pathogens in body tissues

j. treats immune system disorders

k. rheumatoid arthritis

l. life-threatening reaction

m. resistant to invading pathogens

n. a drug that targets microorganisms

EXERCISE 47

Spell each of the complementary terms not built from word parts on pp. 453-454 by having someone dictate them to you.

 To hear and spell the terms select Chapter 10, Chapter Exercises, Spelling. You may type the terms on the screen or write them below in the spaces provided.

☐ Place a check mark in the box if you have completed this exercise using your CD-ROM.

1._____	8._____
2._____	9._____
3._____	10._____
4._____	11._____
5._____	12._____
6._____	13._____
7._____	14._____

Refer to Appendix E for pharmacology terms related to the cardiovascular system and blood.

Abbreviations

ACS	acute coronary syndrome
AFib	atrial fibrillation
AV	atrioventricular
BP	blood pressure
CABG	coronary artery bypass graft
CAD	coronary artery disease
CBC and Diff	complete blood count and differential
CCU	coronary care unit
CHF	congestive heart failure
CPK	creatine phosphokinase
CPR	cardiopulmonary resuscitation
CRP	C-reactive protein
DSA	digital subtraction angiography
DVT	deep vein thrombosis
ECG, EKG	electrocardiogram
ECHO	echocardiogram
HCT	hematocrit
Hgb	hemoglobin

Abbreviations—cont'd

HHD....................	hypertensive heart disease
ICD	implantable cardiac defibrillator
IPG	impedance plethysmography
IV.......................	intravenous
MI	myocardial infarction
PAD....................	peripheral arterial disease
PT	prothrombin time
PTCA..................	percutaneous transluminal coronary angioplasty
RBC....................	red blood cell (erythrocyte)
SPECT.................	single-photon emission computed tomography
TEE....................	transesophageal echocardiogram
WBC	white blood cell (leukocyte)

Refer to Appendix D for a complete list of abbreviations.

EXERCISE 48

Write the meaning of the abbreviation in the blanks.

1. **CAD** _____ _____ _____ has
   received growing interest over the past 20 years. Diagnostic procedures
   for new patients usually begin with an exercise **ECG** _____.
   Patients whose stress tests are borderline usually proceed to noninvasive
   imaging such as **SPECT** _____ _____
   _____ _____ and stress **ECHO** _____.

2. **DVT** _____ _____ _____ is common
   in hospitalized patients. Early detection is important because DVT can
   result in death from a pulmonary embolism. Doppler ultrasound and **IPG**
   _____ _____ are two noninvasive diagnostic pro-
   cedures used to diagnose DVT. MRI and venography may be used as well.

3. The **CBC** _____ _____ _____
   and differential count are a series of automated laboratory tests of the
   peripheral blood that provide a great deal of information about the
   blood and other body organs. Tests performed as part of the CBC are
   RBC _____ _____ _____
   count, **WBC** _____ _____
   _____ count and differential count, **Hgb** _____,
   and **HCT** _____.

4. Standard surgical treatment for CAD includes **CABG** _____
_____ _____ _____. There is a
growth in the use of minimally invasive techniques to treat CAD,
which include transmyocardial laser revascularization and **PTCA**
_____ _____ _____
_____, atherectomy, and stent insertion.

5. Hospitalized patients diagnosed with **MI** _____ _____
are cared for in the **CCU** _____ _____
_____.

6. A sphygmomanometer is used to measure **BP** _____
_____.

7. Diagnosis used to indicate that a patient's heart is unable to pump enough
blood through the body to supply tissues is **CHF** _____
_____ _____.

8. If the patient's heart and/or lungs have ceased to function, the medical team
must begin **CPR** _____ _____.

9. A patient with persistently elevated blood pressure is likely to be diagnosed
with **HHD** _____ _____ _____.

10. When scheduling blood tests for a patient on oral anticoagulant medication,
the doctor is likely to include a **PT** _____ _____.

11. Any interruption of the conduction of electrical impulses from the atria to
the ventricles is called **AV** _____ block.

12. The treatment of **ACS** _____ _____
_____ is aimed at preventing thrombus formation and restoring
blood flow to the occluded coronary artery.

13. Stopping smoking, exercising, and proper diet are important in the medical
management of **PAD** _____ _____
_____.

14. **DSA** _____ _____ _____ is especially
valuable in cardiac applications.

15. The physician ordered a **TEE** _____ _____ to examine the patient's heart structure and function.

16. Two blood tests used in assessing and evaluating cardiovascular diseases
are **CRP** _____ _____ and
CPK _____ _____.

17. A patient experiencing **AFib** _____ _____ may be
referred to an electrophysiologist, a cardiology subspecialist.

18. An **ICD** _____ _____ _____ delivers
an electric shock to convert an arrhythmia back to normal rhythm.

PRACTICAL APPLICATION

EXERCISE **49** *Interact with Medical Documents*

A. Complete the inpatient progress note by writing the medical terms in the blanks. Use the list of definitions with the corresponding numbers on the next page.

University Hospital and Medical Center
4700 North Main Street • Wellness, Arizona 54321 • (987) 555-3210

PATIENT NAME: Natalie Wells   **CASE NUMBER:** 20922-CVR
DATE OF BIRTH: 01/14/19XX   **DATE:** 04/07/20XX

INPATIENT PROGRESS NOTE

CHIEF COMPLAINT: Natalie Wells is a 76-year-old Caucasian woman who was admitted to the hospital for recurrent chest pain.

HISTORY OF PRESENT ILLNESS: The patient has a long history of stable 1. _____ _____.
She had a positive treadmill stress test in 1988. A 2. _____ _____ in 1998 showed reversible 3. _____ . In May 1992 she underwent cataract surgery, and during her postoperative care she developed severe chest pain. An ECG at that time showed ischemic ST changes in the anterior leads. Subsequent coronary 4. _____ revealed a 90% focal 5. _____ left anterior descending coronary artery. The patient then underwent 6. _____ of this lesion. The 90% stenosis was dilated to a 20% stenosis. The patient had an uncomplicated course.

Over the last 10 days the patient has had at least five episodes of chest pain, all relieved by rest or a single nitroglycerin tablet. She had an episode yesterday while gardening, which lasted almost 5 minutes before subsiding after a second nitroglycerin tablet. She went to her 7. _____ office yesterday. 8. _____ was performed, which showed marked anterior T-wave inversion in the anterior leads, and she was immediately sent to this hospital for further evaluation. Atherogenic risk factors for her age include hypercholesterolemia and hypertension; she also smokes one pack of cigarettes per day. She is not a diabetic. Her family history reveals a brother who has had a coronary artery bypass graft.

PHYSICAL EXAM:
On exam today, blood pressure is 138/86. She has tachycardia with a pulse of 120. She is in no acute distress. Her lungs are clear and she has regular rhythm without a murmur. There is no edema or distention of neck veins.

CURRENT MEDICATIONS:
1. Lovastatin 20 mg with evening meal.
2. Enalapril 20 mg bid.
3. Nifedipine 10 mg tid.
4. Nitroglycerin 0.4 mg sublingual prn.

PLAN:
9. _____ _____ with possible coronary stent if necessary.
Serial ECGs, 10. _____ _____, and 11. _____ will be obtained to rule out
12. _____ _____.

_____
Emily Watson, MD

EW/mcm

1. chest pain, occurs when there is an insufficient supply of blood to the heart muscle
2. a nuclear medicine test used to determine blood flow to the myocardium
3. deficient supply of blood to the heart's blood vessels
4. radiographic imaging a blood vessel
5. narrowing
6. surgical repair of a blood vessel
7. physician who studies and treats diseases of the heart
8. process of recording electrical activity of the heart
9. introduction of a catheter into the heart by way of a blood vessel to determine coronary artery disease
10. an enzyme of heart and skeletal muscles
11. a blood test that measures the amount of a certain enzyme approximately 3 hours after necrosis of the heart muscle
12. death of a portion of the myocardial muscle caused by lack of oxygen resulting from an interrupted blood supply

B. Read the progress note and answer the questions following it.

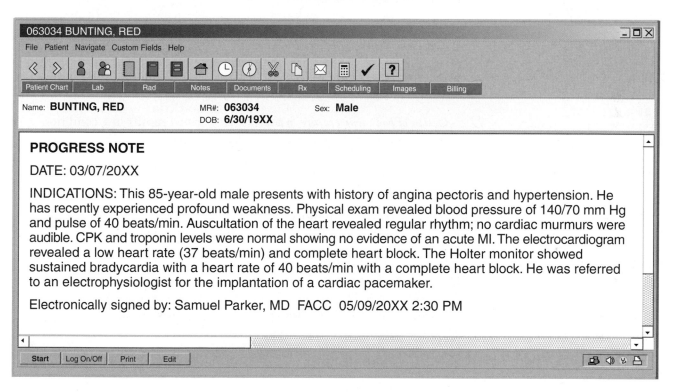

063034 BUNTING, RED

File   Patient   Navigate   Custom Fields   Help

| Patient Chart | Lab | Rad | Notes | Documents | Rx | Scheduling | Images | Billing |

Name: **BUNTING, RED**   MR#: **063034**   Sex: **Male**
DOB: **6/30/19XX**

PROGRESS NOTE

DATE: 03/07/20XX

INDICATIONS: This 85-year-old male presents with history of angina pectoris and hypertension. He has recently experienced profound weakness. Physical exam revealed blood pressure of 140/70 mm Hg and pulse of 40 beats/min. Auscultation of the heart revealed regular rhythm; no cardiac murmurs were audible. CPK and troponin levels were normal showing no evidence of an acute MI. The electrocardiogram revealed a low heart rate (37 beats/min) and complete heart block. The Holter monitor showed sustained bradycardia with a heart rate of 40 beats/min with a complete heart block. He was referred to an electrophysiologist for the implantation of a cardiac pacemaker.

Electronically signed by: Samuel Parker, MD FACC 05/09/20XX 2:30 PM

Start   Log On/Off   Print   Edit

1. The patient had a history of (high or low) BP?

2. Cardiac murmur was ruled out by:
   a. diagnostic imaging test
   b. laboratory test
   c. stethoscope

3. An acute myocardial infarction was ruled out by:
   a. an EKG
   b. an ultrasound test
   c. a laboratory test

4. A cardiac pacemaker is used to:
   a. lower blood pressure
   b. regulate heart rate
   c. treat atrial fibrillation

EXERCISE **50** *Interpret Medical Terms*

To test your understanding of the terms introduced in this chapter, circle the words that correctly complete the sentences. The italicized words refer to the correct answer.

1. *Yellowish, fatty plaque within the arteries* is (**arteriosclerosis, atherosclerosis, aortosclerosis**).

2. *Inflammation of a vein associated with a clot* is called a (**thrombosis, phlebitis, thrombophlebitis**).

3. *Inflammation of the middle muscular layer of the heart* is (**endocarditis, myocarditis, pericarditis**).

4. Another name for a *heart attack* is (**myocardial infarction, coronary fibrillation, angina pectoris**).

5. The *surgical excision of a thickened artery interior* is an (**atherectomy, angioplasty, endarterectomy**).

6. An *acute infection caused by the Epstein-Barr virus* is (**anemia, infectious mononucleosis, rheumatic heart disease**).

7. *Reduction of body temperature to a level below normal* results in a condition called (**hypothermia, hypertension, hyperthermia**).

8. (**Impedance plethysmography, cardiac scan, aortogram**) is used to *determine if a patient has a blood clot in the femoral vein.*

9. *A humming sound* or (**hemorrhage, murmur, auscultation**) originating *in the heart* is sometimes the result of many episodes of rheumatic fever, an inflammatory disease occurring in children.

10. The doctor uses an (**echocardiograph, electrocardiogram, angioscope**) to *visualize the blood vessel* and guide the laser beam to open blocked arteries; this procedure is called (**echocardiography, angioscopy**).

11. The following is *a nuclear medicine test used to diagnose coronary artery disease* (**coronary stent, thallium test, transesophageal echocardiogram**).

12. Each time *the patient came in contact with house dust she immediately began to sneeze and experienced rhinorrhea.* She visited a(n) (**allergist, immunologist, hematologist**) to seek relief from her symptoms.

13. Peanuts are an antigen that can trigger an *exaggerated life-threatening reaction* or (**allergen, anaphylaxis, allergies**).

EXERCISE **51**   *Read Medical Terms in Use*

Practice pronunciation of terms by reading the following medical document. Use the pronunciation key following the medical terms to assist you in saying the word.

To hear these terms select Chapter 10, Chapter Exercises, Read Medical Terms in Use.

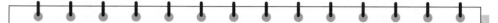

A 55-year-old man presented to his doctor with pain in the calf and swelling in the left foot and ankle. A total of 5 days before, the patient had traveled by air across the country, spending several hours in a sitting position. He has a history of **varicose** (VAR-i-kōs) **veins** (vānz). No previous history of **hypertension** (hī-per-TEN-shun) or **thrombophlebitis** (throm-bō-fle-BĪ-tis) existed. Physical examination revealed an edematous left lower extremity and a tender calf. The pedal **pulse** (puls) was intact. A **Doppler ultrasound** (DOP-ler) (UL-tra-sound) was obtained, which revealed **deep vein thrombosis** (throm-BŌ-sis). The patient was hospitalized and subcutaneous low molecular weight heparin was begun. Concurrently, Coumadin was started and will continue for 6 months. The oral **anticoagulant** (an-tī-cō-AG-ū-lant) therapy will be monitored monthly by **prothrombin** (prō-THROM-bin) **time.**

EXERCISE **52**   *Comprehend Medical Terms in Use*

Test your comprehension of the terms in the previous medical document by circling the correct answer.

1. T   F   A radiographic image was used to diagnose deep vein thrombosis.

2. The patient was diagnosed with:
   a. inflammation of the vein
   b. vascular inflammatory disorder
   c. a clot in a vein in the lower extremity
   d. a clot in the blood vessels of the heart

3. A blood test will be used to determine:
   a. bleeding time
   b. the time it takes for blood to form a clot
   c. the oxygen-carrying capacity of the red blood cell
   d. certain coagulation activity defects

 WEB LINK
For additional information on heart disease, visit the American Heart Association at www.americanheart.org.

CHAPTER REVIEW

◉))) CHAPTER REVIEW ON CD-ROM

Use the CD-ROM that accompanies this textbook to play and practice what you have learned in this chapter. The Chapter Exercises, Practice Activities, Animations, and Games allow you to hear, see, and interact with the chapter content.

Chapter Exercises	**Practice Activities**	**Animations**	**Games**
Exercises in this section of your CD-ROM correlate to exercises in your textbook. You may have completed them as you worked through the chapter.	Practice in study mode, then test your learning in assessment mode. Keep track of your scores from assessment mode if you wish.	☐ Antibiotics ☐ Coronary Artery Bypass Graft ☐ Phagocytosis	☐ Name that Word Part ☐ Term Storm ☐ Term Explorer ☐ Termbusters ☐ Medical Millionaire

Chapter Exercises

Exercises in this section of your CD-ROM correlate to exercises in your textbook. You may have completed them as you worked through the chapter.
☐ Pronunciation
☐ Spelling
☐ Read Medical Terms in Use

Practice Activities

Practice in study mode, then test your learning in assessment mode. Keep track of your scores from assessment mode if you wish.

SCORE
☐ Picture It   _____
☐ Define Word Parts   _____
☐ Build Medical Terms _____
☐ Word Shop   _____
☐ Define Medical Terms _____
☐ Use It   _____
☐ Hear It and Type It: _____
   Clinical Vignettes

Animations
☐ Antibiotics
☐ Coronary Artery Bypass Graft
☐ Phagocytosis
☐ PTCA
☐ Subaortic Stenosis and Echocardiography

Games
☐ Name that Word Part
☐ Term Storm
☐ Term Explorer
☐ Termbusters
☐ Medical Millionaire

REVIEW OF WORD PARTS

Can you define and spell the following word parts?

Combining Forms		**Prefixes**	**Suffixes**
angi/o	myel/o	brady-	-ac
aort/o	phleb/o		-apheresis
arteri/o	plasm/o		-graph
ather/o	splen/o		-odynia
atri/o	therm/o		-penia
cardi/o	thromb/o		-poiesis
ech/o	thym/o		-sclerosis
electr/o	valv/o		
isch/o	valvul/o		
lymphaden/o	ven/o		
lymph/o	ventricul/o		

REVIEW OF TERMS

Can you build, analyze, define, pronounce, and spell the following terms *built from word parts?*

Diseases and Disorders	**Surgical**	**Diagnostic**	**Complementary**
Cardiovascular System	***Cardiovascular System***	***Cardiovascular System***	***Cardiovascular System***
angioma	angioplasty	angiography	atrioventricular (AV)
angiostenosis	atherectomy	angioscope	cardiac
aortic stenosis	endarterectomy	angioscopy	cardiogenic
arteriosclerosis	pericardiocentesis	aortogram	cardiologist
atherosclerosis	phlebectomy	arteriogram	cardiology
bradycardia	phlebotomy	echocardiogram (ECHO)	hypothermia
cardiodynia	valvuloplasty	electrocardiogram (ECG,	intravenous (IV)
cardiomegaly		EKG)	phlebologist
cardiomyopathy	***Lymphatic System***	electrocardiograph	phlebology
cardiovalvulitis	splenectomy	electrocardiography	
endocarditis	splenopexy	venogram	***Blood***
ischemia	thymectomy	venography	hematologist
myocarditis			hematology
pericarditis			hematopoiesis
phlebitis			hemolysis
polyarteritis			hemostasis
tachycardia			myelopoiesis
thrombophlebitis			plasmapheresis
			thrombolysis

Blood
hematoma
multiple myeloma
pancytopenia
thrombosis
thrombus

Lymphatic System
lymphadenitis
lymphadenopathy
lymphoma
splenomegaly
thymoma

Can you define, pronounce, and spell the following terms *not built from word parts?*

Diseases and Disorders	Surgical	Diagnostic	Complementary

Diseases and Disorders

Cardiovascular System

acute coronary syndrome (ACS)
aneurysm
angina pectoris
arrhythmia
atrial fibrillation (AFib)
cardiac arrest
cardiac tamponade
coarctation of the aorta
congenital heart disease
congestive heart failure (CHF)
coronary artery disease (CAD)
coronary occlusion
deep vein thrombosis (DVT)
hypertensive heart disease (HHD)
intermittent claudication
mitral valve stenosis
myocardial infarction (MI)
peripheral arterial disease (PAD)
rheumatic heart disease
varicose veins

Blood

anemia
embolus, *pl.* emboli
hemophilia
leukemia

Lymphatic System

Hodgkin disease
infectious mononucleosis

Surgical

Cardiovascular System

aneurysmectomy
atrial fibrillation ablation
cardiac pacemaker
coronary artery bypass graft (CABG)
coronary stent
embolectomy
femoropopliteal bypass
implantable cardiac defibrillator (ICD)
intracoronary thrombo-lytic therapy
percutaneous transluminal coronary angioplasty (PTCA)

Blood

bone marrow aspiration
bone marrow biopsy
bone marrow transplant

Diagnostic

Cardiovascular System

auscultation
blood pressure (BP)
cardiac catheterization
C-reactive protein (CRP)
creatine phosphokinase (CPK)
digital subtraction angiog-raphy (DSA)
Doppler ultrasound
exercise stress test
homocysteine
impedance plethysmogra-phy (IPG)
lipid profile
percussion
pulse
single-photon emission computed tomography (SPECT)
sphygmomanometer
stethoscope
thallium test
transesophageal echocar-diogram (TEE)
troponin

Blood

coagulation time
complete blood count and differential (CBC and Diff)
hematocrit (HCT)
hemoglobin (Hgb)
prothrombin time (PT)

Complementary

Cardiovascular System

cardiopulmonary resuscita-tion (CPR)
defibrillation
diastole
extracorporeal
extravasation
fibrillation
heart murmur
hypercholesterolemia
hyperlipidemia
hypertension
hypertriglyceridemia
hypotension
lipids
lumen
occlude
systole
vasoconstrictor
vasodilator
venipuncture

Blood

anticoagulant
dyscrasia
hemorrhage

Immune System

allergen
allergist
anaphylaxis
antibodies
antibiotic
antigen
autoimmune disease
immune
immunodeficiency
immunologist
immunology
infection
phagocytosis
vaccine

ANSWERS

Exercise Figures

Exercise Figure

A. 1. blood vessel: angi/o
2. valve: valv/o, valvul/o
3. heart: cardi/o
4. aorta: aort/o
5. artery: arteri/o
6. atrium: atri/o
7. ventricle: ventricul/o

Exercise Figure

B. ather/o/sclerosis

Exercise Figure

C. end/arter/ectomy

Exercise Figure

D. electr/o/cardi/o/gram

Exercise 1

1. e	6. f
2. g	7. d
3. c	8. h
4. i	9. b
5. a	10. j

Exercise 2

1. k	6. j
2. d	7. a
3. b	8. e
4. h	9. c
5. l	10. f

Exercise 3

1. plasma
2. erythrocytes
3. leukocytes
4. platelets
5. platelets
6. serum
7. lymph
8. lymph nodes
9. spleen
10. thymus

Exercise 4

1. to protect the body against pathogens, foreign agents, and abnormal body cells
2. a. spleen
   b. liver
   c. intestinal tract
   d. lymph nodes
   e. bone marrow

3. a. prevention of foreign bodies from entering the body
   b. phagocytosis, inflammation, fever, and activation of protective proteins and natural killer cells
   c. forms specific antibodies to fight infectious agents

Exercise 5

1. heart
2. atrium
3. plasma
4. vessel
5. vein
6. aorta
7. valve
8. spleen
9. thymus gland
10. vein
11. ventricle
12. artery
13. valve
14. lymph, lymph tissue
15. lymph node
16. bone marrow

Exercise 6

1. arteri/o
2. a. phleb/o
   b. ven/o
3. cardi/o
4. atri/o
5. ventricul/o
6. lymph/o
7. aort/o
8. angi/o
9. a. valv/o
   b. valvul/o
10. splen/o
11. plasm/o
12. thym/o
13. lymphaden/o
14. myel/o

Exercise 7

1. sound
2. clot
3. deficiency, blockage
4. heat
5. yellowish, fatty plaque
6. electricity, electrical activity

Exercise 8

1. thromb/o
2. ech/o
3. isch/o
4. ather/o
5. therm/o
6. electr/o

Exercise 9

1. slow
2. instrument used to record; record
3. abnormal reduction in number
4. hardening
5. pain
6. removal
7. formation
8. pertaining to

Exercise 10

1. -poiesis
2. -ac
3. -sclerosis
4. -graph
5. -penia
6. -odynia
7. brady-
8. -apheresis

Exercise 11

Pronunciation Exercise

Exercise 12

1. P   WR   S
   endo/card/itis
   inflammation of the inner (lining) of the heart
2. P   WR   S
   brady/card/ia
   condition of slow heart (rate)
3. WR   CV   S
   cardi/o/megaly
      CF
   enlargement of the heart
4. WR   CV   S
   arteri/o/sclerosis
      CF
   hardening of the arteries
5. WR CV WR   S
   cardi/o/valvul/itis
      CF
   inflammation of the valves of the heart

6. WR   S
myel/oma
(multiple) tumors of the bone marrow

7. P   WR   S
tachy/card/ia
abnormal state of rapid heart (rate)

8. WR CV   S
angi/o/stenosis
   CF
narrowing of blood vessels

9. WR   S
thromb/us
(blood) clot

10. WR   S
isch/emia
deficiency of blood (flow)

11. P   WR   S
peri/card/itis
inflammation of the sac
   surrounding the heart

12. WR   S
cardi/odynia
pain in the heart

13. WR   S
aort/ic stenosis
narrowing, pertaining to the aorta

14. WR   S
thromb/osis
abnormal condition of a (blood) clot

15. WR CV   S
ather/o/sclerosis
   CF
hardening of fatty plaque (deposited
   on the arterial wall)

16. WR CV WR   S
my/o/card/itis
   CF
inflammation of the muscle of the
   heart

17. WR   S
angi/oma
tumor composed of blood vessels

18. WR   S
thym/oma
tumor of the thymus gland

19. WR   S
lymph/oma
tumor of lymphatic tissue

20. WR   S
lymphaden/itis
inflammation of lymph nodes

21. WR CV   S
splen/o/megaly
   CF
enlargement of the spleen

22. WR   S
hemat/oma
tumor of blood

23. P   WR   S
poly/arter/itis
inflammation of many (sites in the)
   arteries

24. WR   CV WR CV S
cardi/o/my/o/pathy
   CF   CF
disease of the heart muscle

25. WR   CV   S
lymphaden/o/pathy
   CF
disease of the lymph nodes

26. WR   CV WR   S
thromb/o/phleb/itis
   CF
inflammation of a vein associated
   with a clot

27. WR   S
phleb/itis
inflammation of a vein

28. P   WR CV S
pan/cyt/o/penia
   CF
abnormal reduction of all (blood)
   cells

Exercise 13

1. myel/oma
2. cardi/o/megaly
3. isch/emia
4. endo/card/itis
5. brady/card/ia
6. arteri/o/sclerosis
7. thromb/osis
8. cardi/odynia
9. my/o/card/itis
10. angi/o/stenosis
11. tachy/card/ia
12. ather/o/sclerosis
13. angi/oma
14. cardi/o/valvul/itis
15. aort/ic stenosis
16. peri/card/itis
17. lymph/oma
18. thym/oma
19. splen/o/megaly
20. hemat/oma
21. lymphaden/itis
22. cardi/o/my/o/pathy
23. poly/arter/itis
24. lymphaden/o/pathy
25. thromb/o/phleb/itis
26. phleb/itis
27. thromb/us
28. pan/cyt/o/penia

Exercise 14

Spelling Exercise; see text p. 413.

Exercise 15

Pronunciation Exercise

Exercise 16

1. coarctation
2. embolus
3. cardiac arrest
4. congenital
5. varicose veins
6. coronary occlusion
7. aneurysm
8. Hodgkin
9. coronary artery disease
10. angina pectoris
11. myocardial infarction
12. atrial fibrillation
13. arrhythmia
14. hypertensive
15. congestive heart failure
16. peripheral arterial disease
17. hemophilia
18. leukemia
19. anemia
20. infectious mononucleosis
21. intermittent claudication
22. cardiac tamponade
23. mitral valve stenosis and rheumatic
    heart disease
24. deep vein thrombosis
25. acute coronary syndrome

Exercise 17

1. d	8. k
2. c	9. g
3. f	10. b
4. e	11. h
5. a	12. l
6. j	13. n
7. i	14. m

Exercise 18

1. i	7. d
2. e	8. k
3. a	9. l
4. h	10. g
5. j	11. c
6. b	12. f

Exercise 19

Spelling Exercise; see text p. 422.

Exercise 20

Pronunciation Exercise

Exercise 21

1. P   WR CV S
   peri/cardi/o/centesis
                  CF
   surgical puncture to aspirate fluid
      from the outer layer of the heart
      (pericardial sac)
2. WR   S
   thym/ectomy
   excision of the thymus gland
3. WR CV S
   angi/o/plasty
        CF
   surgical repair of a blood vessel
4. WR CV S
   splen/o/pexy
         CF
   surgical fixation of the spleen
5. WR   CV S
   valvul/o/plasty
          CF
   surgical repair of a valve
6. P   WR   S
   end/arter/ectomy
   excision within an artery
7. WR CV S
   phleb/o/tomy
         CF
   incision into a vein
8. WR   S
   splen/ectomy
   excision of the spleen
9. WR   S
   phleb/ectomy
   excision of a vein
10. WR   S
    ather/ectomy
    excision of yellowish, fatty plaque

Exercise 22

1. end/arter/ectomy
2. splen/o/pexy
3. valvul/o/plasty
4. phleb/o/tomy
5. thym/ectomy
6. peri/cardi/o/centesis
7. angi/o/plasty
8. splen/ectomy
9. phleb/ectomy
10. ather/ectomy

Exercise 23
Spelling Exercise; see text p. 425.

Exercise 24
Pronunciation Exercise

Exercise 25

1. ablation
2. percutaneous transluminal coronary
   angioplasty
3. cardiac pacemaker
4. blood cells
5. coronary artery bypass graft
6. aneurysmectomy
7. femoropopliteal bypass
8. intracoronary thrombolytic
9. bone marrow transplant
10. embolectomy
11. coronary stent
12. implantable cardiac defibrillator

Exercise 26

1. h   8. c
2. m   9. i
3. k   10. b
4. l   11. j
5. d   12. g
6. e   13. f
7. a

Exercise 27
Spelling Exercise; see text p. 431.

Exercise 28
Pronunciation Exercise

Exercise 29

1. WR CV WR CV S
   electr/o/cardi/o/graph
        CF   CF
   instrument used to record the
      electrical activity of the heart
2. WR CV S
   ven/o/gram
        CF
   radiographic image of the veins (after
      an injection of contrast medium)
3. WR CV S
   angi/o/graphy
        CF
   radiographic imaging of a blood vessel
4. WR CV WR CV S
   ech/o/cardi/o/gram
       CF   CF
   record of the heart by using sound
5. WR CV S
   aort/o/gram
        CF
   radiographic image of the aorta (after
      an injection of contrast medium)
6. WR CV WR CV S
   electr/o/cardi/o/gram
        CF   CF
   record of the electrical activity of the
   heart

7. WR CV S
   arteri/o/gram
         CF
   radiographic image of an artery (after
      an injection of contrast medium)
8. WR CV WR CV S
   electr/o/cardi/o/graphy
        CF   CF
   process of recording the electrical
      activity of the heart
9. WR CV S
   angi/o/scopy
        CF
   visual examination of a blood vessel
10. WR CV   S
    ven/o/graphy
         CF
    radiographic imaging a vein
11. WR CV   S
    angi/o/scope
         CF
    instrument used for visual
       examination of a blood vessel

Exercise 30

1. electr/o/cardi/o/graph
2. arteri/o/gram
3. ven/o/gram
4. angi/o/graphy
5. electr/o/cardi/o/gram
6. ech/o/cardi/o/gram
7. aort/o/gram
8. electr/o/cardi/o/graphy
9. angi/o/scopy
10. ven/o/graphy
11. angi/o/scope

Exercise 31
Spelling Exercise; see text p. 435.

Exercise 32
Pronunciation Exercise

Exercise 33

1. sphygmomanometer
2. coagulation time
3. complete blood count and differential
   count
4. Doppler ultrasound
5. stethoscope
6. blood pressure
7. prothrombin time
8. cardiac catheterization
9. hemoglobin
10. impedance plethysmography
11. thallium test
12. transesophageal echocardiogram
13. single-photon emission computed
    tomography
14. exercise stress test

15. digital subtraction angiography
16. auscultation
17. creatine phosphokinase
18. C-reactive protein
19. pulse
20. homocysteine
21. troponin
22. lipid profile
23. percussion
24. hematocrit

Exercise 34
1. d   7. c
2. l   8. a
3. h   9. e
4. m   10. b
5. g   11. f
6. j   12. i

Exercise 35
1. d   7. e
2. g   8. a
3. b   9. i
4. c   10. j
5. f   11. k
6. h   12. l

Exercise 36
Spelling Exercise; see text pp. 443-444.

Exercise 37
Pronunciation Exercise

Exercise 38
1. P   WR S
   hypo/therm/ia
   condition of (body) temperature that
   is below (normal)
2. WR CV S
   hemat/o/poiesis
        CF
   formation of blood (cells)
3. WR CV S
   cardi/o/logy
        CF
   study of the heart
4. WR CV S
   cardi/o/logist
        CF
   physician who studies and treats
   diseases of the heart
5. WR CV S
   hem/o/lysis
        CF
   dissolution of blood (cells)
6. WR CV S
   hemat/o/logist
        CF
   physician who studies and treats
   diseases of the blood

7. WR S
   cardi/ac
   pertaining to the heart
8. WR CV S
   hemat/o/logy
        CF
   study of the blood
9. WR   S
   plasm/apheresis
   removal of plasma (from withdrawn
   blood)
10. WR CV S
    hem/o/stasis
         CF
    stoppage of bleeding
11. WR CV S
    cardi/o/genic
         CF
    originating in the heart
12. WR CV S
    myel/o/poiesis
         CF
    formation of bone marrow
13. WR CV S
    thromb/o/lysis
         CF
    dissolution of a clot
14. WR CV WR   S
    atri/o/ventricul/ar
         CF
    pertaining to the atrium and ventricle
15. P   WR S
    intra/ven/ous
    pertaining to within the vein
16. WR CV S
    phleb/o/logist
         CF
    physician who studies and treats
    disease of the veins
17. WR CV S
    phleb/o/logy
         CF
    study of veins

Exercise 39
1. cardi/o/logy
2. hemat/o/poiesis
3. hypo/therm/ia
4. hem/o/lysis
5. plasm/apheresis
6. hemat/o/logist
7. cardi/ac
8. cardi/o/logist
9. hemat/o/logy
10. hem/o/stasis
11. myel/o/poiesis

12. cardi/o/genic
13. thromb/o/lysis
14. atri/o/ventricul/ar
15. intra/ven/ous
16. phleb/o/logy
17. phleb/o/logist

Exercise 40
Spelling Exercise; see text p. 447.

Exercise 41
Pronunciation Exercise

Exercise 42
1. vasoconstrictor
2. lumen
3. cardiopulmonary resuscitation
4. diastole
5. fibrillation
6. hypotension
7. extravasation
8. venipuncture
9. systole
10. vasodilator
11. hypertension
12. occlude
13. hypertriglyceridemia
14. hyperlipidemia
15. hemorrhage
16. anticoagulant
17. hypercholesterolemia
18. dyscrasia
19. heart murmur
20. extracorporeal
21. lipids
22. defibrillation

Exercise 43
1. space within a tubelike structure
2. escape of blood from the blood vessel
   into the tissues
3. excessive amount of cholesterol in the
   blood
4. puncture of a vein to remove blood,
   start an intravenous infusion, or in-
   still medication
5. agent or nerve that enlarges the
   blood vessels
6. blood pressure that is above normal
7. emergency procedure consisting of
   artificial ventilation and external cardiac massage
8. phase in the cardiac cycle in which
   ventricles contract
9. blood pressure that is below normal
10. agent or nerve that narrows blood
    vessels
11. cardiac cycle phase in which ventri-
    cles relax

12. rapid, quivering, noncoordinated contractions of the atria and ventricles
13. to close tightly
14. excessive amount of fat in the blood
15. excessive amount of triglycerides in the blood
16. abnormal or pathologic condition of the blood
17. rapid flow of blood
18. agent that slows down the clotting process
19. occurring outside the body
20. humming sound of cardiac or vascular origin
21. fats and fatlike substances that serve as a source of fuel in the body
22. application of electric shock to the myocardium to restore normal heart rhythm

Exercise 44
Spelling Exercise; see text p. 452.

Exercise 45
Pronunciation Exercise

Exercise 46

1. e		8. d	
2. n		9. a	
3. k		10. h	
4. j		11. c	
5. f		12. i	
6. m		13. b	
7. g		14. l	

Exercise 47
Spelling Exercise; see text p. 455.

Exercise 48
1. coronary artery disease; electrocardiogram; single-photon emission computed tomography; echocardiogram
2. deep vein thrombosis; impedance plethysmography
3. complete blood count; red blood cell, white blood cell, hemoglobin, hematocrit
4. coronary artery bypass graft; percutaneous transluminal coronary angioplasty
5. myocardial infarction; coronary care unit
6. blood pressure
7. congestive heart failure
8. cardiopulmonary resuscitation
9. hypertensive heart disease
10. prothrombin time
11. atrioventricular
12. acute coronary syndrome
13. peripheral arterial disease
14. digital subtraction angiography
15. transesophageal echocardiogram
16. C-reactive protein, creatine phosphokinase
17. atrial fibrillation
18. implantable cardiac defibrillator

Exercise 49
A.
  1. angina pectoris
  2. thallium test
  3. ischemia
  4. angiography
  5. stenosis
  6. angioplasty
  7. cardiologist
  8. electrocardiography
  9. cardiac catheterization
  10. creatine phosphokinase
  11. troponin
  12. myocardial infarction

B.
  1. high   3. c
  2. c   4. b

Exercise 50
1. atherosclerosis
2. thrombophlebitis
3. myocarditis
4. myocardial infarction
5. endarterectomy
6. infectious mononucleosis
7. hypothermia
8. impedance plethysmography
9. murmur
10. angioscope, angioscopy
11. thallium test
12. allergist
13. anaphylaxis

Exercise 51
Reading Exercise

Exercise 52
1. *F*, the diagnosis was made with an ultrasound procedure.
2. c
3. d

CHAPTER 11
Digestive System

OUTLINE

ANATOMY, 472

WORD PARTS, 477
Combining Forms, 477
Prefix, 483
Suffix, 483

MEDICAL TERMS, 483
Disease and Disorder Terms, 483
    Built from Word Parts, 483
    Not Built from Word Parts, 489
Surgical Terms, 494
    Built from Word Parts, 494
    Not Built from Word Parts, 501
Diagnostic Terms, 504
    Built from Word Parts, 504
    Not Built from Word Parts, 512
Complementary Terms, 515
    Built from Word Parts, 515
    Not Built from Word Parts, 519
Abbreviations, 523

PRACTICAL APPLICATION, 524
Interact with Medical Documents, 524
Interpret Medical Terms, 527
Read Medical Terms in Use, 528
Comprehend Medical Terms in Use, 529

CHAPTER REVIEW, 529

TABLE 11-1 BARIATRIC SURGERY, 503

OBJECTIVES

Upon completion of this chapter you will be able to:

1. Identify organs and structures of the digestive system.

2. Define and spell word parts related to the digestive system.

3. Define, pronounce, and spell disease and disorder terms related to the digestive system.

4. Define, pronounce, and spell surgical terms related to the digestive system.

5. Define, pronounce, and spell diagnostic terms related to the digestive system.

6. Define, pronounce, and spell complementary terms related to the digestive system.

7. Interpret the meaning of abbreviations related to the digestive system.

8. Interpret, read, and comprehend medical language in simulated medical statements and documents.

ANATOMY

Function

The digestive tract, also known as the **alimentary canal** or the **gastrointestinal tract,** sometimes abbreviated as **GI tract,** is made up of several digestive organs. The organs connect to form a continuous passageway from the mouth to the anus (Figures 11-1, *A* and *B*, and 11-2). With the help of accessory organs, the digestive tract prepares ingested food for use by the body cells through physical and chemical digestion and eliminates the solid waste products from the body.

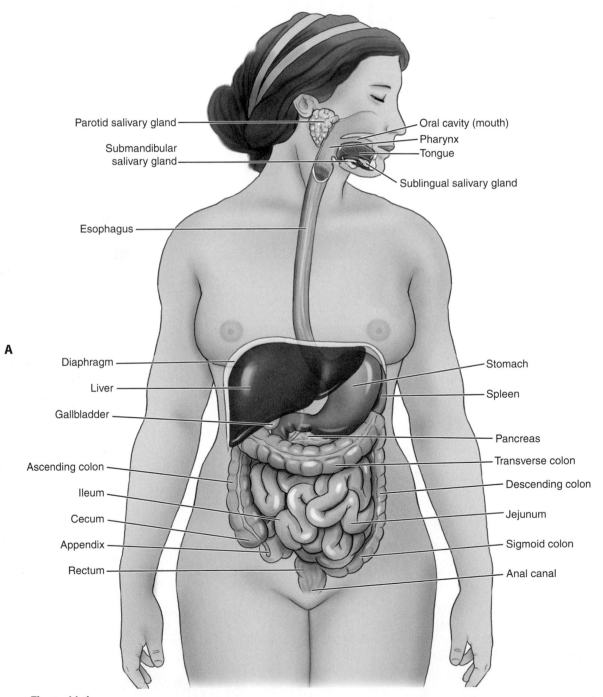

A

Figure 11-1
A, Organs of the digestive system.

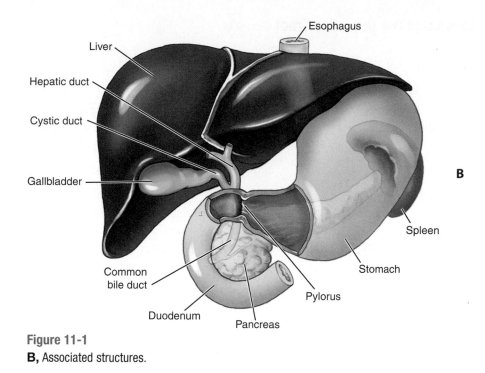

Figure 11-1
B, Associated structures.

Organs of the Digestive Tract

Term	Definition
mouth	opening through which food passes into the body; breaks food into small particles by mastication (chewing) and mixing with saliva
tongue	consists mostly of skeletal muscle; attached in the posterior region of the mouth. It provides movement of food for mastication, directs food to the pharynx for swallowing, and is a major organ for taste and speech.
palate	separates the nasal cavity from the oral cavity
soft palate	posterior portion, not supported by bone
hard palate.	anterior portion, supported by bone
uvula.	soft V-shaped mass that extends from the soft palate; directs food into the throat
pharynx, throat.	performs the swallowing action that passes food from the mouth into the esophagus
esophagus	10-inch (25-cm) tube that extends from the pharynx to the stomach

Hard palate   Soft palate

Uvula   Tongue

Figure 11-2
The oral cavity.

Organs of the Digestive Tract—*cont'd*

Term	Definition
stomach	J-shaped sac that mixes and stores food. It secretes chemicals for digestion and hormones for local communication control
cardia	area around the opening of the esophagus
fundus	uppermost domed portion of the stomach
body	central portion of the stomach
antrum	lower portion of the stomach
pylorus	portion of the stomach that connects to the small intestine
pyloric sphincter	ring of muscle that guards the opening between the stomach and the duodenum
small intestine	20-foot (6-m) canal extending from the pyloric sphincter to the large intestine
duodenum	first 10 to 12 inches (25 cm) of the small intestine
jejunum	second portion of the small intestine, approximately 8 feet (2.4 m) long
ileum	third portion of the small intestine, approximately 11 feet (3.3 m) long, which connects with the large intestine
large intestine	canal that is approximately 5 feet (1.5 m) long and extends from the ileum to the anus (Figure 11-3)
cecum	blind U-shaped pouch that is the first portion of the large intestine (Figure 11-3)
colon	next portion of the large intestine. The colon is divided into four parts: ascending colon, transverse colon, descending colon, and sigmoid colon (Figure 11-3).
rectum	remaining portion of the large intestine, approximately 8 to 10 inches (20 cm) long, extending from the sigmoid colon to the anus
anus	sphincter muscle (ringlike band of muscle fiber that keeps an opening tight) at the end of the digestive tract

ACCESSORY ORGANS

salivary glands	produce saliva, which flows into the mouth
liver	produces bile, which is necessary for the digestion of fats. The liver performs many other functions concerned with digestion and metabolism

DUODENUM is derived from the Latin **duodeni,** meaning **12 each,** a reference to its length. It was named in 240 BC by a Greek physician.

Jejunum is derived from the Latin **jejunus,** meaning **empty;** it was so named because the early anatomists always found it empty.

Ileum is derived from the Greek **eilein,** meaning **to roll,** a reference to the peristaltic waves that move food along the digestive tract. This term was first used in the early part of the seventeenth century.

Term	Definition
bile ducts	passageways that carry bile: the **hepatic duct** is a passageway for bile from the liver, and the **cystic duct** carries bile from the gallbladder. They join to form the **common bile duct,** which conveys bile to the duodenum. Collectively, these passageways are referred to as the **biliary tract.**
gallbladder	small, saclike structure that stores bile
pancreas.	produces pancreatic juice, which helps digest all types of food and secretes insulin for carbohydrate metabolism (see Figure 11-1, *B*)

OTHER STRUCTURES

peritoneum	serous saclike lining of the abdominal and pelvic cavities
appendix.	small pouch, which has no function in digestion, attached to the cecum (also called **vermiform appendix**) (see Figures 11-1 and 11-3)
abdomen.	portion of the body between the thorax and the pelvis

BILIARY SYSTEM
The liver, bile ducts, and gallbladder comprise the biliary system, which creates, transports, stores, and releases bile into the small intestine to facilitate the absorption of fat.

 PANCREAS
is derived from the Greek *pan,* meaning **all,** and *krea,* meaning **flesh.** The pancreas was first described in 300 BC. It was so named because of its fleshy appearance.

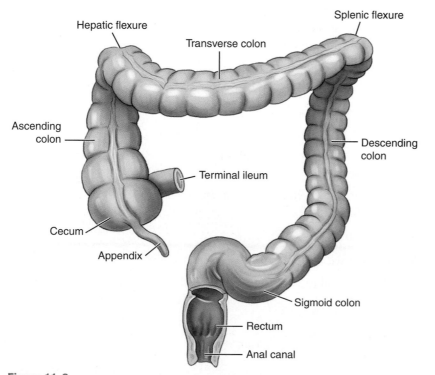

Figure 11-3
Anatomy of the large intestine.

EXERCISE 1

Fill in the blanks with the correct terms.

The digestive tract, also known as the (1) _____ _____, and (2) _____ _____, begins with the mouth, connects with the throat, or (3) _____, and continues on to a 10-inch tube called the (4) _____; this connects with the (5) _____, a J-shaped sac that mixes and stores food.

The small intestine, the next portion of the digestive tract, is made up of three portions. They are called the (6) _____, (7) _____, and (8) _____. The small intestine connects with the first portion of the large intestine, the (9) _____, and then connects with the colon, which is divided into four parts called (10) _____ _____, (11) _____ _____, (12) _____ _____, and (13) _____ _____. The (14) _____ extends from the sigmoid colon to the (15) _____.

EXERCISE 2

Match the definitions in the first column with the correct terms in the second column.

_____ 1. lower portion of the stomach

_____ 2. hangs from the roof of the mouth

_____ 3. produce saliva

_____ 4. produces bile

_____ 5. separates the nasal cavity from the oral cavity

_____ 6. guards the opening between the stomach and the duodenum

_____ 7. secretes insulin for carbohydrate metabolism

_____ 8. small pouch that has no function in digestion

_____ 9. lining of the abdominal and pelvic cavities

_____ 10. portion of the body between the pelvis and thorax

_____ 11. stores bile

_____ 12. uppermost domed portion of the stomach

_____ 13. directs food to the pharynx for swallowing

a. salivary glands

b. pancreas

c. peritoneum

d. uvula

e. gallbladder

f. tongue

g. abdomen

h. liver

i. appendix

j. pyloric sphincter

k. fundus

l. antrum

m. palate

WORD PARTS

Word parts you need to learn to complete this chapter are listed on the following pages. The exercises at the end of each list will help you learn their definitions and spellings.

Combining Forms of Digestive Tract Terms

Combining Form	Definition
an/o	anus
antr/o	antrum
cec/o	cecum
col/o, colon/o	colon (usually denoting the large intestine)
duoden/o	duodenum
enter/o	intestine (usually denoting the small intestine)
esophag/o (NOTE: *esophag/o* was covered in Chapter 9.)	esophagus
gastr/o	stomach
ile/o	ileum
jejun/o	jejunum
or/o, stomat/o	mouth
proct/o, rect/o	rectum
sigmoid/o	sigmoid colon

EXERCISE FIGURE A

Fill in the blanks with combining forms in this diagram of the digestive system.

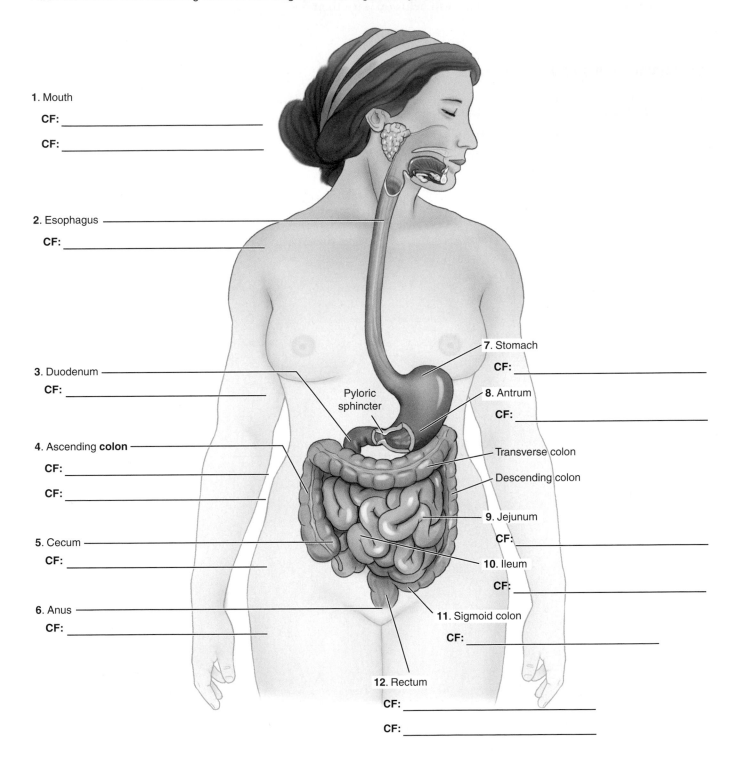

1. Mouth

   CF: _____

   CF: _____

2. Esophagus

   CF: _____

3. Duodenum

   CF: _____

4. Ascending **colon**

   CF: _____

   CF: _____

5. Cecum

   CF: _____

6. Anus

   CF: _____

Pyloric
sphincter

7. Stomach

   CF: _____

8. Antrum

   CF: _____

Transverse colon

Descending colon

9. Jejunum

   CF: _____

10. Ileum

    CF: _____

11. Sigmoid colon

    CF: _____

12. Rectum

    CF: _____

    CF: _____

EXERCISE 3

Write the definitions of the following combining forms.

1. proct/o _____

2. gastr/o _____

3. an/o _____

4. cec/o _____

5. ile/o _____

6. stomat/o _____

7. duoden/o _____

8. col/o _____

9. or/o _____

10. enter/o _____

11. rect/o _____

12. antr/o _____

13. esophag/o _____

14. jejun/o _____

15. sigmoid/o _____

_____

16. colon/o _____

EXERCISE 4

Write the combining form for each of the following terms.

1. cecum _____

2. stomach _____

3. ileum _____

4. jejunum _____

5. sigmoid colon _____

6. esophagus _____

7. rectum   a. _____

    b. _____

8. intestine _____

9. duodenum _____

10. colon   a. _____

    b. _____

11. mouth   a. _____

    b. _____

12. anus _____

13. antrum _____

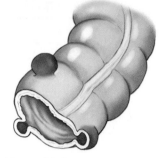

Figure 11-4
Diverticulum of the large intestine.

Combining Forms of the Accessory Organs/Combining Forms Commonly Used with Digestive System Terms

Combining Form	Definition
abdomin/o, celi/o, lapar/o	abdomen (abdominal cavity)
appendic/o	appendix
cheil/o	lip
cholangi/o	bile duct
chol/e (NOTE: the combining vowel is *e*.)	gall, bile
choledoch/o	common bile duct
diverticul/o	diverticulum, or blind pouch, extending from a hollow organ (*pl.* diverticula) (Figure 11-4)
gingiv/o	gum
gloss/o, lingu/o	tongue
hepat/o	liver
herni/o	hernia, or protrusion of an organ through a membrane or cavity wall (Figure 11-5)
palat/o	palate
pancreat/o	pancreas
peritone/o	peritoneum
polyp/o	polyp, small growth
pylor/o (NOTE: *pylor/o* was covered in Chapter 9.)	pylorus, pyloric sphincter
sial/o	saliva, salivary gland
steat/o	fat
uvul/o	uvula

HERNIA
The layman's term for hernia is **rupture.** Types include abdominal, hiatal, or diaphragmatic, inguinal, and umbilical hernia.

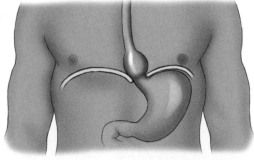

A **B** **C**

Figure 11-5
Types of hernias. **A,** Hiatal. **B,** Inguinal. **C,** Umbilical.

EXERCISE FIGURE B

Fill in the blanks with combining forms in this diagram of the digestive system and associated structures.

1. Palate

    CF: _____

2. Uvula

    CF: _____

3. Tongue

    CF: _____

    CF: _____

4. Gallbladder

    CF: _____ (gall)

    CF: _____ (bladder)

5. Pyloric sphincter

    CF: _____

6. Appendix

    CF: _____

7. Gums

    CF: _____

8. Lips

    CF: _____

9. Salivary glands

    CF: _____

10. Liver

    CF: _____

11. Bile ducts

    CF: _____

12. Common bile duct

    CF: _____

13. Pancreas

    CF: _____

14. Abdomen

    CF: _____

    CF: _____

    CF: _____

EXERCISE 5

Write the definitions of the following combining forms.

1. herni/o _____
2. abdomin/o _____
3. sial/o _____
4. chol/e _____
5. diverticul/o _____
6. gingiv/o _____
7. appendic/o _____
8. gloss/o _____
9. hepat/o _____
10. cheil/o _____
11. peritone/o _____

12. palat/o _____
13. pancreat/o _____
14. lapar/o _____
15. lingu/o _____
16. choledoch/o _____
17. pylor/o _____
18. uvul/o _____
19. cholangi/o _____
20. polyp/o _____
21. celi/o _____
22. steat/o _____

EXERCISE 6

Write the combining form for each of the following.

1. palate _____
2. saliva, salivary gland _____
3. pancreas _____
4. peritoneum _____
5. tongue a. _____
           b. _____
6. gum _____
7. pylorus, pyloric sphincter _____
8. liver _____
9. gall, bile _____
10. abdomen
    a. _____
    b. _____
    c. _____

11. hernia _____
12. diverticulum _____
13. lip _____
14. appendix _____
15. uvula _____
16. bile duct _____
17. common bile duct _____
18. small growth _____
19. fat _____

Prefix

Prefix	Definition
hemi-	half

Suffix

Suffix	Definition
-pepsia	digestion

Refer to Appendix A and Appendix B for a complete listing of word parts.

EXERCISE 7

Write the definition of the following prefix and suffix.

1. -pepsia _____

2. hemi- _____

EXERCISE 8

Write the prefix and suffix for the following definition.

1. digestion   _____

2. half   _____

MEDICAL TERMS

The terms you need to learn to complete this chapter are listed below. The exercises following each list will help you learn the definition and the spelling of each word.

See Appendix J on Evolve for terms relating to nutrition.

Disease and Disorder Terms
Built from Word Parts

The following terms are built from word parts you have already learned and can be translated literally to find their meanings. Further explanation of terms beyond the definition of their word parts, if needed, is included in parentheses.

Term	Definition
appendicitis . . . . (a-*pen*-di-SĪ-tis)	inflammation of the appendix (Exercise Figure C)
cholangioma. . . . . (kō-LAN-jē-ō-ma)	tumor of the bile duct

EXERCISE FIGURE C

Fill in the blanks to complete labeling of the diagram.

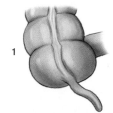

1. Normal appendix.

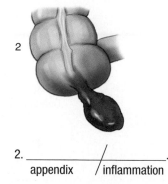

2. _____ / _____.
   appendix   / inflammation

Disease and Disorder Terms—*cont'd*

Built from Word Parts

Term	Definition
cholecystitis . . . . (kō-lē-sis-TĪ-tis)	inflammation of the gallbladder
choledocholithiasis . . . . (kō-led-o-kō-li-THĪ-a-sis)	condition of stones in the common bile duct (Exercise Figure D)
cholelithiasis . . . . (kō-le-li-THĪ-a-sis)	condition of gallstones (Exercise Figure D)
diverticulitis . . . . (dī-ver-tik-ū-LĪ-tis)	inflammation of a diverticulum (see Figure 11-4)
diverticulosis . . . . (dī-ver-tik-ū-LŌ-sis)	abnormal condition of having diverticula (see Figures 11-4 and 11-14, *B*)
esophagitis . . . . (e-sof-a-JĪ-tis)	inflammation of the esophagus
gastritis . . . . (gas-TRĪ-tis)	inflammation of the stomach
gastroenteritis . . . . (*gas*-trō-en-te-RĪ-tis)	inflammation of the stomach and intestines

EXERCISE FIGURE   D

Fill in the blanks to complete labeling of the diagram.

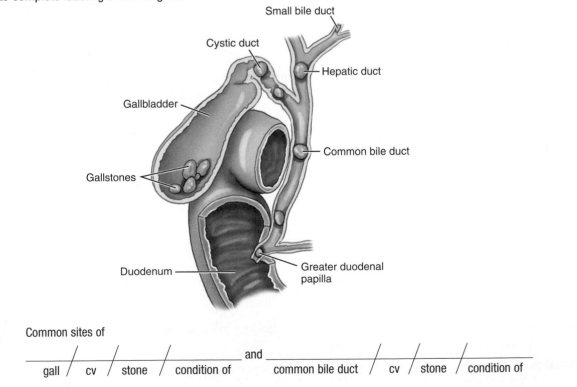

Small bile duct

Cystic duct

Hepatic duct

Gallbladder

Common bile duct

Gallstones

Duodenum

Greater duodenal papilla

Common sites of

_____ / ____ / _____ / _____   and   _____ / ____ / _____ / _____
gall / cv / stone / condition of   common bile duct / cv / stone / condition of

Term	Definition
gastroenterocolitis . . . . (*gas*-trō-*en*-ter-ō-kōl-Ī-tis)	inflammation of the stomach, intestines, and colon
gingivitis . . . . (jin-ji-VĪ-tis)	inflammation of the gums
hepatitis . . . . (hep-a-TĪ-tis)	inflammation of the liver
hepatoma . . . . (hep-a-TŌ-ma)	tumor of the liver
palatitis . . . . (pal-a-TĪ-tis)	inflammation of the palate
pancreatitis . . . . (*pan*-krē-a-TĪ-tis)	inflammation of the pancreas
peritonitis . . . . (per-i-tō-NĪ-tis) (NOTE: the *e* is dropped from the combining form peritone/o.)	inflammation of the peritoneum
polyposis . . . . (pol-i-PŌ-sis)	abnormal condition of (multiple) polyps (in the mucous membrane of the intestine, especially the colon; high potential for malignancy) (Figure 11-6)
proctoptosis . . . . (*prok*-top-TŌ-sis)	prolapse of the rectum
rectocele . . . . (REK-tō-sēl)	protrusion of the rectum
sialolith . . . . (sī-AL-ō-lith)	stone in the salivary gland
steatohepatitis . . . . (*stē*-a-tō-*hep*-a-TĪ-tis)	inflammation of the liver associated with (excess) fat; (often caused by alcohol abuse and over time may cause cirrhosis)
uvulitis . . . . (ū-vū-LĪ-tis)	inflammation of the uvula

NASH
or nonalcoholic **steatohepatitis** may occur in nonalcoholic patients who are obese and/or suffer from type 2 diabetes mellitus.

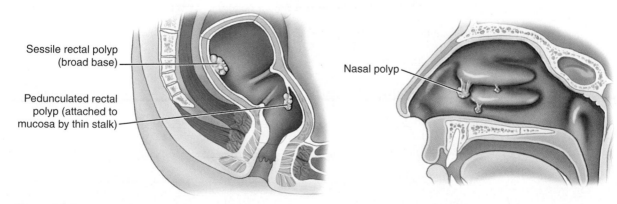

Sessile rectal polyp (broad base)

Pedunculated rectal polyp (attached to mucosa by thin stalk)

Nasal polyp

Figure 11-6
Polyp is a general term used to describe a protruding growth from a mucous membrane. Polyps are commonly found in the nose, uterus, intestines, and urinary bladder.

EXERCISE 9

Practice saying aloud each of the disease and disorder terms built from word parts on pp. 483-485.

 To hear the terms select Chapter 11, Chapter Exercises, Pronunciation.

☐ Place a check mark in the box when you have completed this exercise.

EXERCISE 10

Analyze and define the following terms.

1. cholelithiasis _____

2. diverticulosis _____

3. sialolith _____

4. hepatoma _____

5. uvulitis _____

6. pancreatitis _____

7. proctoptosis _____

8. gingivitis _____

9. gastritis _____

10. rectocele _____

11. palatitis _____

12. hepatitis _____

13. appendicitis _____

14. cholecystitis _____

15. diverticulitis _____

16. gastroenteritis _____

17. gastroenterocolitis _____

18. choledocholithiasis _____

19. cholangioma _____

20. polyposis _____

21. esophagitis _____

22. peritonitis _____

23. steatohepatitis _____

EXERCISE 11

Build disease and disorder terms for the following definitions by using the word parts you have learned.

1. tumor of the liver

   _____ / _____
   WR   S

2. inflammation of the stomach

   _____ / _____
   WR   S

3. stone in the salivary gland

   _____ / CV / _____
   WR   WR

4. inflammation of the appendix

   _____ / _____
   WR   S

5. inflammation of a diverticulum

   _____ / _____
   WR   S

6. inflammation of the gallbladder

   _____ / CV / _____ / _____
   WR   WR   S

7. abnormal condition of having diverticula

   _____ / _____
   WR   S

8. inflammation of the stomach and intestines

   _____ / CV / _____ / _____
   WR   WR   S

9. prolapse of the rectum

   _____ / CV / _____
   WR   S

10. protrusion of the rectum

    _____ / CV / _____
    WR   S

11. inflammation of the uvula

    _____ / _____
    WR   S

12. inflammation of the gums

    _____ / _____
    WR   S

13. inflammation of the liver

    _____ / _____
    WR   S

14. inflammation of the palate

    _____ / _____
    WR   S

15. condition of gallstones

    _____ / CV / _____ / _____
    WR   WR   S

16. inflammation of the liver associated with (excess) fat

    _____ / CV / _____ / _____
    WR   WR   S

17. inflammation of the stomach, intestines, and colon

    _____ / CV / _____ / CV / _____ / _____
    WR   WR   WR   S

18. inflammation of the pancreas

    _____ / _____
    WR   S

19. tumor of the bile duct

_____ / _____
WR   S

20. inflammation of the
esophagus

_____ / _____
WR   S

21. condition of stones in the
common bile duct

_____ / _____ / _____ / _____
WR   CV   WR   S

22. abnormal condition of
(multiple) polyps

_____ / _____
WR   S

23. inflammation of the
peritoneum

_____ / _____
WR   S

EXERCISE 12

Spell each of the disease and disorder terms built from word parts on pp. 483-485 by
having someone dictate them to you.

 To hear and spell the terms select Chapter 11, Chapter Exercises, Spelling. You
may type the terms on the screen or write them below in the spaces provided.

☐ Place a check mark in the box if you have completed this exercise using your CD-ROM.

1._____

2._____

3._____

4._____

5._____

6._____

7._____

8._____

9._____

10._____

11._____

12._____

13. _____

14. _____

15. _____

16. _____

17. _____

18. _____

19. _____

20. _____

21. _____

22. _____

23. _____

Disease and Disorder Terms
Not Built from Word Parts

In some of the following terms, you may recognize word parts you have already learned; however, the full meaning of the terms cannot be discerned by the definition of their word parts.

Term	Definition
adhesion................. (ad-HĒ-zhun)	abnormal growing together of two surfaces that normally are separated. This may occur after abdominal surgery; surgical treatment is called **adhesiolysis** or **adhesiotomy** (Figure 11-7, *A*).
anorexia nervosa .... (*an*-ō-REK-sē-a) (ner-VŌ-sa)	eating disorder characterized by a prolonged refusal to eat, resulting in emaciation, amenorrhea in females, and abnormal fear of becoming obese. It occurs primarily in adolescents and young adults.
bulimia nervosa .... (bū-LĒ-mē-a) (ner-VŌ-sa)	an eating disorder involving gorging with food, followed by induced vomiting or laxative abuse (binging and purging)
cirrhosis .... (sir-RŌ-sis)	chronic disease of the liver with gradual destruction of cells and formation of scar tissue; commonly caused by alcoholism

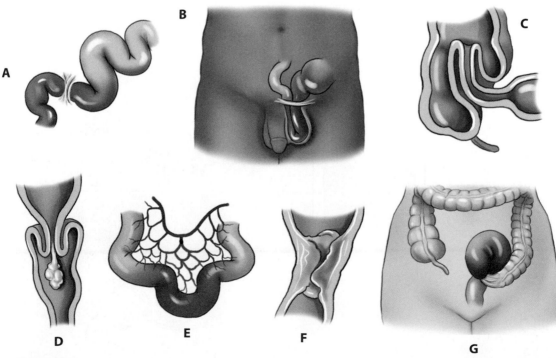

Figure 11-7

Causes of intestinal obstruction. **A,** Adhesions. **B,** Strangulated inguinal hernia. **C,** Ileocecal intussusception. **D,** Intussusception caused by polyps. **E,** Mesenteric vascular occlusion. **F,** Neoplasm. **G,** Volvulus of the sigmoid colon.

Disease and Disorder Terms—*cont'd*

Not Built from Word Parts

Term	Definition
Crohn disease (krōn) (di-ZĒZ)	chronic inflammation of the intestinal tract usually affecting the ileum and characterized by cobblestone ulcerations and the formation of scar tissue that may lead to intestinal obstruction (also called **regional ileitis** or **regional enteritis**.)
duodenal ulcer (*dū*-o-DĒ-nal) (UL-ser)	ulcer in the duodenum (Figure 11-9)
gastric ulcer (GAS-trik) (UL-ser)	ulcer in the stomach (Figure 11-9)
gastroesophageal reflux disease (GERD) (gas-trō-e-sof-a-JĒ-al) (RĒ-fluks) (di-ZĒZ)	the abnormal backward flow of the gastrointestinal contents into the esophagus, causing heartburn and the gradual breakdown of the mucous barrier of the esophagus
hemochromatosis (hē-mō-krō-ma-TŌ-sis)	an iron metabolism disorder that occurs when too much iron is absorbed from food, resulting in excessive deposits of iron in the tissue; can cause congestive heart failure, diabetes, cirrhosis, or cancer of the liver
hemorrhoid (HEM-o-royd)	varicose vein in the rectal area, which may be internal or external (Figure 11-8)

GASTROESOPHAGEAL REFLUX DISEASE (GERD) is a common gastrointestinal disorder. The acidity of the regurgitated stomach contents causes irritation and inflammation of the esophagus (reflux esophagitis). **Barrett esophagus,** cellular changes in the lower esophagus increasing the risk of cancer, may develop as a result of chronic GERD.

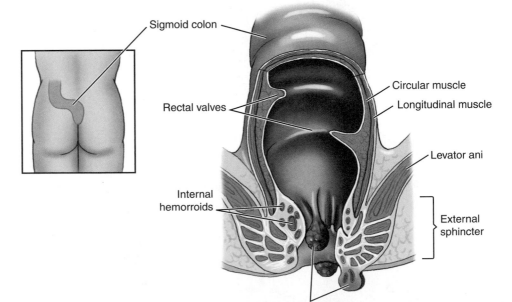

Figure 11-8
Hemorrhoids.

Term	Definition
ileus (IL-ē-us)	obstruction of the intestine, often caused by failure of peristalsis
intussusception (*in*-tu-sus-SEP-shun)	telescoping of a segment of the intestine (Figure 11-7, *C* and *D*)
irritable bowel syndrome (IBS) (IR-i-ta-bl) (BOW-el) (SIN-drōm)	periodic disturbances of bowel function, such as diarrhea and/or constipation, usually associated with abdominal pain
obesity (ō-BĒS-i-tē)	excess of body fat (not body weight)
peptic ulcer (PEP-tik) (UL-ser)	another name for gastric or duodenal ulcer (Figure 11-9)
polyp (POL-ip)	tumorlike growth extending outward from a mucous membrane; usually benign; common sites are in the nose, throat, and intestines (see Figures 11-6 and 11-12)
ulcerative colitis (UL-ser-a-tiv) (kō-LĪ-tis)	inflammation of the colon with the formation of ulcers. The main symptom is bloody diarrhea. An ileostomy may be performed to treat this condition.
volvulus (VOL-vū-lus)	twisting or kinking of the intestine, causing intestinal obstruction (see Figure 11-7, *G*)

EXERCISE 13

Practice saying aloud each of the disease and disorder terms not built from word parts on pp. 489-491.

To hear the terms select Chapter 11, Chapter Exercises, Pronunciation.

☐ Place a check mark in the box when you have completed this exercise.

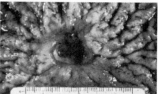

CAM TERM

Hypnotherapy is the use of the power of suggestion and a state of altered consciousness involving focused attention to promote wellness. Studies have demonstrated that hypnosis consistently produces significant results in the treatment of irritable bowel syndrome. Refer to the complementary and alternative therapies appendix on Evolve.

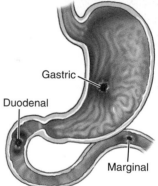

Gastric

Duodenal

Marginal

Figure 11-9
Sites of peptic ulcers.

OBESITY

is when the BMI (body mass index) is greater than 30 kg/m². Overweight is defined as BMI between 25 and 29.9 kg/m². BMI is calculated by dividing weight in kilograms by the square of height in meters (or by dividing weight in pounds by height in inches squared and then multiplying by 703).

EXERCISE 14

Match the definitions in the first column with the correct terms in the second column.

_____ 1. prolonged refusal to eat

_____ 2. chronic disease of the liver

_____ 3. chronic inflammation of the intestinal tract usually affecting the ileum

_____ 4. abnormal growing together of two surfaces

_____ 5. twisted intestine

_____ 6. gastric or duodenal ulcer

_____ 7. telescoping of a segment of the intestine

_____ 8. tumorlike growth

_____ 9. formation of ulcers in the colon

_____ 10. eating disorder involving gorging food, followed by induced vomiting

_____ 11. obstruction of the intestine

_____ 12. periodic disturbance of bowel function

_____ 13. abnormal backward flow of the gastrointestinal contents into the esophagus

_____ 14. excess of body fat

_____ 15. ulcer in the duodenum

_____ 16. ulcer in the stomach

_____ 17. varicose vein in the rectal area

_____ 18. an iron metabolism disorder

a. intussusception

b. cirrhosis

c. gastroesophageal reflux disease

d. volvulus

e. Crohn disease

f. anorexia nervosa

g. peptic ulcer

h. ulcerative colitis

i. irritable bowel syndrome

j. bulimia nervosa

k. polyp

l. obesity

m. ileus

n. adhesion

o. duodenal ulcer

p. gastric ulcer

q. hemorrhoid

r. hemochromatosis

EXERCISE 15

Write the definitions of the following terms.

1. peptic ulcer _____

2. anorexia nervosa _____

3. Crohn disease _____

4. volvulus _____

5. adhesion _____

6. cirrhosis_____

7. intussusception _____

8. gastric ulcer_____

9. duodenal ulcer _____

10. ulcerative colitis _____

11. bulimia nervosa_____

12. hemorrhoid_____

13. polyp _____

14. irritable bowel syndrome_____

15. ileus _____

16. gastroesophageal reflux disease_____

17. obesity _____

18. hemochromatosis _____

EXERCISE 16

Spell each of the disease and disorder terms not built from word parts on pp. 489–491 by having someone dictate them to you.

 To hear and spell the terms select Chapter 11, Chapter Exercises, Spelling. You may type the terms on the screen or write them below in the spaces provided.

☐ Place a check mark in the box if you have completed this exercise using your CD-ROM.

1._____   10. _____

2._____   11. _____

3._____   12. _____

4._____   13. _____

5._____   14. _____

6._____   15. _____

7._____   16. _____

8._____   17. _____

9._____   18. _____

Surgical Terms

Built from Word Parts

The following terms are built from word parts you have already learned and can be translated literally to find their meanings. Further explanation of terms beyond the definition of their word parts, if needed, is included in parentheses.

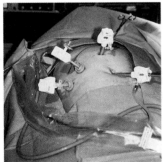

CHOLECYSTECTOMY was first performed in 1882 by a German surgeon. **Laparoscopic cholecystectomy** was first performed in 1987 in France.

Term	Definition
abdominocentesis .... (ab-*dom*-i-nō-sen-TĒ-sis)	surgical puncture to remove fluid from the abdominal cavity (also called **paracentesis**)
abdominoplasty .... (ab-DOM-i-nō-*plas*-tē)	surgical repair of the abdomen
anoplasty .... (Ā-nō-*plas*-tē)	surgical repair of the anus
antrectomy .... (an-TREK-to-mē)	excision of the antrum
appendicectomy .... (a-*pen*-di-SEK-to-mē)	excision of the appendix (also called **appendectomy**)
celiotomy .... (sē-lē-OT-o-mē)	incision into the abdominal cavity
cheilorrhaphy .... (kī-LOR-a-fē)	suture of the lip
cholecystectomy .... (*kō*-le-sis-TEK-to-mē)	excision of the gallbladder (Figure 11-10)
choledocholithotomy .... (kō-*led*-o-kō-li-THOT-o-mē)	incision into the common bile duct to remove a stone
colectomy .... (kō-LEK-to-mē)	excision of the colon
colostomy .... (ko-LOS-to-mē)	creation of an artificial opening into the colon (through the abdominal wall). (Used for the passage of stool. A colostomy, which creates a mouth-like opening on the abdominal wall called a **stoma,** may be permanent or temporary and performed as treatment for bowel obstruction, cancer, or diverticulitis.) (Exercise Figure E)
diverticulectomy .... (*dī*-ver-tik-ū-LEK-to-mē)	excision of a diverticulum

Figure 11-10

Laparoscopic cholecystectomy. CO_2 is used to insufflate the surgical area for better visualization. A small incision is made in the folds of the umbilicus for the insertion of the laparoscope. Three additional small incisions are made for the insertion of operative sheaths to accommodate accessory instrumentation.

EXERCISE FIGURE E

Fill in the blanks to complete labeling of the diagram.

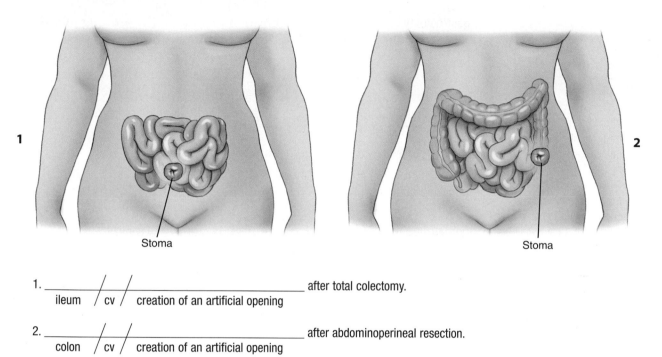

1   2

Stoma   Stoma

1. _____ / __ / _____ after total colectomy.
   ileum   / cv /   creation of an artificial opening

2. _____ / __ / _____ after abdominoperineal resection.
   colon   / cv /   creation of an artificial opening

Term	Definition
enterorrhaphy.............. (en-ter-OR-a-fē)	suture of the intestine
esophagogastroplasty .... (e-*sof*-a-gō-GAS-trō-*plas*-tē)	surgical repair of the esophagus and the stomach
gastrectomy .... (gas-TREK-to-mē)	excision of the stomach (or part of the stomach) (Exercise Figure F)
gastrojejunostomy .... (*gas*-trō-je-jū-NOS-to-mē)	creation of an artificial opening between the stomach and jejunum
gastroplasty .... (GAS-trō-*plas*-tē)	surgical repair of the stomach (Table 11-1)

EXERCISE FIGURE F

Fill in the blanks to label the diagram.

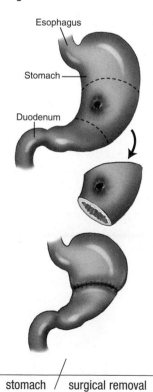

Esophagus

Stomach

Duodenum

_____ / _____
stomach / surgical removal

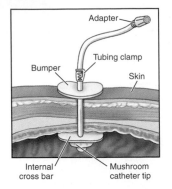

Figure 11-11
Percutaneous endoscopic gastrostomy (PEG) was first described in 1980. It is an alternative to **traditional gastrostomy.** An **endoscope** is used to place a tube in the stomach. Cost and discomfort to the patient are reduced when **PEG** is used instead of traditional gastrostomy.

Surgical Terms—*cont'd*
Built from Word Parts

Term	Definition
gastrostomy . . . . (gas-TROS-to-mē)	creation of an artificial opening into the stomach (through the abdominal wall). (A tube is inserted through the opening for administration of food when swallowing is impossible.) (Figure 11-11)
gingivectomy . . . . (*jin*-ji-VEK-to-mē)	surgical removal of gum (tissue)
glossorrhaphy . . . . (glo-SOR-a-fē)	suture of the tongue
hemicolectomy . . . . (*hem*-ē-kō-LEK-to-mē)	excision of half of the colon
herniorrhaphy . . . . (*her*-nē-OR-a-fē)	suturing of a hernia (for repair)
ileostomy . . . . (il-ē-OS-to-mē)	creation of an artificial opening into the ileum (through the abdominal wall creating a stoma, a mouthlike opening on the abdominal wall). (Used for the passage of stool. It is performed for ulcerative colitis, Crohn disease, or cancer.) (see Exercise Figure E)
laparotomy . . . . (*lap*-a-ROT-o-mē)	incision into the abdomen
palatoplasty . . . . (PAL-a-tō-*plas*-tē)	surgical repair of the palate
polypectomy . . . . (pol-i-PEK-to-mē)	excision of a polyp (Figure 11-12)
pyloromyotomy . . . . (pī-*lor*-ō-mī-OT-o-mē)	incision into the pyloric muscle
pyloroplasty . . . . (pī-LOR-ō-*plas*-tē)	surgical repair of the pylorus
uvulectomy . . . . (ū-vū-LEK-to-mē)	excision of the uvula
uvulopalatopharyngoplasty (UPPP) . . . . (ū-vū-lō-*pal*-a-tō-fa-RING-gō-*plas*-tē)	surgical repair of the uvula, palate, and pharynx (performed to correct obstructive sleep apnea) (see Figure 5-6)

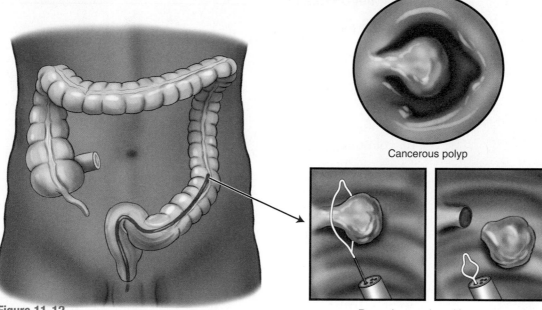

Cancerous polyp

Figure 11-12
Colonoscopy and polypectomy.

Removing a polyp with a snare

EXERCISE 17

Practice saying aloud each of the surgical terms built from word parts on pp. 494-496.

 To hear the terms select Chapter 11, Chapter Exercises, Pronunciation.

☐ Place a check mark in the box when you have completed this exercise.

EXERCISE 18

Analyze and define the following surgical terms.

1. gastrectomy_____

2. esophagogastroplasty _____

3. diverticulectomy_____

4. antrectomy _____

5. palatoplasty _____

6. uvulectomy _____

7. gastrojejunostomy _____

8. cholecystectomy _____

9. colectomy _____

10. colostomy _____

11. pyloroplasty _____

12. anoplasty _____

13. appendicectomy _____

14. cheilorrhaphy _____

15. gingivectomy _____

16. laparotomy _____

17. ileostomy _____

18. gastrostomy _____

19. herniorrhaphy _____

20. glossorrhaphy _____

21. choledocholithotomy _____

22. hemicolectomy _____

23. polypectomy _____

24. enterorrhaphy _____

25. abdominoplasty _____

26. pyloromyotomy _____

27. uvulopalatopharyngoplasty _____

28. celiotomy _____

29. gastroplasty _____

30. abdominocentesis _____

EXERCISE 19

Build surgical terms for the following definitions by using the word parts you have learned.

1. excision of the appendix

   _____ / _____
   WR   S

2. suture of the tongue

   _____ / ___ / _____
   WR   CV   S

3. surgical repair of the esophagus and stomach

   _____ / ___ / _____ / ___ / ___
   WR   CV   WR   CV   S

4. excision of a diverticulum

   _____ / _____
   WR   S

5. artificial opening into the ileum

   _____ / ___ / _____
   WR   CV   S

6. surgical removal of gum tissue

   _____ / _____
   WR   S

7. incision into the abdomen

   _____ / ___ / _____
   WR   CV   S

8. surgical repair of the anus

   _____ / ___ / _____
   WR   CV   S

9. excision of the antrum

   _____ / _____
   WR   S

10. excision of the gallbladder

    _____ / ___ / _____ / _____
    WR   CV   WR   S

11. excision of the colon

    _____ / _____
    WR   S

12. creation of an artificial opening into the colon

    _____ / ___ / _____
    WR   CV   S

13. excision of the stomach

    _____ / _____
    WR   S

14. creation of an artificial opening into the stomach

    _____ / ___ / _____
    WR   CV   S

15. creation of an artificial opening between the stomach and jejunum

_____ / ___ / ___ / ___ / ___
WR   CV   WR   CV   S

16. excision of the uvula

_____ / _____
WR   S

17. surgical repair of the palate

_____ / ___ / _____
WR   CV   S

18. surgical repair of the pylorus

_____ / ___ / _____
WR   CV   S

19. suture of a hernia

_____ / ___ / _____
WR   CV   S

20. suture of the lip

_____ / ___ / _____
WR   CV   S

21. excision of half of the colon

_____ / ___ / _____
P   WR   S

22. incision into the common bile duct to remove a stone

_____ / ___ / ___ / ___ / ___
WR   CV   WR   CV   S

23. excision of a polyp

_____ / _____
WR   S

24. suture of the intestine

_____ / ___ / _____
WR   CV   S

25. surgical repair of the abdomen

_____ / ___ / _____
WR   CV   S

26. incision into the abdominal cavity

_____ / ___ / _____
WR   CV   S

27. incision into the pylorus muscle

_____ / ___ / ___ / ___ / ___
WR   CV   WR   CV   S

28. surgical repair of the uvula, palate, and pharynx

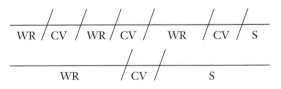

___ / ___ / ___ / ___ / ___ / ___ / ___
WR   CV   WR   CV   WR   CV   S

29. surgical repair of the stomach

_____ / ___ / _____
WR   CV   S

30. surgical puncture to remove fluid from the abdominal cavity

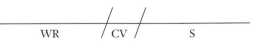

_____ / ___ / _____
WR   CV   S

EXERCISE 20

Spell each of the surgical terms built from word parts on pp. 494-496 by having someone dictate them to you.

 To hear and spell the terms select Chapter 11, Chapter Exercises, Spelling. You may type the terms on the screen or write them below in the spaces provided.

☐ Place a check mark in the box if you have completed this exercise using your CD-ROM.

1. _____   16. _____

2. _____   17. _____

3. _____   18. _____

4. _____   19. _____

5. _____   20. _____

6. _____   21. _____

7. _____   22. _____

8. _____   23. _____

9. _____   24. _____

10. _____   25. _____

11. _____   26. _____

12. _____   27. _____

13. _____   28. _____

14. _____   29. _____

15. _____   30. _____

Surgical Terms

Not Built from Word Parts

In some of the following terms, you may recognize word parts you have already learned; however, the full meaning of the terms cannot be discerned by the definition of their word parts.

Term	Definition
abdominoperineal resection (A&P resection). . . . . (ab-*dom*-i-nō-per-i-NĒ-el) (rē-SEK-shun)	removal of the colon and rectum through both abdominal and perineal approaches; performed to treat colorectal cancer and inflammatory diseases of the lower large intestine. The patient will have a colostomy. (see Exercise Figure E, *2*)

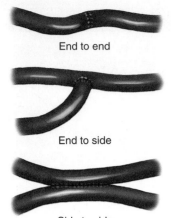

End to end

End to side

Side to side

Figure 11-13
Types of anastomoses.

BARIATRIC
contains the word roots **bar,**
meaning **weight,** and **iatr,**
meaning **treatment.**

Surgical Terms—*cont'd*
Not Built from Word Parts

Term	Definition
anastomosis (*pl.* anastomoses) .... (a-*nas*-to-MŌ-sis)	an opening created by surgically joining two structures, such as blood vessels or bowel segments (Figure 11-13)
bariatric surgery .... (*bar*-ē-AT-rik) (SUR-jer-ē)	surgical reduction of gastric capacity to treat morbid obesity (Table 11-1)
hemorrhoidectomy .... (hem-o-royd-EK-to-mē)	excision of hemorrhoids, the varicosed veins in the rectal region
vagotomy .... (vā-GOT-o-mē)	cutting of certain branches of the vagus nerve, performed with gastric surgery to reduce the amount of gastric acid produced and thus reduce the recurrence of ulcers

EXERCISE 21

Practice saying aloud each of the surgical terms not built from word parts on pp. 501-502.

 To hear the terms select Chapter 11, Chapter Exercises, Pronunciation.

☐ Place a check mark in the box when you have completed this exercise.

EXERCISE 22

Write the term for each of the following definitions.

1. cutting certain branches of the vagus nerve _____

2. opening created by surgically joining two structures _____

3. removal of the colon and rectum _____

4. surgical reduction of gastric capacity to treat morbid obesity _____

5. excision of the varicosed veins in the rectal region _____

TABLE 11-1
Bariatric Surgery

Bariatric surgery may be used to treat morbid obesity for patients with a BMI greater than 40 or those with a BMI greater than 35 associated with a serious medical condition. During surgery, a small stomach pouch is created for the purpose of restricting the amount of food an individual can eat. The following are three types of surgeries performed in the United States.

Roux-en-Y gastric bypass (RYGB)
Creation of a small gastric pouch with drainage of food to the rest of the gastrointestinal tract through a restricted stoma; the duodenum and part of the jejunum are bypassed. RYGB, the most common form of bariatric surgery performed in the United States, restricts food intake and calorie absorption rate.

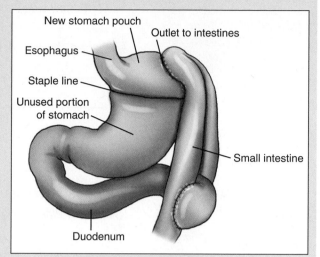

Vertical banded gastroplasty (VBG)
Creation of a small gastric pouch with a vertical line of staples and the connection of a band for the drainage of food into the small intestine; also called stomach stapling.

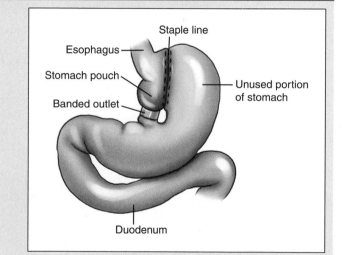

Laparoscopic adjustable gastric banding (LAGB)
Creation of a small gastric pouch by the placement of a band around the upper portion of the stomach; the band can be adjusted to change the size of the stomach through a subcutaneous port.

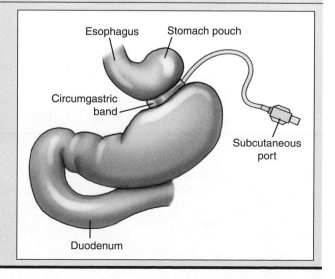

OPERATIVE CHOLANGIOGRAPHY
is performed during surgery to check for residual stones after the removal of the gallbladder. Postoperative cholangiography, also called T-tube cholangiography, is performed in the radiology department after a cholecystectomy, also to check for residual stones. Both use the injection of contrast media into the common bile duct.

COMPUTERIZED TOMOGRAPHY (CT) COLONOGRAPHY,
also called **virtual colonoscopy,** is a new method to test for colon polyps and colon cancer. It involves using a CT scanner and computer software that allows the physician to see the colon in multiple dimensions. It is less invasive than the conventional method of colonoscopy to screen for colon cancer.

CAPSULE ENDOSCOPY,
also known as **camera endoscopy,** was approved for use in 2001 by the Food and Drug Administration. Patients swallow a capsule containing a camera, about the size of a large vitamin pill (Fig 11-15). Pictures are taken by the camera every second as it moves naturally through the digestive tract. The images are recorded on a small device worn around the patient's waist. The recording device is returned to the physician's office after 8 hours. The images are transferred to a computer and examined. The video capsule is expelled in the bowel movement and not retrieved.

Capsule endoscopy replaces the standard endoscopy performed by pushing an endoscopic tube through the small intestine. It is especially helpful in identifying the cause of intestinal bleeding, revealing ulcers in Crohn disease, and diagnosing the causes of abdominal pain.

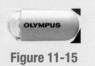

Figure 11-15

EXERCISE 23

Spell each of the surgical terms not built from word parts on pp. 501-502 by having someone dictate them to you.

To hear and spell the terms select Chapter 11, Chapter Exercises, Spelling. You may type the terms on the screen or write them below in the spaces provided.

☐ Place a check mark in the box if you have completed this exercise using your CD-ROM.

1. _____   4. _____

2. _____   5. _____

3. _____

Diagnostic Terms
Built from Word Parts

The following terms are built from word parts you have already learned and can be translated literally to find their meanings. Further explanation of terms beyond the definition of their word parts, if needed, is included in parentheses.

Term	Definition
DIAGNOSTIC IMAGING	
cholangiogram . . . . (kō-LAN-jē-ō-gram)	radiographic image of bile ducts
cholangiography . . . . (kō-*lan*-jē-OG-ra-fē)	radiographic imaging of the bile ducts (after administration of contrast media to outline the ducts)
cholecystogram . . . . (*kō*-le-SIS-tō-gram)	radiographic image of the gallbladder. (Oral cholecystogram is still used to diagnose cholelithiasis, but ultrasound is now the method of choice.) (Exercise Figure G)
CT colonography . . . . (kō-lon-OG-ra-fē)	radiographic imaging of the colon (using a CT scanner and software)
esophagogram . . . . (e-SOF-a-gō-gram)	radiographic image of the esophagus. (Barium is used as contrast media; also called **esophagram** and **barium swallow**)
ENDOSCOPY	
colonoscope . . . . (kō-LON-ō-skōp)	instrument used for visual examination of the colon
colonoscopy . . . . (kō-lon-OS-ko-pē)	visual examination of the colon (see Figures 11-12, 11-14, and 11-16)
endoscope . . . . (EN-dō-skōp)	instrument used for visual examination within a hollow organ

EXERCISE FIGURE G

Fill in the blanks to complete labeling of the diagram.

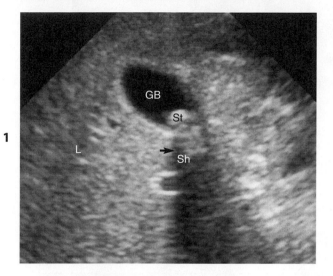

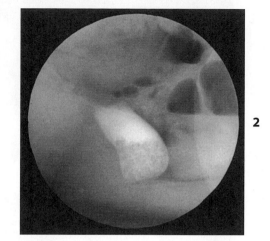

Two types of diagnostic imaging procedures used to evaluate the gallbladder.

1. Abdominal ultrasound showing cholelithiasis.

2. Oral _____ / __ / _____ / __ / _____
    gall / cv / bladder / cv / radiographic image
showing multiple small stones settled at the bottom of the
gallbladder.

Term	Definition
endoscopy . . . . (en-DOS-ko-pē)	visual examination within a hollow organ (see Figure 11-14)
esophagogastroduodenoscopy **(EGD)** . . . . (e-*sof*-a-gō-*gas*-trō-dū- od-e-NOS-ko-pē)	visual examination of the esophagus, stom- ach, and duodenum
esophagoscope . . . . (e-SOF-a-gō-skōp)	instrument for visual examination of the esophagus
esophagoscopy . . . . (e-*sof*-a-GOS-ko-pē)	visual examination of the esophagus
gastroscope . . . . (GAS-trō-skōp)	instrument used for visual examination of the stomach (Exercise Figure H)
gastroscopy . . . . (gas-TROS-ko-pē)	visual examination of the stomach (Exercise Figure H)

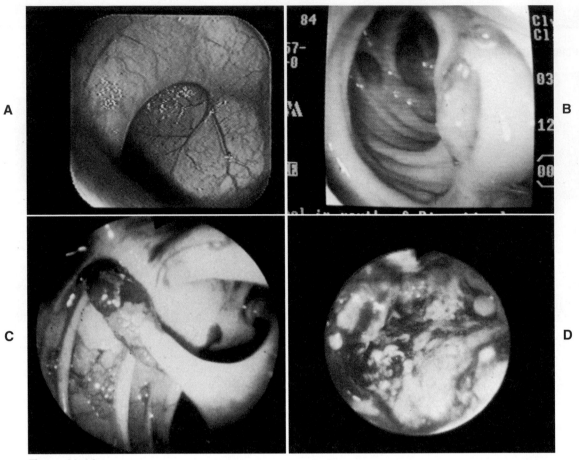

Figure 11-14
Endoscopic views obtained at colonoscopy reveal normal colon **(A)**, diverticulosis **(B)**, colon polyp **(C)**, and colon cancer **(D)**.

Diagnostic Terms—*cont'd*
Built from Word Parts

Term	Definition
laparoscope . . . . (LAP-a-rō-skōp)	instrument used for visual examination of the abdominal cavity. (Also used to perform laparoscopic surgery, a method that sometimes replaces **laparotomy,** open abdominal incisional surgery. Abdominal surgeries performed with a laparoscope include laparoscopic cholecystectomy, laparoscopic herniorrhaphy, laparoscopic appendectomy, and laparoscopic colectomy.) (see Figure 11-10 and Table 8-3)
laparoscopy . . . . (lap-a-ROS-ko-pē)	visual examination of the abdominal cavity
proctoscope . . . . (PROK-tō-skōp)	instrument used for visual examination of the rectum

EXERCISE FIGURE H

Fill in the blanks to complete labeling of the diagram.

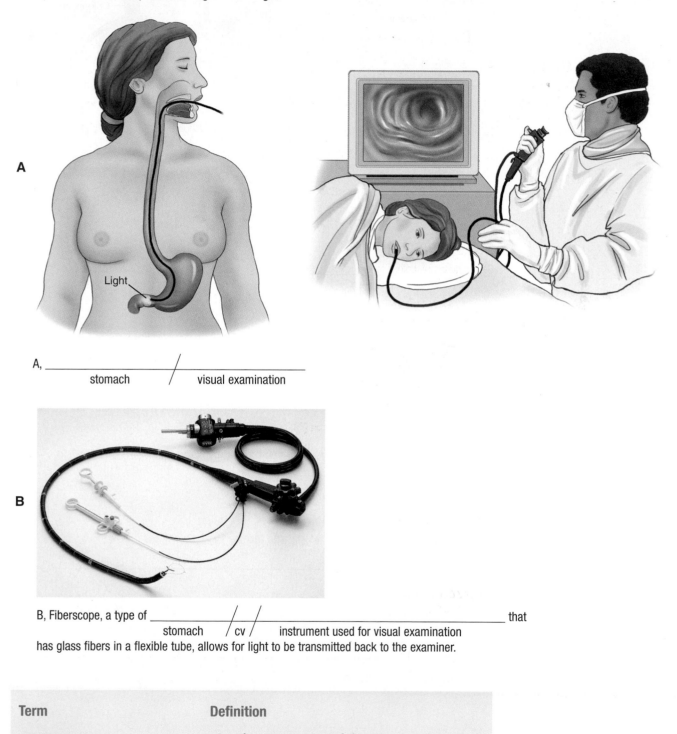

A, _____ / _____
      stomach   visual examination

B, Fiberscope, a type of _____ / ____ / _____ that
                     stomach / cv / instrument used for visual examination
has glass fibers in a flexible tube, allows for light to be transmitted back to the examiner.

Term	Definition
proctoscopy .... (prok-TOS-ko-pē)	visual examination of the rectum
sigmoidoscope .... (sig-MOY-dō-skōp)	instrument used for visual examination of the sigmoid colon
sigmoidoscopy .... (*sig*-moy-DOS-ko-pē)	visual examination of the sigmoid colon (Figure 11-16)

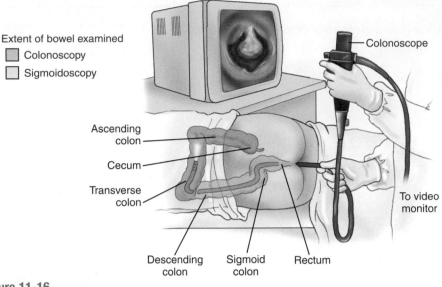

Figure 11-16
Sigmoidoscopy, colonoscopy.

EXERCISE 24

Practice saying aloud each of the diagnostic terms built from word parts on pp. 504-507.

 To hear the terms select Chapter 11, Chapter Exercises, Pronunciation.

☐ Place a check mark in the box when you have completed this exercise.

EXERCISE 25

Analyze and define the following diagnostic terms.

1. esophagoscope _____

2. esophagoscopy _____

3. gastroscope _____

4. gastroscopy _____

5. proctoscope_____

6. proctoscopy_____

7. endoscope _____

8. endoscopy _____

9. sigmoidoscope _____

10. sigmoidoscopy _____

11. cholecystogram_____

12. cholangiogram _____

13. esophagogastroduodenoscopy_____

14. colonoscope _____

15. laparoscope_____

16. colonoscopy _____

17. laparoscopy_____

18. CT colonography_____

19. esophagogram_____

20. cholangiography_____

EXERCISE 26

Build diagnostic terms that correspond to the following definitions by using the word parts you have learned.

1. visual examination within a
   hollow organ

2. instrument used for visual
   examination of the stomach

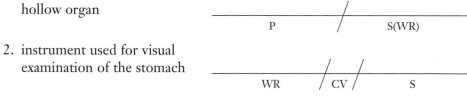

3. instrument used for visual examination of the rectum

_____ / _____ / _____
  WR   CV   S

4. instrument used for visual examination of the sigmoid colon

_____ / _____ / _____
  WR   CV   S

5. radiographic image of the gallbladder

_____ / _____ / _____ / _____ / _____
  WR   CV   WR   CV   S

6. instrument used for visual examination within a hollow organ

_____ / _____
    P   S(WR)

7. instrument used for visual examination of the esophagus

_____ / _____ / _____
  WR   CV   S

8. visual examination of the rectum

_____ / _____ / _____
  WR   CV   S

9. visual examination of the esophagus

_____ / _____ / _____
  WR   CV   S

10. visual examination of the sigmoid colon

_____ / _____ / _____
  WR   CV   S

11. radiographic image of bile ducts

_____ / _____ / _____
  WR   CV   S

12. visual examination of the stomach

_____ / _____ / _____
  WR   CV   S

13. instrument used for visual examination of the abdominal cavity

_____ / _____ / _____
  WR   CV   S

14. visual examination of the esophagus, stomach, and duodenum

_____ / _____ / _____ / _____ / _____ / _____ / _____
 WR   CV   WR   CV   WR   CV   S

15. visual examination of the colon

_____ / _____ / _____
  WR   CV   S

16. visual examination of the
    abdominal cavity

    _____ / ___ / _____
    WR   CV   S

17. instrument used for visual
    examination of the colon

    _____ / ___ / _____
    WR   CV   S

18. radiographic imaging of
    the colon   CT

    _____ / ___ / _____
    WR   CV   S

19. radiographic imaging of
    the bile ducts

    _____ / ___ / _____
    WR   CV   S

20. radiographic image of the
    esophagus

    _____ / ___ / _____
    WR   CV   S

EXERCISE 27

Spell each of the diagnostic terms built from word parts on pp. 504-507 by having someone dictate them to you.

 To hear and spell the terms select Chapter 11, Chapter Exercises, Spelling. You may type the terms on the screen or write them below in the spaces provided.

☐ Place a check mark in the box if you have completed this exercise using your CD-ROM.

1. _____
2. _____
3. _____
4. _____
5. _____
6. _____
7. _____
8. _____
9. _____
10. _____

11. _____
12. _____
13. _____
14. _____
15. _____
16. _____
17. _____
18. _____
19. _____
20. _____

Diagnostic Terms
Not Built from Word Parts

In some of the following terms, you may recognize word parts you have already learned; however, the full meaning of the terms cannot be discerned by the definition of their word parts.

Term	Definition
DIAGNOSTIC IMAGING	
abdominal ultrasonography . . . (ab-DOM-i-nal) (*ul*-tra-so-NOG-ra-fē)	process of recording images of internal organs using high-frequency sound waves produced by a transducer placed directly on the skin covering the abdominal cavity. Images may be viewed on a monitor and/or recorded for later use. The size and structure of organs such as the liver, gallbladder, bile ducts, and pancreas can be visualized. Liver cysts, abscesses, tumors, gallstones, an enlarged pancreas, and pancreatic tumors may be detected (Exercise Figure G).
barium enema (BE) . . . . (BAR-ē-um) (EN-e-ma)	series of radiographic images taken of the large intestine after a barium enema has been administered rectally (also called **lower GI series**) (Figure 11-17)
upper GI (gastrointestinal) series	series of radiographic images taken of the stomach and duodenum after barium has been swallowed
ENDOSCOPY	
endoscopic retrograde cholangiopancreatography (ERCP) . . . . (en-dō-SKOP-ic) (RET-rō-grād) (kō-*lan*-jē-ō-*pan*-krē-a-TOG-rah-fē)	radiographic examination of the biliary tract and pancreatic ducts with contrast media, fluoroscopy, and endoscopy (Figure 11-18)
endoscopic ultrasound (EUS) . . . . (en-dō-SKOP-ic) (UL-tra-sound)	a procedure using an endoscope fitted with an ultrasound probe that provides images of layers of the intestinal wall; used to detect tumors and cystic growths and for staging of malignant tumors
LABORATORY	
fecal occult blood test (FOBT) . . . . (FĒ-kl) (o-KULT) (blud)	a test to detect occult blood in feces. It is used to screen for colon cancer or polyps. Occult blood refers to blood that is present but can only be viewed microscopically (also called **guaiac test**).

ABDOMINAL ULTRASOUND is replacing the use of the cholecystogram to diagnose the presence of cholelithiasis.

ENDOSCOPIC RETROGRADE CHOLANGIOPANCREATOGRAPHY (ERCP) was first performed in 1968. ERCP is used to evaluate obstructions, pancreatic cancer, and unexplained pancreatitis. It is used to diagnose stone diseases, strictures, and pancreatic neoplasms.

Term	Definition
Helicobacter pylori (H. pylori) antibodies test . . . . (hel-i-kō-BAK-ter) (pī-LŌ-rē) (AN-ti-bod-ēs)	a blood test to determine the presence of *H. pylori* bacteria. The bacteria can be found in the lining of the stomach and can cause peptic ulcers. Tests for *H. pylori* are also performed on biopsy specimens and by breath test.

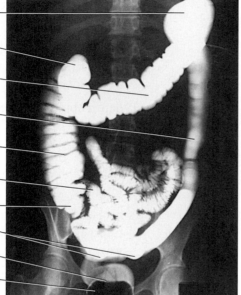

Left (splenic) colic flexure
Right (hepatic) colic flexure
Transverse colon
Descending colon
Ascending colon
Terminal ileum
Cecum
Sigmoid
Rectum
Air-filled retention tip

Figure 11-17
Barium enema.

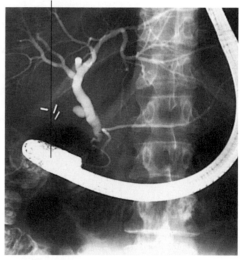

Endoscope

Figure 11-18
Endoscopic retrograde cholangiopancreatography (ERCP) is used to diagnose biliary and pancreatic pathologic conditions.

EXERCISE 28

Practice saying aloud each of the diagnostic terms not built from word parts on pp. 512-513.

 To hear the terms select Chapter 11, Chapter Exercises, Pronunciation.

☐ Place a check mark in the box when you have completed this exercise.

EXERCISE 29

Write definitions for the following terms.

1. upper GI series _____

2. barium enema _____

3. endoscopic retrograde cholangiopancreatography _____

_____

4. endoscopic ultrasound _____

5. *Helicobacter pylori* antibodies test _____

6. fecal occult blood test _____

7. abdominal ultrasonography _____

EXERCISE 30

Match the procedures in the first column with their correct definitions in the second column.

_____ 1. fecal occult blood test

_____ 2. barium enema

_____ 3. *Helicobacter pylori* antibodies test

_____ 4. upper GI series

_____ 5. endoscopic retrograde cholangiopancreatography

_____ 6. abdominal ultrasonography

_____ 7. endoscopic ultrasound

a. used to diagnose peptic ulcers

b. radiographic image of the stomach and duodenum

c. provides images of layers of the intestinal wall

d. detects blood in feces

e. radiographic image of the esophagus

f. radiographic image of the large intestine

g. process of recording images of internal organs by using sound waves

h. examination of biliary tract and pancreatic ducts

EXERCISE 31

Spell each of the diagnostic terms not built from word parts on pp. 512-513 by having someone dictate them to you.

 To hear and spell the terms select Chapter 11, Chapter Exercises, Spelling. You may type the terms on the screen or write them below in the spaces provided.

☐ Place a check mark in the box if you have completed this exercise using your CD-ROM.

1. _____

2. _____

3. _____

4. _____

5. _____

6. _____

7. _____

Complementary Terms
Built from Word Parts

The following terms are built from word parts you have already learned and can be translated literally to find their meanings. Further explanation of terms beyond the definition of their word parts, if needed, is included in parentheses.

Term	Definition
abdominal (ab-DOM-i-nal)	pertaining to the abdomen
anal (Ā-nal)	pertaining to the anus
aphagia (a-FĀ-ja)	without swallowing (the inability to)
colorectal (kō-lō-REK-tal)	pertaining to the colon and rectum
dyspepsia (dis-PEP-sē-a)	difficult digestion (often used to describe GI symptoms)
dysphagia (dis-FĀ-ja)	difficult swallowing
gastrodynia (*gas*-trō-DIN-ē-a)	pain in the stomach
gastroenterologist (*gas*-trō-en-ter-OL-o-jist)	a physician who studies and treats diseases of the stomach and intestines (GI tract and accessory organs)
gastroenterology (*gas*-trō-en-ter-OL-o-jē)	study of the stomach and intestines (a branch of medicine that deals with treating diseases of the GI tract and accessory organs)
gastromalacia (*gas*-trō-ma-LĀ-sha)	softening of the stomach
glossopathy (glos-OP-a-thē)	disease of the tongue
ileocecal (*il*-ē-ō-SĒ-kal)	pertaining to the ileum and cecum
nasogastric (*nā*-zō-GAS-trik)	pertaining to the nose and stomach
oral (OR-al)	pertaining to the mouth
pancreatic (*pan*-krē-AT-ik)	pertaining to the pancreas
peritoneal (*per*-i-tō-NĒ-al)	pertaining to the peritoneum
proctologist (prok-TOL-o-jist)	physician who studies and treats diseases of the rectum
proctology (prok-TOL-o-jē)	study of the rectum (a branch of medicine that deals with disorders of the rectum and anus)

Complementary Terms—*cont'd*

Built from Word Parts

Term	Definition
rectal . . . . (REK-tal)	pertaining to the rectum
steatorrhea . . . . (*stē*-a-tō-RĒ-a)	discharge of fat (excessive amount of fat in the stool, causing frothy, foul-smelling fecal matter usually associated with the malabsorption of fat in conditions such as chronic pancreatitis and celiac disease)
steatosis . . . . (*stē*-a-tō-sis)	abnormal condition of fat (increased fat at the cellular level often affecting the liver)
stomatogastric . . . . (*stō*-ma-tō-GAS-trik)	pertaining to the mouth and stomach
sublingual . . . . (sub-LING-gwal)	pertaining to under the tongue

EXERCISE 32

Practice saying aloud each of the complementary terms built from word parts on pp. 515-516.

To hear the terms select Chapter 11, Chapter Exercises, Pronunciation.

☐ Place a check mark in the box when you have completed this exercise.

EXERCISE 33

Analyze and define the following complementary terms.

1. aphagia _____

2. dyspepsia _____

3. anal _____

4. dysphagia _____

5. glossopathy _____

6. ileocecal _____

7. oral _____

8. stomatogastric _____

9. gastromalacia _____

10. pancreatic _____

11. gastrodynia _____

12. peritoneal _____

13. steatosis _____

14. sublingual _____

15. proctology _____

16. nasogastric _____

17. abdominal _____

18. proctologist _____

19. gastroenterology _____

20. gastroenterologist _____

21. colorectal _____

22. rectal _____

23. steatorrhea _____

EXERCISE 34

Build the complementary terms for the following definitions by using the word parts you have learned.

1. disease of the tongue

     _____ / __ / _____
        WR   CV   S

2. without swallowing (the inability to)

     _____ / _____
        P   S(WR)

3. pertaining to under the tongue

     _____ / _____ / _____
        P   WR   S

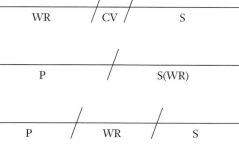

4. pertaining to the nose and the stomach

     _____ / __ / _____ / _____
       WR   CV   WR   S

5. pertaining to the mouth and the stomach

     _____ / __ / _____ / _____
       WR   CV   WR   S

6. pertaining to the anus

     _____ / _____
       WR   S

7. pertaining to the peritoneum

     _____ / _____
       WR   S

8. pertaining to the abdomen

     _____ / _____
       WR   S

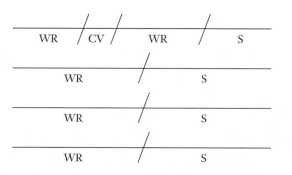

9. difficult swallowing

        _____ / _____
             P   S(WR)

10. pertaining to the ileum and cecum

        _____ / CV / _____ / S
         WR   WR

11. softening of the stomach

        _____ / CV / S
         WR

12. pain in the stomach

        _____ / S
         WR

13. physician who studies and treats diseases of the rectum

        _____ / CV / S
         WR

14. difficult digestion

        _____ / S(WR)
         P

15. pertaining to the pancreas

        _____ / S
         WR

16. study of the rectum

        _____ / CV / S
         WR

17. discharge of fat

        _____ / CV / S
         WR

18. pertaining to the mouth

        _____ / S
         WR

19. physician who studies and treats diseases of the stomach and intestines

        _____ / CV / WR / CV / S
         WR

20. study of the stomach and intestines

        _____ / CV / WR / CV / S
         WR

21. pertaining to the colon and rectum

        _____ / CV / WR / S
         WR

22. pertaining to the rectum

        _____ / S
         WR

23. abnormal condition of fat

        _____ / S
         WR

EXERCISE 35

Spell each of the complementary terms built from word parts on pp. 515-516 by having someone dictate them to you.

To hear and spell the terms select Chapter 11, Chapter Exercises, Spelling. You may type the terms on the screen or write them below in the spaces provided.

☐ Place a check mark in the box if you have completed this exercise using your CD-ROM.

1._____   13._____

2._____   14._____

3._____   15._____

4._____   16._____

5._____   17._____

6._____   18._____

7._____   19._____

8._____   20._____

9._____   21._____

10._____   22._____

11._____   23._____

12._____

Complementary Terms
Not Built from Word Parts

In some of the following terms, you may recognize word parts you have already learned; however, the full meaning of the terms cannot be discerned by the definition of their word parts.

Term	Definition
ascites . . . . (a-SĪ-tēz)	abnormal collection of fluid in the peritoneal cavity (Figure 11-19)
diarrhea . . . . (dī-a-RĒ-a) (NOTE: diarrhea is composed of *dia-*, meaning through, and *-rrhea*, meaning flow.)	frequent discharge of liquid stool
dysentery . . . . (DIS-en-ter-ē)	disorder that involves inflammation of the intestine (usually the large intestine) associated with diarrhea and abdominal pain

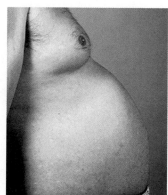

Figure 11-19
Ascites.

Complementary Terms—*cont'd*
Not Built from Word Parts

Term	Definition
emesis (EM-e-sis)	expelling matter from the stomach through the mouth (also called **vomiting** or **vomitus**)
feces (FĒ-sēz)	waste from the digestive tract expelled through the rectum (also called **stool** or **fecal matter**)
flatus (FLĀ-tus)	gas in the digestive tract or expelled through the anus
gastric lavage (GAS-trik) (la-VOZH)	washing out of the stomach
gavage (ga-VOZH)	process of feeding a person through a nasogastric tube
hematemesis (hē-ma-TEM-e-sis)	vomiting of blood
hematochezia (hē-ma-tō-KĒ-zha)	passage of bloody feces
melena (me-LĒ-na)	black, tarry stool that contains digested blood; usually a result of bleeding in the upper GI tract
nausea (NAW-zē-a)	urge to vomit
peristalsis (per-i-STAL-sis)	involuntary wavelike contractions that propel food along the digestive tract
reflux (RĒ-fluks)	abnormal backward flow. In esophageal reflux, the stomach contents flow back into the esophagus.
stoma (STŌ-ma)	surgical opening between an organ and the surface of the body, such as the opening established in the abdominal wall by colostomy, ileostomy, or a similar operation. Stoma may also refer to an opening created between body structures or between portions of the intestines. (see Exercise Figure E)
vomiting (VOM-it-ing)	expelling matter from the stomach through the mouth (also called **vomitus** or **emesis**)

EXERCISE 36

Practice saying aloud each of the complementary terms not built from word parts on pp. 519-520.

 To hear the terms select Chapter 11, Chapter Exercises, Pronunciation.

☐ Place a check mark in the box when you have completed this exercise.

EXERCISE 37

Match the definitions in the first column with the correct terms in the second column.

_____	1. abnormal collection of fluid	a.	hematemesis
_____	2. expelling matter from the stomach	b.	flatus
_____	3. feeding a person through a tube	c.	gastric lavage
_____	4. washing out of the stomach	d.	reflux
_____	5. urge to vomit	e.	vomiting, emesis
_____	6. frequent discharge of liquid stool	f.	gavage
_____	7. waste expelled from the rectum	g.	melena
_____	8. vomiting of blood	h.	dysentery
_____	9. abnormal backward flow	i.	diarrhea
_____	10. inflammation of the intestine associated with diarrhea and abdominal pain	j.	peristalsis
		k.	feces
_____	11. gas expelled through the anus	l.	nausea
_____	12. involuntary wavelike contractions	m.	ascites
_____	13. black, tarry stools	n.	hematochezia
_____	14. surgical opening between an organ and the surface of the body	o.	stoma
_____	15. passage of bloody feces		

EXERCISE 38

Write definitions for each of the following terms.

1. ascites _____

2. gavage _____

3. gastric lavage_____

4. feces_____

5. nausea _____

6. vomiting _____

7. dysentery _____

8. diarrhea _____

9. flatus _____

10. reflux _____

11. hematemesis _____

12. peristalsis _____

13. melena _____

14. stoma _____

15. hematochezia _____

16. emesis _____

EXERCISE 39

Spell each of the complementary terms not built from word parts on pp. 519-520 by having someone dictate them to you.

 To hear and spell the terms select Chapter 11, Chapter Exercises, Spelling. You may type the terms on the screen or write them below in the spaces provided.

☐ Place a check mark in the box if you have completed this exercise using your CD-ROM.

1. _____   9. _____

2. _____   10. _____

3. _____   11. _____

4. _____   12. _____

5. _____   13. _____

6. _____   14. _____

7. _____   15. _____

8. _____   16. _____

Refer to Appendix J (on the Evolve website) for a list of nutritional terms and Appendix E (at the back of the book) for pharmacology terms related to the digestive system.

Abbreviations

A&P resection..............	abdominoperineal resection
BE........................	barium enema
EGD.......................	esophagogastroduodenoscopy
ERCP......................	endoscopic retrograde cholangiopancrea-tography
EUS.......................	endoscopic ultrasound
FOBT......................	fecal occult blood test
GERD......................	gastroesophageal reflux disease
GI	gastrointestinal
H. pylori	*Helicobacter pylori*
IBS	irritable bowel syndrome
N&V.......................	nausea and vomiting
PEG......................	percutaneous endoscopic gastrostomy
UGI	upper gastrointestinal
UPPP......................	uvulopalatopharyngoplasty

Refer to Appendix D for a complete list of abbreviations.

EXERCISE 40

Write the meaning of the following abbreviations.

1. ERCP _____ _____ _____

2. EUS _____ _____

3. N&V _____ _____ _____

4. IBS _____ _____ _____

5. PEG _____ _____ _____

6. UGI _____ _____

7. UPPP _____

8. GERD _____ _____ _____

9. GI _____

10. *H. pylori* _____ _____

11. BE _____ _____

12. EGD _____

13. A&P resection _____ _____

14. FOBT _____ _____ _____ _____

PRACTICAL APPLICATION

EXERCISE **41** *Interact with Medical Documents*

A. Complete the endoscopy report by writing the medical terms in the blanks. Use the list of definitions with the corresponding numbers.

University Hospital and Medical Center
4700 North Main Street • Wellness, Arizona 54321 • (987) 555-3210

PATIENT NAME: Ruth Clifton   **CASE NUMBER:** 77721-DIG
DATE OF BIRTH: 09/15/19XX   **DATE:** 12/27/20XX

ENDOSCOPY REPORT

CASE HISTORY: This is a 40-year-old African American woman who was referred to the 1. _____ clinic for evaluation. Patient reports 2. _____ and vomiting with upper abdominal pain. She has also had a problem with 3. _____ but denies any 4. _____ or 5. _____. She has not used any alcohol or salicylates. She is currently taking several medications but they are not known for ulcerogenic side effects.

PROCEDURE: 6. _____: The patient was given 2 mg of intravenous Versed along with lidocaine spray to the pharynx. After the patient was placed in the left lateral decubitus position, the Olympus 7. _____ was passed into the esophagus without difficulty. The esophagus in its entirety was essentially free of mucosal abnormalities. No evidence of 8. _____. The stomach was entered and some gastric juices were aspirated. The esophagus, cardia, and body of the stomach were free of abnormalities. A biopsy of the gastric mucosa was taken for 9. _____. In the distal antral area some mild erythematous changes were noted. The pylorus had normal peristaltic activity. The first part of the duodenum, however, revealed evidence of ulcerations, both anterosuperiorly as well as posteroinferiorly, with surrounding erythema. These 10. _____ were less than 1 cm in size. The second part of the duodenum was free of mucosal abnormalities. Withdrawing the scope confirmed the findings upon entry. The patient tolerated the procedure quite well and recovered uneventfully.

Vital signs will be taken every half hour for the next 2 hours.

POSTPROCEDURAL DIAGNOSIS:
11. _____
12. _____ _____

_____
Jesus Garcia, MD

JG/mcm

---

1. visual examination within a hollow organ
2. urge to vomit
3. difficult digestion
4. vomiting of blood
5. black, tarry stool that contains digested blood
6. visual examination of the esophagus, stomach, and duodenum
7. instrument used for visual examination of the stomach
8. abnormal backward flow
9. abbreviation for *Helicobacter pylori*
10. eroded sores
11. inflammation of the stomach
12. ulcers in the duodenum

EXERCISE 41   *Interact with Medical Documents—cont'd*

B. Read the radiology report and answer the questions following it.

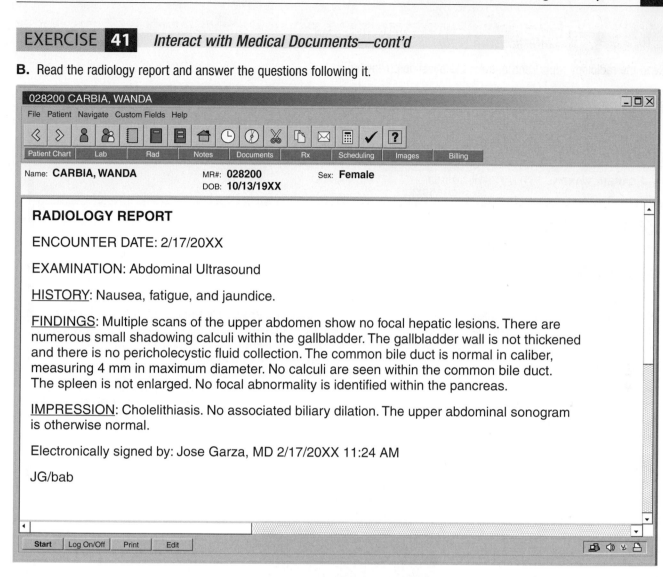

1. The exam included which diagnostic procedure:
   a. radiographic imaging of the colon with computerized tomography
   b. radiographic imaging of the bile ducts after administration of contrast media
   c. use of an endoscope fitted with an ultrasound probe to obtain images of layers of the intestinal wall
   d. recording images of organs with sound waves produced by a transducer placed directly on the skin

2. The patient's symptoms included:
   a. expelling matter from the stomach through the mouth
   b. condition characterized by a yellow tinge to the skin
   c. bluish discoloration of the skin
   d. erythroderma

3. The examination revealed the presence of:
   a. stones within the gallbladder
   b. stones within the common bile duct
   c. lesions in the liver
   d. inflammation of the pancreas

4. "Biliary dilation" would most likely refer to:
   a. inflammation of the pancreas
   b. the presence of fluid in the upper abdomen
   c. choledocholithiasis
   d. widening of the bile ducts or gallbladder

EXERCISE **41** *Interact with Medical Documents—cont'd*

C. Read the radiology report and answer the questions following it.

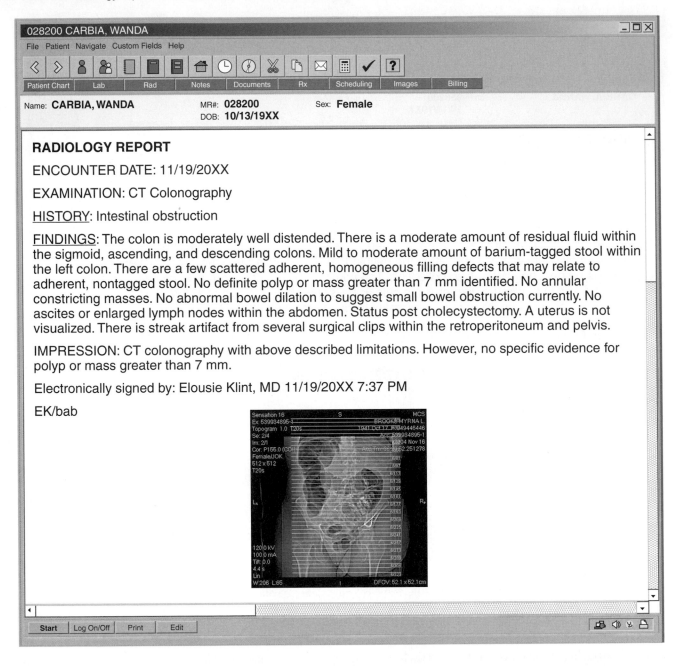

```
028200 CARBIA, WANDA                                          _ □ ✕
File  Patient  Navigate  Custom Fields  Help
```

| Patient Chart | Lab | Rad | Notes | Documents | Rx | Scheduling | Images | Billing |

Name: **CARBIA, WANDA**   MR#: **028200**   Sex: **Female**
DOB: **10/13/19XX**

RADIOLOGY REPORT

ENCOUNTER DATE: 11/19/20XX

EXAMINATION: CT Colonography

HISTORY: Intestinal obstruction

FINDINGS: The colon is moderately well distended. There is a moderate amount of residual fluid within the sigmoid, ascending, and descending colons. Mild to moderate amount of barium-tagged stool within the left colon. There are a few scattered adherent, homogeneous filling defects that may relate to adherent, nontagged stool. No definite polyp or mass greater than 7 mm identified. No annular constricting masses. No abnormal bowel dilation to suggest small bowel obstruction currently. No ascites or enlarged lymph nodes within the abdomen. Status post cholecystectomy. A uterus is not visualized. There is streak artifact from several surgical clips within the retroperitoneum and pelvis.

IMPRESSION: CT colonography with above described limitations. However, no specific evidence for polyp or mass greater than 7 mm.

Electronically signed by: Elousie Klint, MD 11/19/20XX 7:37 PM

EK/bab

| Start | Log On/Off | Print | Edit |

1. No ascites indicates:
   a. no fluid accumulation in the peritoneal cavity
   b. no inflammation of the intestine associated with diarrhea and abdominal pain
   c. no residual fluid within the sigmoid colon
   d. no kinking of the intestine

2. The CT colonography was performed:
   a. before excision of the colon
   b. after excision of the appendix
   c. before creation of an artificial opening into the colon
   d. after excision of the gallbladder

3. The report most clearly suggests that the intestinal obstruction was probably *not* caused by a(n):
   a. adhesion
   b. volvulus
   c. intussusception
   d. polyp or mass

EXERCISE 42 *Interpret Medical Terms*

To test your understanding of the terms introduced in this chapter, circle the words that correctly complete the sentences. The italicized words refer to the correct answer.

1. Mr. E. was admitted to the hospital with a diagnosis of *gallstones*, or (**cholelithiasis, cholecystitis, sialolithiasis**).

2. An abdominal ultrasound confirmed the admitting diagnosis, and Mr. E. is now scheduled for a laparoscopic *excision of the gallbladder*, or (**cholecystostomy, cholecystectomy, colectomy**).

3. The plural spelling of the term meaning *opening created by surgically joining two structures* is (**anastomoses, anastomosis, anastomosices**).

4. The patient was diagnosed with a condition including the symptom of *inflammation of the colon and formation of ulcers*, called (**cirrhosis, ulcerative colitis, peptic ulcer**).

5. A *prolapse of the rectum* is (**rectocele, intussusception, proctoptosis**).

6. An *abnormal growing together of two surfaces* is (**anastomosis, adhesion, amniocentesis**).

7. Three surgical procedures that may be performed on a patient with peptic ulcers are (1) *excision of the stomach*, or (**gastrotomy, gastrostomy, gastrectomy**); (2) *surgical repair of the pylorus*, or (**pyloroplasty, cheilorrhaphy, gastrojejunostomy**); and (3) *cutting of certain branches of the vagus nerve*, or (**colostomy, vagotomy, gingivectomy**).

8. *Difficult digestion* is (**dyspepsia, dysphagia, gastrodynia**).

9. *Feeding* a person *through a gastric tube* is called (**lavage, gavage, gastrostomy**).

10. The *surgical procedure to remove the colon and rectum and create an artificial opening into the colon* are (**colectomy and colostomy, abdominoperineal resection and colostomy, abdominoperineal resection and ileostomy**).

11. To rule out cancer of the colon, the doctor performed a diagnostic procedure to *visually examine the colon* or (**colonoscopy, colonoscope, colostomy**).

12. The doctor diagnosed the patient as having *an obstruction of the intestine* or (**polyp, irritable bowel syndrome, ileus**).

13. The following test is used to screen for colon cancer (**fecal occult blood test, *Helicobacter pylori* antibodies test, upper GI series**).

14. (**Stoma, Stomata, Stomaes**) is the plural spelling of the term meaning *surgical opening between an organ and the surface of the body.*

 WEB LINK
For more information about diseases and disorders of the digestive system and the latest treatments available, please visit the National Digestive Diseases Information Clearing House at http://digestive.niddlc.nih.gov.

EXERCISE **43** *Read Medical Terms in Use*

Practice pronunciation of terms by reading the following discussion. Use the pronunciation key following the medical term to assist you in saying the word.

 To hear these terms select Chapter 11, Chapter Exercises, Read Medical Terms in Use.

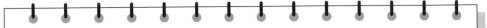

COLORECTAL CANCER

Colorectal (kō-lō-REK-tal) cancer begins in the colon or rectum and is the second leading cause of cancer deaths in the United States. Most are adenocarcinomas that originate as a benign, adenomatous **polyp** (POL-ip).

Many people have no symptoms until the tumor is quite advanced, and symptoms vary depending on the location of the tumor. Warning signs are altered bowel habits, **rectal** (REK-tal) bleeding, **abdominal** (ab-DOM-i-nal) cramps, **flatus** (FLĀ-tus) and bloating, iron deficiency anemia, and weight loss.

Screening and diagnostic tests for colorectal cancer include digital rectal examination, **fecal** (FĒ-kl) **occult** (o-KULT) blood test, **sigmoidoscopy** (*sig*-moy-DOS-ko-pē), **colonoscopy** (kō-lon-OS-ko-pē), and **barium** (BAR-ē-um) **enema** (EN-e-ma). As well as being an important diagnostic tool, colonoscopy may be used for biopsy and for the removal of **polyps.** To perform a **polypectomy** (pol-i-PEK-to-mē), a braided wire snare is inserted into the **colonoscope** (kō-LON-ō-skōp). A snare loop, like a noose, is placed around the stem of the polyp. With electrosurgical power attached to the snare, the polyp is detached. The polyp is removed from the colon for histologic examination.

For cancer beyond the early stage, conventional surgery is the main treatment. The type of surgery depends on the location and stage of the tumor. Types of surgeries performed are left or right-sided **hemicolectomy** (*hem*-ē-kō-LEK-to-mē) with **anastomosis** (a-*nas*-to-MŌ-sis), sigmoid **colectomy** (kō-LEK-to-mē), and **abdominoperineal** (ab-*dom*-i-nō-*per*-i-NĒ-el) **resection** with **colostomy** (ko-LOS-to-mē).

EXERCISE 44   *Comprehend Medical Terms in Use*

Test your comprehension of terms in the previous medical discussion by circling the correct answer.

1. Which of the following is used for diagnosing colorectal cancer?

   a. visual exam of the stomach

   b. series of radiographic images of the small intestine

   c. visual exam of the colon

   d. radiographic image of the esophagus

2. T   F   A polypectomy may be performed during a colonoscopy.

3. T   F   Depending on the location of the tumor, a surgical treatment for colorectal cancer may be performed that creates an opening between the colon and abdominal wall for the passage of stool.

4. T   F   Vomiting blood is a warning sign for colorectal cancer.

CHAPTER REVIEW

CHAPTER REVIEW ON CD-ROM

Use the CD-ROM that accompanies this textbook to play and practice what you have learned in this chapter. The Chapter Exercises, Practice Activities, Animations, and Games allow you to hear, see, and interact with the chapter content.

Chapter Exercises	**Practice Activities**	**Animations**	**Games**
Exercises in this section of your CD-ROM correlate to exercises in your textbook. You may have completed them as you worked through the chapter.	Practice in study mode, and then test your learning in assessment mode. Keep track of your scores from assessment mode if you wish.	☐ Cirrhosis ☐ Digestive Tract ☐ Diverticulitis ☐ ERCP	☐ Name that Word Part ☐ Term Storm ☐ Term Explorer ☐ Termbusters ☐ Medical Millionaire

Chapter Exercises

Exercises in this section of your CD-ROM correlate to exercises in your textbook. You may have completed them as you worked through the chapter.

☐ Pronunciation
☐ Spelling
☐ Read Medical Terms in Use

Practice Activities

SCORE

☐ Picture It   _____
☐ Define Word Parts   _____
☐ Build Medical Terms   _____
☐ Word Shop   _____
☐ Define Medical Terms   _____
☐ Use It   _____
☐ Hear It and Type It: _____
    Clinical Vignettes

REVIEW OF WORD PARTS

Can you define and spell the following word parts?

Combining Forms			Prefix	Suffix
abdomin/o	duoden/o	palat/o	hemi-	-pepsia
an/o	enter/o	pancreat/o		
antr/o	esophag/o	peritone/o		
appendic/o	gastr/o	polyp/o		
cec/o	gingiv/o	proct/o		
celi/o	gloss/o	pylor/o		
cheil/o	hepat/o	rect/o		
cholangi/o	herni/o	sial/o		
chol/e	ile/o	sigmoid/o		
choledoch/o	jejun/o	steat/o		
col/o	lapar/o	stomat/o		
colon/o	lingu/o	uvul/o		
diverticul/o	or/o			

REVIEW OF TERMS

Can you build, analyze, define, pronounce, and spell the following terms *built from word parts*?

Diseases and Disorders	Surgical	Diagnostic	Complementary
appendicitis	abdominocentesis	cholangiogram	abdominal
cholangioma	abdominoplasty	cholangiography	anal
cholecystitis	anoplasty	cholecystogram	aphagia
choledocholithiasis	antrectomy	colonoscope	colorectal
cholelithiasis	appendicectomy	colonoscopy	dyspepsia
diverticulitis	celiotomy	CT colonography	dysphagia
diverticulosis	cheilorrhaphy	endoscope	gastrodynia
esophagitis	cholecystectomy	endoscopy	gastroenterologist
gastritis	choledocholithotomy	esophagogastroduodenoscopy	gastroenterology
gastroenteritis	colectomy	(EGD)	gastromalacia
gastroenterocolitis	colostomy	esophagogram	glossopathy
gingivitis	diverticulectomy	esophagoscope	ileocecal
hepatitis	enterorrhaphy	esophagoscopy	nasogastric
hepatoma	esophagogastroplasty	gastroscope	oral
palatitis	gastrectomy	gastroscopy	pancreatic
pancreatitis	gastrojejunostomy	laparoscope	peritoneal
peritonitis	gastroplasty	laparoscopy	proctologist
polyposis	gastrostomy	proctoscope	proctology
proctoptosis	gingivectomy	proctoscopy	rectal
rectocele	glossorrhaphy	sigmoidoscope	steatorrhea
sialolith	hemicolectomy	sigmoidoscopy	steatosis
steatohepatitis	herniorrhaphy		stomatogastric
uvulitis	ileostomy		sublingual
	laparotomy		
	palatoplasty		
	polypectomy		
	pyloromyotomy		
	pyloroplasty		
	uvulectomy		
	uvulopalatopharyngoplasty		
	(UPPP)		

Can you define, pronounce, and spell the following terms *not built from word parts?*

Diseases and Disorders	**Surgical**	**Diagnostic**	**Complementary**
adhesion	abdominoperineal resection (A&P resection)	abdominal ultrasonography	ascites
anorexia nervosa		barium enema (BE)	diarrhea
bulimia nervosa	anastomosis	endoscopic retrograde cholan-	dysentery
cirrhosis	(*pl.* anastomoses)	giopancreatography (ERCP)	emesis
Crohn disease	bariatric surgery	endoscopic ultrasound (EUS)	feces
duodenal ulcer	hemorrhoidectomy	fecal occult blood test (FOBT)	flatus
gastric ulcer	vagotomy	*Helicobacter pylori* antibodies	gastric lavage
gastroesophageal reflux		test	gavage
disease (GERD)		upper GI (gastrointestinal)	hematemesis
hemochromatosis		series	hematochezia
hemorrhoid			melena
ileus			nausea
intussusception			peristalsis
irritable bowel syndrome			reflux
(IBS)			stoma
obesity			vomiting
peptic ulcer			
polyp			
ulcerative colitis			
volvulus			

ANSWERS

Exercise Figures

Exercise Figure
A.
1. mouth: or/o, stomat/o
2. esophagus: esophag/o
3. duodenum: duoden/o
4. colon: col/o, colon/o
5. cecum: cec/o
6. anus: an/o
7. stomach: gastr/o
8. antrum: antr/o
9. jejunum: jejun/o
10. ileum: ile/o
11. sigmoid colon: sigmoid/o
12. rectum: proct/o, rect/o

Exercise Figure
B.
1. palate: palat/o
2. uvula: uvul/o
3. tongue: gloss/o, lingu/o
4. gallbladder: chol/e (gall), cyst/o (bladder)
5. pyloric sphincter: pylor/o
6. appendix: appendic/o
7. gum: gingiv/o
8. lip: cheil/o
9. salivary glands: sial/o
10. liver: hepat/o
11. bile duct: cholangi/o
12. common bile duct: choledoch/o
13. pancreas: pancreat/o
14. abdomen: abdomin/o, celi/o, lapar/o

Exercise Figure
C. 2. appendic/itis

Exercise Figure
D. chol/e/lith/iasis, choledoch/o/lith/iasis

Exercise Figure
E.
1. ile/o/stomy
2. col/o/stomy

Exercise Figure
F. gastr/ectomy

Exercise Figure
G. 2. chol/e/cyst/o/gram

Exercise Figure
H. A. gastr/o/scopy
   B. gastr/o/scope

Exercise 1
1. alimentary canal
2. gastrointestinal tract
3. pharynx
4. esophagus
5. stomach
6. duodenum
7. jejunum
8. ileum
9. cecum
10. ascending colon
11. transverse colon
12. descending colon
13. sigmoid colon
14. rectum
15. anus

Exercise 2
1. l
2. d
3. a
4. h
5. m
6. j
7. b
8. i
9. c
10. g
11. e
12. k
13. f

Exercise 3
1. rectum
2. stomach
3. anus
4. cecum
5. ileum
6. mouth
7. duodenum
8. colon
9. mouth
10. intestine
11. rectum
12. antrum
13. esophagus
14. jejunum
15. sigmoid colon
16. colon

Exercise 4
1. cec/o
2. gastr/o
3. ile/o
4. jejun/o
5. sigmoid/o
6. esophag/o
7. a. rect/o
   b. proct/o
8. enter/o
9. duoden/o
10. a. col/o
    b. colon/o
11. a. or/o
    b. stomat/o
12. an/o
13. antr/o

Exercise 5
1. hernia
2. abdomen
3. saliva, salivary gland
4. gall, bile
5. diverticulum
6. gum

Exercise 1 (continued)
7. appendix
8. tongue
9. liver
10. lip
11. peritoneum
12. palate
13. pancreas
14. abdomen
15. tongue
16. common bile duct
17. pylorus, pyloric sphincter
18. uvula
19. bile duct
20. polyp, small growth
21. abdomen
22. fat

Exercise 6
1. palat/o
2. sial/o
3. pancreat/o
4. peritone/o
5. a. gloss/o
   b. lingu/o
6. gingiv/o
7. pylor/o
8. hepat/o
9. chol/e
10. a. abdomin/o
    b. celi/o
    c. lapar/o
11. herni/o
12. diverticul/o
13. cheil/o
14. appendic/o
15. uvul/o
16. cholangi/o
17. choledoch/o
18. polyp/o
19. steat/o

Exercise 7
1. digestion
2. half

Exercise 8
1. -pepsia
2. hemi-

Exercise 9
Pronunciation Exercise

Exercise 10

1. WR CV WR S
   chol/e/lith/iasis
      CF
   condition of gallstones
2. WR   S
   diverticul/osis
   abnormal condition of having
      diverticula
3. WR CV WR
   sial/o/lith
      CF
   stone in the salivary gland
4. WR   S
   hepat/oma
   tumor of the liver
5. WR   S
   uvul/itis
   inflammation of the uvula
6. WR   S
   pancreat/itis
   inflammation of the pancreas
7. WR CV S
   proct/o/ptosis
      CF
   prolapse of the rectum
8. WR   S
   gingiv/itis
   inflammation of the gums
9. WR   S
   gastr/itis
   inflammation of the stomach
10. WR CV S
    rect/o/cele
       CF
    protrusion of the rectum
11. WR   S
    palat/itis
    inflammation of the palate
12. WR   S
    hepat/itis
    inflammation of the liver
13. WR   S
    appendic/itis
    inflammation of the appendix
14. WR CV WR S
    chol/e/cyst/itis
       CF
    inflammation of the gallbladder
15. WR   S
    diverticul/itis
    inflammation of a diverticulum
16. WR CV WR S
    gastr/o/enter/itis
       CF
    inflammation of the stomach
       and intestines

17. WR CV WR CV WR S
    gastr/o/enter/o/col/itis
       CF   CF
    inflammation of the stomach,
       intestines, and colon
18. WR   CV WR S
    choledoch/o/lith/iasis
          CF
    condition of stones in the common
       bile duct
19. WR   S
    cholangi/oma
    tumor of the bile duct
20. WR   S
    polyp/osis
    abnormal condition of (multiple)
       polyps
21. WR   S
    esophag/itis
    inflammation of the esophagus
22. WR   S
    periton/itis
    inflammation of the peritoneum
23. WR CV WR S
    steat/o/hepat/itis
       CF
    inflammation of the liver associated
       with (excess) fat

Exercise 11

1. hepat/oma
2. gastr/itis
3. sial/o/lith
4. appendic/itis
5. diverticul/itis
6. chol/e/cyst/itis
7. diverticul/osis
8. gastr/o/enter/itis
9. proct/o/ptosis
10. rect/o/cele
11. uvul/itis
12. gingiv/itis
13. hepat/itis
14. palat/itis
15. chol/e/lith/iasis
16. steat/o/hepat/itis
17. gastr/o/enter/o/col/itis
18. pancreat/itis
19. cholangi/oma
20. esophag/itis
21. choledoch/o/lith/iasis
22. polyp/osis
23. periton/itis

Exercise 12
Spelling Exercise; see text p. 488.

Exercise 13
Pronunciation Exercise

Exercise 14

1. f   10. j
2. b   11. m
3. e   12. i
4. n   13. c
5. d   14. l
6. g   15. o
7. a   16. p
8. k   17. q
9. h   18. r

Exercise 15

1. another name for gastric or duodenal
   ulcer
2. eating disorder characterized by a
   prolonged refusal to eat
3. chronic inflammation of the intestinal
   tract usually affecting the ileum
4. twisting or kinking of the intestine
5. abnormal growing together of two
   surfaces that normally are separated
6. chronic disease of the liver with gradual destruction of cells
7. telescoping of segment of the
   intestine
8. ulcer in the stomach
9. ulcer in the duodenum
10. inflammation of the colon with the
    formation of ulcers
11. eating disorder involving gorging
    food followed by induced vomiting
12. varicose vein in the rectal area
13. tumorlike growth extending out from
    a mucous membrane
14. disturbance of bowel function
15. obstruction of the intestine, often
    caused by failure of peristalsis
16. abnormal backward flow of the gas-
    trointestinal contents into the
    esophagus
17. excess body fat
18. an iron metabolism disorder

Exercise 16
Spelling Exercise; see text p. 493.

Exercise 17
Pronunciation Exercise

Exercise 18

1. WR   S
   gastr/ectomy
   excision of the stomach
2. WR   CV WR CV S
   esophag/o/gastr/o/plasty
        CF   CF
   surgical repair of the esophagus and
      the stomach

3. WR   S
    diverticul/ectomy
    excision of a diverticulum

4. WR   S
    antr/ectomy
    excision of the antrum

5. WR CV S
    palat/o/plasty
        CF
    surgical repair of the palate

6. WR   S
    uvul/ectomy
    excision of the uvula

7. WR CV WR CV S
    gastr/o/jejun/o/stomy
       CF   CF
    creation of an artificial opening be-
        tween the stomach and the jejunum

8. WR CV WR   S
    chol/e/cyst/ectomy
        CF
    excision of the gallbladder

9. WR   S
    col/ectomy
    excision of the colon

10. WR CV S
    col/o/stomy
        CF
    creation of an artificial opening into
        the colon

11. WR CV S
    pylor/o/plasty
        CF
    surgical repair of the pylorus

12. WR CV S
    an/o/plasty
       CF
    surgical repair of the anus

13. WR   S
    appendic/ectomy
    excision of the appendix

14. WR CV S
    cheil/o/rrhaphy
        CF
    suture of the lip

15. WR   S
    gingiv/ectomy
    surgical removal of gum (tissue)

16. WR CV S
    lapar/o/tomy
        CF
    incision into the abdomen

17. WR CV S
    ile/o/stomy
        CF
    creation of an artificial opening into
        the ileum

18. WR CV S
    gastr/o/stomy
        CF
    creation of an artificial opening into
        the stomach

19. WR CV S
    herni/o/rrhaphy
        CF
    suturing of a hernia

20. WR CV S
    gloss/o/rrhaphy
        CF
    suture of the tongue

21. WR   CV WR CV S
    choledoch/o/lith/o/tomy
            CF   CF
    incision into the common bile duct
        to remove a stone

22. P WR S
    hemi/col/ectomy
    excision of half of the colon

23. WR   S
    polyp/ectomy
    excision of a polyp

24. WR CV S
    enter/o/rrhaphy
        CF
    suture of the intestine

25. WR   CV S
    abdomin/o/plasty
            CF
    surgical repair of the abdomen

26. WR CV WR CV S
    pylor/o/my/o/tomy
        CF   CF
    incision into the pylorus muscle

27. WR CV WR CV WR CV S
    uvul/o/palat/o/pharyng/o/plasty
        CF   CF   CF
    surgical repair of the uvula, palate,
        and pharynx

28. WR CV S
    celi/o/tomy
        CF
    incision into the abdominal cavity

29. WR CV S
    gastr/o/plasty
        CF
    surgical repair of the stomach

30. WR   CV S
    abdomin/o/centesis
            CF
    surgical puncture to remove fluid
        from the abdominal cavity

Exercise 19
1. appendic/ectomy
2. gloss/o/rrhaphy
3. esophag/o/gastr/o/plasty
4. diverticul/ectomy
5. ile/o/stomy
6. gingiv/ectomy
7. lapar/o/tomy
8. an/o/plasty
9. antr/ectomy
10. chol/e/cyst/ectomy
11. col/ectomy
12. col/o/stomy
13. gastr/ectomy
14. gastr/o/stomy
15. gastr/o/jejun/o/stomy
16. uvul/ectomy
17. palat/o/plasty
18. pylor/o/plasty
19. herni/o/rrhaphy
20. cheil/o/rrhaphy
21. hemi/col/ectomy
22. choledoch/o/lith/o/tomy
23. polyp/ectomy
24. enter/o/rrhaphy
25. abdomin/o/plasty
26. celi/o/tomy
27. pylor/o/my/o/tomy
28. uvul/o/palat/o/pharyng/o/plasty
29. gastr/o/plasty
30. abdomin/o/centesis

Exercise 20
Spelling Exercise; see text p. 501.

Exercise 21
Pronunciation Exercise

Exercise 22
1. vagotomy
2. anastomosis
3. abdominoperineal resection
4. bariatric surgery
5. hemorrhoidectomy

Exercise 23
Spelling Exercise; see text p. 504.

Exercise 24
Pronunciation Exercise

Exercise 25
1. WR   CV S
    esophag/o/scope
            CF
    instrument used for visual
        examination of the esophagus

2.   WR   CV   S
esophag/o/scopy
　　　CF
visual examination of the esophagus

3.   WR   CV   S
gastr/o/scope
　　　CF
instrument used for visual
　　examination of the stomach

4.   WR   CV   S
gastr/o/scopy
　　　CF
visual examination of the stomach

5.   WR   CV   S
proct/o/scope
　　　CF
instrument used for visual
　　examination of the rectum

6.   WR   CV   S
proct/o/scopy
　　　CF
visual examination of the rectum

7.   P   S(WR)
endo/scope
instrument used for visual
　　examination within a hollow organ

8.   P   S(WR)
endo/scopy
visual examination within a hollow
　　organ

9.   WR   CV   S
sigmoid/o/scope
　　　CF
instrument used for visual
　　examination of the sigmoid colon

10.   WR   CV   S
sigmoid/o/scopy
　　　CF
visual examination of the sigmoid colon

11.   WR   CV WR CV   S
chol/e/cyst/o/gram
　　CF　　CF
radiographic image of the gallbladder

12.   WR   CV   S
cholangi/o/gram
　　　CF
radiographic image of bile ducts

13.   WR   CV WR CV   WR   CV   S
esophag/o/gastr/o/duoden/o/scopy
　　CF　　　CF　　　CF
visual examination of the esophagus,
　　stomach, and duodenum

14.   WR   CV   S
colon/o/scope
　　　CF
instrument used for visual
　　examination of the colon

15.   WR   CV   S
lapar/o/scope
　　　CF
instrument used for visual
　　examination of the abdominal cavity

16.   WR   CV   S
colon/o/scopy
　　　CF
visual examination of the colon

17.   WR   CV   S
lapar/o/scopy
　　　CF
visual examination of the abdominal
　　cavity

18.　　　WR   CV   S
CT colon/o/graphy
　　　　CF
radiographic imaging of the colon

19.   WR   CV   S
esophag/o/gram
　　　CF
radiographic image of the esophagus

20.   WR   CV   S
cholangi/o/graphy
　　　CF
radiographic imaging of the bile
　　ducts

Exercise 26

1. endo/scopy
2. gastr/o/scope
3. proct/o/scope
4. sigmoid/o/scope
5. chol/e/cyst/o/gram
6. endo/scope
7. esophag/o/scope
8. proct/o/scopy
9. esophag/o/scopy
10. sigmoid/o/scopy
11. cholangi/o/gram
12. gastr/o/scopy
13. lapar/o/scope
14. esophag/o/gastr/o/duoden/o/scopy
15. colon/o/scopy
16. lapar/o/scopy
17. colon/o/scope
18. colon/o/scopy
19. cholangi/o/graphy
20. esophag/o/gram

Exercise 27
Spelling Exercise; see text p. 511.

Exercise 28
Pronunciation Exercise

Exercise 29
1. series of radiographic images taken of
　the stomach and duodenum after bar-
　ium has been swallowed
2. series of radiographic images taken of
　the large intestine after a barium en-
　ema has been administered
3. radiographic examination of the biliary
　tract and pancreatic ducts
4. an endoscope fitted with an ultrasound
　probe providing images of layers of
　the intestinal wall
5. a blood test to determine the presence
　of *Helicobacter pylori* bacteria, a cause
　of peptic ulcers
6. a test to detect fecal occult blood
7. process of recording images of internal
　organs using sound waves

Exercise 30
1. d
2. f
3. a
4. b
5. h
6. g
7. c

Exercise 31
Spelling Exercise; see text p. 514.

Exercise 32
Pronunciation Exercise

Exercise 33
1.   P   S(WR)
a/phagia
without swallowing (inability to)

2.   P   S(WR)
dys/pepsia
difficult digestion

3.   WR   S
an/al
pertaining to the anus

4.   P   S(WR)
dys/phagia
difficult swallowing

5.   WR   CV   S
gloss/o/pathy
　　　CF
disease of the tongue

6. WR CV WR S
   ile/o/cec/al
   CF
   pertaining to the ileum and cecum

7. WR S
   or/al
   pertaining to the mouth

8. WR CV WR S
   stomat/o/gastr/ic
   CF
   pertaining to the mouth and stomach

9. WR CV S
   gastr/o/malacia
   CF
   softening of the stomach

10. WR S
    pancreat/ic
    pertaining to the pancreas

11. WR S
    gastr/odynia
    pain in the stomach

12. WR S
    peritone/al
    pertaining to the peritoneum

13. WR S
    steat/osis
    abnormal condition of fat

14. P WR S
    sub/lingu/al
    pertaining to under the tongue

15. WR CV S
    proct/o/logy
    CF
    study of the rectum

16. WR CV WR S
    nas/o/gastr/ic
    CF
    pertaining to the nose and stomach

17. WR S
    abdomin/al
    pertaining to the abdomen

18. WR CV S
    proct/o/logist
    CF
    physician who studies and treats
    diseases of the rectum

19. WR CV WR CV S
    gastr/o/enter/o/logy
    CF   CF
    study of the stomach and intestines

20. WR CV WR CV S
    gastr/o/enter/o/logist
    CF   CF
    physician who studies and treats
    diseases of the stomach and
    intestines

21. WR CV WR S
    col/o/rect/al
    CF
    pertaining to the colon and rectum

22. WR S
    rect/al
    pertaining to the rectum

23. WR CV S
    steat/o/rrhea
    CF
    discharge of fat

Exercise 34
1. gloss/o/pathy
2. a/phagia
3. sub/lingu/al
4. nas/o/gastr/ic
5. stomat/o/gastr/ic
6. an/al
7. peritone/al
8. abdomin/al
9. dys/phagia
10. ile/o/cec/al
11. gastr/o/malacia
12. gastr/odynia
13. proct/o/logist
14. dys/pepsia
15. pancreat/ic
16. proct/o/logy
17. steat/o/rrhea
18. or/al
19. gastr/o/enter/o/logist
20. gastr/o/enter/o/logy
21. col/o/rect/al
22. rect/al
23. steat/osis

Exercise 35
Spelling Exercise; see text p. 519.

Exercise 36
Pronunciation Exercise

Exercise 37
1. m	9. d
2. e	10. h
3. f	11. b
4. c	12. j
5. l	13. g
6. i	14. o
7. k	15. n
8. a	

Exercise 38
1. abnormal collection of fluid in the
   peritoneal cavity
2. process of feeding a person through a
   nasogastric tube
3. washing out of the stomach
4. waste from the digestive tract expelled through the rectum
5. urge to vomit
6. expelling matter from the stomach
   through the mouth
7. disorder that involves inflammation
   of the intestine
8. frequent discharge of liquid stool
9. gas expelled through the anus
10. abnormal backward flow
11. vomiting of blood
12. involuntary wavelike contractions
    that propel food along the digestive
    tract
13. black, tarry stools that contain di-
    gested blood
14. surgical opening between an organ
    and the surface of the body
15. passage of bloody feces
16. expelling matter from the stomach
    through the mouth

Exercise 39
Spelling Exercise; see text p. 522.

Exercise 40
1. endoscopic retrograde cholangiopancreatography
2. endoscopic ultrasound
3. nausea and vomiting
4. irritable bowel syndrome
5. percutaneous endoscopic gastrostomy
6. upper gastrointestinal
7. uvulopalatopharyngoplasty
8. gastroesophageal reflux disease
9. gastrointestinal
10. *Helicobacter pylori*
11. barium enema
12. esophagogastroduodenoscopy
13. abdominoperineal resection
14. fecal occult blood test

Exercise 41

A.
1. endoscopy
2. nausea
3. dyspepsia
4. hematemesis
5. melena
6. esophagogastroduodenoscopy
7. gastroscope
8. reflux
9. *H. pylori*
10. ulcers
11. gastritis
12. duodenal ulcers

B.
1. d
2. b
3. a
4. d

C.
1. a
2. d
3. d

Exercise 42

1. cholelithiasis
2. cholecystectomy
3. anastomoses
4. ulcerative colitis
5. proctoptosis
6. adhesion
7. gastrectomy, pyloroplasty, vagotomy
8. dyspepsia
9. gavage
10. abdominal perineal resection and colostomy
11. colonoscopy
12. ileus
13. fecal occult blood test
14. stomata

Exercise 43

Reading Exercise

Exercise 44

1. c
2. *T*
3. *T*
4. *F,* vomiting blood is not a warning sign of colorectal cancer.

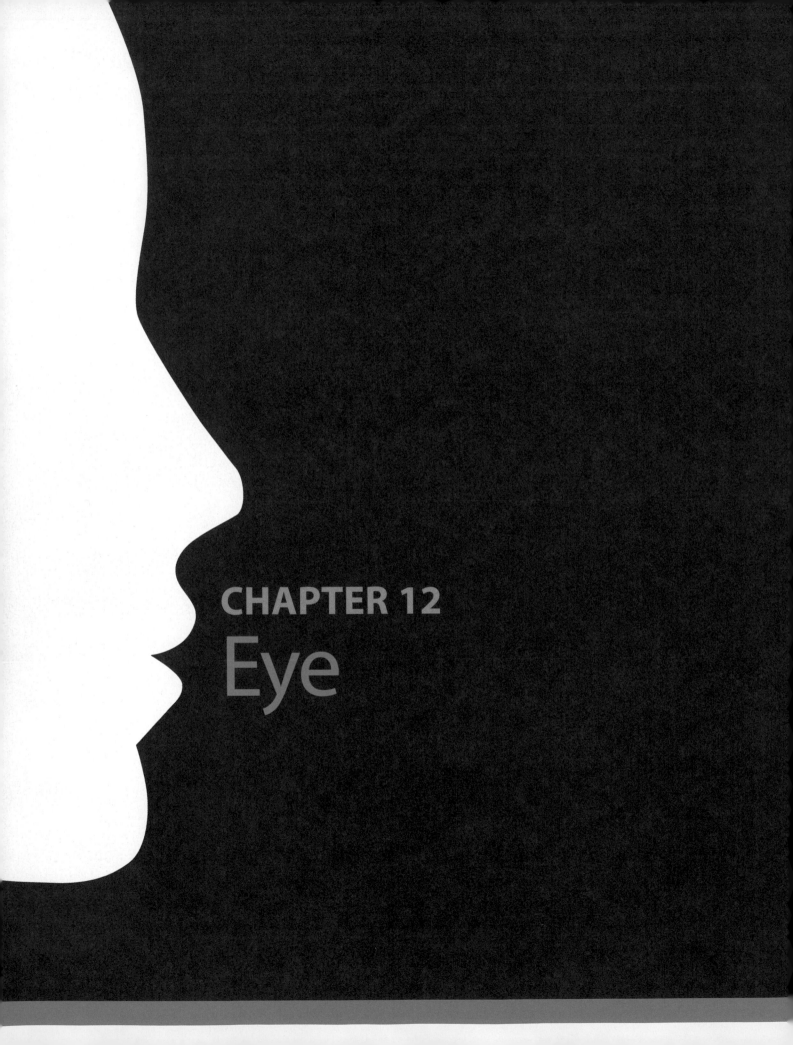

CHAPTER 12
Eye

OUTLINE

ANATOMY, 540

WORD PARTS, 543
Combining Forms, 543
Prefixes and Suffixes, 546

MEDICAL TERMS, 547
Disease and Disorder Terms, 547
    Built from Word Parts, 547
    Not Built from Word Parts, 551
Surgical Terms, 555
    Built from Word Parts, 555
    Not Built from Word Parts, 558
Diagnostic Terms, 561
    Built from Word Parts, 561
Complementary Terms, 563
    Built from Word Parts, 563
    Not Built from Word Parts, 566
Abbreviations, 568

PRACTICAL APPLICATION, 569
Interact with Medical Documents, 569
Interpret Medical Terms, 571
Read Medical Terms in Use, 571
Comprehend Medical Terms in Use, 572

CHAPTER REVIEW, 572

OBJECTIVES

Upon completion of this chapter you will be able to:

1. Identify organs and structures of the eye.

2. Define and spell word parts related to the eye.

3. Define, pronounce, and spell disease and disorder terms related to the eye.

4. Define, pronounce, and spell surgical terms related to the eye.

5. Define, pronounce, and spell diagnostic terms related to the eye.

6. Define, pronounce, and spell complementary terms related to the eye.

7. Interpret the meaning of abbreviations related to the eye.

8. Interpret, read, and comprehend medical language in simulated medical statements and documents.

ANATOMY

Function

The eyes are organs of vision and are located in a bony protective cavity of the skull called the **orbit.** Only a small portion of the eye is visible from the exterior (Figure 12-1).

Structures of the Eye

Term	Definition
sclera	outer protective layer of the eye; the portion seen on the anterior portion of the eyeball is referred to as the **white of the eye**
cornea	transparent anterior part of the sclera, which is in front of the aqueous humor and lies over the iris
choroid	middle layer of the eye, which is interlaced with many blood vessels
iris	the pigmented muscular structure that allows light to pass through
pupil	opening in the center of the iris
lens	lies directly behind the pupil. Its function is to focus and bend light.
retina	innermost layer of the eye, which contains the vision receptors (see Figure 12-2)
aqueous humor	watery liquid found in the anterior cavity of the eye
vitreous humor	jellylike substance found behind the lens in the posterior cavity of the eye that maintains its shape
meibomian glands	oil glands found in the upper and lower edges of the eyelids that help lubricate the eye
lacrimal glands and ducts	produce and drain tears
optic nerve	carries visual impulses from the retina to the brain
conjunctiva	mucous membrane lining the eyelids and covering the anterior portion of the sclera

IRIS was the special messenger of the Queen of Heaven according to Greek mythology. In this role she passed from heaven to earth over the rainbow while dressed in rainbow hues. Her name was applied to the **circular eye muscle** because of its varied colors.

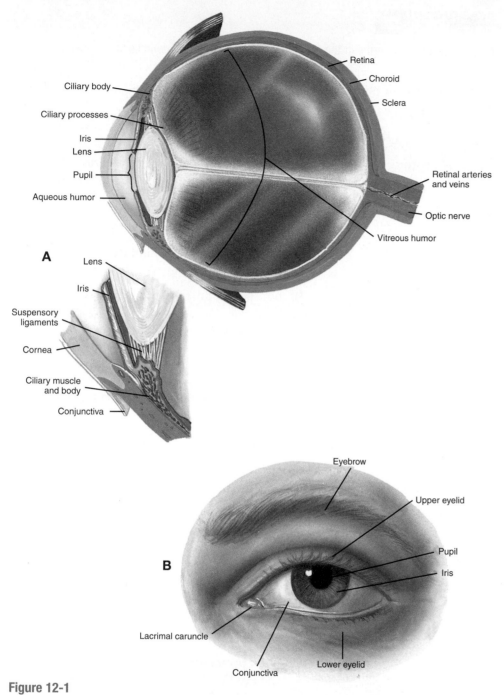

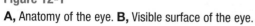

Figure 12-1
A, Anatomy of the eye. **B,** Visible surface of the eye.

EXERCISE 1

Match the anatomic terms in the first column with the correct definitions in the second column.

_____ 1. aqueous humor

_____ 2. choroid

_____ 3. conjunctiva

_____ 4. cornea

_____ 5. iris

_____ 6. lacrimal glands

_____ 7. lens

a. lies directly behind the pupil

b. the pigmented muscular structure

c. middle layer of the eye

d. watery liquid found in the anterior cavity of the eye

e. produce tears

f. mucous membrane lining the eyelids

g. jellylike substance behind the lens and in the posterior cavity

h. transparent anterior part of the sclera

EXERCISE 2

Match the anatomic terms in the first column with the correct definitions in the second column.

_____ 1. meibomian glands

_____ 2. optic nerve

_____ 3. orbit

_____ 4. pupil

_____ 5. retina

_____ 6. sclera

_____ 7. vitreous humor

a. outer protective layer of the eye

b. innermost layer of the eye

c. jellylike substance found behind the lens and in the posterior cavity of the eye

d. oil glands in eyelids that help lubricate the eye

e. opening in the center of the iris

f. carries visual impulses from the retina to the brain

g. middle layer of the eye

h. bony protective cavity of the skull in which the eye lies

WORD PARTS

Combining Forms of the Eye

Word parts you need to learn to complete this chapter are listed on the following pages. The exercises at the end of each list will help you learn their definitions and spellings.

Combining Form	Definition
blephar/o	eyelid
conjunctiv/o	conjunctiva
cor/o, core/o, pupill/o .... (NOTE: pupil has one *l*; the combining form has two *l*s.)	pupil
corne/o, kerat/o .... (NOTE: *kerat/o* also means *hard* or *horny tissue*; see Chapter 4.)	cornea
dacry/o, lacrim/o	tear, tear duct
irid/o, ir/o	iris
ocul/o, ophthalm/o	eye
opt/o.....................	vision
retin/o....................	retina
scler/o....................	sclera

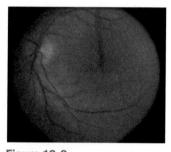

Figure 12-2
Ophthalmoscopic view of the retina.

Spelling Ophthalm
Look closely at the spelling of the word root **ophthalm**. Medical terms containing **ophthalm** are often misspelled by omitting the first h. **ph** gives the **f** sound followed by the sound of **thal.** Think pronunciation when spelling terms that contain **ophthalm,** as in ophthalmology (of(ph)-thal-MOL-ō-jē).

EXERCISE 3

Write the definitions of the following combining forms.

1. ocul/o _____

2. blephar/o _____

3. corne/o _____

4. lacrim/o _____

5. retin/o _____

6. pupill/o _____

7. scler/o _____

8. irid/o _____

9. conjunctiv/o _____

10. cor/o _____

11. ophthalm/o _____

12. kerat/o _____

13. ir/o _____

14. core/o _____

15. opt/o _____

16. dacry/o _____

EXERCISE FIGURE A

Diagrams of the eye. Fill in the blanks with combining forms.

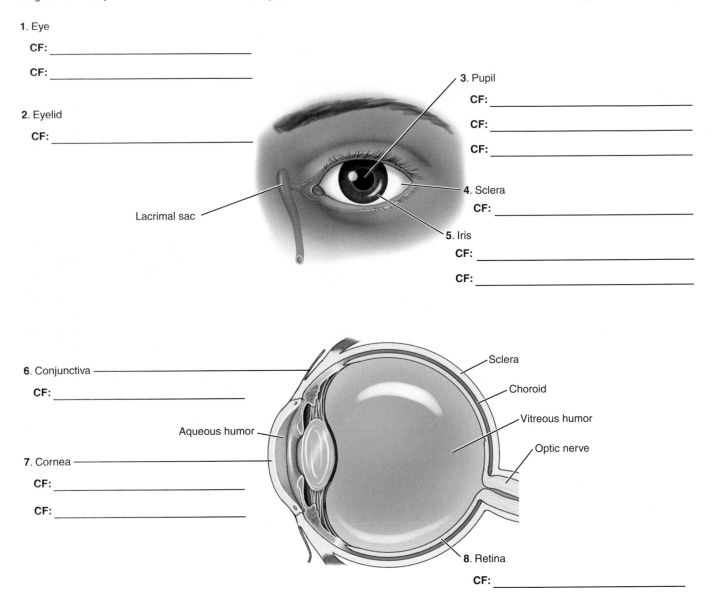

1. Eye

    CF: _____

    CF: _____

2. Eyelid

    CF: _____

3. Pupil

    CF: _____

    CF: _____

    CF: _____

4. Sclera

    CF: _____

5. Iris

    CF: _____

    CF: _____

Lacrimal sac

6. Conjunctiva

    CF: _____

Aqueous humor

7. Cornea

    CF: _____

    CF: _____

Sclera

Choroid

Vitreous humor

Optic nerve

8. Retina

    CF: _____

EXERCISE 4

Write the combining form for each of the following terms.

1. eye   a. _____   6. pupil   a. _____

               b. _____   b. _____

2. cornea   a. _____   c. _____

               b. _____   7. sclera   _____

3. conjunctiva   _____   8. retina   _____

4. tear, tear duct   a. _____   9. iris   a. _____

               b. _____   b. _____

5. eyelid   _____   10. vision   _____

Combining Forms Commonly Used with the Eye

Combining Form	Definition
cry/o	cold
dipl/o	two, double
phot/o	light
ton/o	tension, pressure

EXERCISE 5

Write the definitions of the following combining forms.

1. ton/o _____   3 cry/o _____

2. phot/o _____   4. dipl/o _____

EXERCISE 6

Write the combining form for each of the following.

1. cold _____   3. two, double _____

2. tension, pressure _____   4. light _____

Prefixes and Suffixes

Prefixes	Definition
bi-, bin-....................	two

Suffixes	Definitions
-opia.....................	vision (condition)
-phobia..................	abnormal fear of or aversion to specific things
-plegia	paralysis

Refer to Appendix A and Appendix B for a complete listing of word parts.

EXERCISE 7

Write the definition of the following prefixes and suffixes.

1. -opia _____

2. bi- _____

3. -plegia _____

4. -phobia _____

5. bin- _____

EXERCISE 8

Write the prefixes or suffixes for each of the following definitions.

1. paralysis _____

2. two   a. _____

                       b. _____

3. abnormal fear of or
   aversion to specific things _____

4. vision (condition) _____

MEDICAL TERMS

The terms you need to learn to complete this chapter are listed on the following pages. The exercises following each list will help you learn the definition and the spelling of each word.

Disease and Disorder Terms
Built from Word Parts

The following terms are built from word parts you have already learned and can be translated literally to find their meanings. Further explanation of terms beyond the definition of their word parts, if needed, is included in parentheses.

Term	Definition
blepharitis . . . . (*blef*-a-RĪ-tis)	inflammation of the eyelid (Exercise Figure B)
blepharoptosis . . . . (*blef*-ar-op-TŌ-sis)	drooping of the eyelid (Exercise Figure C) (commonly called **ptosis**)
conjunctivitis . . . . (kon-*junk*-ti-VĪ-tis)	inflammation of the conjunctiva (commonly called **pinkeye**)
dacryocystitis . . . . (*dak*-rē-ō-sis-TĪ-tis)	inflammation of the tear (lacrimal) sac (Exercise Figure D)
diplopia . . . . (di-PLŌ-pē-a)	double vision
endophthalmitis . . . . (en-dof-thal-MĪ-tis) (NOTE: the *o* in *endo* is dropped.)	inflammation within the eye
iridoplegia . . . . (*īr*-i-dō-PLĒ-ja)	paralysis of the iris
iritis . . . . (*ī*-RĪ-tis)	inflammation of the iris
keratitis . . . . (ker-a-TĪ-tis)	inflammation of the cornea
keratomalacia . . . . (*ker*-a-tō-ma-LĀ-sha)	softening of the cornea (usually a bilateral condition associated with vitamin A deficiency)
leukocoria . . . . (lū-kō-KŌ-rē-a)	condition of white pupil
oculomycosis . . . . (*ok*-ū-lō-mī-KŌ-sis)	abnormal condition of the eye caused by a fungus
ophthalmalgia . . . . (*of*-thal-MAL-ja)	pain in the eye
ophthalmoplegia . . . . (of-thal-mō-PLĒ-ja)	paralysis of the eye (muscle)
photophobia . . . . (*fō*-tō-FŌ-bē-a)	abnormal fear of (sensitivity to) light

EXERCISE FIGURE B

Fill in the blanks to complete labeling of this diagram.

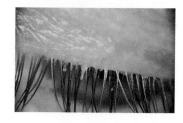

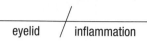

eyelid / inflammation

with thickened lids and crusts around the lashes.

EXERCISE FIGURE C

Fill in the blanks to label the diagram.

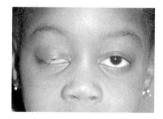

eyelid / cv / drooping

EXERCISE FIGURE D

Fill in the blanks to label the diagram.

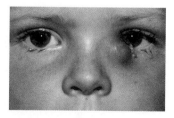

tear / cv / sac /inflammation

Disease and Disorder Terms—*cont'd*
Built from Word Parts

Term	Definition
retinoblastoma . . . . (ret-i-nō-blas-TŌ-ma)	tumor arising from a developing retinal cell (a congenital, malignant tumor)
retinopathy . . . . (*ret*-i-NOP-a-thē)	(any noninflammatory) disease of the retina (such as diabetic retinopathy)
sclerokeratitis . . . . (*sklēr*-ō-ker-a-TĪ-tis)	inflammation of the sclera and the cornea
scleromalacia . . . . (*sklēr*-ō-ma-LĀ-sha)	softening of the sclera
xerophthalmia . . . . (*zēr*-of-THAL-mē-a)	condition of dry eye (conjunctiva and cornea) (caused by vitamin A deficiency)

EXERCISE   9

Practice saying aloud each of the disease and disorder terms built from word parts on pp. 547-548.

To hear the terms select Chapter 12, Chapter Exercises, Pronunciation.

☐ Place a check mark in the box when you have completed this exercise.

EXERCISE   10

Analyze and define the following terms.

1. sclerokeratitis _____

2. ophthalmalgia _____

3. blepharoptosis _____

4. diplopia _____

5. conjunctivitis _____

6. leukocoria _____

7. iridoplegia _____

8. scleromalacia _____

9. photophobia _____

10. blepharitis _____

11. oculomycosis _____

12. dacryocystitis _____

13. endophthalmitis _____

14. iritis _____

15. retinoblastoma _____

16. keratitis _____

17. ophthalmoplegia _____

18. retinopathy _____

19. xerophthalmia _____

20. keratomalacia _____

EXERCISE 11

Build disease and disorder terms for the following definitions by using the word parts you have learned.

1. inflammation of the conjunctiva _____ / _____
                 WR   S

2. abnormal eye condition caused by a fungus
   _____ / _____ / _____ / _____
     WR   CV   WR   S

3. pain in the eye
   _____ / _____
        WR   S

4. double vision
   _____ / _____
        WR   S

5. inflammation of the eyelid
   _____ / _____
        WR   S

6. condition of white pupil
   _____ / _____ / _____ / _____
     WR   CV   WR   S

7. paralysis of the iris
   _____ / _____ / _____
     WR   CV   S

8. drooping of the eyelid
   _____ / _____ / _____
     WR   CV   S

9. inflammation of the iris
   _____ / _____
        WR   S

10. tumor arising from a developing retinal cell
    _____ / _____ / _____ / _____
      WR   CV   WR   S

11. softening of the sclera
    _____ / _____ / _____
      WR   CV   S

12. inflammation of a tear (lacrimal) sac
    _____ / _____ / _____ / _____
      WR   CV   WR   S

13. inflammation of the sclera
    and cornea

    _____ / _____ / _____ / _____
    WR   / CV /   WR   /   S

14. abnormal fear of (sensitivity
    to) light

    _____ / _____ / _____
    WR   / CV /   S

15. inflammation of the cornea

    _____ / _____
    WR   /   S

16. disease of the retina

    _____ / _____ / _____
    WR   / CV /   S

17. inflammation within the eye

    _____ / _____ / _____
    P   /   WR   /   S

18. paralysis of the eye (muscle)

    _____ / _____ / _____
    WR   / CV /   S

19. condition of dry eye

    _____ / _____ / _____
    WR   /   WR   /   S

20. softening of the cornea

    _____ / _____ / _____
    WR   / CV /   S

EXERCISE 12

Spell each of the disease and disorder terms built from word parts on pp. 547-548 by having someone dictate them to you.

 To hear and spell the terms select Chapter 12, Chapter Exercises, Spelling. You may type the terms on the screen or write them below in the spaces provided.

☐ Place a check mark in the box if you have completed this exercise using your CD-ROM.

1. _____   11. _____

2. _____   12. _____

3. _____   13. _____

4. _____   14. _____

5. _____   15. _____

6. _____   16. _____

7. _____   17. _____

8. _____   18. _____

9. _____   19. _____

10. _____   20. _____

Disease and Disorder Terms
Not Built from Word Parts

In some of the following terms, you may recognize word parts you have already learned; however, the full meaning of the terms cannot be discerned by the definition of their word parts.

Term	Definition
amblyopia . . . . (*am*-ble-Ō-pē-a)	reduced vision in one eye caused by disuse or misuse associated with strabismus, unequal refractive errors, or otherwise impaired vision. The brain suppresses images from the impaired eye to avoid double vision (also called **lazy eye**).
astigmatism (Ast) . . . . (a-STIG-ma-tizm)	defective curvature of the refractive surface of the eye (Figure 12-3, *C*)
cataract . . . . (KAT-a-rakt)	clouding of the lens of the eye (Figure 12-4)
chalazion . . . . (ka-LĀ-zē-on)	obstruction of an oil gland of the eyelid (also called **meibomian cyst**) (Figure 12-5)
detached retina . . . . (RET-in-a)	separation of the retina from the choroid in back of the eye (Figure 12-6)
emmetropia (Em) . . . . (em-e-TRŌ-pē-a)	normal refractive condition of the eye

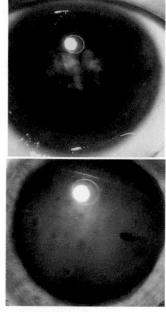

Figure 12-4
A, Snowflake cataract.
B, Senile cataract.

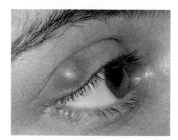

Figure 12-5
Chalazion (right upper eyelid).

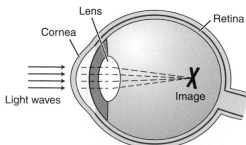

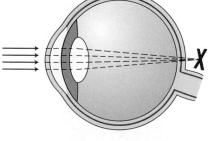

A. Myopia (nearsightedness)

B. Hyperopia (farsightedness)

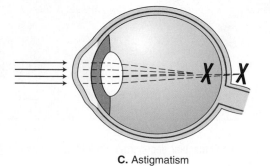

C. Astigmatism

Figure 12-3
Refraction errors.

GLAUCOMA
is composed of the Greek
glaukos, meaning
blue-gray or **sea green,** and
oma, meaning a morbid condition. The term was given to any
condition in which gray or green
replaced the black in the pupil.

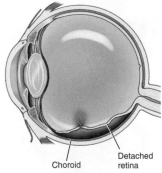

Figure 12-6
Detached retina. Vitreous fluid has
seeped through a break in the
retina, causing the choroid coat
and retina to separate.

CAM TERM
Light therapy is the
therapeutic use of ultraviolet, colored, and laser lights to reestab-
lish the body's natural rhythm,
reduce pain and depression, and
improve other health conditions.
One type of light therapy, photodynamic therapy, has demonstrated repeated success in
treating a variety of ophthalmic
conditions, including age-related
macular degeneration, intraocular tumors, and eyelid basali-
oma. Refer to the complementary
and alternative therapies appendix on Evolve.

AGE-RELATED MACULAR
DEGENERATION (ARMD)
is the leading cause of legal
blindness in persons older than
65 years. Onset occurs between
the ages of 50 and 60 (see
Figure 12-7).

Disease and Disorder Terms—*cont'd*
Not Built from Word Parts

Term	Definition
glaucoma . . . . (glaw-KŌ-ma)	eye disorder characterized by optic nerve damage usually caused by the abnormal increase of intraocular pressure (IOP). If not treated it will lead to blindness.
hyperopia . . . . (hī-per-Ō-pē-a)	farsightedness (Figure 12-3, *B*)
macular degeneration . . . . (MAC-ū-lar)	a progressive deterioration of the portion of the retina called the **macula lutea,** result-ing in loss of central vision (Figure 12-7)
myopia . . . . (mī-Ō-pē-a)	nearsightedness (see Figure 12-3, *A*)
nyctalopia . . . . (nik-ta-LŌ-pē-a)	poor vision at night or in faint light (also called **night blindness**)
nystagmus . . . . (nis-TAG-mus)	involuntary, jerking movements of the eyes
pinguecula . . . . (ping-GWEH-kū-la)	yellowish mass on the conjunctiva that may be related to exposure to ultraviolet light, dry climates, and dust. A pinguec-ula that spreads onto the cornea becomes a **pterygium.**
presbyopia . . . . (*pres*-bē-Ō-pē-a)	impaired vision as a result of aging

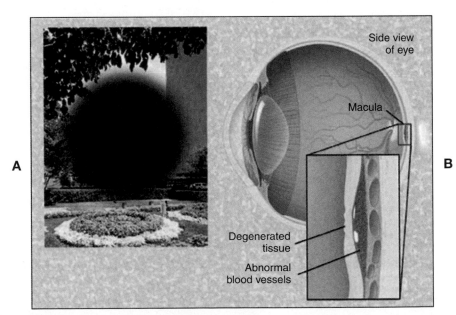

Figure 12-7
A, How a patient with age-related macular degeneration might see the world. **B,** Wet macular degen-eration with new blood vessels.

Term	Definition
pterygium................. (te-RIJ-ē-um)	thin tissue growing into the cornea from the conjunctiva, usually caused from sun exposure
retinitis pigmentosa .... (ret-i-NĪ-tis) (pig-men-TŌ-sa)	hereditary, progressive disease marked by night blindness with atrophy and retinal pigment changes
strabismus .... (stra-BIZ-mus)	abnormal condition of squint or crossed eyes caused by the visual axes not meeting at the same point
sty..................... (stī)	infection of an oil gland of the eyelid (Figure 12-8) (also spelled **stye** and also called **hordeolum**)

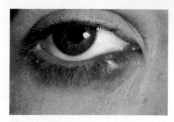

Figure 12-8
Sty, stye, or hordeolum.

EXERCISE 13

Practice saying aloud each of the disease and disorder terms not built from word parts on pp. 551-553.

To hear the terms select Chapter 12, Chapter Exercises, Pronunciation.

☐ Place a check mark in the box when you have completed this exercise.

EXERCISE 14

Fill in the blanks with the correct terms.

1. Another name for nearsightedness is _____.

2. Impaired vision as a result of aging is _____.

3. The abnormal condition of squinted or crossed eyes caused by visual axes not meeting at the same point is called _____.

4. An obstruction of an oil gland of the eyelid is called a(n) _____.

5. A defective curvature of the refractive surface of the eye causes a condition known as _____.

6. _____ is the name given to involuntary, jerking movements of the eye.

7. A clouding of the lens of the eye is called a(n) _____.

8. _____ is the name given to an infection of the oil gland of the eyelids.

9. A disorder usually caused by the abnormal increase of intraocular pressure is _____.

10. A(n) _____ _____ is a separation of the retina from the choroid in the back of the eye.

11. Another name for farsightedness is _____.

12. Normal refractive condition of the eye is called _____.

13. _____ _____ is a hereditary, progressive disease causing night blindness with retinal pigment changes and atrophy.

14. Another name for night blindness is _____.

15. A thin tissue growing into the cornea from the conjunctiva is called a(n) _____.

16. _____ _____ is the progressive deterioration of the macula lutea.

17. Another name for lazy eye is _____.

18. _____ may be related to exposure to ultraviolet light, dry climates, and dust and may spread onto the cornea to become a pterygium.

EXERCISE 15

Match the terms in the first column with the correct definitions in the second column.

_____ 1. astigmatism

_____ 2. cataract

_____ 3. chalazion

_____ 4. detached retina

_____ 5. glaucoma

_____ 6. myopia

_____ 7. nystagmus

_____ 8. hyperopia

_____ 9. presbyopia

_____ 10. strabismus

_____ 11. sty

_____ 12. pterygium

_____ 13. retinitis pigmentosa

_____ 14. nyctalopia

_____ 15. emmetropia

_____ 16. macular degeneration

_____ 17. pinguecula

_____ 18. amblyopia

a. infection of an oil gland of the eyelid

b. deterioration of the macula lutea

c. crossed eyes or squinting caused by visual axes not meeting at the same point

d. involuntary, jerking movements of the eye

e. impaired vision caused by aging

f. defective curvature of the refractive surface of the eye

g. normal refractive condition of the eye

h. clouding of a lens of the eye

i. hereditary progressive disease marked by night blindness

j. nearsightedness

k. obstruction of an oil gland of the eye

l. usually caused from sun exposure

m. eye disorder characterized by optic nerve damage

n. separation of the retina from the choroid in the back of the eye

o. poor vision at night or in faint light

p. farsightedness

q. double vision

r. yellow mass on the conjunctiva

s. reduced vision in one eye caused by disuse or misuse

EXERCISE 16

Spell each of the disease and disorder terms not built from word parts on pp. 551-553 by having someone dictate them to you.

 To hear and spell the terms select Chapter 12, Chapter Exercises, Spelling. You may type the terms on the screen or write them below in the spaces provided.

☐ Place a check mark in the box if you have completed this exercise using your CD-ROM.

1._____   10._____

2._____   11._____

3._____   12._____

4._____   13._____

5._____   14._____

6._____   15._____

7._____   16._____

8._____   17._____

9._____   18._____

Surgical Terms

Built from Word Parts

The following terms are built from word parts you have already learned and can be translated literally to find their meanings. Further explanation of terms beyond the definition of their word parts, if needed, is included in parentheses.

Term	Definition
blepharoplasty (BLEF-a-rō-*plas*-tē)	surgical repair of the eyelid
cryoretinopexy (*krī-ō*-RE-tin-ō-pek-sē)	surgical fixation of the retina by using extreme cold (carbon dioxide)
dacryocystorhinostomy (*dak*-rē-ō-*sis*-tō-rī-NOS-to-mē)	creation of an artificial opening between the tear (lacrimal) sac and the nose (to restore drainage into the nose when the nasolacrimal duct is obstructed or obliterated)
dacryocystotomy (*dak*-rē-ō-sis-TOT-o-mē)	incision into the tear (lacrimal) sac
iridectomy (ir-i-DEK-to-mē)	excision (of part) of the iris
iridotomy (ir-i-DOT-o-mē)	incision into the iris

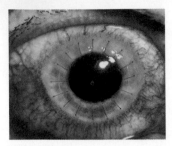

Figure 12-9
Appearance of eye after
keratoplasty.

Surgical Terms—*cont'd*
Built from Word Parts

Term	Definition
keratoplasty . . . . (KER-a-tō-*plas*-tē)	surgical repair of the cornea (corneal transplant) (Figure 12-9)
sclerotomy . . . . (skle-ROT-o-mē)	incision into the sclera

EXERCISE 17

Practice saying aloud each of the surgical terms built from word parts on pp. 555-556.

 To hear the terms select Chapter 12, Chapter Exercises, Pronunciation.

☐ Place a check mark in the box when you have completed this exercise.

EXERCISE 18

Analyze and define the following surgical terms.

1. keratoplasty _____

2. sclerotomy _____

3. dacryocystotomy _____

4. cryoretinopexy _____

5. blepharoplasty _____

6. iridectomy _____

7. dacryocystorhinostomy _____

8. iridotomy _____

EXERCISE 19

Build surgical terms for the following definitions by using the word parts you have learned.

1. creation of an artificial opening between the tear (lacrimal) sac and the nose

   ___ / ___ / ___ / ___ / ___ / ___ / ___
   WR / CV / WR / CV / WR / CV / S

2. excision of the iris

   ___ / ___
   WR / S

3. surgical repair of the cornea

   ___ / ___ / ___
   WR / CV / S

4. incision of the sclera

   ___ / ___ / ___
   WR / CV / S

5. incision into the iris

   ___ / ___ / ___
   WR / CV / S

6. surgical repair of the eyelid

   ___ / ___ / ___
   WR / CV / S

7. surgical fixation of the retina by a method using extreme cold

   ___ / ___ / ___ / ___ / ___
   WR / CV / WR / CV / S

8. incision into the (lacrimal) tear sac

   ___ / ___ / ___ / ___ / ___
   WR / CV / WR / CV / S

EXERCISE 20

Spell each of the surgical terms built from word parts on pp. 555-556 by having someone dictate them to you.

To hear and spell the terms select Chapter 12, Chapter Exercises, Spelling. You may type the terms on the screen or write them below in the spaces provided.

☐ Place a check mark in the box if you have completed this exercise using your CD-ROM.

1. _____   5. _____

2. _____   6. _____

3. _____   7. _____

4. _____   8. _____

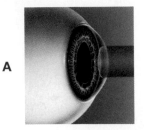

A

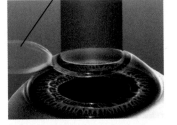

Flap of cornea

B

Figure 12-10
Excimer laser treatments for near-sightedness. **A, PRK** (photorefractive keratectomy): removes tissue from the surface of the cornea. **B, LASIK** (laser-assisted in situ keratomileusis): reshapes corneal tissue below the surface of the cornea. The Excimer laser was invented in the early 1980s. It is a computer-controlled ultraviolet beam of light that reshapes the cornea. It has replaced **RK** (radial keratotomy), a surgery in which spokelike incisions are made to reshape the cornea.

WEB LINK
To learn more about refractive surgery and corneal modification, visit the American Optometric Association's Web site at www.aoa.org.

Surgical Terms

Not Built from Word Parts

In some of the following terms, you may recognize word parts you have already learned; however, the full meaning of the terms cannot be discerned by the definition of their word parts.

Term	Definition
enucleation................. (ē-*nū*-klē-Ā-shun)	surgical removal of the eyeball (also, the removal of any organ that comes out clean and whole)
LASIK (laser-assisted in situ keratomileusis).............. (LĀ-sik)	a laser procedure that reshapes the corneal tissue beneath the surface of the cornea to correct astigmatism, hyperopia, and myopia. LASIK is a combination of Excimer laser and lamellar keratoplasty. It differs from PRK in that it reshapes corneal tissue beneath the surface rather than on the surface (Figure 12-10, *B*).
phacoemulsification.......... (fa-kō-ē-mul-si-fi-KĀ-shun)	method to remove cataracts in which an ultrasonic needle probe breaks up the lens, which is then aspirated
PRK (photorefractive keratectomy)............... (fō-tō-rē-FRAK-tiv) (ker-a-TEK-to-mē)	a procedure for the treatment of nearsightedness in which an Excimer laser is used to reshape (flatten) the corneal surface by removing a portion of the cornea (Figure 12-10, *A*)
retinal photocoagulation....... (RET-in-al) (fō-tō-kō-*ag*-ū-LĀ-shun)	a procedure to repair tears in the retina by use of an intense, precisely focused light beam, which causes coagulation of the tissue protein

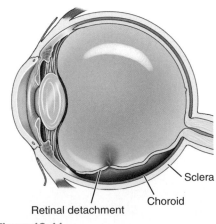

Retinal detachment   Choroid   Sclera

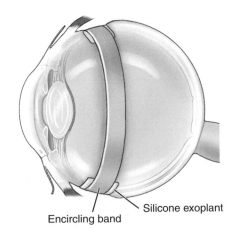

Encircling band   Silicone exoplant

Figure 12-11
Scleral buckling. A surgical procedure to repair a detached retina.

Term	Definition
scleral buckling . . . . (SKLER-al) (BUK-ling)	a procedure to repair a detached retina. A strip of sclera is resected, or a fold is made in the sclera. An exoplant is used to hold and buckle the sclera (Figure 12-11).
trabeculectomy. . . . . (tra-bek-ū-LEK-to-mē)	surgical creation of a drain to reduce intra-ocular pressure (used to treat glaucoma)
vitrectomy. . . . . (vi-TREK-to-mē)	surgical removal of all or part of the vitre-ous humor (used to treat diabetic reti-nopathy)

EXERCISE 21

Practice saying aloud each of the surgical terms not built from word parts on pp. 558-559.

To hear the terms select Chapter 12, Chapter Exercises, Pronunciation.

☐ Place a check mark in the box when you have completed this exercise.

EXERCISE 22

Fill in the blank with the correct terms.

1. The procedure performed to repair tears in the retina is called

   _____ _____.

2. Surgical removal of an eyeball is called a(n)_____.

3. _____ is the name given to the procedure that breaks up the lens with ultrasound and then aspirates it.

4. A procedure using the Excimer laser and lamellar keratoplasty to correct hyperopia, myopia, and astigmatism is called _____.

5. _____ is the surgical creation of a drain to reduce intraocular pressure.

6. An operation to repair a detached retina in which the sclera is folded or resected and an exoplant is used to buckle and hold the sclera is called

   _____ _____.

7. Surgery to remove vitreous humor from the eye is called _____.

8. _____ is a procedure for the treatment of nearsightedness in which an Excimer laser is used to reshape the corneal surface.

EXERCISE 23

Match the terms in the first column with their correct definitions in the second column.

_____ 1. LASIK

_____ 2. enucleation

_____ 3. trabeculectomy

_____ 4. retinal photocoagulation

_____ 5. phacoemulsification

_____ 6. scleral buckling

_____ 7. vitrectomy

_____ 8. PRK

a. procedure to repair tears in the retina

b. surgical creation of a permanent drain to reduce intraocular pressure

c. procedure for the treatment of near-sightedness in which an Excimer laser is used to reshape the corneal surface

d. procedure in which the lens is broken up by ultrasound and aspirated

e. procedure used to correct astigmatism, nearsightedness, and farsightedness by reshaping tissue beneath the corneal surface

f. surgical removal of an eyeball

g. surgical removal of vitreous humor

h. operation in which a cataract is lifted from the eye with an extremely cold probe

i. detached retina surgery in which the sclera is folded and an exoplant is used to buckle and hold the sclera

j. surgical incision of the sclera

EXERCISE 24

Spell each of the surgical terms not built from word parts on pp. 558-559 by having someone dictate them to you.

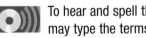 To hear and spell the terms select Chapter 12, Chapter Exercises, Spelling. You may type the terms on the screen or write them below in the spaces provided.

☐ Place a check mark in the box if you have completed this exercise using your CD-ROM.

1. _____

2. _____

3. _____

4. _____

5. _____

6. _____

7. _____

8. _____

Diagnostic Terms
Built from Word Parts

The following terms are built from word parts you have already learned and can be translated literally to find their meanings. Further explanation of terms beyond the definition of their word parts, if needed, is included in parentheses.

Term	Definition
DIAGNOSTIC IMAGING	
fluorescein angiography...... (flō-RES-ēn) (an-jē-OG-ra-fē)	(photographic) process of recording blood vessels (of the eye with fluorescing dye)
OPHTHALMIC EVALUATION	
keratometer .... (*ker*-a-TOM-e-ter)	instrument used to measure (the curvature of) the cornea (used for fitting contact lenses)
ophthalmoscope........... (of-THAL-mō-skōp)	instrument used for visual examination (the interior) of the eye (Figure 12-12)
ophthalmoscopy........... (*of*-thal-MOS-ko-pē)	visual examination of the eye
optometry................ (op-TOM-e-trē)	measurement of vision (visual acuity and the prescribing of corrective lenses)
pupillometer.............. (pū-pil-OM-e-ter)	instrument used to measure (the diameter of) the pupil
pupilloscope.............. (pū-PIL-ō-skōp)	instrument used for visual examination of the pupil
retinoscopy............... (*ret*-i-NOS-ko-pē)	visual examination of the retina
tonometer................ (ton-OM-e-ter)	instrument used to measure pressure (within the eye, used to diagnose glaucoma)
tonometry................ (ton-OM-e-trē)	measurement of pressure (within the eye)

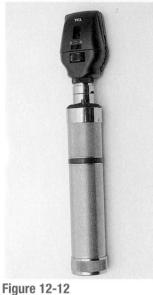

Figure 12-12
Ophthalmoscope.

EXERCISE 25

Practice saying aloud each of the diagnostic terms built from word parts above.

 To hear the terms select Chapter 12, Chapter Exercises, Pronunciation.

☐ Place a check mark in the box when you have completed this exercise.

EXERCISE 26

Analyze and define the following diagnostic terms.

1. pupilloscope _____

2. optometry _____

3. ophthalmoscope _____

4. tonometry _____

5. pupillometer _____

6. tonometer _____

7. keratometer _____

8. ophthalmoscopy _____

9. (fluorescein) angiography _____

10. retinoscopy _____

EXERCISE 27

Build diagnostic terms that correspond to the following definitions by using the word parts you have learned.

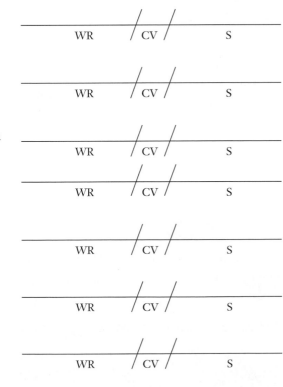

1. measurement of pressure
   (within the eye)

   _____/___/_____
   WR   CV   S

2. instrument used to measure
   (the diameter of) the pupil

   _____/___/_____
   WR   CV   S

3. instrument used to measure
   (the curvature of) the cornea

   _____/___/_____
   WR   CV   S

4. measurement of vision

   _____/___/_____
   WR   CV   S

5. instrument used for visual
   examination of the eye

   _____/___/_____
   WR   CV   S

6. instrument used to measure
   pressure (within the eye)

   _____/___/_____
   WR   CV   S

7. instrument used for visual
   examination of the pupil

   _____/___/_____
   WR   CV   S

8. visual examination of the eye

_____ / _____ / _____
WR   CV   S

9. process of recording blood vessels (of the eye with fluorescing dye)

fluorescein _____ / _____ / _____
WR   CV   S

10. visual examination of the retina

_____ / _____ / _____
WR   CV   S

EXERCISE 28

Spell each of the diagnostic terms built from word parts on p. 561 by having someone dictate them to you.

 To hear and spell the terms select Chapter 12, Chapter Exercises, Spelling. You may type the terms on the screen or write them below in the spaces provided.

☐ Place a check mark in the box if you have completed this exercise using your CD-ROM.

1._____   6. _____

2._____   7. _____

3._____   8. _____

4._____   9. _____

5._____   10. _____

Complementary Terms

Built from Word Parts

The following terms are built from word parts you have already learned and can be translated literally to find their meanings. Further explanation of terms beyond the definition of their word parts, if needed, is included in parentheses.

Term	Definition
binocular.................... (bin-OK-ū-lar)	pertaining to two or both eyes
corneal.................... (KOR-nē-al)	pertaining to the cornea
intraocular................. (_in_-tra-OK-ū-lar)	pertaining to within the eye
lacrimal.................... (LAK-ri-mal)	pertaining to tears
nasolacrimal............... (_nā_-zō-LAK-ri-mal)	pertaining to the nose and tear ducts
ophthalmic................ (of-THAL-mik)	pertaining to the eye

Complementary Terms—*cont'd*
Built from Word Parts

Term	Definition
ophthalmologist . . . . (*of*-thal-MOL-o-jist)	physician who studies and treats diseases of the eye
ophthalmology (Ophth) . . . . (*of*-thal-MOL-o-jē)	study of the eye (a branch of medicine that deals with treating diseases of the eye)
ophthalmopathy . . . . (*of*-thal-MOP-a-thē)	(any) disease of the eye
optic . . . . (OP-tik)	pertaining to vision
pupillary . . . . (PŪ-pi-lar-ē)	pertaining to the pupil
retinal . . . . (RET-i-nal)	pertaining to the retina

EXERCISE 29

Practice saying aloud each of the complementary terms built from word parts on pp. 563-564.

To hear the terms select Chapter 12, Chapter Exercises, Pronunciation.

☐ Place a check mark in the box when you have completed this exercise.

EXERCISE 30

Analyze and define the following complementary terms.

1. ophthalmology _____

2. binocular _____

3. lacrimal _____

4. pupillary _____

5. ophthalmologist _____

6. corneal _____

7. ophthalmic _____

8. nasolacrimal _____

9. optic _____

10. intraocular _____

11. retinal _____

12. ophthalmopathy _____

EXERCISE **31**

Build the complementary terms for the following definitions by using the word parts you have learned.

1. study of the eye

 _____ / _____ / _____
 WR   CV   S

2. pertaining to two or both eyes

 _____ / _____ / _____
 P   WR   S

3. pertaining to the retina

 _____ / _____
 WR   S

4. pertaining to within the eye

 _____ / _____ / _____
 P   WR   S

5. physician who studies and treats diseases of the eye

 _____ / _____ / _____
 WR   CV   S

6. pertaining to tears

 _____ / _____
 WR   S

7. pertaining to vision

 _____ / _____
 WR   S

8. pertaining to the eye

 _____ / _____
 WR   S

9. pertaining to the cornea

 _____ / _____
 WR   S

10. pertaining to the nose and tear ducts

 _____ / _____ / _____ / _____
 WR   CV   WR   S

11. disease of the eye

 _____ / _____ / _____
 WR   CV   S

12. pertaining to the pupil

 _____ / _____
 WR   S

EXERCISE 32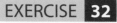

Spell each of the complementary terms built from word parts on pp. 563-564 by having someone dictate them to you.

 To hear and spell the terms select Chapter 12, Chapter Exercises, Spelling. You may type the terms on the screen or write them below in the spaces provided.

☐ Place a check mark in the box if you have completed this exercise using your CD-ROM.

1. _____	7. _____
2. _____	8. _____
3. _____	9. _____
4. _____	10. _____
5. _____	11. _____
6. _____	12. _____

Complementary Terms

Not Built from Word Parts

In some of the following terms, you may recognize word parts you have already learned; however, the full meaning of the terms cannot be discerned by the definition of their word parts.

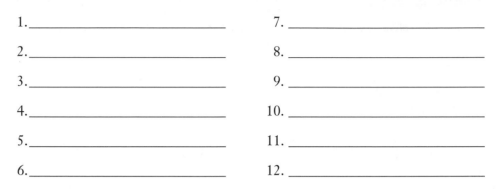

Term	Definition
miotic . . . . (mī-OT-ik)	agent that constricts the pupil
mydriatic . . . . (*mid*-rē-AT-ik)	agent that dilates the pupil
optician . . . . (op-TISH-in)	a specialist who fills prescriptions for lenses (cannot prescribe lenses)
optometrist . . . . (op-TOM-e-trist)	a health professional who prescribes corrective lenses and/or eye exercises
visual acuity (VA) . . . . (VIZH-ū-al) (a-KŪ-i-tē)	sharpness of vision for either distance or near

OPTOMETRIST
is derived from the Greek
optikos, meaning
sight, and **metron,** meaning
measure. Literally, an optometrist is a person who measures sight.

EXERCISE 33

Practice saying aloud each of the complementary terms not built from word parts above.

 To hear the terms select Chapter 12, Chapter Exercises, Pronunciation.

☐ Place a check mark in the box when you have completed this exercise.

EXERCISE 34

Write the definitions for the following complementary terms.

1. optometrist _____

2. mydriatic _____

3. visual acuity _____

4. miotic _____

5. optician _____

EXERCISE 35

Fill in the blanks with the correct terms.

1. An agent that dilates a pupil is a(n) _____.

2. An agent that constricts a pupil is a(n) _____.

3. A health professional who prescribes corrective lenses and/or eye exercises is a(n) _____.

4. Another term for sharpness of vision is _____ _____.

5. A specialist who fills prescriptions for lenses but who cannot prescribe lenses is a(n) _____.

EXERCISE 36

Spell each of the complementary terms not built from word parts on p. 566 by having someone dictate them to you.

 To hear and spell the terms select Chapter 12, Chapter Exercises, Spelling. You may type the terms on the screen or write them below in the spaces provided.

☐ Place a check mark in the box if you have completed this exercise using your CD-ROM.

1. _____   4. _____

2. _____   5. _____

3. _____

Abbreviations

ARMD	age-related macular degeneration
Ast	astigmatism
Em	emmetropia
IOP	intraocular pressure
Ophth	ophthalmology
VA	visual acuity

EXERCISE 37

Write the meaning of the following abbreviations in the spaces provided.

1. VA _____ _____

2. Ast _____

3. IOP _____ _____

4. Em _____

5. Ophth _____

6. ARMD _____ _____ _____

PRACTICAL APPLICATION

EXERCISE **38**   *Interact with Medical Documents*

A. Complete the progress note by writing the medical terms in the blanks. Use the list of definitions with the corresponding numbers.

University Hospital and Medical Center
4700 North Main Street • Wellness, Arizona 54321 • (987) 555-3210

PATIENT NAME: William Graves   **CASE NUMBER:** 20066-OPH
DATE OF BIRTH: 06/27/19XX   **DATE:** 04/05/20XX

PROGRESS NOTE

SUBJECTIVE: Mr. Graves is a 66-year-old white male here today for his annual 1. _____ exam. He has no current complaints. He has a family history of 2. _____ in his brother. He has a history of hypertension and type 2 diabetes mellitus. A 3. _____ was removed from his right eye 5 years ago.

Current Medications: Glyburide 5 mg bid and Lopressor 50 mg bid.

Allergies: None.

OBJECTIVE:
Visual Acuities: Aided: right eye 20/25 left eye 20/30-1 both eyes 20/25
                   Unaided: right eye 20/100 left eye 20/80-1 both eyes 20/80

Externals: 2 mm 4. _____ right eye. PERLA (pupils equal and reactive to light and accommodation). EOMI (extraocular movements intact).

Ophthalmoscopic: Lens: left eye showed early cortical spokes
                   Disk: margins normal
                   Cup-to-disk ratio: 0.2 both eyes
                   Fundus: Within normal limits, including DVM
                   Refraction: right eye-1.00-0.50 × 90 20/20, left eye-1.25-0.25 × 90 20/20
                   Tonometry: 14 mm Hg/right eye, 13 mm Hg/left eye

Visual Field: Full

ASSESSMENT: Patient has compound myopic 5. _____ and 6. _____ with diabetic 7. _____ and grade II hypertension. He also shows an early 8. _____ in the left eye.

PLAN: Provide prescription for corrective lenses. See patient for follow-up visit in 6 months to reevaluate diabetic retinopathy and cataract. Counseled patient to report any sudden changes in vision.

Milli Bentley, MD

MB/mcm

---

1. study of the eye
2. eye disorder characterized by optic nerve damage usually caused by the abnormal increase of intraocular pressure
3. thin tissue growing into the cornea from the conjunctiva
4. drooping of eyelid
5. defective curvature of the refractive surface of the eye
6. impaired vision as a result of aging
7. (any noninflammatory) disease of the retina
8. clouding of the lens of the eye

B. Read the following case study and answer the questions that follow.

Case Study

Patient Profile: This 70-year-old woman was admitted to the hospital for surgical treatment of chronic, poorly controlled **glaucoma** and for **cataract** extraction.

Subjective: The patient reported a progressive loss of **visual acuity** in her right eye; she complained of headaches and problems with glare (particularly at night) and said she perceives halos around lights.

Objective: Vision testing and physical examination (i.e., **ophthalmoscopy,** slit lamp microscopy, and **tonometry**) revealed acuity (unaided) of 10/100 for the right eye and 20/60 for the left eye. Opacification of right lens was evident, as was moderate **corneal** edema.

Therapeutic Management: After a **mydriatic** agent was applied to the right pupil, a combined procedure **phacoemulsification** of the cataract and **trabeculectomy** with releasable sutures (to minimize **IOP**) was performed with the patient under local anesthesia. The patient tolerated the procedure well and returned to her room wearing a 12-hour collagen shield on the treated eye.

1. Vision testing and physical examination of the patient revealed opacification of the right lens, confirming the need for:
   a. PRK
   b. phacoemulsification
   c. scleral buckling
   d. enucleation

2. Application of a mydriatic agent would:
   a. reduce tears
   b. produce tears
   c. constrict the pupil
   d. dilate the pupil

3. A trabeculectomy was performed because the patient had a history of:
   a. abnormal condition of crossed eyes
   b. disorder characterized by optic nerve damage, usually caused by abnormal increased ocular pressure
   c. nearsightedness
   d. a progressive deterioration of a portion of the retina

4. The abbreviation IOP stands for:
   a. both eyes
   b. normal vision
   c. intraocular pressure
   d. iris outer pupil

EXERCISE 39   *Interpret Medical Terms*

To test your understanding of the terms introduced in this chapter, circle the words that correctly complete the sentences. The italicized words refer to the correct answer.

1. The patient's *pupils* needed to be *dilated*; therefore the doctor requested that a (**miotic, mydriatic, miopic**) medication be placed in each eye.

2. A person with a *defective curvature of the refractive surface* of the eye has a(n) (**astigmatism, glaucoma, strabismus**).

3. The doctor diagnosed the patient with the *clouded lens* of the eye as having a(n) (**nystagmus, astigmatism, cataract**).

4. To *measure the pressure within the patient's eye*, the physician used a(n) (**pupillometer, tonometer, keratometer**).

5. A person who is *farsighted* has (**hyperopia, myopia, diplopia**).

6. An *obstruction of the oil gland of the eyelid* is called a (**sty, chalazion, conjunctivitis**).

7. A patient with an *involuntary jerking movement of the eyes* has a condition known as (**astigmatism, strabismus, nystagmus**).

8. The name of the *surgery performed to create a permanent drain to reduce intraocular pressure* is (**trabeculectomy, strabotomy, phacoemulsification**).

9. The doctor ordered a *photographic imaging of the blood vessels of the eye* or a(n) (**ophthalmoscopy, fluorescein angiography, optometer**).

10. *Condition of dry eye* (**oculomycosis, ophthalmoplegia, xerophthalmia**) begins with *night blindness* (**nyctalopia, photophobia, diplopia**) and may progress to *softening of the cornea* (**iridoplegia, keratomalacia, sclerokeratitis**).

EXERCISE 40   *Read Medical Terms in Use*

Practice pronunciation of terms by reading the following medical document. Use the pronunciation key following the medical terms to help you say the word.

 To hear these terms select Chapter 12, Chapter Exercises, Read Medical Terms in Use.

An elderly gentleman visited his **ophthalmologist** (*of*-thal-MOL-o-jist) because of decreased vision. A **tonometry** (ton-OM-e-trē) examination showed borderline readings. **Visual acuity** (VIZH-ū-al) (a-KŪ-i-tē) measurement indicated a mild degree of **myopia** (mī-Ō-pē–a) and **presbyopia** (*pres*-bē-Ō-pē-a). A diagnosis of **glaucoma** (glaw-KŌ-ma) is suspect in this case and Timoptic eye drops were prescribed, one drop daily.

A **cataract** (KAT-a-rakt) of the right eye was found. Lens implant surgery will be performed when the cataract matures sufficiently. Approximately 5 years ago the patient had a **detached retina** (RET-i-na) of the left eye. A **scleral buckling** (SKLER-al) (BUK-ling) procedure was performed and was successful in halting the process of retinal detachment.

EXERCISE **41**   *Comprehend Medical Terms in Use*

Test your comprehension of terms in the previous medical document by circling the correct answer.

1. T   F   The ophthalmologist used an instrument to measure pressure within the patient's eyes to assist in the diagnosis of abnormally increased intraocular pressure.

2. Visual acuity measurement indicated:
   a. farsightedness and impaired vision as a result of aging
   b. nearsightedness and impaired vision as a result of aging
   c. poor night vision and farsightedness
   d. poor night vision and impaired vision because of aging

3. Timoptic eye drops were prescribed to address symptoms most likely caused by:
   a. inflammation of the cornea
   b. optic nerve damage caused by abnormally increased IOP
   c. separation of the retina from the choroid
   d. clouding of the lens of the eye

4. T   F   A scleral buckling procedure was used to correct clouding of the lens in the right eye.

CHAPTER REVIEW

◉)) CHAPTER REVIEW ON CD-ROM

Use the CD-ROM that accompanies this textbook to play and practice what you have learned in this chapter. The Chapter Exercises, Practice Activities, Animations, and Games allow you to hear, see, and interact with the chapter content.

Chapter Exercises	**Practice Activities**	**Animations**	**Games**
Exercises in this section of your CD-ROM correlate to exercises in your textbook. You may have completed them as you worked through the chapter.	Practice in study mode, then test your learning in assessment mode. Keep track of your scores from assessment mode if you wish.	☐ Anatomy of the Eye ☐ Aqueous and Vitreous Humor	☐ Name that Word Part ☐ Term Storm ☐ Term Explorer ☐ Termbusters ☐ Medical Millionaire

	SCORE
☐ Pronunciation	
☐ Spelling	
☐ Read Medical Terms in Use	
☐ Picture It	_____
☐ Define Word Parts	_____
☐ Build Medical Terms	_____
☐ Word Shop	_____
☐ Define Medical Terms	_____
☐ Use It	_____
☐ Hear It and Type It: Clinical Vignettes	_____

REVIEW OF WORD PARTS

Can you define and spell the following word parts?

Combining Forms		Prefixes	Suffixes
blephar/o	kerat/o	bi-	-opia
conjunctiv/o	lacrim/o	bin-	-phobia
cor/o	ocul/o		-plegia
core/o	ophthalm/o		
corne/o	opt/o		
cry/o	phot/o		
dacry/o	pupill/o		
dipl/o	retin/o		
irid/o	scler/o		
ir/o	ton/o		

REVIEW OF TERMS

Can you build, analyze, define, pronounce, and spell the following terms *built from word parts?*

Diseases and Disorders	Surgical	Diagnostic	Complementary
blepharitis	blepharoplasty	fluorescein angiography	binocular
blepharoptosis	cryoretinopexy	keratometer	corneal
conjunctivitis	dacryocystorhinostomy	ophthalmoscope	intraocular
dacryocystitis	dacryocystotomy	ophthalmoscopy	lacrimal
diplopia	iridectomy	optometry	nasolacrimal
endophthalmitis	iridotomy	pupillometer	ophthalmic
iridoplegia	keratoplasty	pupilloscope	ophthalmologist
iritis	sclerotomy	retinoscopy	ophthalmology (Ophth)
keratitis		tonometer	ophthalmopathy
keratomalacia		tonometry	optic
leukocoria			pupillary
oculomycosis			retinal
ophthalmalgia			
ophthalmoplegia			
photophobia			
retinoblastoma			
retinopathy			
sclerokeratitis			
scleromalacia			
xerophthalmia			

Can you define, pronounce, and spell the following terms *not built from word parts?*

Diseases and Disorders		Surgical	Complementary
amblyopia	myopia	enucleation	miotic
astigmatism (Ast)	nyctalopia	LASIK (laser-assisted in situ	mydriatic
cataract	nystagmus	keratomileusis)	optician
chalazion	pinguecula	phacoemulsification	optometrist
detached retina	presbyopia	PRK (photorefractive	visual acuity (VA)
emmetropia (Em)	pterygium	keratectomy)	
glaucoma	retinitis pigmentosa	retinal photocoagulation	
hyperopia	strabismus	scleral buckling	
macular degeneration	sty (hordeolum)	trabeculectomy	
		vitrectomy	

ANSWERS

Exercise Figures

Exercise Figure

A. 1. eye: ocul/o, ophthalm/o
2. eyelid: blephar/o
3. pupil: cor/o, core/o, pupill/o
4. sclera: scler/o
5. iris: irid/o, ir/o
6. conjunctiva: conjunctiv/o
7. cornea: corne/o, kerat/o
8. retina: retin/o

Exercise Figure

B. blephar/itis

Exercise Figure

C. blephar/o/ptosis

Exercise Figure

D. dacry/o/cyst/itis

Exercise 1

1. d	5. b
2. c	6. e
3. f	7. a
4. h	

Exercise 2

1. d	5. b
2. f	6. a
3. h	7. c
4. e	

Exercise 3

1. eye	9. conjunctiva
2. eyelid	10. pupil
3. cornea	11. eye
4. tear, tear duct	12. cornea
5. retina	13. iris
6. pupil	14. pupil
7. sclera	15. vision
8. iris	16. tear, tear duct

Exercise 4

1. a. ocul/o
   b. ophthalm/o
2. a. corne/o
   b. kerat/o
3. conjunctiv/o
4. a. dacry/o
   b. lacrim/o
5. blephar/o
6. a. cor/o
   b. core/o
   c. pupill/o
7. scler/o
8. retin/o
9. a. irid/o
   b. ir/o
10. opt/o

Exercise 5

1. tension, pressure	3. cold
2. light	4. two, double

Exercise 6

1. cry/o	3. dipl/o
2. ton/o	4. phot/o

Exercise 7

1. vision (condition)
2. two
3. paralysis
4. abnormal fear of or aversion to specific things
5. two

Exercise 8

1. -plegia
2. a. bi-
   b. bin-
3. -phobia
4. -opia

Exercise 9

Pronunciation Exercise

Exercise 10

1. WR CV WR S
   scler/o/kerat/itis
   ⁀CF
   inflammation of the sclera and the cornea
2. WR S
   ophthalm/algia
   pain in the eye
3. WR CV S
   blephar/o/ptosis
   ⁀CF
   drooping of the eyelid
4. WR S
   dipl/opia
   double vision
5. WR S
   conjunctiv/itis
   inflammation of the conjunctiva
6. WR CV WR S
   leuk/o/cor/ia
   ⁀CF
   condition of white pupil
7. WR CV S
   irid/o/plegia
   ⁀CF
   paralysis of the iris

8. WR CV S
   scler/o/malacia
   ⁀CF
   softening of the sclera
9. WR CV S
   phot/o/phobia
   ⁀CF
   abnormal fear of (sensitivity to) light
10. WR S
    blephar/itis
    inflammation of the eyelid
11. WR CV WR S
    ocul/o/myc/osis
    ⁀CF
    abnormal condition of the eye caused by a fungus
12. WR CV WR S
    dacry/o/cyst/itis
    ⁀CF
    inflammation of the tear (lacrimal) sac
13. P WR S
    end/ophthalm/itis
    inflammation within the eye
14. WR S
    ir/itis
    inflammation of the iris
15. WR CV WR S
    retin/o/blast/oma
    ⁀CF
    tumor arising from a developing retinal cell
16. WR S
    kerat/itis
    inflammation of the cornea
17. WR CV S
    ophthalm/o/plegia
    ⁀CF
    paralysis of the eye (muscles)
18. WR CV S
    retin/o/pathy
    ⁀CF
    disease of the retina
19. WR WR S
    xer/ophthalm/ia
    condition of dry eye
20. WR CV S
    kerat/o/malacia
    ⁀CF
    softening of the cornea

Exercise 11
1. conjunctiv/itis
2. ocul/o/myc/osis
3. ophthalm/algia
4. dipl/opia
5. blephar/itis
6. leuk/o/cor/ia
7. irid/o/plegia
8. blephar/o/ptosis
9. ir/itis
10. retin/o/blast/oma
11. scler/o/malacia
12. dacry/o/cyst/itis
13. scler/o/kerat/itis
14. phot/o/phobia
15. kerat/itis
16. retin/o/pathy
17. end/ophthalm/itis
18. ophthalm/o/plegia
19. xer/ophthalm/ia
20. kerat/o/malacia

Exercise 12
Spelling Exercise; see text p. 550.

Exercise 13
Pronunciation Exercise

Exercise 14
1. myopia
2. presbyopia
3. strabismus
4. chalazion
5. astigmatism
6. nystagmus
7. cataract
8. sty (hordeolum)
9. glaucoma
10. detached retina
11. hyperopia
12. emmetropia
13. retinitis pigmentosa
14. nyctalopia
15. pterygium
16. macular degeneration
17. amblyopia
18. pinguecula

Exercise 15
1. f   10. c
2. h   11. a
3. k   12. l
4. n   13. i
5. m   14. o
6. j   15. g
7. d   16. b
8. p   17. r
9. e   18. s

Exercise 16
Spelling Exercise; see text p. 555.

Exercise 17
Pronunciation Exercise

Exercise 18
1. WR CV S
   kerat/o/plasty
        CF
   surgical repair of the cornea
2. WR CV S
   scler/o/tomy
        CF
   incision into the sclera
3. WR CV WR CV S
   dacry/o/cyst/o/tomy
        CF   CF
   incision into the tear sac
4. WRCV WR CV S
   cry/o/retin/o/pexy
       CF   CF
   surgical fixation of the retina by
       using extreme cold
5. WR CV S
   blephar/o/plasty
         CF
   surgical repair of the eyelid
6. WR   S
   irid/ectomy
   excision of the iris
7. WR CV WR CV WR CV S
   dacry/o/cyst/o/rhin/o/stomy
        CF   CF   CF
   creation of an artificial opening
       between the tear (lacrimal) sac and
       the nose
8. WR CV S
   irid/o/tomy
        CF
   incision into the iris

Exercise 19
1. dacry/o/cyst/o/rhin/o/stomy
2. irid/ectomy
3. kerat/o/plasty
4. scler/o/tomy
5. irid/o/tomy
6. blephar/o/plasty
7. cry/o/retin/o/pexy
8. dacry/o/cyst/o/tomy

Exercise 20
Spelling Exercise; see text p. 557.

Exercise 21
Pronunciation Exercise

Exercise 22
1. retinal photocoagulation
2. enucleation
3. phacoemulsification
4. LASIK
5. trabeculectomy
6. scleral buckling
7. vitrectomy
8. PRK

Exercise 23
1. e   5. d
2. f   6. i
3. b   7. g
4. a   8. c

Exercise 24
Spelling Exercise; see text p. 560.

Exercise 25
Pronunciation Exercise

Exercise 26
1. WR CV S
   pupill/o/scope
         CF
   instrument used for visual
       examination of the pupil
2. WR CV S
   opt/o/metry
        CF
   measurement of vision (visual acuity
       and the prescribing of corrective
       lenses)
3. WR CV S
   ophthalm/o/scope
            CF
   instrument used for visual
       examination of the eye
4. WR CV S
   ton/o/metry
        CF
   measurement of pressure (within the
       eye)
5. WR CV S
   pupill/o/meter
         CF
   instrument used to measure the pupil
       (diameter)
6. WR CV S
   ton/o/meter
        CF
   instrument used to measure pressure
       (within the eye)

7. WR CV S
   kerat/o/meter
   CF
   instrument used to measure (the
   curvature of) the cornea

8. WR CV S
   ophthalm/o/scopy
   CF
   visual examination of the eye

9. WR CV S
   (fluorescein) angi/o/graphy
   CF
   process of recording blood vessels
   (of the eye with fluorescing dye)

10. WR CV S
    retin/o/scopy
    CF
    visual examination of the retina

Exercise 27
1. ton/o/metry
2. pupill/o/meter
3. kerat/o/meter
4. opt/o/metry
5. ophthalm/o/scope
6. ton/o/meter
7. pupill/o/scope
8. ophthalm/o/scopy
9. fluorescein angi/o/graphy
10. retin/o/scopy

Exercise 28
Spelling Exercise; see text p. 563.

Exercise 29
Pronunciation Exercise

Exercise 30
1. WR CV S
   ophthalm/o/logy
   CF
   study of the eye

2. P WR S
   bin/ocul/ar
   pertaining to two or both eyes

3. WR S
   lacrim/al
   pertaining to tears

4. WR S
   pupill/ary
   pertaining to the pupil

5. WR CV S
   ophthalm/o/logist
   CF
   physician who studies and treats
   diseases of the eye

6. WR S
   corne/al
   pertaining to the cornea

7. WR S
   ophthalm/ic
   pertaining to the eye

8. WRCV WR S
   nas/o/lacrim/al
   CF
   pertaining to the nose and tear ducts

9. WR S
   opt/ic
   pertaining to vision

10. P WR S
    intra/ocul/ar
    pertaining to within the eye

11. WR S
    retin/al
    pertaining to the retina

12. WR CV S
    ophthalm/o/pathy
    CF
    disease of the eye

Exercise 31
1. ophthalm/o/logy
2. bin/ocul/ar
3. retin/al
4. intra/ocul/ar
5. ophthalm/o/logist
6. lacrim/al
7. opt/ic
8. ophthalm/ic
9. corne/al
10. nas/o/lacrim/al
11. ophthalm/o/pathy
12. pupill/ary

Exercise 32
Spelling Exercise; see text p. 566.

Exercise 33
Pronunciation Exercise

Exercise 34
1. a health professional who prescribes
   corrective lenses and/or eye exercises
2. agent that dilates the pupil
3. sharpness of vision
4. agent that constricts the pupil
5. a specialist who fills prescriptions for
   lenses

Exercise 35
1. mydriatic
2. miotic
3. optometrist
4. visual acuity
5. optician

Exercise 36
Spelling Exercise; see text p. 567.

Exercise 37
1. visual acuity
2. astigmatism
3. intraocular pressure
4. emmetropia
5. ophthalmology
6. age-related macular degeneration

Exercise 38
A. 1. ophthalmology
   2. glaucoma
   3. pterygium
   4. blepharoptosis
   5. astigmatism
   6. presbyopia
   7. retinopathy
   8. cataract

B. 1. b
   2. d
   3. b
   4. c

Exercise 39
1. mydriatic
2. astigmatism
3. cataract
4. tonometer
5. hyperopia
6. chalazion
7. nystagmus
8. trabeculectomy
9. fluorescein angiography
10. xerophthalmia, nyctalopia,
    keratomalacia

Exercise 40
Reading Exercise

Exercise 41
1. *T*
2. b
3. b
4. *F*, scleral buckling was used to correct
   a detached retina and not a cataract.

NOTES

CHAPTER 13
Ear

OUTLINE

ANATOMY, 580

WORD PARTS, 582
Combining Forms, 582

MEDICAL TERMS, 584
Disease and Disorder Terms, 584
Built from Word Parts, 584
Not Built from Word Parts, 587
Surgical Terms, 590
Built from Word Parts, 590
Diagnostic Terms, 592
Built from Word Parts, 592
Complementary Terms, 595
Built from Word Parts, 595
Abbreviations, 597

PRACTICAL APPLICATION, 598
Interact with Medical Documents, 598
Interpret Medical Terms, 600
Read Medical Terms in Use, 600
Comprehend Medical Terms in Use, 601

CHAPTER REVIEW, 601

OBJECTIVES

Upon completion of this chapter you will be able to:

1. Identify organs and structures of the ear.

2. Define and spell word parts related to the ear.

3. Define, pronounce, and spell disease and disorder terms related to the ear.

4. Define, pronounce, and spell surgical terms related to the ear.

5. Define, pronounce, and spell diagnostic terms related to the ear.

6. Define, pronounce, and spell complementary terms related to the ear.

7. Interpret the meaning of abbreviations related to the ear.

8. Interpret, read, and comprehend medical language in simulated medical statements and documents.

ANATOMY

Function

The two functions of the ear are to hear and to provide the sense of balance. The ear is made up of three parts: the *external* ear, the *middle* ear, and the *inner* ear, also called the *labyrinth* (Figure 13-1). We hear because sound waves vibrate through the ear where they are transformed into nerve impulses that are then carried to the brain.

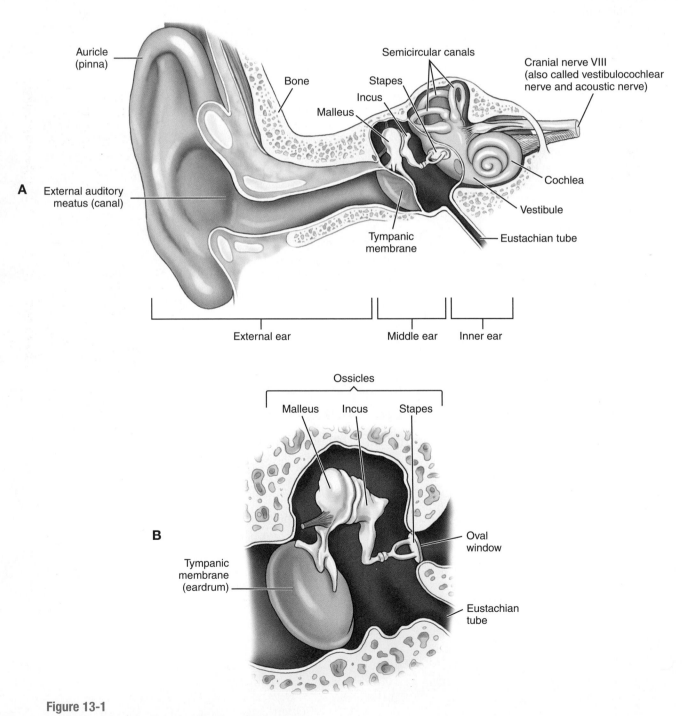

Figure 13-1
A, Gross anatomy of the ear. **B,** The middle ear.

Structures of the Ear

Term	Definition
external ear	
auricle (pinna)	external structure located on both sides of the head. The auricle directs sound waves into the external auditory meatus.
external auditory meatus (canal).	short tube that ends at the tympanic membrane. The inner part lies within the temporal bone of the skull and contains the glands that secrete earwax (cerumen).
middle ear	
tympanic membrane (eardrum)	semitransparent membrane that separates the external auditory meatus and the middle ear cavity. The tympanic membrane transmits sound vibrations to the ossicles (Figure 13-2).
eustachian tube	connects the middle ear and the pharynx. It equalizes air pressure on both sides of the eardrum.
ossicles	bones of the middle ear that carry sound vibrations. The ossicles are composed of the **malleus** (hammer), **incus** (anvil), and stapes (stirrup). The stapes connects to the **oval window**, which transmits the sound vibrations to the cochlea of the inner ear.
labyrinth (inner ear)	bony spaces within the temporal bone of the skull. It contains the cochlea, semicircular canals, and vestibule.
cochlea.	is snail-shaped and contains the organ of hearing. The cochlea connects to the oval window in the middle ear.
semicircular canals and vestibule.	contains receptors and endolymph that help the body maintain its sense of balance (equilibrium)
mastoid bone and cells	located in the skull bone behind the external auditory meatus

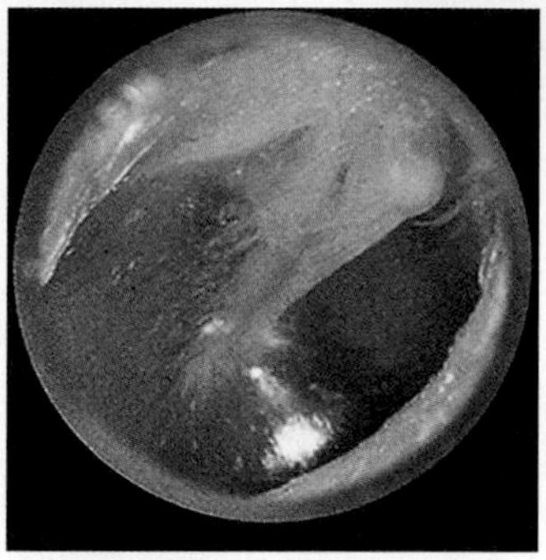

Figure 13-2
Normal tympanic membrane.

TYMPANIC MEMBRANE
is derived from the Greek **tympanon,** meaning **drum,** because of its resemblance to a drum or tambourine.

STAPES
is Latin for **stirrup.** The anatomic stapes was so named for its stirruplike shape.

EXERCISE 1

Match the anatomic terms in the first column with the correct definitions in the second column.

_____ 1. auricle

_____ 2. cochlea

_____ 3. eustachian tube

_____ 4. external auditory meatus

_____ 5. labyrinth

_____ 6. mastoid bone

_____ 7. ossicles

_____ 8. oval window

_____ 9. semicircular canals and vestibule

_____ 10. tympanic membrane

a. contains receptors and endolymph, which help maintain equilibrium

b. equalizes air pressure on both sides of the eardrum

c. separates the external auditory meatus and middle ear cavity

d. malleus, incus, and stapes

e. transmits sound vibration to the inner ear

f. contains glands that secrete earwax

g. external structure located on each side of the head

h. bony spaces within the temporal bone

i. relays messages to the brain

j. contains the organ of hearing

k. located in the skull behind the external auditory meatus

WORD PARTS

Word parts you need to learn to complete this chapter are listed below. The exercises at the end of each list will help you learn their definitions and spellings.

Combining Forms of the Ear

Combining Form	Definition
audi/o	hearing
aur/i, aur/o, ot/o	ear
cochle/o	cochlea
labyrinth/o	labyrinth (inner ear)
mastoid/o	mastoid bone
myring/o	tympanic membrane (eardrum)
staped/o	stapes (middle ear bone)
tympan/o	tympanic membrane (eardrum), middle ear
vestibul/o	vestibule

Refer to Appendixes A and B for a complete list of word parts.

EXERCISE FIGURE A

Fill in the blanks with combining forms in this diagram of the ear.

1. Ear

    CF: _____

    CF: _____

    CF: _____

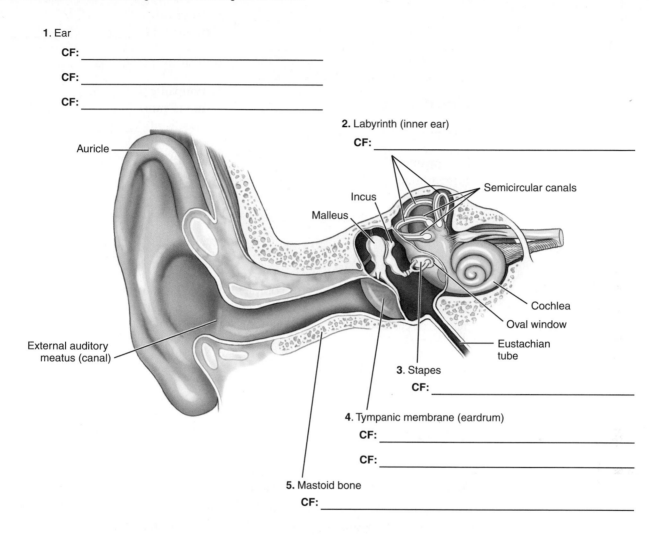

2. Labyrinth (inner ear)

    CF: _____

Auricle

Incus

Malleus

Semicircular canals

Cochlea

Oval window

Eustachian tube

3. Stapes

    CF: _____

External auditory meatus (canal)

4. Tympanic membrane (eardrum)

    CF: _____

    CF: _____

5. Mastoid bone

    CF: _____

EXERCISE 2

Write the definitions of the following combining forms.

1. staped/o _____

2. mastoid/o _____

3. audi/o _____

4. aur/i, aur/o, ot/o _____

5. tympan/o _____

6. vestibul/o _____

7. labyrinth/o _____

8. myring/o _____

9. cochle/o _____

EXERCISE **3**

Write the combining form for each of the following terms.

1. ear   a. _____

                 b. _____

                 c. _____

2. mastoid bone _____

3. stapes _____

4. tympanic membrane (eardrum), middle ear _____

5. labyrinth (inner ear) _____

6. hearing _____

7. tympanic membrane (eardrum) _____

8. cochlea _____

9. vestibule _____

MEDICAL TERMS

The terms you need to learn to complete this chapter are listed on the following pages. The exercises following each list will help you learn the definition and spelling of each word.

Disease and Disorder Terms

Built from Word Parts

The following terms are built from word parts you have already learned and can be translated literally to find their meanings. Further explanation of terms beyond the definition of their word parts, if needed, is included in parentheses.

Term	Definition
labyrinthitis .... (*lab*-i-rin-THĪ-tis)	inflammation of the labyrinth (inner ear) (also called **vestibular neuritis**)
mastoiditis .... (*mas*-toyd-Ī-tis)	inflammation of the mastoid bone
myringitis .... (mir-in-JĪ-tis)	inflammation of the tympanic membrane (eardrum)
otalgia .... (ō-TAL-ja)	pain in the ear
otomastoiditis .... (ō-tō-*mas*-toyd-Ī-tis)	inflammation of the ear and the mastoid bone
otomycosis .... (ō-tō-mī-KŌ-sis)	abnormal condition of fungus in the ear (usually affects the external auditory meatus)
otopyorrhea .... (ō-tō-pī-ō-RĒ-a)	discharge of pus from the ear

Term	Definition
otorrhea .... (ō-tō-RĒ-a)	discharge from the ear (may be serous, bloody, consisting of pus, or containing cerebrospinal fluid)
otosclerosis .... (ō-tō-skle-RŌ-sis)	hardening of the ear (stapes) (caused by irregular bone development and resulting in hearing loss)
tympanitis................. (tim-pan-Ī-tis)	inflammation of the middle ear (also called **otitis media**) (Figure 13-3)

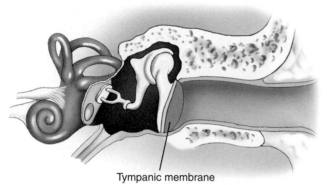

Tympanic membrane

Figure 13-3
Otitis media. Signs include bulging, perforated, reddened, or retracted tympanic membrane.

EXERCISE 4

Practice saying aloud each of the disease and disorder terms built from word parts on pp. 584-585.

 To hear the terms select Chapter 13, Chapter Exercises, Pronunciation.

☐ Place a check mark in the box when you have completed this exercise.

EXERCISE 5

Analyze and define the following terms.

1. otomycosis _____

2. tympanitis _____

3. otomastoiditis _____

4. otalgia _____

5. labyrinthitis _____

6. myringitis _____

7. otosclerosis _____

8. mastoiditis_____

9. otopyorrhea _____

10. otorrhea_____

EXERCISE 6

Build disease and disorder terms for the following definitions with the word parts you have learned.

1. inflammation of the tympanic membrane

2. discharge of pus from the ear

3. inflammation of the mastoid bone

4. pain in the ear

5. hardening of the ear (stapes)

6. abnormal condition of fungus in the ear

7. inflammation of the ear and the mastoid bone

8. inflammation of the labyrinth

9. inflammation of the middle ear

10. discharge from the ear

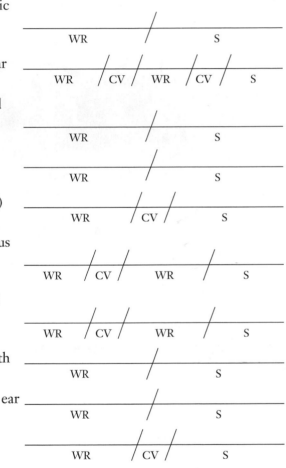

EXERCISE 7

Spell each of the disease and disorder terms built from word parts on pp. 584-585 by having someone dictate them to you.

 To hear and spell the terms select Chapter 13, Chapter Exercises, Spelling. You may type the terms on the screen or write them below in the spaces provided.

☐ Place a check mark in the box if you have completed this exercise using your CD-ROM.

1. _____   6. _____

2. _____   7. _____

3. _____   8. _____

4. _____   9. _____

5. _____   10. _____

Disease and Disorder Terms

Not Built from Word Parts

In some of the following terms, you may recognize word parts you have already learned; however, the full meaning of the terms cannot be discerned by the definition of their word parts.

Term	Definition
acoustic neuroma............ (a-KOOS-tik) (nū-RŌ-ma)	benign tumor within the auditory canal growing from the acoustic nerve (cranial nerve VIII, vestibulocochlear nerve); may cause hearing loss and may damage structures of the cerebellum as it grows
ceruminoma................ (se-roo-mi-NŌ-ma)	tumor of a gland that secretes earwax (cerumen)
cholesteatoma .... (ko-le-STĒ-a-tō-ma)	cystlike mass composed of epithelial cells and cholesterol occurring in the middle ear; may be associated with chronic otitis media
Ménière disease............ (me-NYĀR) (di-ZĒZ)	chronic disease of the inner ear characterized by dizziness, ringing in the ear, and hearing loss
otitis externa............... (ō-TĪ-tis) (eks-TER-na)	inflammation of the outer ear (Figure 13-4)
otitis media (OM) .... (ō-TĪ-tis) (MĒ-dē-a)	inflammation of the middle ear (see Figure 13-3)
presbycusis .... (prez-bi-KŪ-sis)	hearing impairment in old age

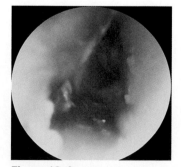

Figure 13-4
Otitis externa.

Disease and Disorder Terms—*cont'd*
Not Built from Word Parts

Term	Definition
tinnitus .... (tin-NĪ-tus)	ringing in the ears
vertigo. .... (VER-ti-gō)	a sense that either one's own body (subjective vertigo) or the environment (objective vertigo) is revolving; may indicate inner ear disease

EXERCISE 8

Practice saying aloud each of the disease and disorder terms not built from word parts on pp. 587-588.

 To hear the terms select Chapter 13, Chapter Exercises, Pronunciation.

☐ Place a check mark in the box when you have completed this exercise.

EXERCISE 9

Fill in the blanks with the correct terms.

1. The patient reported that her body seemed to be revolving, or _____, and ringing in the ears, or _____.

2. A chronic ear disease characterized by dizziness, ringing in the ears, and hearing loss is called _____ disease.

3. Inflammation of the middle ear is called _____ _____.

4. _____ is the name given to a tumor of a gland that secretes earwax.

5. _____ _____ means inflammation of the outer ear.

6. A benign tumor arising from the acoustic nerve is called a(n) _____ _____.

7. _____ is hearing impairment in old age.

8. _____ may be associated with chronic otitis media.

EXERCISE 10

Match the terms in the first column with the correct definitions in the second column.

_____ 1. vertigo

_____ 2. ceruminoma

_____ 3. tinnitus

_____ 4. Ménière disease

_____ 5. otitis externa

_____ 6. acoustic neuroma

_____ 7. otitis media

_____ 8. presbycusis

_____ 9. cholesteatoma

a. inflammation of the middle ear

b. tumor of a gland that secretes earwax

c. chronic ear problem characterized by vertigo, tinnitus, and hearing loss

d. benign tumor arising from the acoustic nerve

e. sense of revolving of one's own body or the environment

f. hardening of the oval window

g. ringing in the ears

h. inflammation of the outer ear

i. hearing impairment in old age

j. mass composed of epithelial cells and cholesterol

EXERCISE 11

Spell each of the disease and disorder terms not built from word parts on pp. 587-588 by having someone dictate them to you.

To hear and spell the terms select Chapter 13, Chapter Exercises, Spelling. You may type the terms on the screen or write them below in the spaces provided.

☐ Place a check mark in the box if you have completed this exercise using your CD-ROM.

1. _____

2. _____

3. _____

4. _____

5. _____

6. _____

7. _____

8. _____

9. _____

Surgical Terms

Built from Word Parts

The following terms are built from word parts you have already learned and can be translated literally to find their meanings. Further explanation of terms beyond the definition of their word parts, if needed, is included in parentheses.

Term	Definition
cochlear implant............ (KŌK-lē-ar) (IM-plant)	pertaining to the cochlea implant (surgically inserted prosthetic device that uses electrical currents to stimulate the auditory nerve and provide hearing)
labyrinthectomy .... (*lab*-i-rin-THEK-to-mē)	excision of the labyrinth
mastoidectomy.............. (*mas*-toy-DEK-to-mē)	excision of the mastoid bone
mastoidotomy............... (*mas*-toy-DOT-o-mē)	incision into the mastoid bone
myringoplasty............... (mi-RING-gō-*plas*-tē)	surgical repair of the tympanic membrane
myringotomy................ (mir-ing-GOT-o-mē)	incision into the tympanic membrane (performed to release pus or fluid and relieve pressure in the middle ear) (also called **tympanocentesis**) (Exercise Figure B)
stapedectomy............... (stā-pe-DEK-to-mē)	excision of the stapes (performed to restore hearing in cases of otosclerosis; the stapes is replaced by a prosthesis) (Figure 13-5)
tympanoplasty .... (TIM-pa-nō-*plas*-tē)	surgical repair (of the hearing mechanism) of the middle ear (including the tympanic membrane and the ossicles)

EXERCISE FIGURE B

Fill in the blanks to complete labeling of the diagram.

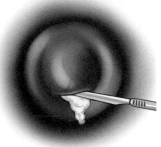

tympanic / cv / incision membrane

is performed to release pus from the middle ear through the tympanic membrane to treat acute otitis media.

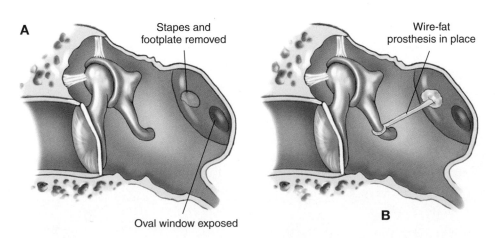

Figure 13-5
Stapedectomy. **A,** Stapes is removed. **B,** Prosthesis is in place.

EXERCISE 12

Practice saying aloud each of the surgical terms built from word parts on p. 590.

To hear the terms select Chapter 13, Chapter Exercises, Pronunciation.

☐ Place a check mark in the box when you have completed this exercise.

EXERCISE 13

Analyze and define the following surgical terms.

1. mastoidectomy _____

2. myringotomy _____

3. labyrinthectomy _____

4. mastoidotomy _____

5. tympanoplasty _____

6. myringoplasty _____

7. stapedectomy _____

8. cochlear implant _____

EXERCISE 14

Build surgical terms for the following definitions by using the word parts you have learned.

1. incision into the mastoid bone
   _____ / ____ / _____
   WR   CV   S

2. excision of the labyrinth
   _____ / _____
   WR   S

3. surgical repair (of the hearing mechanism) of the middle ear
   _____ / ____ / _____
   WR   CV   S

4. excision of the mastoid bone
   _____ / _____
   WR   S

5. incision into the tympanic membrane
   _____ / ____ / _____
   WR   CV   S

6. surgical repair of the tympanic membrane
   _____ / ____ / _____
   WR   CV   S

7. excision of the stapes
   _____ / _____
   WR   S

8. pertaining to the cochlea
   _____ / _____ implant
   WR   S

EXERCISE 15

Spell each of the surgical terms built from word parts on p. 590 by having someone dictate them to you.

 To hear and spell the terms select Chapter 13, Chapter Exercises, Spelling. You may type the terms on the screen or write them below in the spaces provided.

☐ Place a check mark in the box if you have completed this exercise using your CD-ROM.

1. _____ 5. _____

2. _____ 6. _____

3. _____ 7. _____

4. _____ 8. _____

Diagnostic Terms

Built from Word Parts

The following terms are built from word parts you have already learned and can be translated literally to find their meanings. Further explanation of terms beyond the definition of their word parts, if needed, is included in parentheses.

Term	Definition
audiogram (AW-dē-ō-gram)	(graphic) record of hearing (Figure 13-6)
audiometer (*aw*-dē-OM-e-ter)	instrument used to measure hearing
audiometry (*aw*-dē-OM-e-trē)	measurement of hearing
otoscope (Ō-tō-skōp)	instrument used for visual examination of the ear
otoscopy (ō-TOS-ko-pē)	visual examination of the ear
tympanometer (*tim*-pa-NOM-e-ter)	instrument used to measure middle ear (function)
tympanometry (tim-pa-NOM-e-trē)	measurement (of movement) of the tympanic membrane

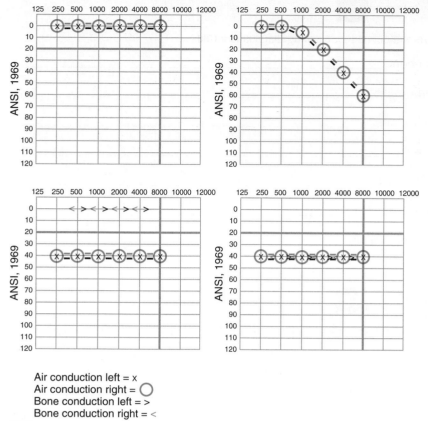

Air conduction left = x
Air conduction right = ◯
Bone conduction left = >
Bone conduction right = <

Figure 13-6

Audiogram. Although hearing is within normal limits, the results of this audiologic evaluation indicate a mild hearing loss in the left ear.

EXERCISE 16

Practice saying aloud each of the diagnostic terms built from word parts on p. 592.

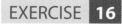 To hear the terms select Chapter 13, Chapter Exercises, Pronunciation.

☐ Place a check mark in the box when you have completed this exercise.

EXERCISE 17

Analyze and define the following diagnostic terms.

1. otoscope_____

2. audiometry _____

3. audiogram _____

4. otoscopy _____

5. audiometer _____

6. tympanometry_____

7. tympanometer_____

EXERCISE 18

Build diagnostic terms that correspond to the following definitions by using the word parts you have learned.

1. measurement (of movement)
   of the tympanic membrane

2. instrument used to measure
   hearing

3. visual examination of the ear

4. (graphic) record of hearing

5. instrument used for visual
   examination of the ear

6. measurement of hearing

7. instrument used to measure
   middle ear (function)

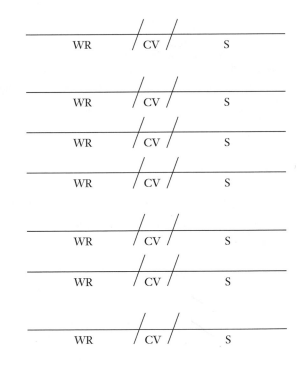

EXERCISE 19

Spell each of the diagnostic terms built from word parts on p. 592 by having someone dictate them to you.

 To hear and spell the terms select Chapter 13, Chapter Exercises, Spelling. You may type the terms on the screen or write them below in the spaces provided.

☐ Place a check mark in the box if you have completed this exercise using your CD-ROM.

1. _____   5. _____

2. _____   6. _____

3. _____   7. _____

4. _____

Complementary Terms

Built from Word Parts

The following terms are built from word parts you have already learned and can be translated literally to find their meanings. Further explanation of terms beyond the definition of their word parts, if needed, is included in parentheses.

Term	Definition
audiologist (*aw*-dē-OL-o-jist)	one who studies and specializes in hearing
audiology (*aw*-dē-OL-o-jē)	study of hearing
aural (AW-rul)	pertaining to the ear
cochlear (KOK-lē-ar)	pertaining to the cochlea
otologist (ō-TOL-o-jist)	physician who studies and treats diseases of the ear
otology (ō-TOL-o-jē)	study of the ear (a branch of medicine that deals with diseases of the ear)
otorhinolaryngologist (ō-tō-*rī*-nō-*lar*-ing-GOL-o-jist)	physician who studies and treats diseases of the ear, nose, and larynx (throat) (also called **otolaryngologist**)
vestibular (ves-TIB-ū-lar)	pertaining to the vestibule
vestibulocochlear (ves-*tib*-ū-lo-KOK-lē-ar)	pertaining to the vestibule and the cochlea

EXERCISE 20

Practice saying aloud each of the complementary terms built from word parts on p. 595.

 To hear the terms select Chapter 13, Chapter Exercises, Pronunciation.

☐ Place a check mark in the box when you have completed this exercise.

EXERCISE 21

Analyze and define the following complementary terms.

1. otology _____

2. audiologist _____

3. otorhinolaryngologist _____

4. audiology _____

5. otologist _____

6. aural _____

7. cochlear _____

8. vestibular _____

9. vestibulocochlear _____

EXERCISE 22

Build the complementary terms for the following definitions by using the word parts you have learned.

1. study of hearing

     _____ / _____ / _____
           WR   CV   S

2. physician who studies and treats diseases of the ear, nose, and larynx (throat)

     _____ / __ / _____ / __ / _____ / __ / __
      WR / CV / WR / CV / WR / CV / S

3. study of the ear

     _____ / _____ / _____
           WR   CV   S

4. one who studies and specializes in hearing

     _____ / _____ / _____
           WR   CV   S

5. physician who studies and treats diseases of the ear

     _____ / _____ / _____
           WR   CV   S

6. pertaining to the ear

     _____ / _____
           WR   S

7. pertaining to the vestibule
   and the cochlea

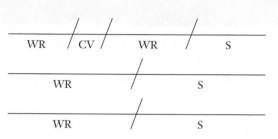

   _____ / ___ / _____ / ___
   WR   / CV /   WR   /   S

8. pertaining to the vestibule

   _____ / _____
        WR   /   S

9. pertaining to the cochlea

   _____ / _____
        WR   /   S

EXERCISE 23

Spell each of the complementary terms built from word parts on p. 595 by having someone dictate them to you.

To hear and spell the terms select Chapter 13, Chapter Exercises, Spelling. You may type the terms on the screen or write them below in the spaces provided.

☐ Place a check mark in the box if you have completed this exercise using your CD-ROM.

1. _____   6. _____

2. _____   7. _____

3. _____   8. _____

4. _____   9. _____

5. _____

Abbreviations

AOM	acute otitis media
EENT.....................	eyes, ears, nose, and throat
ENT......................	ears, nose, throat
OM	otitis media

EXERCISE 24

Write the meaning of the following abbreviations.

1. ENT _____ _____ _____

2. EENT _____ _____ _____ and
   _____

3. OM _____ _____

4. AOM _____ _____ _____

PRACTICAL APPLICATION

EXERCISE 25 *Interact with Medical Documents*

A. Complete the progress note by writing the medical terms in the blanks. Use the list of definitions with the corresponding numbers.

University Hospital and Medical Center
4700 North Main Street • Wellness, Arizona 54321 • (987) 555-3210

PATIENT NAME: Jimmy Tohe
DATE OF BIRTH: 03/04/19XX

CASE NUMBER: 99665-AUD
DATE: 09/04/20XX

PROGRESS NOTE

SUBJECTIVE DATA: Jimmy Tohe is a 62-year-old Native American male, appearing younger than his stated age. He was brought into the 1. _____ clinic by his daughter, who states that he is unable to hear what is being said to him by family members. She states that this problem has existed for at least 30 years but that it appears to be getting markedly worse. The patient states he had several episodes of ear infections as a child and young adult. He denies any 2. _____ or 3. _____.

OBJECTIVE DATA: Temperature, 99.4. Pulse, 72. Respirations, 20. Blood pressure, 136/76. Weight, 162 pounds. Patient ambulates without difficulty. Alert and oriented ×3. 4. _____ reveals scarring of the tympanic membranes bilaterally. Auditory canals appear normal bilaterally. Patient states he is allergic to Demerol.

ASSESSMENT:
1. Severe loss of hearing bilaterally, probably caused by 5._____ _____ as a child.
2. Recent exacerbation of hearing loss most likely attributable to 6. _____.

PLAN:
1. Patient referred to 7. _____ for complete 8. _____ workup.

Bridey McKeegan, MD

BM/mcm

---

1. abbreviation for ears, nose, and throat
2. ringing in the ears
3. a sense of one's own body or the environment revolving
4. visual examination of the ear

5. inflammation of the middle ear
6. hearing impairment in old age
7. one who studies and specializes in hearing
8. measurement of hearing

B. Read the clinical notes report and answer the questions following it.

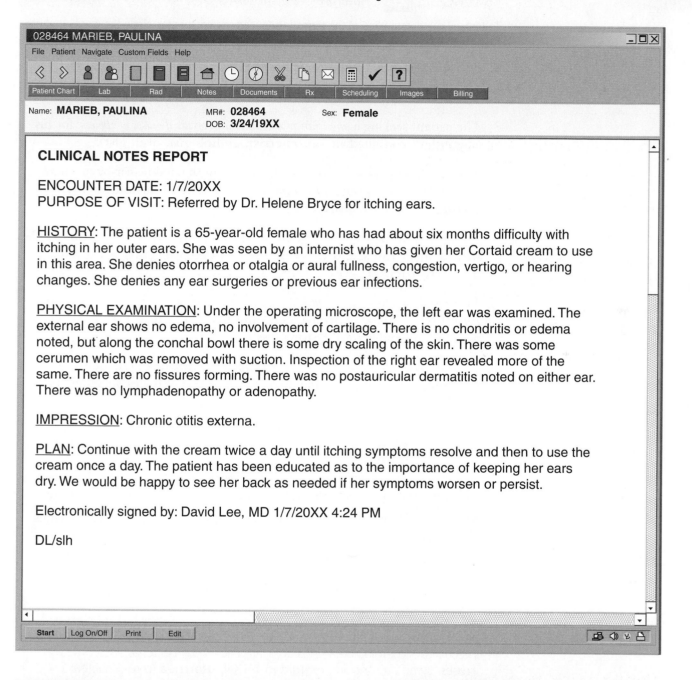

1. The patient has been experiencing:
   a. itchiness
   b. hearing loss
   c. otalgia
   d. vertigo

2. In the patient's left ear, suction removed:
   a. scaling
   b. cerumen
   c. chondritis
   d. otorrhea

3. The patient's condition has been diagnosed as chronic:
   a. abnormal condition of fungus in the ear
   b. inflammation of the tympanic membrane
   c. hardening of the stapes
   d. inflammation of the outer ear

EXERCISE **26** *Interpret Medical Terms*

To test your understanding of the terms introduced in this chapter, circle the words that correctly complete the sentences. The italicized phrase is the definition of the term.

1. *Inflammation of the eardrum* is (**labyrinthitis, mastoiditis, myringitis**).

2. The patient reported *ringing in the ears,* or (**tinnitus, vertigo, tympanitis**).

3. The patient seeking a *physician who studies and treats diseases of the ear* for his labyrinthitis consulted an (**optometrist, audiologist, otologist**).

4. The physician planned to release the pus from the middle ear by making an *incision in the tympanic membrane,* or performing a (**mastoidotomy, myringotomy, labyrinthectomy**).

5. Tinnitus, hearing loss, and vertigo in *chronic disease of the inner ear* (**mastoiditis, Ménière disease, presbycusis**) usually occur in episodes that can last for several days.

6. Manifestations of *benign tumor within the auditory canal growing from cranial nerve VIII* (**acoustic neuroma, ceruminoma, cholesteatoma**) often begin with tinnitus and gradual hearing loss.

7. A *cystlike mass composed of epithelial cells and cholesterol* (**acoustic neuroma, ceruminoma, cholesteatoma**) may destroy adjacent bones, including the ossicles.

EXERCISE **27** *Read Medical Terms in Use*

Practice pronunciation of terms by reading the following information on acute otitis media. Use the pronunciation key following the medical term to assist you in saying the words.

 To hear these terms select Chapter 13, Chapter Exercises, Read Medical Terms in Use.

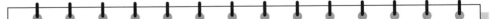

ACUTE OTITIS MEDIA
Acute otitis media (ō-TĪ-tis) (MĒ-dia) is one of the most common pediatric infections. Most middle ear infections are caused by bacteria, and some by viruses. Symptoms include **otalgia** (ō-TAL-ja), **otorrhea** (ō-tō-RĒ-a), ear pulling, and irritability. The tympanic membrane will be bulging, red in color, with a thickened appearance and reduced translucency. Antibiotics may be ordered if the infection does not resolve on its own. If unresponsive to antibiotic treatment, a **myringotomy** (mir-ing-GOT-o-mē) may be performed to identify the causative pathogen, allowing for the appropriate antibiotic treatment to be prescribed.

EXERCISE 28   *Comprehend Medical Terms in Use*

Test your comprehension of terms in the previous passage by answering T for true and F for false.

_____ 1. Inflammation of the outer ear is one of the most common pediatric infections.

_____ 2. Pain and discharge from the ear are symptoms of acute otitis media.

_____ 3. Surgical repair of the tympanic membrane may be performed to identify causative organisms.

CHAPTER REVIEW

CHAPTER REVIEW ON CD-ROM

Use the CD-ROM that accompanies this textbook to play and practice what you have learned in this chapter. The Chapter Exercises, Practice Activities, Animations, and Games allow you to hear, see, and interact with the chapter content.

Chapter Exercises

Exercises in this section of your CD-ROM correlate to exercises in your textbook. You may have completed them as you worked through the chapter.
☐ Pronunciation
☐ Spelling
☐ Read Medical Terms in Use

Practice Activities

Practice in study mode, then test your learning in assessment mode. Keep track of your scores from assessment mode if you wish.

                               SCORE
☐ Picture It   _____
☐ Define Word Parts   _____
☐ Build Medical Terms   _____
☐ Word Shop   _____
☐ Define Medical Terms   _____
☐ Use It   _____
☐ Hear It and Type It: _____
   Clinical Vignettes

Animations
☐ None for this chapter.

Games
☐ Name that Word Part
☐ Term Storm
☐ Term Explorer
☐ Termbusters
☐ Medical Millionaire

REVIEW OF WORD PARTS

Can you define and spell the following word parts?

Combining Forms

audi/o	myring/o
aur/i	ot/o
aur/o	staped/o
cochle/o	tympan/o
labyrinth/o	vestibul/o
mastoid/o	

REVIEW OF TERMS

Can you build, analyze, define, pronounce, and spell the following terms *built from word parts?*

Diseases and Disorders	Surgical	Diagnostic	Complementary
labyrinthitis	cochlear implant	audiogram	audiologist
mastoiditis	labyrinthectomy	audiometer	audiology
myringitis	mastoidectomy	audiometry	aural
otalgia	mastoidotomy	otoscope	cochlear
otomastoiditis	myringoplasty	otoscopy	otologist
otomycosis	myringotomy	tympanometer	otology
otopyorrhea	stapedectomy	tympanometry	otorhinolaryngologist
otorrhea	tympanoplasty		vestibular
otosclerosis			vestibulocochlear
tympanitis			

Can you define, pronounce, and spell the following terms *not built from word parts?*

Diseases and Disorders

acoustic neuroma
ceruminoma
cholesteatoma
Ménière disease
otitis externa
otitis media (OM)
presbycusis
tinnitus
vertigo

ANSWERS

Exercise Figures

Exercise Figure

A. 1. ear: aur/i, aur/o, ot/o
2. labyrinth: labyrinth/o
3. stapes: staped/o
4. tympanic membrane: myring/o, tympan/o
5. mastoid bone: mastoid/o

Exercise Figure

B. myring/o/tomy

Exercise 1

1. g	6. k
2. j	7. d
3. b	8. e
4. f	9. a
5. h	10. c

Exercise 2

1. stapes
2. mastoid bone
3. hearing
4. ear
5. tympanic membrane (eardrum), middle ear
6. vestibule
7. labyrinth
8. tympanic membrane (eardrum)
9. cochlea

Exercise 3

1. a. aur/i
   b. aur/o
   c. ot/o
2. mastoid/o
3. staped/o
4. tympan/o
5. labyrinth/o
6. audi/o
7. myring/o
8. cochle/o
9. vestibul/o

Exercise 4

Pronunciation Exercise

Exercise 5

1. WR CV WR S
   ot/o/myc/osis
   CF
   abnormal condition of fungus in the ear

2. WR S
   tympan/itis
   inflammation of the middle ear

3. WR CV WR S
   ot/o/mastoid/itis
   CF
   inflammation of the ear and the mastoid bone

4. WR S
   ot/algia
   pain in the ear

5. WR S
   labyrinth/itis
   inflammation of the labyrinth

6. WR S
   myring/itis
   inflammation of the tympanic membrane

7. WR CV S
   ot/o/sclerosis
   CF
   hardening of the ear (stapes)

8. WR S
   mastoid/itis
   inflammation of the mastoid bone

9. WR CV WR CV S
   ot/o/py/o/rrhea
   CF   CF
   discharge of pus from the ear

10. WR CV S
    ot/o/rrhea
    CF
    discharge from the ear

Exercise 6

1. myring/itis
2. ot/o/py/o/rrhea
3. mastoid/itis
4. ot/algia
5. ot/o/sclerosis
6. ot/o/myc/osis
7. ot/o/mastoid/itis
8. labyrinth/itis
9. tympan/itis
10. ot/o/rrhea

Exercise 7

Spelling Exercise; see text p. 587.

Exercise 8

Pronunciation Exercise

Exercise 9

1. vertigo; tinnitus
2. Ménière
3. otitis media
4. ceruminoma
5. otitis externa
6. acoustic neuroma
7. presbycusis
8. cholesteatoma

Exercise 10

1. e	6. d
2. b	7. a
3. g	8. i
4. c	9. j
5. h	

Exercise 11

Spelling Exercise; see text p. 589.

Exercise 12

Pronunciation Exercise

Exercise 13

1. WR S
   mastoid/ectomy
   excision of the mastoid bone

2. WR CV S
   myring/o/tomy
   CF
   incision into the tympanic membrane

3. WR S
   labyrinth/ectomy
   excision of the labyrinth

4. WR CV S
   mastoid/o/tomy
   CF
   incision into the mastoid bone

5. WR CV S
   tympan/o/plasty
   CF
   surgical repair of the middle ear

6. WR CV S
   myring/o/plasty
   CF
   surgical repair of the tympanic membrane

7. WR S
   staped/ectomy
   excision of the stapes

8. WR S
   cochle/ar implant
   pertaining to the cochlea implant

Exercise 14
1. mastoid/o/tomy
2. labyrinth/ectomy
3. tympan/o/plasty
4. mastoid/ectomy
5. myring/o/tomy
6. myring/o/plasty
7. staped/ectomy
8. cochle/ar implant

Exercise 15
Spelling Exercise; see text p. 592.

Exercise 16
Pronunciation Exercise

Exercise 17
1. WR CV S
   ot/o/scope
      CF
   instrument used for the visual
      examination of the ear
2. WR CV S
   audi/o/metry
      CF
   measurement of hearing
3. WR CV S
   audi/o/gram
      CF
   (graphic) record of hearing
4. WR CV S
   ot/o/scopy
      CF
   visual examination of the ear
5. WR CV S
   audi/o/meter
      CF
   instrument used to measure hearing
6. WR CV S
   tympan/o/metry
      CF
   measurement (of movement) of the
      tympanic membrane
7. WR CV S
   tympan/o/meter
      CF
   instrument used to measure middle
      ear (function)

Exercise 18
1. tympan/o/metry
2. audi/o/meter
3. ot/o/scopy
4. audi/o/gram
5. ot/o/scope
6. audi/o/metry
7. tympan/o/meter

Exercise 19
Spelling Exercise; see text p. 595.

Exercise 20
Pronunciation Exercise

Exercise 21
1. WR CV S
   ot/o/logy
      CF
   study of the ear
2. WR CV S
   audi/o/logist
      CF
   one who studies and specializes in
      hearing
3. WR CV WR CV WR CV S
   ot/o/rhin/o/laryng/o/logist
      CF   CF   CF
   physician who studies and treats
      diseases of the ear, nose, and larynx
      (throat)
4. WR CV S
   audi/o/logy
      CF
   study of hearing
5. WR CV S
   ot/o/logist
      CF
   physician who studies and treats
      diseases of the ear
6. WR S
   aur/al
   pertaining to the ear
7. WR S
   cochle/ar
   pertaining to the cochlea
8. WR S
   vestibul/ar
   pertaining to the vestibule
9. WR CV WR S
   vestibul/o/cochle/ar
      CF
   pertaining to the vestibule and cochlea

Exercise 22
1. audi/o/logy
2. ot/o/rhin/o/laryng/o/logist
3. ot/o/logy
4. audi/o/logist
5. ot/o/logist
6. aur/al
7. vestibul/o/cochle/ar
8. vestibul/ar
9. cochle/ar

Exercise 23
Spelling Exercise; see text p. 597.

Exercise 24
1. ears, nose, throat
2. eyes, ears, nose, and throat
3. otitis media
4. acute otitis media

Exercise 25
A. 1. ENT
   2. tinnitus
   3. vertigo
   4. otoscopy
   5. otitis media
   6. presbycusis
   7. audiologist
   8. audiometry

B. 1. a
   2. b
   3. d

Exercise 26
1. myringitis
2. tinnitus
3. otologist
4. myringotomy
5. Ménière disease
6. acoustic neuroma
7. cholesteatoma

Exercise 27
Reading Exercise

Exercise 28
1. *F*, inflammation of the middle ear
   (otitis media) is the most common
   pediatric infection.
2. *T*
3. *F*, myringotomy, incision into the
   tympanic membrane would be
   performed.

NOTES

CHAPTER 14

Musculoskeletal System

OUTLINE

ANATOMY, 608

WORD PARTS, 620
Combining Forms, 620
Prefixes, 627
Suffixes, 628

MEDICAL TERMS, 629
Disease and Disorder Terms, 629
    Built from Word Parts, 629
    Not Built from Word Parts, 636
Surgical Terms, 643
    Built from Word Parts, 643
Diagnostic Terms, 650
    Built from Word Parts, 650
Complementary Terms, 653
    Built from Word Parts, 653
    Not Built from Word Parts, 660
Abbreviations, 662

PRACTICAL APPLICATION, 664
Interact with Medical Documents, 664
Interpret Medical Terms, 666
Read Medical Terms in Use, 667
Comprehend Medical Terms in Use, 667
Use Plural Endings, 668

CHAPTER REVIEW, 668

TABLE 14-1 TYPES OF ARTHROPLASTY, 644

TABLE 14-2 PROCEDURES FOR TREATMENT OF COMPRESSION FRACTURES CAUSED BY OSTEOPOROSIS, 646

TABLE 14-3 DIAGNOSTIC IMAGING PROCEDURES USED FOR THE MUSCULOSKELETAL SYSTEM, 652

OBJECTIVES

Upon completion of this chapter you will be able to:

1. Identify organs and structures of the musculoskeletal system.

2. Identify and define types of body movement.

3. Define and spell word parts related to the musculoskeletal system.

4. Define, pronounce, and spell disease and disorder terms related to the musculoskeletal system.

5. Define, pronounce, and spell surgical terms related to the musculoskeletal system.

6. Define, pronounce, and spell diagnostic terms related to the musculoskeletal system.

7. Define, pronounce, and spell complementary terms related to the musculoskeletal system.

8. Interpret the meaning of abbreviations related to the musculoskeletal system.

9. Interpret, read, and comprehend medical language in simulated medical statements and documents.

ANATOMY

The musculoskeletal system is made up of muscles, bones (Figure 14-1), and joints. The body contains 206 bones (Figure 14-2 and Figure 14-3, *A* and *B*) and more than 600 muscles. Joints are located any place that two or more bones meet.

Function

The functions of the muscular system are movement, posture, joint stability, and heat production. The functions of the skeletal system are to provide a framework for the body, protect the soft body parts such as the brain, store calcium, and produce blood cells.

Bone Structure

Term	Definition
periosteum	outermost layer of the bone, made up of fibrous tissue
compact bone.	dense, hard layers of bone tissue that lie underneath the periosteum
cancellous (spongy) bone.	contains little spaces like a sponge and is encased in the layers of compact bone

PERIOSTEUM is composed of the prefix **peri-,** meaning **surrounding,** and the word root **oste,** meaning **bone.**

 DIAPHYSIS comes from the Greek **diaphusis,** meaning **state of growing between.**

 EPIPHYSIS has been used in the English language since the 1600s and retains the meaning given to it by a Greco-Roman physician. It means a **portion of bone attached for a time to another bone by a cartilage, but that later combines with the principal bone.** During the period of growth, the epiphysis is separated from the main portion of the bone by cartilage.

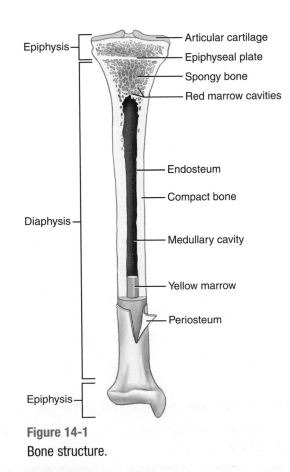

Epiphysis — Articular cartilage
— Epiphyseal plate
— Spongy bone
— Red marrow cavities
— Endosteum
— Compact bone
Diaphysis — — Medullary cavity
— Yellow marrow
— Periosteum
Epiphysis —

Figure 14-1
Bone structure.

Term	Definition
endosteum	membranous lining of the hollow cavity of the bone
diaphysis	shaft of the long bones (Figure 14-1)
epiphysis (*pl.* epiphyses)	end of each long bone (Figure 14-1)
bone marrow	material found in the cavities of bones
red marrow.	thick, blood-like material found in flat bones and the ends of long bones; location of blood cell formation.
yellow marrow	soft, fatty material found in the medullary cavity of long bones

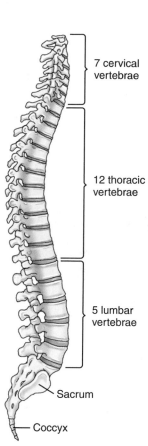

ENDOSTEUM
is composed of the prefix **endo-,** meaning **within,** and the word root **oste,** meaning **bone.**

7 cervical vertebrae

12 thoracic vertebrae

5 lumbar vertebrae

Sacrum

Coccyx

Figure 14-2
Vertebral column.

Skeletal Bones

Term	Definition
maxilla	upper jawbone
mandible.	lower jawbone
vertebral column	made up of bones called **vertebrae** *(pl.)* or **vertebra** *(sing.)* through which the spinal cord runs. The vertebral column protects the spinal cord, supports the head, and provides a point of attachment for ribs and muscles (Figure 14-2).
cervical vertebrae (C1 to C7)	first set of seven bones, forming the neck
thoracic vertebrae (T1 to T12)	second set of 12 vertebrae. They articulate with the 12 pairs of ribs to form the outward curve of the spine.
lumbar vertebrae (L1 to L5)	third set of five larger vertebrae, which forms the inward curve of the spine
sacrum	next five vertebrae, which fuse together to form a triangular bone positioned between the two hip bones
coccyx	four vertebrae fused together to form the tailbone
lamina (*pl.* laminae)	part of the vertebral arch
clavicle	collarbone
scapula.	shoulder blade
acromion process.	extension of the scapula, which forms the high point of the shoulder
sternum	breastbone
xiphoid process	lower portion of the sternum
humerus	upper arm bone

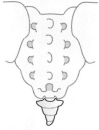

Coccyx is derived from the Greek word *cuckoo* because of its resemblance to a cuckoo's beak.

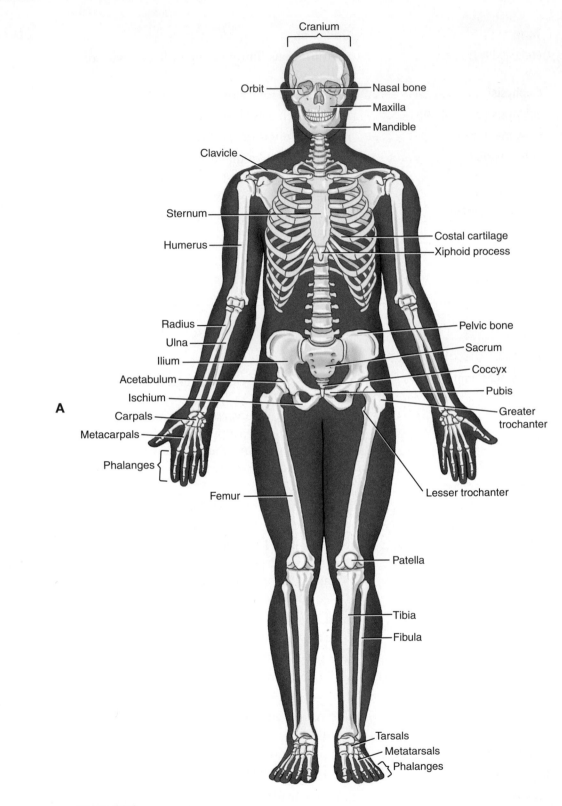

Figure 14-3
A, Anterior view of the skeleton.

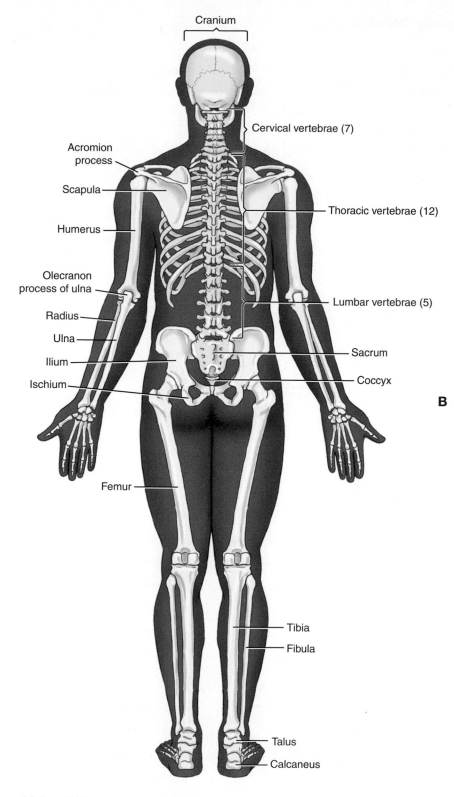

Figure 14-3, cont'd
B, Posterior view of the skeleton.

Skeletal Bones—*cont'd*

Term	Definition
ulna and radius.............	lower arm bones
olecranon process	projection at the upper end of the ulna that forms the bony point of the elbow
carpal bones................	wrist bones
metacarpal bones...........	hand bones
phalanges (*sing.* phalanx)	finger and toe bones
pelvic bone, hip bone	made up of three bones fused together
ischium.................	lower, rear portion on which one sits
ilium...................	upper, wing-shaped part on each side
pubis..................	anterior portion of the pelvic bone
acetabulum................	large socket in the pelvic bone for the head of the femur
femur	upper leg bone
tibia and fibula.............	lower leg bones
patella (*pl.* patellae)	kneecap
tarsal bones	ankle bones
calcaneus.................	heel bone
metatarsal bones	foot bones

EXERCISE 1

Match the definitions in the first column with the correct terms in the second column.

_____ 1. shaft of a long bone

_____ 2. hard layer of bone tissue

_____ 3. outermost layer of bone

_____ 4. found in bone cavities

_____ 5. lining of the bone cavity

_____ 6. end of each long bone

_____ 7. contains little spaces

_____ 8. socket in the pelvic bone

_____ 9. heel bone

_____ 10. part of the arch of the vertebra

a. lamina

b. cancellous bone

c. acetabulum

d. diaphysis

e. endometrium

f. calcaneus

g. epiphysis

h. periosteum

i. compact bone

j. endosteum

k. bone marrow

EXERCISE 2

Write the name of the bone to match the definition.

1. shoulder blade   _____

2. breastbone   _____

3. lower jawbone   _____

4. collarbone   _____

5. upper arm bone   _____

6. lower arm bones   a. _____

                           b. _____

7. ankle bones   _____

8. finger, toe bones   _____

9. foot bones   _____

10. hand bones   _____

11. upper leg bone   _____

12. lower leg bones   a. _____

                            b. _____

13. kneecap   _____

14. neck   _____ _____

15. third set of vertebrae   _____

16. anterior portion of the pelvic bone   _____

17. five vertebrae fused together   _____

18. lower rear portion of the pelvic bone   _____

19. tailbone   _____

20. upper, wing-shaped part of the pelvic bone   _____

21. wrist bones   _____

Joints

Joints, also called **articulations**, hold our bones together and make movement possible (in most joints) (Figure 14-4).

Term	Definition
articular cartilage............	smooth layer of gristle covering the contacting surface of joints
meniscus	crescent-shaped cartilage found in the knee
intervertebral disk	cartilaginous pad found between the vertebrae in the spine
pubic symphysis............	cartilaginous joint at which two pubic bones fuse together
synovia	fluid secreted by the synovial membrane and found in joint cavities
bursa (*pl.* bursae)...........	fluid-filled sac that allows for easy movement of one part of a joint over another
ligament	flexible, tough band of fibrous connective tissue that attaches one bone to another at a joint
tendon...................	band of fibrous connective tissue that attaches muscle to bone
aponeurosis	strong sheet of tissue that acts as a tendon to attach muscles to bone

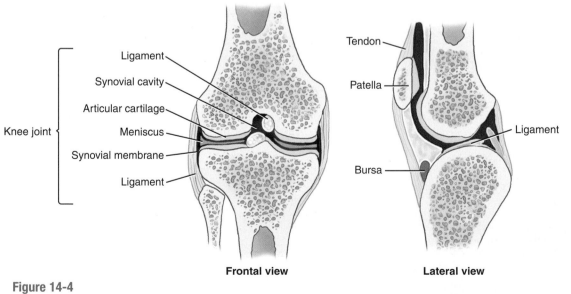

Frontal view   **Lateral view**

Figure 14-4
Knee joint.

Muscles

Term	Definition
skeletal muscles (also known as *striated muscles*).........	attached to bones by tendons and make body movement possible. Skeletal muscles produce action by pulling and by working in pairs. They are also known as **voluntary muscles** because we have control over these muscles (Figure 14-5, *A* and *B*, and Figure 14-6).
smooth muscles (also known as *unstriated muscles*)........	located in internal organs such as the walls of blood vessels and the digestive tract. They are also called **involuntary muscles** because they respond to impulses from the autonomic nerves and are not controlled voluntarily (see Figure 14-6).
cardiac muscle (known as *myocardium*)...............	forms most of the wall of the heart. Its involuntary contraction produces the heartbeat (see Figure 14-6).

EXERCISE 3

Match the definitions in the first column with the correct terms in the second column.

_____ 1. attaches muscle to bone	a.	skeletal muscles
_____ 2. fluid-filled sac	b.	aponeurosis
_____ 3. smooth layer of gristle	c.	bursa
_____ 4. voluntary muscles	d.	smooth muscles
_____ 5. fluid	e.	cartilage
_____ 6. located in the internal organs	f.	intervertebral disk
_____ 7. attaches bone to bone	g.	cardiac muscles
_____ 8. cartilage found in the knee	h.	ligament
_____ 9. pubic bone joint	i.	meniscus
_____ 10. acts as a tendon	j.	periosteum
_____ 11. found between each vertebra	k.	pubic symphysis
_____ 12. produces heartbeat	l.	synovia
	m.	tendon

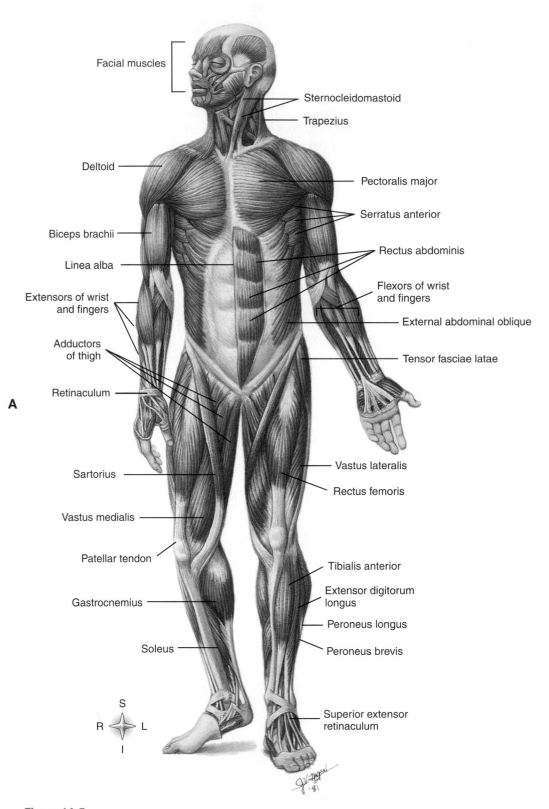

Facial muscles

Sternocleidomastoid

Trapezius

Deltoid

Pectoralis major

Serratus anterior

Biceps brachii

Rectus abdominis

Linea alba

Flexors of wrist
and fingers

Extensors of wrist
and fingers

External abdominal oblique

Adductors
of thigh

Tensor fasciae latae

Retinaculum

A

Sartorius

Vastus lateralis

Rectus femoris

Vastus medialis

Patellar tendon

Tibialis anterior

Gastrocnemius

Extensor digitorum
longus

Peroneus longus

Soleus

Peroneus brevis

S

R ✛ L

I

Superior extensor
retinaculum

Figure 14-5
A, Anterior view of the muscular system.

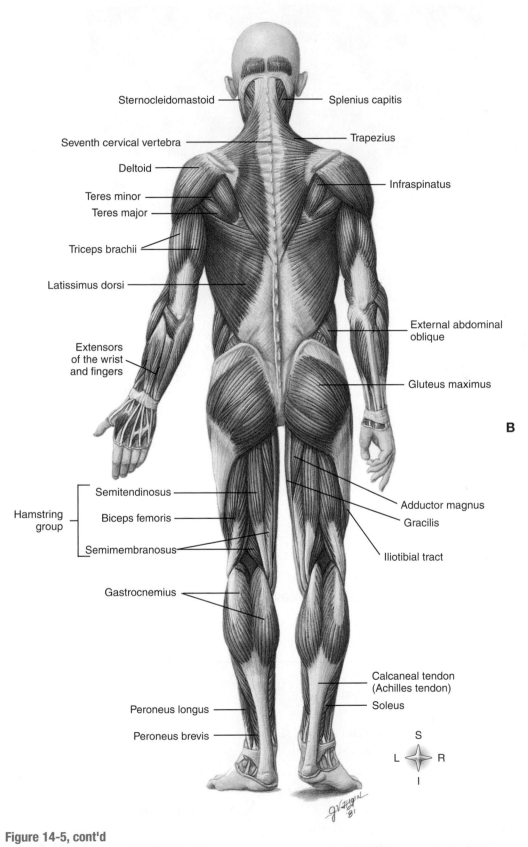

Figure 14-5, cont'd
B, Posterior view of the muscular system.   *Continued*

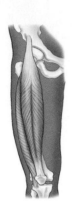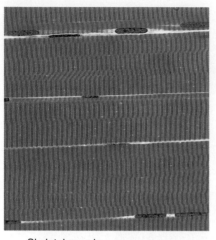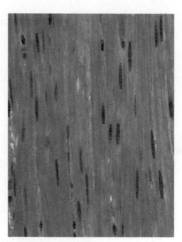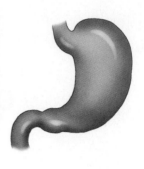

Skeletal muscle

Smooth muscle

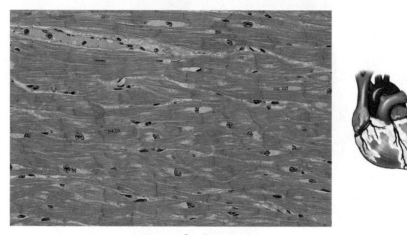

Cardiac muscle

Figure 14-6
Types of muscle tissue.

Types of Body Movement

Bones and muscles work together to produce various types of body movement. Some are listed below (Figure 14-7).

Term	Definition
abduction (ab-DUK-shun)	movement of drawing away from the middle
adduction (ad-DUK-shun)	movement of drawing toward the middle
inversion (in-VER-zhun)	turning inward
eversion (ē-VER-zhun)	turning outward
extension (ek-STEN-shun)	movement in which a limb is placed in a straight position
flexion (FLEK-shun)	movement in which a limb is bent

Term	Definition
pronation .... (prō-NĀ-shun)	movement that turns the palm down
supination................. (sū-pi-NĀ-shun)	movement that turns the palm up
rotation .... (rō-TĀ-shun)	turning around its own axis

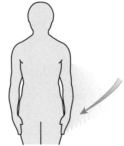

Adduction   Abduction   Rotation

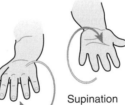

Pronation   Supination

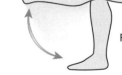

Eversion   Inversion

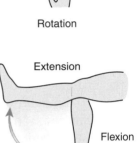

Extension

Flexion

Figure 14-7
Types of body movements.

EXERCISE 4

Write the definitions of the following terms.

1. abduction _____

2. pronation_____

3. supination _____

4. rotation _____

5. extension _____

6. eversion _____

7. adduction _____

8. flexion _____

9. inversion _____

EXERCISE　5

Match the terms in the first column with the correct definitions in the second column.

_____ 1. abduction
_____ 2. adduction
_____ 3. pronation
_____ 4. rotation
_____ 5. eversion
_____ 6. extension
_____ 7. flexion
_____ 8. inversion
_____ 9. supination

a. movement in which the limb is placed in a straight position

b. movement that turns the palm up

c. turning outward

d. drawing toward the middle

e. conveying toward the center

f. turning inward

g. movement in which the limb is bent

h. drawing away from the middle

i. movement that turns the palm down

j. turning around its own axis

WORD PARTS

At first glance the number of word parts introduced in this chapter may seem overwhelming, but notice that many of them are names for bones already learned in the anatomic section. The definitions of the word parts include both anatomic terms and commonly used words. For example, both *carpal* and *wrist bone* are given as the definition of the combining form *carp/o*. Word parts you need to learn to complete this chapter are listed on the following pages. The exercises at the end of each list will help you learn their definitions and spellings.

Combining Forms of the Musculoskeletal System

METACARPUS literally means **beyond the wrist.** It is composed of the prefix **meta-,** meaning **beyond,** and **carpus,** meaning **wrist.**

Combining Form	Definition
carp/o	carpals (wrist bones)
clavic/o, clavicul/o	clavicle (collarbone)
cost/o	rib
crani/o	cranium (skull)
femor/o	femur (upper leg bone)
fibul/o	fibula (lower leg bone) (perone/o is also a word root for fibula)
humer/o	humerus (upper arm bone)
ili/o	ilium
ischi/o	ischium
lumb/o	loin, lumbar region of the spine
mandibul/o	mandible (lower jawbone)

Combining Form	Definition
maxill/o..................	maxilla (upper jawbone)
patell/o..................	patella (kneecap)
pelv/i, pelv/o.............. (NOTE: both *i* and *o* may be used as the connecting vowel with *pelvis*)	pelvis, pelvic bone (also covered in Chapter 9)
phalang/o.................	phalanges (finger or toe bones)
pub/o....................	pubis
rachi/o...................	spine, vertebral column
radi/o...................	radius (lower arm bone)
sacr/o...................	sacrum
scapul/o.................	scapula (shoulder blade)
spondyl/o, vertebr/o........	vertebra
stern/o..................	sternum (breastbone)
tars/o...................	tarsals (ankle bones)
tibi/o...................	tibia (lower leg bone)
uln/o...................	ulna (lower arm bone)

EXERCISE 6

Write the definitions of the following combining forms.

1. clavic/o _____

2. cost/o _____

3. crani/o _____

4. femor/o _____

5. clavicul/o _____

6. humer/o _____

7. ili/o _____

8. ischi/o _____

9. carp/o _____

10. fibul/o _____

11. mandibul/o _____

12. lumb/o _____

13. pelv/o _____

EXERCISE FIGURE A

Fill in the blanks with combining forms in this diagram of the skeleton, anterior view.

7. Cranium
CF: _____

8. Maxilla
CF: _____

1. Mandible
CF: _____

9. Clavicle
CF: _____
CF: _____

Humerus

2. Sternum
CF: _____

10. Ribs
CF: _____

Vertebral column

Pelvis

Radius

Ulna

Carpals

Metacarpals

3. Phalanges
CF: _____

11. Femur
CF: _____

4. Patella
CF: _____

Knee joint

12. Fibula
CF: _____

13. Tibia
CF: _____

5. Tarsals
CF: _____

Metatarsals

6. Phalanges
CF: _____

EXERCISE FIGURE B

Fill in the blanks with combining forms in this diagram of the skeleton, posterior view, and the pelvis.

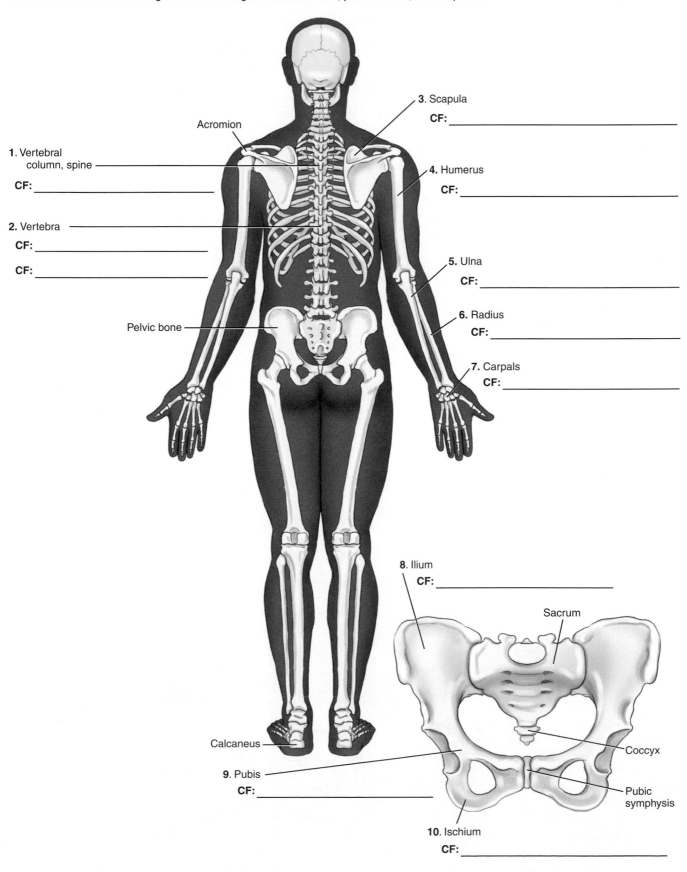

3. Scapula

CF: _____

Acromion

1. Vertebral
column, spine

CF: _____

4. Humerus

CF: _____

2. Vertebra

CF: _____

CF: _____

5. Ulna

CF: _____

6. Radius

CF: _____

Pelvic bone

7. Carpals

CF: _____

8. Ilium

CF: _____

Sacrum

Calcaneus

Coccyx

9. Pubis

CF: _____

Pubic
symphysis

10. Ischium

CF: _____

EXERCISE 7

Write the combining form for each of the following terms.

1. clavicle a. _____
   b. _____

2. rib _____

3. cranium _____

4. femur _____

5. humerus _____

6. carpals _____

7. ischium _____

8. fibula _____

9. ilium _____

10. mandible _____

11. loin, lumbar region of the spine _____

12. pelvis, pelvic bone
    a. _____
    b. _____

EXERCISE 8

Write the definitions of the following combining forms.

1. rachi/o _____

2. patell/o _____

3. spondyl/o _____

4. maxill/o _____

5. phalang/o _____

6. uln/o _____

7. radi/o _____

8. tibi/o _____

9. pub/o _____

10. tars/o _____

11. scapul/o _____

12. stern/o _____

13. vertebr/o _____

14. sacr/o _____

EXERCISE 9

Write the combining form for each of the following terms.

1. maxilla _____

2. ulna _____

3. radius _____

4. tibia _____

5. pubis _____

6. tarsals _____

7. vertebra a. _____
   b. _____

8. sternum _____

9. scapula _____

10. patella _____

11. phalanges _____

12. sacrum _____

13. vertebral column, spine _____

Combining Forms of Joints

Combining Form	Definition
aponeur/o..................	aponeurosis
arthr/o....................	joint
burs/o....................	bursa (cavity)
chondr/o..................	cartilage
disk/o....................	intervertebral disk
menisc/o..................	meniscus (crescent)
synovi/o..................	synovia, synovial membrane
ten/o, tend/o, tendin/o........	tendon

DISK
is from the Greek
diskos, meaning flat
plate. A variant spelling, ***disc,***
is also used, though chiefly in
ophthalmology.

▌ EXERCISE FIGURE **C**

Fill in the blanks with combining forms on these diagrams of the knee joint.

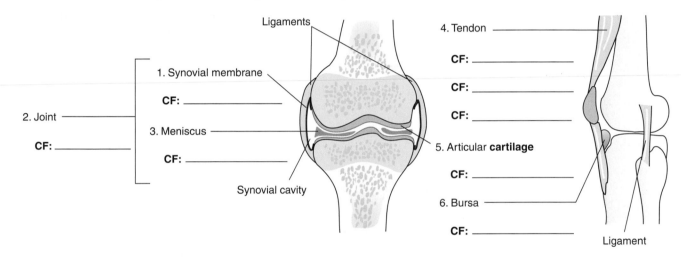

EXERCISE 10

Write the definitions of the following combining forms.

1. arthr/o _____ 6. ten/o _____

2. aponeur/o _____ 7. burs/o _____

3. menisc/o _____ 8. tend/o _____

4. tendin/o_____ 9. synovi/o_____

5. chondr/o _____ 10. disk/o_____

EXERCISE 11

Write the combining form for each of the following terms.

1. meniscus   _____
2. aponeurosis   _____
3. joint   _____
4. cartilage   _____
5. tendon   a. _____

      b. _____

      c. _____

6. bursa   _____
7. synovia, synovial membrane   _____
8. intervertebral disk   _____

Combining Forms Commonly Used with Musculoskeletal System Terms

Combining Form	Definition
ankyl/o	crooked, stiff, bent
kinesi/o	movement, motion
kyph/o	hump
lamin/o	lamina (thin, flat plate or layer)
lord/o	bent forward
myel/o . . . . (NOTE: *myel/o* also means **spinal cord;** see Chapter 15.)	bone marrow (also covered in Chapter 10)
my/o, myos/o . . . . (NOTE: *my/o* was introduced in Chapter 2.)	muscle
oste/o	bone
petr/o . . . . (NOTE: *lith/o*, also a combining form for **stone,** was introduced in Chapter 6.)	stone
scoli/o	crooked, curved

EXERCISE 12

Write the definitions of the following combining forms.

1. my/o _____

2. petr/o _____

3. kinesi/o _____

4. oste/o _____

5. lamin/o _____

6. myel/o _____

7. kyph/o _____

8. ankyl/o _____

9. scoli/o _____

10. myos/o _____

11. lord/o _____

EXERCISE 13

Write the combining form for each of the following.

1. muscle   a. _____

                 b. _____

2. stone   _____

3. movement, motion   _____

4. bone   _____

5. lamina   _____

6. bone marrow   _____

7. hump   _____

8. crooked, stiff, bent   _____

9. crooked, curved   _____

10. bent forward   _____

Prefixes

Prefix	Definition
inter-	between
supra-	above
sym-, syn-	together, joined

EXERCISE 14

Write the definition of the following prefixes.

1. supra- _____

2. sym-, syn- _____

3. inter- _____

EXERCISE 15

Write the prefix for each of the following definitions.

1. together, joined   a. _____

                 b. _____

2. between   _____

3. above   _____

Suffixes

Suffix	Definition
-asthenia	weakness
-clasia, -clasis, -clast	break
-desis	surgical fixation, fusion
-physis	growth
-schisis	split, fissure

EXERCISE 16

Write the definitions of the following suffixes.

1. -physis _____

2. -clasis _____

3. -desis _____

4. -clast _____

5. -schisis _____

6. -clasia _____

7. -asthenia _____

EXERCISE 17

Write the suffix for each of the following definitions.

1. growth   _____

2. weakness   _____

3. break   a. _____

           b. _____

           c. _____

4. surgical fixation, fusion _____

5. split, fissure _____

MEDICAL TERMS

Disease and Disorder Terms

Built from Word Parts

The following terms are built from word parts you have already learned and can be translated literally to find their meanings. Further explanation of terms beyond the definition of their word parts, if needed, is included in parentheses.

Term	Definition
ankylosis................. (an-ki-LŌ-sis)	abnormal condition of stiffness (often referring to fixation of a joint, such as the result of chronic rheumatoid arthritis)
arthritis.................. (ar-THRĪ-tis)	inflammation of a joint. (The most common forms of arthritis are osteoarthritis and rheumatoid arthritis.) (Figure 14-8)

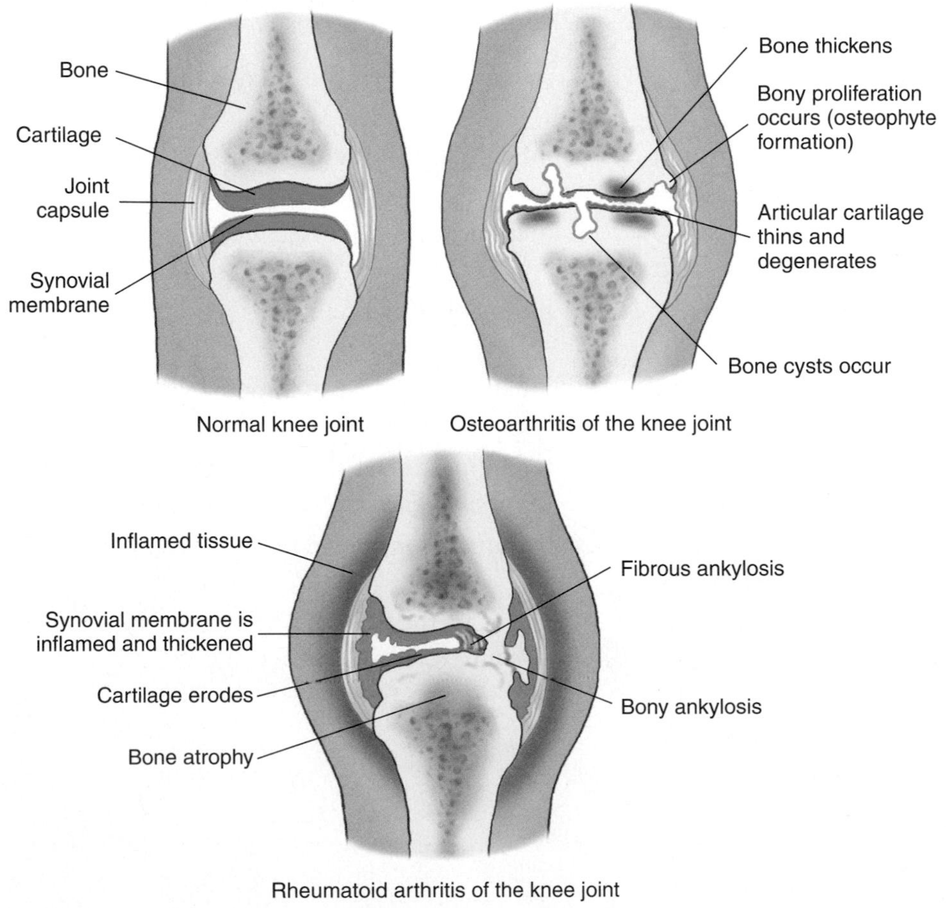

Normal knee joint

Osteoarthritis of the knee joint

Rheumatoid arthritis of the knee joint

Figure 14-8
Normal and arthritic knee joints.

Disease and Disorder Terms—*cont'd*
Built from Word Parts

Term	Definition
bursitis . . . . (ber-SĪ-tis)	inflammation of a bursa
chondromalacia . . . . (*kon*-drō-ma-LĀ-sha)	softening of cartilage
cranioschisis. . . . . (*krā*-nē-OS-ki-sis)	fissure of the skull (congenital)
diskitis . . . . (dis-KĪ-tis)	inflammation of an intervertebral disk (also called **discitis**)
fibromyalgia . . . . (*fī*-brō-mī-AL-ja)	pain in the fibrous tissues and muscles (a common condition characterized by widespread pain and stiffness of muscles, fatigue, and disturbed sleep)
kyphosis . . . . (kī-FŌ-sis)	abnormal condition of a hump (of the thoracic spine) (also called **hunchback** or **humpback**) (Exercise Figure D)
lordosis. . . . . (lōr-DŌ-sis)	abnormal condition of bending forward (forward curvature of the lumbar spine) (also called **swayback**) (Exercise Figure D)
maxillitis. . . . . (*mak*-si-LĪ-tis)	inflammation of the maxilla
meniscitis. . . . . (*men*-i-SĪ-tis)	inflammation of a meniscus
myasthenia. . . . . (*mī*-as-THĒ-nē-a)	muscle weakness
myeloma. . . . . (*mī*-e-LŌ-ma)	tumor of the bone marrow (malignant)
osteitis . . . . (*os*-tē-Ī-tis)	inflammation of the bone
osteoarthritis (OA). . . . . (*os*-tē-ō-ar-THRĪ-tis)	inflammation of the bone and joint (Figure 14-8)
osteochondritis. . . . . (*os*-tē-ō-kon-DRĪ-tis)	inflammation of the bone and cartilage
osteofibroma . . . . (*os*-tē-ō-fī-BRŌ-ma)	tumor of the bone and fibrous tissue (benign)
osteomalacia . . . . (*os*-tē-ō-ma-LĀ-sha)	softening of bones

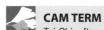

CAM TERM
Tai Chi, often referred to as "meditation in motion," is an ancient Chinese art using slow movements and focused breathing to support mental and physical health. Studies indicate significant improvement in upper and lower body strength, balance, and flexibility in the elderly with Tai Chi practice.

Term	Definition
osteomyelitis (os-tē-ō-*mī*-e-LĪ-tis)	inflammation of the bone and bone marrow (caused by bacterial infection)
osteopenia (os-tē-ō-PĒ-nē-a)	abnormal reduction of bone mass (caused by inadequate replacement of bone lost to normal bone lysis and can lead to osteoporosis)
osteopetrosis (os-tē-ō-pe-TRŌ-sis)	abnormal condition of stonelike bones (marblelike bones caused by increased formation of bone)
osteosarcoma (os-tē-ō-sar-KŌ-ma)	malignant tumor of the bone
polymyositis (*pol*-ē-mī-ō-SĪ-tis)	inflammation of many muscles
rachischisis (ra-KIS-ki-sis)	fissure of the vertebral column (congenital) (also called **spina bifida**) (see Exercise Figure C in Chapter 15)
rhabdomyolysis (*rab*-dō-mī-OL-i-sis)	dissolution of striated muscle (The severity of the condition and the degree of weakness and pain vary. Some causes of the illness are trauma, extreme exertion, and drug toxicity; in severe cases renal failure can result.)
scoliosis (*skō*-lē-Ō-sis)	abnormal (lateral) curve (of the spine) (Exercise Figure D)
spondylarthritis (*spon*-dil-ar-THRĪ-tis)	inflammation of the vertebral joints
spondylosis (*spon*-di-LŌ-sis)	abnormal condition of the vertebra (a general term used to describe changes to the spine from osteoarthritis or ankylosis)
synoviosarcoma (si-*nō*-vē-ō-sar-KŌ-ma)	malignant tumor of the synovial membrane
tendinitis (*ten*-di-NĪ-tis)	inflammation of a tendon (also spelled **tendonitis**)
tenosynovitis (*ten*-ō-*sin*-ō-VĪ-tis) (NOTE: the *i* in *synovi* is dropped because the suffix begins with an *i*.)	inflammation of the tendon and synovial membrane

Fill in the blanks to label the diagram.

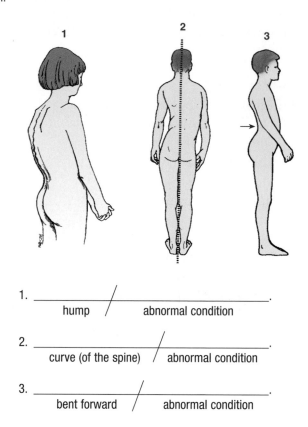

1. _____ / _____ .
   hump   abnormal condition

2. _____ / _____ .
   curve (of the spine)   abnormal condition

3. _____ / _____ .
   bent forward   abnormal condition

EXERCISE 18

Practice saying aloud each of the disease and disorder terms built from word parts on pp. 629-631.

 To hear the terms select Chapter 14, Chapter Exercises, Pronunciation.

☐ Place a check mark in the box when you have completed this exercise.

EXERCISE 19

Analyze and define the following disease and disorder terms.

1. osteitis _____

2. osteomyelitis _____

3. osteopetrosis _____

4. osteomalacia _____

5. osteochondritis _____

6. osteofibroma _____

7. arthritis _____

8. rhabdomyolysis _____

9. myeloma _____

10. tendinitis _____

11. osteopenia _____

12. spondylosis _____

13. bursitis _____

14. spondylarthritis _____

15. ankylosis _____

16. kyphosis _____

17. scoliosis _____

18. cranioschisis _____

19. maxillitis _____

20. meniscitis _____

21. rachischisis _____

22. myasthenia _____

23. osteosarcoma _____

24. chondromalacia _____

25. synoviosarcoma _____

26. tenosynovitis _____

27. polymyositis _____

28. diskitis _____

29. lordosis _____

30. osteoarthritis _____

31. fibromyalgia _____

EXERCISE 20

Build disease and disorder terms for the following definitions with the word parts you have learned.

1. inflammation of the bone and cartilage

   _____ / ___ / _____ / ___
   WR   CV   WR   S

2. tumor of the bone and fibrous tissue

   _____ / ___ / _____ / ___
   WR   CV   WR   S

3. inflammation of a joint

   _____ / ___
   WR   S

4. dissolution of striated muscle

   _____ / ___ / _____ / ___ / ___
   WR   CV   WR   CV   S

5. tumor of the bone marrow

   _____ / ___
   WR   S

6. inflammation of a tendon

   _____ / ___
   WR   S

7. abnormal condition of the vertebra

   _____ / ___
   WR   S

8. abnormal reduction of bone mass

   _____ / ___ / ___
   WR   CV   S

9. inflammation of the bursa

   _____ / ___
   WR   S

10. inflammation of the vertebral joints

    _____ / _____ / ___
    WR   WR   S

11. abnormal condition of stiffness

    _____ / ___
    WR   S

12. abnormal condition of a hump (of the thoracic spine)

    _____ / ___
    WR   S

13. abnormal (lateral) curve of the spine

    _____ / ___
    WR   S

14. fissure of the skull

    _____ / ___ / ___
    WR   CV   S

15. inflammation of the maxilla

    _____ / ___
    WR   S

16. inflammation of the meniscus

    _____ / ___
    WR   S

17. fissure of the vertebral column   _____ / _____
                                              WR   S

18. muscle weakness   _____ / _____
                             WR   S

19. inflammation of the bone   _____ / _____
                                      WR   S

20. inflammation of the bone
    and bone marrow   _____ / ____ / _____ / _____
                        WR   CV   WR   S

21. abnormal condition of
    stonelike bones (marblelike
    bones)   _____ / ____ / _____ / _____
               WR   CV   WR   S

22. softening of bones   _____ / ____ / _____
                           WR   CV   S

23. inflammation of the tendon
    and synovial membrane   _____ / ____ / _____ / _____
                              WR   CV   WR   S

24. malignant tumor of the
    synovial membrane   _____ / ____ / _____
                          WR   CV   S

25. malignant tumor of the bone   _____ / ____ / _____
                                    WR   CV   S

26. softening of cartilage   _____ / ____ / _____
                               WR   CV   S

27. inflammation of an
    intervertebral disk   _____ / _____
                               WR   S

28. inflammation of many muscles   _____ / _____ / _____
                                      P   WR   S

29. abnormal condition of bending
    forward   _____ / _____
                   WR   S

30. inflammation of the bone
    and joint   _____ / ____ / _____ / _____
                  WR   CV   WR   S

31. pain in the fibrous tissues
    and muscles   _____ / ____ / _____ / _____
                    WR   CV   WR   S

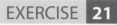

EXERCISE 21

Spell each of the disease and disorder terms built from word parts on pp. 629-631 by having someone dictate them to you.

To hear and spell the terms select Chapter 14, Chapter Exercises, Spelling. You may type the terms on the screen or write them below in the spaces provided.

☐ Place a check mark in the box if you have completed this exercise using your CD-ROM.

1._____
2._____
3._____
4._____
5._____
6._____
7._____
8._____
9._____
10._____
11._____
12._____
13._____
14._____
15._____
16._____

17._____
18._____
19._____
20._____
21._____
22._____
23._____
24._____
25._____
26._____
27._____
28._____
29._____
30._____
31._____

Disease and Disorder Terms

Not Built from Word Parts

In some of the following terms, you may recognize word parts you have already learned; however, the full meaning of the terms cannot be discerned by the definition of their word parts.

ANKYLOSING SPONDYLITIS was first described in 1884 by Adolf von Strümpell (1853–1925). It became known as **Strümpell-Marie disease** after von Strümpell and French physician Pierre Marie.

Term	Definition
ankylosing spondylitis . . . . (ang-ki-LŌ-sing) (*spon*-di-LĪ-tis)	form of arthritis that first affects the spine and adjacent structures and that, as it progresses, causes a forward bend of the spine (also called **Strümpell-Marie arthritis** or **disease,** or **rheumatoid spondylitis**)

Term	Definition
bunion.................... (BUN-yun)	abnormal enlargement of the joint at the base of the great toe. It is a common problem, often hereditary or caused by poorly fitted shoes (also called **hallux valgus**) (Figure 14-9).
carpal tunnel syndrome (CTS) ... (KAR-pl) (TUN-el) (SIN-drōm)	a common nerve entrapment disorder of the wrist caused by compression of the median nerve. Symptoms include pain and paresthesia in portions of the hand and fingers (Figure 14-10).
Colles fracture .... (KOL-ēz) (FRAK-chur)	a type of wrist fracture. The fracture is at the lower end of the radius, the distal fragment being displaced backward.
exostosis................... (ek-sos-TŌ-sis)	abnormal benign growth on the surface of a bone (also called **spur**)
fracture (fx)................. (FRAK-chūr)	broken bone (Figure 14-11)

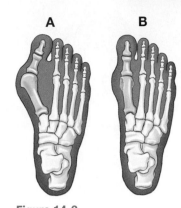

Figure 14-9
A, Bunion. **B,** Following a bunionectomy.

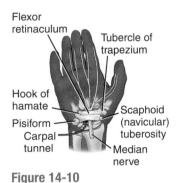

Figure 14-10
Structures involved with carpal tunnel syndrome, which is caused by compression of the median nerve. **Palmar uniportal endoscopic carpal tunnel release,** also called **Mirza,** is used surgically to treat this condition.

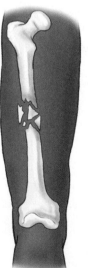

Comminuted fracture

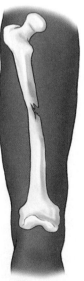

Greenstick fracture

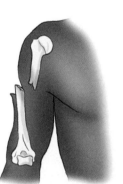

Compound fracture   Impacted fracture

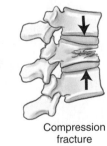

Radius

Colles fracture

Compression fracture

Figure 14-11
Types of fractures.

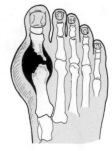

Figure 14-12
Gout.

Disease and Disorder Terms—*cont'd*
Not Built from Word Parts

Term	Definition
gout . . . . (gowt)	disease in which an excessive amount of uric acid in the blood causes sodium urate crystals (**tophi**) to be deposited in the joints, especially that of the great toe, producing arthritis (Figure 14-12)
herniated disk. . . . . (HER-nē-āt-ed) (disk)	rupture of the intervertebral disk cartilage, which allows the contents to protrude through it, putting pressure on the spinal nerve roots (also called **slipped disk, ruptured disk, herniated intervertebral disk,** or **herniated nucleus pulposus [HNP]**) (Figure 14-13, *A*)
Lyme disease . . . . (līm) (di-ZĒZ)	an infection caused by a bacteria *(Borrelia burgdorferi)* carried by deer ticks and transmitted to humans by the bite of an infected tick. Symptoms, caused by the body's immune response to the bacteria, vary and may include a rash at the site of the tick bite and flulike symptoms such as fever, headache, joint pain, and fatigue. Lyme disease was first reported in Lyme, Conn., in 1975. The primary treatment is antibiotics. Left untreated, Lyme disease can mimic several musculoskeletal diseases mentioned in this chapter (Figure 14-14).

Herniated
nucleus pulposus

A

B

Figure 14-13
A, Herniated disk. **B,** Percutaneous diskectomy.

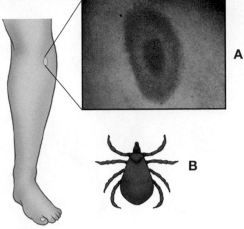

Figure 14-14

A, Target lesion of Lyme disease. **B,** Tick that causes Lyme disease.

ROTATOR CUFF INJURIES AND REPAIR
The rotator cuff of the shoulder stabilizes the head of the humerus during shoulder abduction (see Figure 14-7). Degenerative changes, repetitive motions, or falls can cause tears in older adults, and trauma may cause tears in young adults. Symptoms include shoulder pain and the inability to maintain abduction of the arm at the shoulder. If conservative treatments such as physical therapy, drugs, and heat/cold applications are not effective, surgical treatment, most commonly referred to as **rotator cuff repair,** is performed.

REPETITIVE MOTION SYNDROME
is an increasingly common and somewhat controversial diagnosis in which pain develops in the hand and forearm in the course of normal work activities. Permanent injury is not common. This condition is also referred to as **repetitive strain syndrome.**

Term	Definition
muscular dystrophy (MD) (MUS-kū-lar) (DIS-tro-fē)	group of hereditary diseases characterized by degeneration of muscle and weakness
myasthenia gravis (MG) (*mī*-as-THĒ-nē-a) (GRA-vis)	chronic disease characterized by muscle weakness and thought to be caused by a defect in the transmission of impulses from nerve to muscle cell. The face, larynx, and throat are frequently affected; no true paralysis of the muscles exists.
osteoporosis (*os*-tē-ō-po-RŌ-sis)	abnormal loss of bone density occurring predominantly in postmenopausal women, which can lead to an increase in fractures of the ribs, thoracic and lumbar vertebrae, hips, and wrists (Figure 14-15)
rheumatoid arthritis (RA) (RŪ-ma-toid) (ar-THRĪ-tis)	a chronic systemic disease characterized by autoimmune inflammatory changes in the connective tissue throughout the body (see Figure 14-8)
spinal stenosis (SPĪ-nal) (ste-NŌ-sis)	narrowing of the spinal canal with compression of nerve roots. The condition is either congenital or due to spinal degeneration. Symptoms are pain radiating to the thigh or lower legs and numbness or tingling in the lower extremities (Figure 14-16).
spondylolisthesis (*spon*-di-lō-lis-THĒ-sis)	forward slipping of one vertebra over another (Figure 14-16)

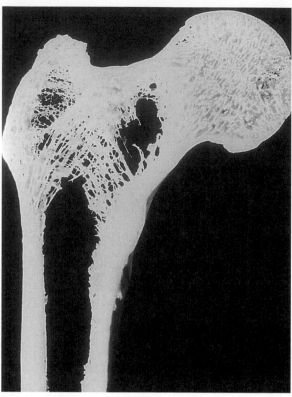

Figure 14-15
This thin section of the femur shows the loss of bone seen in patients with osteoporosis. Fractures can occur from normal trauma because the bone is porous and brittle.

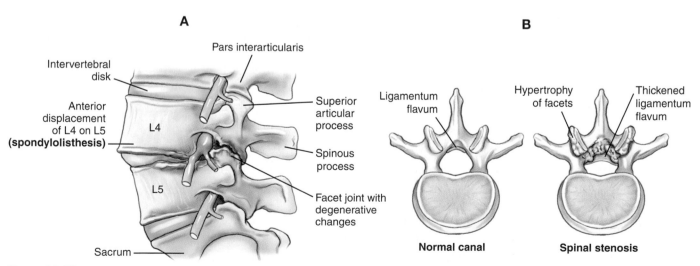

Figure 14-16
A, Spondylolisthesis showing degenerative changes in the disk and joint. **B,** Spinal stenosis. Spondylolisthesis may occur with or without spinal stenosis.

EXERCISE 22

Practice saying aloud each of the disease and disorder terms not built from word parts on pp. 636-639.

 To hear the terms select Chapter 14, Chapter Exercises, Pronunciation.

☐ Place a check mark in the box when you have completed this exercise.

EXERCISE 23

Write the term for each of the following definitions.

1. abnormal benign growth
   on the surface of a bone   _____

2. group of hereditary diseases
   characterized by degeneration
   of muscle and weakness   _____ _____

3. chronic disease characterized
   by muscle weakness and
   thought to be caused by a
   defect in the transmission
   of impulses from nerve to
   muscle cell   _____ _____

4. abnormal enlargement
   of the joint at the base
   of the great toe   _____

5. form of arthritis that first
   affects the spine and adjacent
   structures   _____ _____

6. disease in which an excessive
   amount of uric acid in the
   blood causes sodium urate
   crystals (tophi) to be
   deposited in the joints   _____

7. rupture of the intervertebral
   disk cartilage, which allows
   the contents to protrude
   through it, putting pressure
   on the spinal nerve roots   a. _____ _____

         b. _____ _____

         c. _____ _____

         d. _____ _____ _____

         e. _____ _____ _____

8. broken bone _____

9. abnormal loss of bone density _____

10. a disorder of the wrist caused
    by compression of the
    median nerve   _____ _____ _____

11. a type of fractured wrist   _____ _____

12. form of arthritis characterized
    by inflammatory changes in
    the connective tissue
    throughout the body   _____ _____

13. forward slipping of one
    vertebra over another   _____

14. an infection transmitted
    to humans by a deer tick   _____ _____

15. narrowing of the spinal
    column with compression
    of nerve roots   _____ _____

EXERCISE 24

Write the definitions of the following terms.

1. exostosis _____

2. muscular dystrophy _____

3. myasthenia gravis _____

4. bunion _____

5. ankylosing spondylitis _____

6. osteoporosis _____

7. gout _____

8. herniated disk, slipped disk, ruptured disk _____

9. fracture _____

10. carpal tunnel syndrome _____

11. Colles fracture _____

12. rheumatoid arthritis _____

13. Lyme disease _____

14. spondylolisthesis _____

15. spinal stenosis _____

COLLES FRACTURE
was first described in
1814 by Irish surgeon and
anatomist **Abraham Colles**
(1773–1843). In 1804 Colles
was appointed Professor of
Anatomy and Surgery at the
Irish College of Surgeons.

EXERCISE 25

Spell each of the disease and disorder terms not built from word parts on pp. 636-639 by having someone dictate them to you.

 To hear and spell the terms select Chapter 14, Chapter Exercises, Spelling. You may type the terms on the screen or write them below in the spaces provided.

☐ Place a check mark in the box if you have completed this exercise using your CD-ROM.

1. _____   9. _____

2. _____   10. _____

3. _____   11. _____

4. _____   12. _____

5. _____   13. _____

6. _____   14. _____

7. _____   15. _____

8. _____

Surgical Terms

Built from Word Parts

The following terms are built from word parts you have already learned and can be translated literally to find their meanings. Further explanation of terms beyond the definition of their word parts, if needed, is included in parentheses.

Term	Definition
aponeurorrhaphy . . . . (*ap*-ō-nū-ROR-a-fē)	suture of an aponeurosis
arthrocentesis. . . . . (*ar*-thrō-sen-TĒ-sis)	surgical puncture of a joint to aspirate fluid
arthroclasia. . . . . (*ar*-thrō-KLĀ-zha)	(surgical) breaking of a (stiff) joint
arthrodesis . . . . (*ar*-thrō-DĒ-sis)	surgical fixation of a joint (also called joint fusion)
arthroplasty . . . . (AR-thrō-*plas*-tē)	surgical repair of a joint (Table 14-1)
bursectomy. . . . . (bur-SEK-to-mē)	excision of a bursa
carpectomy. . . . . (kar-PEK-to-mē)	excision of a carpal bone
chondrectomy. . . . . (kon-DREK-to-mē)	excision of a cartilage

TABLE 14-1
Types of Arthroplasty

Total hip replacement arthroplasty (THA) is indicated for degenerative joint disease or rheumatoid arthritis. The operation commonly involves replacement of the hip joint with a metallic femoral head and a plastic-coated acetabulum.

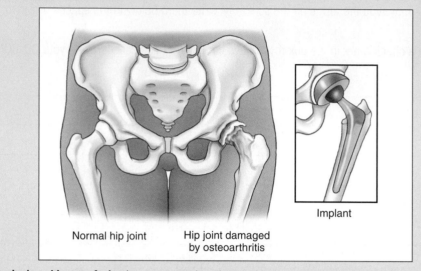

Normal hip joint   Hip joint damaged by osteoarthritis   Implant

Birmingham hip resurfacing is a new procedure that provides an option for younger, active patients needing a total hip arthroplasty. The procedure, recently approved by the Food and Drug Administration, requires the removal of a few millimeters of bone from the femoral head instead of the removal of the entire femoral head required in total hip arthroplasty. A metal cap is then placed on top of the femur, and smooth metal is placed in the acetabulum.

Total knee joint replacement arthroplasty is designed to replace worn surfaces of the knee joint. Various prostheses are used.

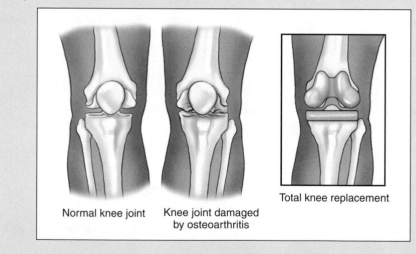

Normal knee joint   Knee joint damaged by osteoarthritis   Total knee replacement

Metatarsal arthroplasty is used to treat deformities associated with rheumatoid arthritis or hallux valgus and to treat painful or unstable joints.

Surgical Terms—*cont'd*
Built from Word Parts

Term	Definition
chondroplasty . . . . (KON-drō-*plas*-tē)	surgical repair of a cartilage
costectomy . . . . (kos-TEK-to-mē)	excision of a rib
cranioplasty . . . . (KRĀ-nē-ō-*plas*-tē)	surgical repair of the skull
craniotomy . . . . (*krā*-nē-OT-o-mē)	incision of the skull (as for surgery of the brain)
diskectomy . . . . (dis-KEK-to-mē)	excision of an intervertebral disk (a portion of the disk is removed to relieve pressure on nerve roots) (also spelled **discectomy**) (see Figure 14-13, *B*)
laminectomy . . . . (*lam*-i-NEK-to-mē)	excision of a lamina (often performed to relieve pressure on the nerve roots in the lower spine caused by a herniated disk and other conditions)
maxillectomy . . . . (*mak*-si-LEK-to-mē)	excision of the maxilla
meniscectomy . . . . (*men*-i-SEK-to-mē)	excision of the meniscus (performed for a torn cartilage)
myorrhaphy . . . . (mī-OR-a-fē)	suture of a muscle
ostectomy . . . . (os-TEK-to-mē) (NOTE: the *e* is dropped from oste.)	excision of bone
osteoclasis . . . . (*os*-tē-OK-la-sis)	(surgical) breaking of a bone (to correct a deformity)
patellectomy . . . . (*pat*-e-LEK-to-mē)	excision of the patella
phalangectomy . . . . (fal-an-JEK-to-mē)	excision of a finger or toe bone
rachiotomy . . . . (*rā*-kē-OT-o-mē)	incision into the vertebral column
spondylosyndesis . . . . (*spon*-di-lō-sin-DĒ-sis) (NOTE: the prefix *syn*- appears in the middle of the term.)	fusing together of the vertebrae (spinal fusion)

PERCUTANEOUS DISKECTOMY
is an endoscopic procedure that uses fluoroscopy to guide insertion of a nucleotome into the affected spinal disk and remove the thick, sticky nucleus of the disk. This allows the disk to soften and contract, relieving the severe low back and leg pain.

Surgical Terms—*cont'd*

Built from Word Parts

Term	Definition
synovectomy. . . . . (sin-ō-VEK-to-mē) (NOTE: the *i* in *synovi* is dropped because the suffix begins with a vowel.)	excision of the synovial membrane (of a joint)
tarsectomy . . . . (tar-SEK-to-mē)	excision of (one or more) tarsal bones
tenomyoplasty . . . . (*ten*-ō-MĪ-ō-*plas*-tē)	surgical repair of the tendon and muscle
tenorrhaphy . . . . (ten-NOR-a-fē)	suture of a tendon
vertebroplasty. . . . . (VER-te-brō-*plas*-tē)	surgical repair of the vertebra (Table 14-2)

TABLE 14-2

Procedures for Treatment of Compression Fractures Caused by Osteoporosis

Percutaneous vertebroplasty (PV) is a minimally invasive operation in which an interventional radiologist places a needle through the skin into the damaged vertebra. A special liquid cement called polymethylmethacrylate is injected into the area through the needle to fill the holes left by osteoporosis. The liquid takes 20 minutes to harden, sealing and stabilizing the fracture and relieving pain. Vertebroplasties were first performed in 1984 and are currently being performed in select health care centers in the United States.

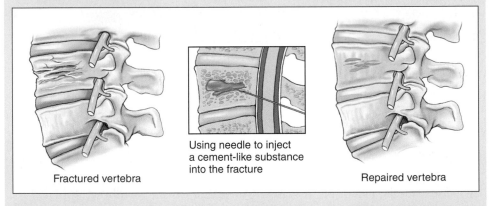

Fractured vertebra

Using needle to inject a cement-like substance into the fracture

Repaired vertebra

Kyphoplasty was approved in 1998 by the Food and Drug Administration. Kyphoplasty is similar to vertebroplasty except a balloonlike device is used to expand the compressed vertebra before the cement is injected.

EXERCISE **26**

Practice saying aloud each of the surgical terms built from word parts on pp. 643-646.

To hear the terms select Chapter 14, Chapter Exercises, Pronunciation.

☐ Place a check mark in the box when you have completed this exercise.

EXERCISE **27**

Analyze and define the following surgical terms.

1. osteoclasis _____

2. ostectomy _____

3. arthroclasia _____

4. arthrodesis_____

5. arthroplasty_____

6. chondrectomy_____

7. chondroplasty _____

8. myorrhaphy _____

9. tenomyoplasty_____

10. tenorrhaphy _____

11. costectomy _____

12. patellectomy _____

13. aponeurorrhaphy _____

14. carpectomy _____

15. phalangectomy _____

16. meniscectomy_____

17. spondylosyndesis _____

18. laminectomy_____

19. bursectomy _____

20. craniotomy _____

21. cranioplasty_____

22. maxillectomy _____

23. rachiotomy _____

24. tarsectomy _____

25. synovectomy _____

26. diskectomy _____

27. vertebroplasty _____

28. arthrocentesis _____

EXERCISE 28

Build surgical terms for the following definitions by using the word parts you have learned.

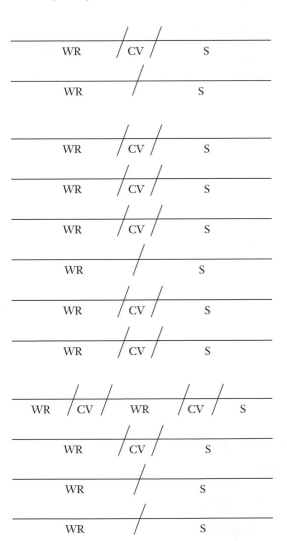

1. (surgical) breaking of a bone
   (to correct a deformity)

   _____ / _____ / _____
   WR   CV   S

2. excision of bone

   _____ / _____
   WR   S

3. (surgical) breaking of a
   (stiff) joint

   _____ / _____ / _____
   WR   CV   S

4. surgical fixation of a joint

   _____ / _____ / _____
   WR   CV   S

5. surgical repair of a joint

   _____ / _____ / _____
   WR   CV   S

6. excision of cartilage

   _____ / _____
   WR   S

7. surgical repair of cartilage

   _____ / _____ / _____
   WR   CV   S

8. suture of a muscle

   _____ / _____ / _____
   WR   CV   S

9. surgical repair of a tendon
   and muscle

   _____ / _____ / _____ / _____ / _____
   WR   CV   WR   CV   S

10. suture of a tendon

    _____ / _____ / _____
    WR   CV   S

11. excision of a rib

    _____ / _____
    WR   S

12. excision of the patella

    _____ / _____
    WR   S

13. suture of an aponeurosis

_____ / _____ / _____
WR   CV   S

14. excision of a carpal bone

_____ / _____
WR   S

15. excision of a finger or toe bone

_____ / _____
WR   S

16. excision of a meniscus

_____ / _____
WR   S

17. fusing together of the vertebrae

_____ / _____ / _____ / _____
WR   CV   P   S

18. excision of a lamina

_____ / _____
WR   S

19. excision of a bursa

_____ / _____
WR   S

20. incision of the skull

_____ / _____ / _____
WR   CV   S

21. surgical repair of the skull

_____ / _____ / _____
WR   CV   S

22. excision of the maxilla

_____ / _____
WR   S

23. incision of the vertebral column

_____ / _____ / _____
WR   CV   S

24. excision of (one or more) tarsal bones

_____ / _____
WR   S

25. excision of the synovial membrane

_____ / _____
WR   S

26. excision of an intervertebral disk

_____ / _____
WR   S

27. surgical repair of the vertebra

_____ / _____ / _____
WR   CV   S

28. surgical puncture of a joint to aspirate fluid

_____ / _____ / _____
WR   CV   S

EXERCISE 29

Spell each of the surgical terms built from word parts on pp. 643-646 by having someone dictate them to you.

 To hear and spell the terms select Chapter 14, Chapter Exercises, Spelling. You may type the terms on the screen or write them below in the spaces provided.

☐ Place a check mark in the box if you have completed this exercise using your CD-ROM.

1._____   15._____

2._____   16._____

3._____   17._____

4._____   18._____

5._____   19._____

6._____   20._____

7._____   21._____

8._____   22._____

9._____   23._____

10._____   24._____

11._____   25._____

12._____   26._____

13._____   27._____

14._____   28._____

Diagnostic Terms

Built from Word Parts

The following terms are built from word parts you have already learned and can be translated literally to find their meanings. Further explanation of terms beyond the definition of their word parts, if needed, is included in parentheses.

Term	Definition
DIAGNOSTIC IMAGING	
arthrography............. (ar-THROG-ra-fē)	radiographic imaging of a joint (with contrast media). (Magnetic resonance imaging [MRI] has mostly replaced arthrography as the imaging technique for diarthrodial [movable] joints such as the knee, wrist, hip, and shoulder. Arthrography is still used for specialized functions such as when metal is present in the body.)

Term	Definition
ENDOSCOPY	
arthroscopy................ (ar-THROS-ko-pē)	visual examination of a joint (used for a diarthrodial [movable] joint) (Exercise Figure E)
OTHER	
electromyogram (EMG)........ (ē-*lek*-trō-MĪ-ō-gram)	record of the (intrinsic) electrical activity in a (skeletal) muscle (Figure 14-17)

Practice saying aloud each of the diagnostic terms built from word parts on pp. 650-651.

EXERCISE 30

To hear the terms select Chapter 14, Chapter Exercises, Pronunciation.

☐ Place a check mark in the box when you have completed this exercise.

EXERCISE 31

Analyze and define the following diagnostic terms.

1. electromyogram _____

2. arthrography _____

3. arthroscopy _____

EXERCISE 32

Build diagnostic terms for the following definitions using word parts you have learned.

1. radiographic imaging
   of a joint _____ / _____ / _____
   WR   CV   S

2. visual examination of a joint _____ / _____ / _____
   WR   CV   S

3. record of the electrical
   activity of a muscle _____ / _____ / _____ / _____ / _____
   WR / CV / WR / CV / S

Fill in the blanks to complete labeling of the diagram.

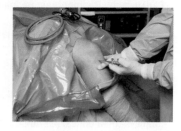

_____ / _____ / _____
joint / cv / visual
examination

of the knee performed for diagnostic purposes or for surgical repair of ligaments or meniscus.

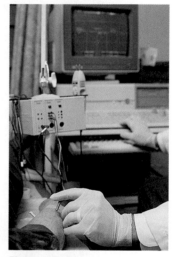

Figure 14-17
Patient having an electromyogram (EMG) of the forearm.

TABLE 14-3

Diagnostic Imaging Procedures Used for the Musculoskeletal System

The following diagnostic imaging procedures are commonly used for diagnosing diseases, fractures, strains, and other conditions of the musculoskeletal system.

Radiography (radiographic imaging) of the bones and joints is used to identify fractures or tumors, monitor healing, or identify abnormal structures (see Figure 14-18).

Computed tomography (CT) of the bones and joints gives accurate definition of bone structure and demonstrates subtle changes such as linear fractures (Figure 14-19).

Magnetic resonance imaging (MRI) is used to evaluate the ligaments of the knee, spinal stenosis, spinal cord defects, and degenerative disk changes (Figure 14-20).

Bone scan (nuclear medicine test) is used to detect the presence of metastatic disease of the bone and to monitor degenerative bone disease (Figure 14-21).

Single-photon emission computed tomography (SPECT) of the bone is an even more sensitive nuclear method for detecting bone abnormalities.

Bone densitometry is a method of determining the density of bone by radiographic techniques used to diagnose osteoporosis. **DEXA (dual-energy X-ray absorptiometry)** is commonly used for this test.

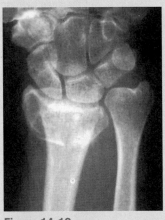

Figure 14-18
Radiograph showing a Colles fracture.

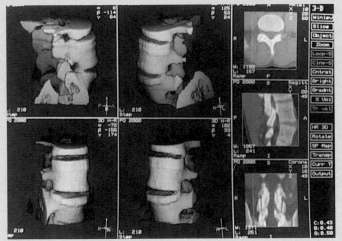

Figure 14-19
CT scan showing three-dimensional reconstruction images of the lumbar spine.

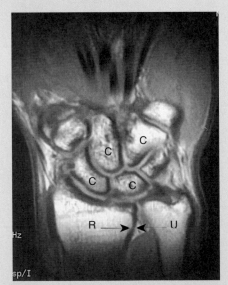

Figure 14-20
Coronal MRI of the wrist. Marrow within the carpal bones *(C)*, radius *(R)*, and ulna *(U)*.

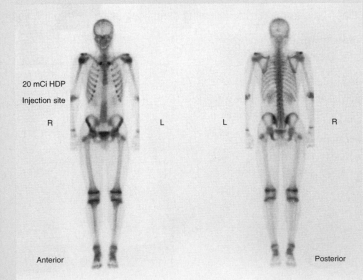

Figure 14-21
Whole-body nuclear medicine bone scan.

EXERCISE 33

Spell each of the diagnostic terms built from word parts on pp. 650-651 by having someone dictate them to you.

 To hear and spell the terms select Chapter 14, Chapter Exercises, Spelling. You may type the terms on the screen or write them below in the spaces provided.

☐ Place a check mark in the box if you have completed this exercise using your CD-ROM.

1. _____   3. _____

2. _____

Complementary Terms

Built from Word Parts

The following terms are built from word parts you have already learned and can be translated literally to find their meanings. Further explanation of terms beyond the definition of their word parts, if needed, is included in parentheses.

Term	Definition
athralgia .... (ar-THRAL-ja)	pain in the joint
atrophy .... (AT-ro-fē)	without development (wasting)
bradykinesia .... (brad-ē-ki-NĒ-zha)	slow movement
carpal .... (CAR-pal)	pertaining to the wrist
cranial .... (KRĀ-nē-al)	pertaining to the cranium
dyskinesia .... (*dis*-ki-NĒ-zha)	difficult movement
dystrophy .... (DIS-tro-fē)	abnormal development
femoral .... (FEM-or-al)	pertaining to the femur
humeral .... (HŪ-mer-al)	pertaining to the humerus
hyperkinesia .... (*hī*-per-ki-NĒ-zha)	excessive movement (overactive)
hypertrophy .... (hī-PER-tro-fē)	excessive development
iliofemoral .... (*il*-ē-ō-FEM-or-al)	pertaining to the ilium and femur

Complementary Terms—cont'd

Built from Word Parts

Term	Definition
intercostal................. (in-ter-KOS-tal)	pertaining to between the ribs
intervertebral .... (*in*-ter-VER-te-bral)	pertaining to between the vertebrae
intracranial................. (*in*-tra-KRĀ-nē-al)	pertaining to within the cranium
ischiofibular .... (*is*-kē-ō-FIB-ū-lar)	pertaining to the ischium and fibula
ischiopubic................. (*is*-kē-ō-PŪ-bik)	pertaining to the ischium and pubis
lumbar .... (LUM-bar)	pertaining to the loins (the part of the back between the thorax and pelvis)
lumbocostal .... (lum-bō-KOS-tal)	pertaining to the loins and the ribs
lumbosacral .... (lum-bō-SĀ-kral)	pertaining to the lumbar regions (loin) and the sacrum
osteoblast................. (OS-tē-ō-blast)	developing bone (cell)
osteocyte .... (OS-tē-ō-sīt)	bone cell
osteonecrosis.............. (*os*-tē-ō-ne-KRŌ-sis)	abnormal death of bone (tissues)
pelvic .... (PEL-vik)	pertaining to the pelvis
pelvisacral .... (pel-vi-SĀ-kral)	pertaining to the pelvis and the sacrum
pubic..................... (PŪ-bik)	pertaining to the pubis
pubofemoral .... (*pū*-bō-FEM-or-al)	pertaining to the pubis and femur
sacral .... (SĀ-kral)	pertaining to the sacrum
sternoclavicular .... (*ster*-nō-kla-VIK-ū-lar)	pertaining to the sternum and clavicle
sternoid .... (STER-noyd)	resembling the sternum
subcostal .... (sub-KOS-tal)	pertaining to below the rib
submandibular .... (*sub*-man-DIB-ū-lar)	pertaining to below the mandible

Term	Definition
submaxillary (sub-MAK-si-*lar*-ē)	pertaining to below the maxilla
subscapular (sub-SKAP-ū-lar)	pertaining to below the scapula
substernal (sub-STER-nal)	pertaining to below the sternum
suprapatellar (sū-pra-pa-TEL-ar)	pertaining to above the patella
suprascapular (*sū*-pra-SKAP-ū-lar)	pertaining to above the scapula
symphysis (SIM-fi-sis)	growing together (as in symphysis pubis)
vertebrocostal (*ver*-te-brō-KOS-tal)	pertaining to the vertebrae and ribs

EXERCISE 34

Practice saying aloud each of the complementary terms built from word parts on pp. 653-655.

 To hear the terms select Chapter 14, Chapter Exercises, Pronunciation.

☐ Place a check mark in the box when you have completed this exercise.

EXERCISE 35

Analyze and define the following complementary terms.

1. symphysis _____

2. femoral _____

3. humeral _____

4. intervertebral _____

5. hyperkinesia _____

6. dyskinesia _____

7. bradykinesia _____

8. intracranial _____

9. sternoclavicular _____

10. iliofemoral _____

11. ischiofibular _____

12. submaxillary _____

13. ischiopubic _____

14. submandibular _____

15. pubofemoral _____

16. suprascapular _____

17. subcostal _____

18. vertebrocostal _____

19. subscapular _____

20. osteoblast _____

21. osteocyte _____

22. osteonecrosis _____

23. sternoid _____

24. arthralgia _____

25. carpal _____

26. lumbar _____

27. lumbocostal _____

28. lumbosacral _____

29. sacral _____

30. pubic _____

31. substernal _____

32. suprapatellar _____

33. dystrophy _____

34. atrophy _____

35. hypertrophy _____

36. intercostal _____

37. cranial _____

38. pelvic _____

39. pelvisacral _____

EXERCISE 36

Build the complementary terms for the following definitions by using the word parts you have learned.

1. growing together

  _____ / _____
         P   S(WR)

2. pertaining to the femur

  _____ / _____
         WR   S

3. pertaining to the humerus

  _____ / _____
         WR   S

4. pertaining to between the vertebrae

  _____ / _____ / _____
         P   WR   S

5. excessive movement (overactivity)

  _____ / _____ / _____
         P   WR   S

6. difficult movement

  _____ / _____ / _____
         P   WR   S

7. slow movement

  _____ / _____ / _____
         P   WR   S

8. pertaining to within the cranium

  _____ / _____ / _____
         P   WR   S

9. pertaining to the sternum and clavicle

  _____ / _____ / _____ / _____
       WR   CV   WR   S

10. pertaining to the ilium and femur

  _____ / _____ / _____ / _____
       WR   CV   WR   S

11. pertaining to the ischium and fibula

  _____ / _____ / _____ / _____
       WR   CV   WR   S

12. pertaining to below the maxilla

  _____ / _____ / _____
         P   WR   S

13. pertaining to the ischium and pubis

  _____ / _____ / _____ / _____
       WR   CV   WR   S

14. pertaining to below the mandible

  _____ / _____ / _____
         P   WR   S

15. pertaining to the pubis and femur

  _____ / _____ / _____ / _____
       WR   CV   WR   S

16. pertaining to above the scapula _____ / _____ / _____
                                            P   WR   S

17. pertaining to below the rib

    ___P___ / ___WR___ / ___S___

18. pertaining to the vertebrae and ribs

    ___WR___ / CV / ___WR___ / ___S___

19. pertaining to below the scapula

    ___P___ / ___WR___ / ___S___

20. developing bone (cell)

    ___WR___ / CV / ___WR___

21. bone cell

    ___WR___ / CV / ___S___

22. abnormal death of bone (tissues)

    ___WR___ / CV / ___WR___ / ___S___

23. resembling the sternum

    ___WR___ / ___S___

24. pain in the joint

    ___WR___ / ___S___

25. pertaining to the wrist

    ___WR___ / ___S___

26. pertaining to the sacrum

    ___WR___ / ___S___

27. pertaining to the loins

    ___WR___ / ___S___

28. pertaining to the pubis

    ___WR___ / ___S___

29. pertaining to the lumbar region (loin) and the sacrum

    ___WR___ / CV / ___WR___ / ___S___

30. pertaining to the loins and ribs

    ___WR___ / CV / ___WR___ / ___S___

31. pertaining to below the sternum

    ___P___ / ___WR___ / ___S___

32. pertaining to above the patella

    ___P___ / ___WR___ / ___S___

33. abnormal development

    ___P___ / ___S(WR)___

34. without development

    ___P___ / ___S(WR)___

35. excessive development

    ___P___ / ___S(WR)___

36. pertaining to the cranium

    ___WR___ / ___S___

37. pertaining to between the ribs

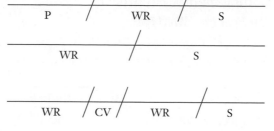

         P   WR   S

38. pertaining to the pelvis

        WR   S

39. pertaining to the pelvis
and sacrum

      WR   CV   WR   S

EXERCISE 37

Spell each of the complementary terms built from word parts on pp. 653-655 by having someone dictate them to you.

 To hear and spell the terms select Chapter 14, Chapter Exercises, Spelling. You may type the terms on the screen or write them below in the spaces provided.

☐ Place a check mark in the box if you have completed this exercise using your CD-ROM.

1. _____
2. _____
3. _____
4. _____
5. _____
6. _____
7. _____
8. _____
9. _____
10. _____
11. _____
12. _____
13. _____
14. _____
15. _____
16. _____
17. _____
18. _____
19. _____
20. _____

21. _____
22. _____
23. _____
24. _____
25. _____
26. _____
27. _____
28. _____
29. _____
30. _____
31. _____
32. _____
33. _____
34. _____
35. _____
36. _____
37. _____
38. _____
39. _____

Complementary Terms
Not Built from Word Parts

In some of the following terms, you may recognize word parts you have already learned; however, the full meaning of the terms cannot be discerned by the definition of their word parts.

Term	Definition
chiropodist, podiatrist......... (ki-ROP-o-dist) (pō-DĪ-a-trist)	specialist in treating and diagnosing diseases and disorders of the foot, including medical and surgical treatment
chiropractic................. (*kī*-rō-PRAK-tik)	system of therapy that consists of manipulation of the vertebral column
chiropractor .... (KĪ-rō-prac-tor)	specialist in chiropractic
crepitus................... (KREP-i-tus)	the crackling sound heard when two bones rub against each other or grating caused by the rubbing together of dry surfaces of a joint. (Crepitus is also used to describe the crackling sound heard with pneumonia or the sound heard from the discharge of gas from the bowel.) (also called **crepitation**)
orthopedics (ortho)........... (*or*-thō-PĒ-diks)	branch of medicine dealing with the study and treatment of diseases and abnormalities of the musculoskeletal system
orthopedist .... (*or*-thō-PĒ-dist)	physician who specializes in orthopedics
orthotics .... (or-THOT-iks)	making and fitting of orthopedic appliances, such as arch supports, used to support, align, prevent, or correct deformities
orthotist .... (or-THOT-ist)	a person who specializes in orthotics
osteopath .... (OS-tē-ō-path)	physician who specializes in osteopathy
osteopathy .... (*os*-tē-OP-a-thē)	system of medicine that uses the usual forms of diagnosis and treatment but places greater emphasis on the role of the relation between body organs and the musculoskeletal system; manipulation may be used in addition to other treatments
prosthesis (*pl.* prostheses)..... (pros-THĒ-sis) (pros-THĒ-sēz)	an artificial substitute for a missing body part such as a leg, eye, or total hip replacement

EXERCISE 38

Practice saying aloud each of the complementary terms not built from word parts on p. 660.

To hear the terms select Chapter 14, Chapter Exercises, Pronunciation.

☐ Place a check mark in the box when you have completed this exercise.

EXERCISE 39

Match the definitions in the first column with the correct terms in the second column.

____	1. specialist in manipulation of the vertebral column	a.	chiropodist
____	2. branch of medicine dealing with treatment of diseases of the musculoskeletal system	b.	chiropractic
		c.	chiropractor
____	3. physician who places emphasis on manipulation	d.	osteopath
		e.	osteopathy
____	4. foot specialist	f.	orthopedics
____	5. substitute for a body part	g.	orthopedist
____	6. system of therapy	h.	podiatrist
____	7. system of medicine	i.	orthotics
____	8. making of orthopedic appliances	j.	prosthesis
____	9. skilled in orthotics	k.	orthotist
____	10. crackling or grating sound	l.	crepitus
____	11. physician who treats diseases and disorders of the musculoskeletal system		

EXERCISE 40

Write the definitions of the following.

1. chiropractor _____

2. chiropractic _____

3. orthopedics _____

4. orthopedist _____

5. chiropodist _____

6. podiatrist _____

7. osteopath _____

8. osteopathy _____

9. orthotics _____

10. prosthesis _____

11. orthotist _____

12. crepitus _____

EXERCISE **41**

Spell each of the complementary terms not built from word parts on p. 660 by having someone dictate them to you.

 To hear and spell the terms select Chapter 14, Chapter Exercises, Spelling. You may type the terms on the screen or write them below in the spaces provided.

☐ Place a check mark in the box if you have completed this exercise using your CD-ROM.

1._____   7._____

2._____   8._____

3._____   9._____

4._____   10._____

5._____   11._____

6._____   12._____

Refer to Appendix E for pharmacology terms related to the musculoskeletal system.

Abbreviations

C1-C7	cervical vertebrae
CTS	carpal tunnel syndrome
EMG	electromyogram
fx.	fracture
HNP.	herniated nucleus pulposus
L1-L5	lumbar vertebrae
MD	muscular dystrophy
MG	myasthenia gravis
OA.	osteoarthritis
ortho.	orthopedics
RA.	rheumatoid arthritis
T1-T12	thoracic vertebrae
THA.	total hip arthroplasty

Refer to Appendix D for a complete list of abbreviations.

EXERCISE 42

Write the meaning of the abbreviations in the following sentences.

1. Vertebrae make up the bones of the spinal column. **C1 to C7** _____ _____ are the first set that form the neck. The second set **T1 to T12** _____ _____ articulate with the 12 pairs of ribs that form the outward curve of the spine. **L1 to L5** _____ _____, the third set, are larger and form the inward curve of the spine.

2. Patients with **RA** _____ _____ often are obese and may experience muscle atrophy, and weakness because of inactivity.

3. Approximately 27% of Americans have **OA** _____; as the population ages this figure is expected to increase.

4. Acquired **MG** _____ _____ most often affects women and the onset occurs at any age. It is an acquired autoimmune disorder.

5. **EMG** _____ is used to evaluate patients with localized or diffuse muscle weakness, such as polymyositis.

6. **CTS** _____ _____ _____ is a common condition in which, for various reasons, the median nerve in the wrist becomes compressed, causing numbness and pain.

7. Nine types of **MD** _____ _____ have been identified. Because symptoms of the disease are similar to other muscular disorders, diagnosis is often difficult.

8. **HNP** _____ _____ _____ may also be referred to as slipped or ruptured disk or herniated intervertebral disk.

9. **THA** _____ _____ _____ is used to treat severe osteoarthritis of the hip joints.

PRACTICAL APPLICATION

EXERCISE 43 *Interact with Medical Documents*

Complete the operative report by writing the medical terms in the blanks. Use the list of definitions with the corresponding numbers.

University Hospital and Medical Center
4700 North Main Street • Wellness, Arizona 54321 • (987) 555-3210

PATIENT NAME: William McBride   **CASE NUMBER:** 10003-MKL
DATE OF BIRTH: 12/04/19XX   **DATE:** 04/30/20XX

OPERATIVE REPORT

HISTORY: William McBride is a 55-year-old African American male who reports pain in his left knee when walking and golfing. He states that his knees have "been painful" for many years since he quit playing semiprofessional hockey, but the pain has become much more severe in the last 6 months. He was admitted to the Medical Center's Outpatient 1. _____ Center for an 2. _____ of his left knee.

PREOPERATIVE DIAGNOSIS: Degenerative 3. _____ of the left knee, with possible tear of the 4. _____ meniscus.

OPERATIVE REPORT: After induction of spinal anesthetic, the patient was positioned on the operating table, and a tourniquet was applied over the upper left thigh. After positioning the leg in a circumferential holder, the end of the table was flexed to allow the leg to hang freely. The patient's left leg was prepped and draped in the usual manner. After exsanguination of the leg with an Esmarch bandage, the tourniquet was inflated to 300 mm Hg. The knee was inspected by anterolateral and anteromedial parapatellar portholes.

FINDINGS: The synovium in the 5. _____ pouch showed moderate to severe inflammatory changes with villi formation and hyperemia. The undersurface of the patella showed loss of normal articular cartilage on the lateral patellar facet with exposed bone in that area and moderate to severe 6. _____ of the medial facet. Similar changes were noted in the intercondylar groove. In the medial compartment, the patient had smooth articular cartilage on the femur and moderate chondromalacia of the tibial plateau. The medial meniscus appeared normal with no evidence of tears and a smooth articular surface on the femoral condyle. No additional 7. _____ being identified.

The tourniquet was then released and the knee flushed with lactated Ringer solution until the bleeding slowed. The wounds were Steri-Stripped closed, a sterile bandage with an external Ace wrap applied, and the patient returned to the postoperative recovery area in stable condition. The patient tolerated the procedure well.

POSTOPERATIVE DIAGNOSIS: Degenerative arthritis with mild chondromalacia of the left knee.

Martin Spencer, DO

MS/mcm

1. branch of medicine dealing with the study and treatment of diseases and abnormalities of the musculoskeletal system
2. visual examination of a joint
3. inflammation of a joint
4. toward the middle or midline
5. pertaining to above the patella
6. softening of the cartilage
7. study of (body changes caused by) disease

B. Read the chart note and answer the questions following it.

011107 TAFT, GRACE   _ □ X

File Patient Navigate Custom Fields Help

| Patient Chart | Lab | Rad | Notes | Documents | Rx | Scheduling | Images | Billing |

Name: **TAFT, GRACE**   MR#: **011107**   Sex: **Female**
DOB: **10/17/19XX**

CLINICAL NOTE

ENCOUNTER DATE: 04/02/20XX

HISTORY: This 67-year-old woman is seen for a follow up visit in Orthopedics. She was seen one week ago in the Emergency Department for treatment of Colles fracture of the right wrist. The patient is postmenopausal with a history of cigarette smoking.

PHYSICAL EXAMINATION: The patient is 5'5" tall and weighs 117 lbs. The examination of the right forearm and hand reveals normal color with minimal swelling. Further skeletal evaluation reveals mild dorsal kyphosis.

DIAGNOSTIC STUDIES: Bone-mineral density measurement shows evidence of osteoporosis.

IMPRESSION: Healing distal radial fracture and osteoporosis.

RECOMMENDATIONS: The patient was advised to continue immobilization of the right forearm for another three weeks. Calcium and vitamin D therapy were recommended. Fosamax was prescribed as treatment for her osteoporosis. A follow-up visit is scheduled in three weeks.

Electronically signed by: Maxwell S. Kline, MD 04/02/20XX 4:30 PM

MSK/kew

| Start | Log On/Off | Print | Edit |

---

1. Physical evaluation of the patient revealed:
   a. an abnormal condition of bending forward
   b. an abnormal condition of stiffness
   c. an abnormal hump of the thoracic spine
   d. an abnormal lateral curve of the spine

2. The patient received a diagnosis of:
   a. softening of the cartilage
   b. abnormal reduction of bone mass
   c. stonelike (marblelike) bones
   d. abnormal loss of bone density

To test your understanding of the terms introduced in this chapter, circle the words that correctly complete the sentences. The italicized words refer to the correct answer.

1. The medical term for *hunchback* is (**kyphosis, ankylosis, scoliosis**).

2. The medical term for *excision of cartilage* is (**carpectomy, chondrectomy, costectomy**).

3. *Difficult movement* is (**hyperkinesia, bradykinesia, dyskinesia**).

4. Vitamin D deficiency in adults may cause *osteomalacia*, or (**muscle weakness, marblelike bones, softening of bones**).

5. The *surgical breaking of a bone* to correct a deformity is called (**osteoclasis, arthroclasia, osteoplasty**).

6. The medical term that means *pertaining to below the rib* is (**subscapular, subcostal, substernal**).

7. The medical term for *growing together* is (**diaphysis, epiphysis, symphysis**).

8. A(n) (**orthopedist, podiatrist, chiropractor**) is *competent to treat* a person with a *fractured femur.*

9. (**Osteoporosis, osteopetrosis, osteomyelitis**) is the *abnormal loss of bone density.*

10. A common *disorder of the wrist caused by compression of the median nerve* is called (**lordosis, carpal tunnel syndrome, synoviosarcoma**).

11. Some patients who are taking statin drugs to lower their cholesterol levels may experience a rather rare side effect, *dissolution of striated muscle*, or (**spondylosis, rhabdomyolysis, spondylolisthesis**).

12. During an examination of the patient's left knee, *a crackling sound* (**osteopenia, exostosis, crepitus**) was noted, during flexion, extension, and range of motion of the joint.

EXERCISE 45   *Read Medical Terms in Use*

Practice the pronunciation of terms by reading the following statements. Use the pronunciation key following the medical terms to assist you in saying the word.

 To hear these terms select Chapter 14, Chapter Exercises, Read Medical Terms in Use.

1. The **orthopedist** (or-thō-PĒ-dist) recommended Mr. Jones have an **arthrodesis** (ar-thrō-DĒ-sis) to reduce pain caused from an ankle **fracture** (FRAK-chur) he sustained several years ago.
2. Mrs. Brown severed a tendon by accidentally walking through a glass patio door. A **tenorrhaphy** (ten-OR-a-fē) was performed to repair the tendon.
3. An **electromyogram** (e-*lek*-trō-MĪ-ō-gram) can assist the physician in diagnosing **muscular dystrophy** (MUS-kū-lar) (DIS-trō-fē). **Atrophy** (AT-rō-fē) frequently occurs in patients with this disease.
4. Adjective forms of medical terms are used by health professionals to indicate areas of the body that describe anatomic locations, areas of pain, sites of injections, locations of lesions, and so forth. Below are some examples.
   a. **cranial** (KRĀ-nē-al) laceration
   b. **intercostal** (in-ter-KOS-tal) muscles
   c. pain in the **subcostal** (sub-KOS-tal) region
   d. herniation of an **intervertebral** (in-ter-VER-te-bral) disk
   e. **intracranial** (in-tra-KRĀ-nē-al) pressure
   f. **femoral** (FEM-or-al) artery
   g. strain of the **ischiopubic** (is-kē-ō-PŪ-bik) area
   h. degenerative disease of the **sternoclavicular** (*ster*-nō-kla-VIK-ū-lar) joint

EXERCISE 46   *Comprehend Medical Terms in Use*

Test your comprehension of terms in the previous statements by circling the correct answer.

1. T F   A specialist in treating and diagnosing disorders of the foot recommended Mr. Jones for surgical fixation of the ankle joint.

2. A record of electrical activity of muscles is used in the diagnosis of:
   a. an abnormal benign growth on the surface of the body
   b. a group of hereditary diseases involving muscular degeneration and weakness
   c. wrist fracture
   d. form of arthritis that causes a forward bend of the spine

WEB LINK
For additional information on arthritis, visit the Arthritis Foundation at www.arthritis.org.

3. Which of the following is true for statements in number 4?
   a. herniation within the vertebra
   b. degenerative disease of the joint between the scapula and collarbone
   c. laceration of the wrist
   d. pain below the ribs

EXERCISE **47** *Use Plural Endings*

Circle the correct singular or plural term to match the context of the sentence.

1. The (**epiphysis, epiphyses**) are the enlarged ends of the long bone.
2. The distal (**phalanx, phalanges**) of the ring finger was fractured.
3. Osteoporosis was present in four lumbar (**vertebrae, vertebra**).
4. A (**prosthesis, prostheses**) was implanted in the left hip.
5. Many synovial joints contain (**bursa, bursae**).

CHAPTER REVIEW

CHAPTER REVIEW ON CD-ROM

Use the CD-ROM that accompanies this textbook to play and practice what you have learned in this chapter. The Chapter Exercises, Practice Activities, Animations, and Games allow you to hear, see, and interact with the chapter content.

Chapter Exercises	**Practice Activities**	**Animations**	**Games**
Exercises in this section of your CD-ROM correlate to exercises in your textbook. You may have completed them as you worked through the chapter.	Practice in study mode, then test your learning in assessment mode. Keep track of your scores from assessment mode if you wish.	☐ Spinal Structure	☐ Name that Word Part
			☐ Term Storm
			☐ Term Explorer
			☐ Termbusters
			☐ Medical Millionaire

Chapter Exercises
Exercises in this section of your CD-ROM correlate to exercises in your textbook. You may have completed them as you worked through the chapter.
☐ Pronunciation
☐ Spelling
☐ Read Medical Terms in Use

Practice Activities
Practice in study mode, then test your learning in assessment mode. Keep track of your scores from assessment mode if you wish.

SCORE
☐ Picture It _____
☐ Define Word Parts _____
☐ Build Medical Terms _____
☐ Word Shop _____
☐ Define Medical Terms _____
☐ Use It _____
☐ Hear It and Type It: _____
   Clinical Vignettes

Animations
☐ Spinal Structure

Games
☐ Name that Word Part
☐ Term Storm
☐ Term Explorer
☐ Termbusters
☐ Medical Millionaire

CHAPTER REVIEW

REVIEW OF WORD PARTS

Can you define and spell the following word parts?

Combining Forms

ankyl/o	disk/o	lumb/o	petr/o	synovi/o
aponeur/o	femor/o	mandibul/o	phalang/o	tars/o
arthr/o	fibul/o	maxill/o	pub/o	ten/o
burs/o	humer/o	menisc/o	rachi/o	tend/o
carp/o	ili/o	my/o	radi/o	tendin/o
chondr/o	ischi/o	myel/o	sacr/o	tibi/o
clavic/o	kinesi/o	myos/o	scapul/o	uln/o
clavicul/o	kyph/o	oste/o	scoli/o	vertebr/o
cost/o	lamin/o	patell/o	spondyl/o	
crani/o	lord/o	pelv/i	stern/o	
		pelv/o		

Prefixes

inter-
supra-
sym-
syn-

Suffixes

-asthenia
-clasia
-clasis
-clast
-desis
-physis
-schisis

REVIEW OF TERMS

Can you build, analyze, define, pronounce, and spell the following terms *built from word parts?*

Diseases and Disorders

ankylosis
arthritis
bursitis
chondromalacia
cranioschisis
diskitis
fibromyalgia
kyphosis
lordosis
maxillitis
meniscitis
myasthenia
myeloma
osteitis
osteoarthritis (OA)
osteochondritis
osteofibroma
osteomalacia
osteomyelitis
osteopenia
osteopetrosis
osteosarcoma
polymyositis
rachischisis
rhabdomyolysis
scoliosis
spondylarthritis
spondylosis
synoviosarcoma
tendinitis
tenosynovitis

Surgical

aponeurorrhaphy
arthrocentesis
arthroclasia
arthrodesis
arthroplasty
bursectomy
carpectomy
chondrectomy
chondroplasty
costectomy
cranioplasty
craniotomy
diskectomy
laminectomy
maxillectomy
meniscectomy
myorrhaphy
ostectomy
osteoclasis
patellectomy
phalangectomy
rachiotomy
spondylosyndesis
synovectomy
tarsectomy
tenomyoplasty
tenorrhaphy
vertebroplasty

Diagnostic

arthrography
arthroscopy
electromyogram
  (EMG)

Complementary

arthralgia
atrophy
bradykinesia
carpal
cranial
dyskinesia
dystrophy
femoral
humeral
hyperkinesia
hypertrophy
iliofemoral
intercostal
intervertebral
intracranial
ischiofibular
ischiopubic
lumbar
lumbocostal
lumbosacral

osteoblast
osteocyte
osteonecrosis
pelvic
pelvisacral
pubic
pubofemoral
sacral
sternoclavicular
sternoid
subcostal
submandibular
submaxillary
subscapular
substernal
suprapatellar
suprascapular
symphysis
vertebrocostal

Can you define, pronounce, and spell the following terms *not built from word parts?*

Types of Body Movements

abduction
adduction
inversion
eversion
extension
flexion
pronation
supination
rotation

Diseases and Disorders

ankylosing spondylitis
bunion
carpal tunnel syndrome (CTS)
Colles fracture
exostosis
fracture (fx)
gout
herniated disk
Lyme disease
muscular dystrophy (MD)
myasthenia gravis (MG)
osteoporosis
rheumatoid arthritis (RA)
spinal stenosis
spondylolisthesis

Complementary

chiropodist
chiropractic
chiropractor
crepitus
orthopedics (ortho)
orthopedist
orthotics
orthotist
osteopath
osteopathy
podiatrist
prosthesis

ANSWERS

Exercise Figures

Exercise Figure

A.
1. mandible: mandibul/o
2. sternum: stern/o
3. phalanges: phalang/o
4. patella: patell/o
5. tarsals: tars/o
6. phalanges: phalang/o
7. cranium: crani/o
8. maxilla: maxill/o
9. clavicle: clavic/o, clavicul/o
10. ribs: cost/o
11. femur: femor/o
12. fibula: fibul/o
13. tibia: tibi/o

Exercise Figure

B.
1. a. vertebral column, spine: rachi/o
2. vertebra: spondyl/o, vertebr/o
3. scapula: scapul/o
4. humerus: humer/o
5. ulna: uln/o
6. radius: radi/o
7. carpals: carp/o
8. ilium: ili/o
9. pubis: pub/o
10. ischium: ischi/o

Exercise Figure

C.
1. synovial membrane: synovi/o
2. joint: arthr/o
3. meniscus: menisc/o
4. tendon: ten/o, tend/o, tendin/o
5. cartilage: chondr/o
6. bursa: burs/o

Exercise Figure

D.
1. kyph/osis
2. scoli/osis
3. lord/osis

Exercise Figure

E. arthr/o/scopy

Exercise 1

1. d
2. i
3. h
4. k
5. j
6. g
7. b
8. c
9. f
10. a

Exercise 2

1. scapula
2. sternum
3. mandible
4. clavicle
5. humerus
6. a. ulna
   b. radius
7. tarsals
8. phalanges
9. metatarsals
10. metacarpals
11. femur
12. a. fibula
    b. tibia
13. patella
14. cervical vertebrae
15. lumbar
16. pubis
17. sacrum
18. ischium
19. coccyx
20. ilium
21. carpals

Exercise 3

1. m
2. c
3. e
4. a
5. l
6. d
7. h
8. i
9. k
10. b
11. f
12. g

Exercise 4

1. movement of drawing away from the middle
2. movement that turns the palm down
3. movement that turns the palm up
4. turning around its own axis
5. movement in which a limb is placed in a straight position
6. turning outward
7. movement of drawing toward the middle
8. movement in which a limb is bent
9. turning inward

Exercise 5

1. h
2. d
3. i
4. j
5. c
6. a
7. g
8. f
9. b

Exercise 6

1. clavicle
2. rib
3. cranium (skull)
4. femur
5. clavicle
6. humerus
7. ilium
8. ischium
9. carpals
10. fibula
11. mandible
12. loin, lumbar region
13. pelvis, pelvic bone

Exercise 7

1. a. clavicul/o
   b. clavic/o
2. cost/o
3. crani/o
4. femor/o
5. humer/o
6. carp/o
7. ischi/o
8. fibul/o
9. ili/o
10. mandibul/o
11. lumb/o
12. a. pelv/i
    b. pelv/o

Exercise 8

1. vertebral column, spine
2. patella
3. vertebra
4. maxilla
5. phalanges
6. ulna
7. radius
8. tibia
9. pubis
10. tarsals
11. scapula
12. sternum
13. vertebra
14. sacrum

Exercise 9

1. maxill/o
2. uln/o
3. radi/o
4. tibi/o
5. pub/o
6. tars/o
7. a. vertebr/o
   b. spondyl/o
8. stern/o
9. scapul/o
10. patell/o
11. phalang/o
12. sacr/o
13. rachi/o

Exercise 10

1. joint
2. aponeurosis
3. meniscus
4. tendon
5. cartilage
6. tendon
7. bursa
8. tendon
9. synovia, synovial membrane
10. intervertebral disk

Exercise 11

1. menisc/o
2. aponeur/o
3. arthr/o
4. chondr/o
5. a. tendin/o
   b. ten/o
   c. tend/o
6. burs/o
7. synovi/o
8. disk/o

Exercise 12
1. muscle
2. stone
3. movement, motion
4. bone
5. lamina
6. bone marrow
7. hump
8. crooked, stiff, bent
9. crooked, curved
10. muscle
11. bent forward

Exercise 13
1. a. my/o
   b. myos/o
2. petr/o
3. kinesi/o
4. oste/o
5. lamin/o
6. myel/o
7. kyph/o
8. ankyl/o
9. scoli/o
10. lord/o

Exercise 14
1. above
2. together, joined
3. between

Exercise 15
1. a. syn-
   b. sym-
2. inter-
3. supra-

Exercise 16
1. growth
2. break
3. surgical fixation, fusion
4. break
5. split, fissure
6. break
7. weakness

Exercise 17
1. -physis
2. -asthenia
3. a. -clasis
   b. -clast
   c. -clasia
4. -desis
5. -schisis

Exercise 18
Pronunciation Exercise

Exercise 19
1. WR S
   oste/itis
   inflammation of the bone
2. WR CV WR S
   oste/o/myel/itis
        CF
   inflammation of the bone and bone marrow
3. WR CV WR S
   oste/o/petr/osis
        CF
   abnormal condition of stonelike bones (marblelike bones)
4. WR CV S
   oste/o/malacia
        CF
   softening of bones

5. WR CV WR S
   oste/o/chondr/itis
        CF
   inflammation of the bone and cartilage
6. WR CV WR S
   oste/o/fibr/oma
        CF
   tumor of the bone and fibrous tissue
7. WR S
   arthr/itis
   inflammation of a joint
8. WR CVWRCV S
   rhabd/o/my/o/lysis
        CF   CF
   dissolution of striated muscle
9. WR S
   myel/oma
   tumor of the bone marrow
10. WR S
   tendin/itis
   inflammation of a tendon
11. WR CV S
   oste/o/penia
        CF
   abnormal reduction of bone (mass)
12. WR S
   spondyl/osis
   abnormal condition of the vertebra
13. WR S
   burs/itis
   inflammation of the bursa
14. WR WR S
   spondyl/arthr/itis
   inflammation of the vertebral joints
15. WR S
   ankyl/osis
   abnormal condition of stiffness
16. WR S
   kyph/osis
   abnormal condition of a hump (of the thoracic spine)
17. WR S
   scoli/osis
   abnormal (lateral) curve (of the spine)
18. WR CV S
   crani/o/schisis
        CF
   fissure of the skull
19. WR S
   maxill/itis
   inflammation of the maxilla
20. WR S
   menisc/itis
   inflammation of the meniscus
21. WR S
   rachi/schisis
   fissure of the vertebral column

22. WR S
   my/asthenia
   muscle weakness
23. WR CV S
   oste/o/sarcoma
        CF
   malignant tumor of the bone
24. WR CV S
   chondr/o/malacia
        CF
   softening of cartilage
25. WR CV S
   synovi/o/sarcoma
        CF
   malignant tumor of the synovial membrane
26. WR CV WR S
   ten/o/synov/itis
        CF
   inflammation of the tendon and synovial membrane
27. P WR S
   poly/myos/itis
   inflammation of many muscles
28. WR S
   disk/itis
   inflammation of an intervertebral disk
29. WR S
   lord/osis
   abnormal condition of bending forward
30. WR CV WR S
   oste/o/arthr/itis
        CF
   inflammation of bone and joint
31. WR CV WR S
   fibr/o/my/algia
        CF
   pain in the fibrous tissues and muscles

Exercise 20
1. oste/o/chondr/itis
2. oste/o/fibr/oma
3. arthr/itis
4. rhabd/o/my/o/lysis
5. myel/oma
6. tendin/itis
7. spondyl/osis
8. oste/o/penia
9. burs/itis
10. spondyl/arthr/itis
11. ankyl/osis
12. kyph/osis
13. scoli/osis
14. crani/o/schisis
15. maxill/itis
16. menisc/itis

17. rachi/schisis
18. my/asthenia
19. oste/itis
20. oste/o/myel/itis
21. oste/o/petr/osis
22. oste/o/malacia
23. ten/o/synov/itis
24. synovi/o/sarcoma
25. oste/o/sarcoma
26. chondr/o/malacia
27. disk/itis
28. poly/myos/itis
29. lord/osis
30. oste/o/arthr/itis
31. fibr/o/my/algia

Exercise 21
Spelling Exercise; see text p. 636.

Exercise 22
Pronunciation Exercise

Exercise 23
1. exostosis
2. muscular dystrophy
3. myasthenia gravis
4. bunion
5. ankylosing spondylitis
6. gout
7. a. herniated disk
   b. slipped disk
   c. ruptured disk
   d. herniated nucleus pulposus
   e. herniated intervertebral disk
8. fracture
9. osteoporosis
10. carpal tunnel syndrome
11. Colles fracture
12. rheumatoid arthritis
13. spondylolisthesis
14. Lyme disease
15. spinal stenosis

Exercise 24
1. abnormal benign growth on the surface of a bone
2. group of hereditary diseases characterized by degeneration of muscle and weakness
3. chronic disease characterized by muscle weakness and thought to be caused by a defect in the transmission of impulses from nerve to muscle cell
4. abnormal enlargement of the joint at the base of the great toe
5. form of arthritis that first affects the spine and adjacent structures
6. abnormal loss of bone density

7. disease in which an excessive amount of uric acid in the blood causes sodium urate crystals (tophi) to be deposited in the joints
8. rupture of the intervertebral disk cartilage, which allows the contents to protrude through it, putting pressure on the spinal nerve roots
9. broken bone
10. a disorder of the wrist caused by compression of the median nerve
11. a type of fractured wrist
12. a chronic systemic disease characterized by inflammatory changes in the connective tissue throughout the body
13. an infection transmitted to humans by deer ticks
14. forward slipping of one vertebra over another
15. narrowing of the spinal column with compression of nerve roots

Exercise 25
Spelling Exercise; see text p. 643.

Exercise 26
Pronunciation Exercise

Exercise 27
1. WR CV S
   oste/o/clasis
        CF
   (surgical) breaking of a bone
2. WR   S
   ost/ectomy
   excision of bone
3. WR CV S
   arthr/o/clasia
        CF
   (surgical) breaking of a (stiff) joint
4. WR CV S
   arthr/o/desis
        CF
   surgical fixation of a joint
5. WR CV S
   arthr/o/plasty
        CF
   surgical repair of a joint
6. WR   S
   chondr/ectomy
   excision of a cartilage
7. WR CV S
   chondr/o/plasty
        CF
   surgical repair of a cartilage

8. WR CV   S
   my/o/rrhaphy
        CF
   suture of a muscle
9. WR CV WR CV S
   ten/o/my/o/plasty
        CF   CF
   surgical repair of the tendon and muscle
10. WR CV   S
    ten/o/rrhaphy
         CF
    suture of a tendon
11. WR   S
    cost/ectomy
    excision of a rib
12. WR   S
    patell/ectomy
    excision of the patella
13. WR CV S
    aponeur/o/rrhaphy
         CF
    suture of an aponeurosis
14. WR   S
    carp/ectomy
    excision of a carpal bone
15. WR   S
    phalang/ectomy
    excision of a finger or toe bone
16. WR   S
    menisc/ectomy
    excision of the meniscus
17. WR CV P   S
    spondyl/o/syn/desis
         CF
    fusing together of the vertebrae
18. WR   S
    lamin/ectomy
    excision of the lamina
19. WR   S
    burs/ectomy
    excision of a bursa
20. WR CV S
    crani/o/tomy
         CF
    incision into the skull
21. WR CV S
    crani/o/plasty
         CF
    surgical repair of the skull
22. WR   S
    maxill/ectomy
    excision of the maxilla
23. WR CV S
    rachi/o/tomy
         CF
    incision into the vertebral column

24. WR   S
    tars/ectomy
    excision of (one or more) tarsal bones
25. WR   S
    synov/ectomy
    excision of the synovial membrane
26. WR   S
    disk/ectomy
    excision of an intervertebral disk
27. WR CV S
    vertebr/o/plasty
        CF
    surgical repair of a vertebra
28. WR CV S
    arthr/o/centesis
         CF
    surgical puncture of a joint to
        aspirate fluid

Exercise 28
1. oste/o/clasis
2. ost/ectomy
3. arthr/o/clasia
4. arthr/o/desis
5. arthr/o/plasty
6. chondr/ectomy
7. chondr/o/plasty
8. my/o/rrhaphy
9. ten/o/my/o/plasty
10. ten/o/rrhaphy
11. cost/ectomy
12. patell/ectomy
13. aponeur/o/rrhaphy
14. carp/ectomy
15. phalang/ectomy
16. menisc/ectomy
17. spondyl/o/syn/desis
18. lamin/ectomy
19. burs/ectomy
20. crani/o/tomy
21. crani/o/plasty
22. maxill/ectomy
23. rachi/o/tomy
24. tars/ectomy
25. synov/ectomy
26. disk/ectomy
27. vertebr/o/plasty
28. arthr/o/centesis

Exercise 29
Spelling Exercise; see text p. 650.

Exercise 30
Pronunciation Exercise

Exercise 31
1. WR CV WRCV S
   electr/o/my/o/gram
        CF   CF
   record of the electrical activity in a
       muscle

2. WR CV S
   arthr/o/graphy
        CF
   radiographic imaging of a joint
3. WR CV S
   arthr/o/scopy
        CF
   visual examination of a joint

Exercise 32
1. arthr/o/gram
2. arthr/o/scopy
3. electr/o/my/o/gram

Exercise 33
Spelling Exercise; see text p. 653.

Exercise 34
Pronunciation Exercise

Exercise 35
1. P   S(WR)
   sym/physis
   growing together
2. WR S
   femor/al
   pertaining to the femur
3. WR S
   humer/al
   pertaining to the humerus
4. P   WR   S
   inter/vertebr/al
   pertaining to between the vertebrae
5. P   WR S
   hyper/kinesi/a
   excessive movement (overactivity)
6. P   WR S
   dys/kinesi/a
   difficult movement
7. P   WR S
   brady/kinesi/a
   slow movement
8. P   WR S
   intra/crani/al
   pertaining to within the cranium
9. WR CV WR   S
   stern/o/clavicul/ar
        CF
   pertaining to the sternum and clavicle
10. WRCV WR S
    ili/o/femor/al
        CF
    pertaining to the ilium and femur
11. WR CV WR S
    ischi/o/fibul/ar
         CF
    pertaining to the ischium and fibula

12. P   WR   S
    sub/maxill/ary
    pertaining to below the maxilla
13. WR CV WR S
    ischi/o/pub/ic
         CF
    pertaining to the ischium and pubis
14. P   WR   S
    sub/mandibul/ar
    pertaining to below the mandible
15. WR CV WR S
    pub/o/femor/al
        CF
    pertaining to the pubis and femur
16. P   WR   S
    supra/scapul/ar
    pertaining to above the scapula
17. P   WR S
    sub/cost/al
    pertaining to below the rib
18. WR   CV WR S
    vertebr/o/cost/al
         CF
    pertaining to the vertebrae and ribs
19. P   WR   S
    sub/scapul/ar
    pertaining to below the scapula
20. WR CV WR
    oste/o/blast
        CF
    developing bone (cell)
21. WR CV S
    oste/o/cyte
        CF
    bone cell
22. WR CV WR   S
    oste/o/necr/osis
         CF
    abnormal death of bone (tissues)
23. WR   S
    stern/oid
    resembling the sternum
24. WR   S
    arthr/algia
    pain in the joint
25. WR S
    carp/al
    pertaining to the wrist
26. WR S
    lumb/ar
    pertaining to the loins
27. WR CV WR S
    lumb/o/cost/al
         CF
    pertaining to the loins and to the ribs

28. WR CV WR S
 lumb/o/sacr/al
   CF
 pertaining to the lumbar region (loin)
   and the sacrum
29. WR S
 sacr/al
 pertaining to the sacrum
30. WR S
 pub/ic
 pertaining to the pubis
31. P WR S
 sub/stern/al
 pertaining to below the sternum
32. P WR S
 supra/patell/ar
 pertaining to above the patella
33. P S(WR)
 dys/trophy
 abnormal development
34. P S(WR)
 a/trophy
 without development
35. P S(WR)
 hyper/trophy
 excessive development
36. P WR S
 inter/cost/al
 pertaining to between the ribs
37. WR S
 crani/al
 pertaining to the cranium
38. WR S
 pelv/ic
 pertaining to the pelvis
39. WR CV WR S
 pelv/i/sacr/al
   CF
 pertaining to the pelvis and sacrum

Exercise 36
1. sym/physis
2. femor/al
3. humer/al
4. inter/vertebr/al
5. hyper/kinesi/a
6. dys/kinesi/a
7. brady/kinesi/a
8. intra/crani/al
9. stern/o/clavicul/ar
10. ili/o/femor/al
11. ischi/o/fibul/ar
12. sub/maxill/ary
13. ischi/o/pub/ic
14. sub/mandibul/ar
15. pub/o/femor/al
16. supra/scapul/ar
17. sub/cost/al
18. vertebr/o/cost/al
19. sub/scapul/ar
20. oste/o/blast

21. oste/o/cyte
22. oste/o/necr/osis
23. stern/oid
24. arthr/algia
25. carp/al
26. sacr/al
27. lumb/ar
28. pub/ic
29. lumb/o/sacr/al
30. lumb/o/cost/al
31. sub/stern/al
32. supra/patell/ar
33. dys/trophy
34. a/trophy
35. hyper/trophy
36. crani/al
37. inter/cost/al
38. pelv/ic
39. pelv/i/sacr/al

Exercise 37
Spelling Exercise; see text p. 659.

Exercise 38
Pronunciation Exercise

Exercise 39
1. c
2. f
3. d
4. a, h
5. j
6. b
7. e
8. i
9. k
10. l
11. g

Exercise 40
1. specialist in chiropractic
2. system of therapy that consists of manipulation of the vertebral column
3. branch of medicine dealing with the
 study and treatment of diseases and
 abnormalities of the musculoskeletal
 system
4. physician who specializes in
 orthopedics
5. specialist in treating and diagnosing
 foot diseases and disorders
6. specialist in treating and diagnosing
 diseases and disorders of the foot
7. physician who specializes in osteopathy
8. system of medicine in which emphasis
 is on the relation between body organs
 and the musculoskeletal system
9. making and fitting of orthopedic
 appliances
10. an artificial substitute for a missing
 body part
11. a person who is skilled in orthotics
12. crackling sound heard when two
 bones rub against each other or grat-
 ing caused by rubbing together of dry
 surfaces

Exercise 41
Spelling Exercise; see text p. 662.

Exercise 42
1. cervical vertebrae; thoracic vertebrae;
 lumbar vertebrae
2. rheumatoid arthritis
3. osteoarthritis
4. myasthenia gravis
5. electromyogram
6. carpal tunnel syndrome
7. muscular dystrophy
8. herniated nucleus pulposus
9. total hip replacement

Exercise 43
A. 1. orthopedic
  2. arthroscopy
  3. arthritis
  4. medial
  5. suprapatellar
  6. chondromalacia
  7. pathology

B. 1. c
  2. d

Exercise 44
1. kyphosis
2. chondrectomy
3. dyskinesia
4. softening of bones
5. osteoclasis
6. subcostal
7. symphysis
8. orthopedist
9. osteoporosis
10. carpal tunnel syndrome
11. rhabdomyolysis
12. crepitus

Exercise 45
Reading Exercise

Exercise 46
1. *F*, an orthopedist and not a podiatrist
 is treating Mr. Jones.
2. b
3. d

Exercise 47
1. epiphyses
2. phalanx
3. vertebrae
4. prosthesis
5. bursae

CHAPTER 15

Nervous System and Behavioral Health

OUTLINE

ANATOMY, 678

WORD PARTS, 683
Combining Forms, 683
Suffixes, 687

MEDICAL TERMS, 688
Disease and Disorder Terms, 688
    Built from Word Parts, 688
    Not Built from Word Parts, 693
Surgical Terms, 699
    Built from Word Parts, 699
Diagnostic Terms, 701
    Built from Word Parts, 701
    Not Built from Word Parts, 703
Complementary Terms, 706
    Built from Word Parts, 706
    Not Built from Word Parts, 711
Behavioral Health Terms, 715
    Built from Word Parts, 715
    Not Built from Word Parts, 718
Abbreviations, 721

PRACTICAL APPLICATION, 723
Interact with Medical Documents, 723
Interpret Medical Terms, 725
Read Medical Terms in Use, 726
Comprehend Medical Terms in Use, 726

CHAPTER REVIEW, 727

OBJECTIVES

Upon completion of this chapter you will be able to:

1. Identify organs and structures of the nervous system.

2. Define and spell word parts related to the nervous system.

3. Define, pronounce, and spell disease and disorder terms related to the nervous system.

4. Define, pronounce, and spell surgical terms related to the nervous system.

5. Define, pronounce, and spell diagnostic terms related to the nervous system.

6. Define, pronounce, and spell complementary terms related to the nervous system.

7. Define, pronounce, and spell behavioral health terms.

8. Interpret the meaning of abbreviations related to the nervous system.

9. Interpret, read, and comprehend medical language in simulated medical statements and documents.

ANATOMY

Function

The nervous system and the endocrine system cooperate in regulating and controlling the activities of the other body systems.

The nervous system may be divided into two parts: the *central nervous system* (CNS) and the *peripheral nervous system* (PNS) (Figures 15-1 and 15-2). The central nervous system consists of the brain and spinal cord. The peripheral nervous system is made up of cranial nerves, which carry impulses between the brain and neck and head, and spinal nerves, which carry messages between the spinal cord and abdomen, limbs, and chest.

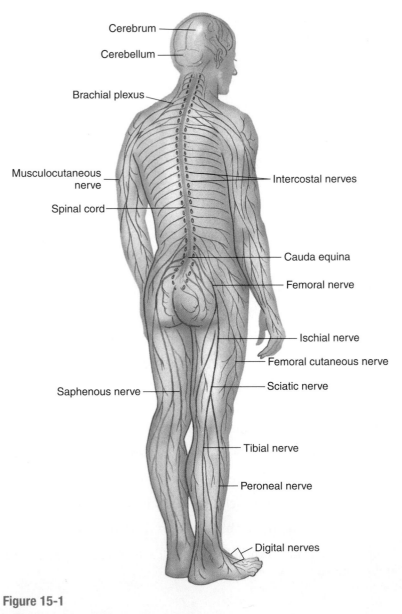

Figure 15-1

Simplified view of the nervous system.

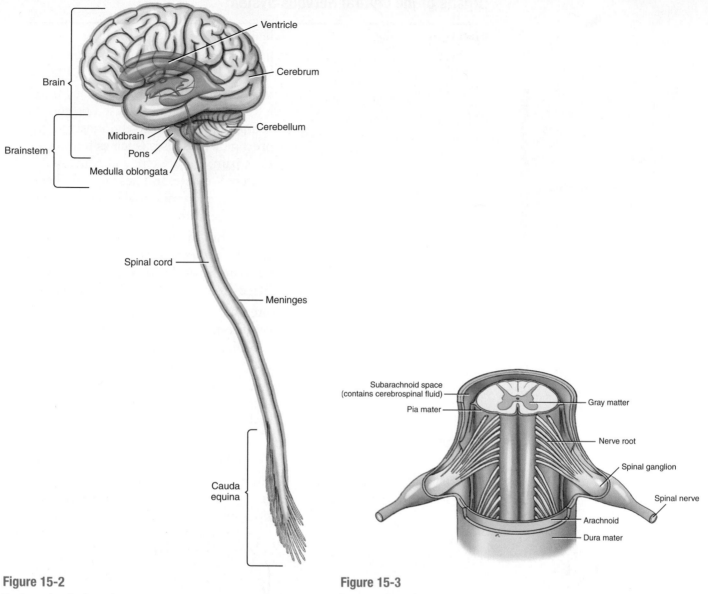

Figure 15-2
Brain and spinal cord.

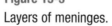

Figure 15-3
Layers of meninges.

Organs of the Central Nervous System

 CEREBELLUM was named in the third century BC by Erasistratus, who also named the cerebrum. *Cerebellum* literally means **little brain** and is the diminutive of **cerebrum**, meaning **brain.** Although it was named long ago, its function was not understood until the nineteenth century.

Term	Definition
brain	major portion of the central nervous system (Figure 15-2)
cerebrum	largest portion of the brain, divided into left and right hemispheres. The cerebrum controls the skeletal muscles, interprets general senses (such as temperature, pain, and touch), and contains centers for sight and hearing. Intellect, memory, and emotional reactions also take place in the cerebrum.
ventricles	spaces within the brain that contain a fluid called *cerebrospinal fluid.* The cerebrospinal fluid flows through the subarachnoid space around the brain and spinal cord.
cerebellum	located under the posterior portion of the cerebrum. Its function is to assist in the coordination of skeletal muscles and to maintain balance (also called **hindbrain**).
brainstem	stemlike portion of the brain that connects with the spinal cord. Ten of the 12 cranial nerves originate in the brainstem.
pons	literally means *bridge.* It connects the cerebrum with the cerebellum and brainstem.
medulla oblongata	located between the pons and spinal cord. It contains centers that control respiration, heart rate, and the muscles in the blood vessel walls, which assist in determining blood pressure.

Term	Definition
midbrain	most superior portion of the brainstem
cerebrospinal fluid (CSF)	clear, colorless fluid contained in the ventricles that flows through the subarachnoid space around the brain and spinal cord. It cushions the brain and spinal cord from shock, transports nutrients, and clears metabolic waste.
spinal cord	passes through the vertebral canal extending from the medulla oblongata to the level of the second lumbar vertebra. The spinal cord conducts nerve impulses to and from the brain and initiates reflex action to sensory information without input from the brain.
meninges	three layers of membrane that cover the brain and spinal cord (Figure 15-3)
dura mater	tough outer layer of the meninges
arachnoid	delicate middle layer of the meninges. The arachnoid membrane is loosely attached to the pia mater by weblike fibers, which allow for the *subarachnoid space*.
pia mater	thin inner layer of the meninges

MENINGES were first named by a Persian physician in the tenth century. When translated into Latin, they became **dura mater,** meaning **hard mother** (because it is a tough membrane), and **pia mater,** meaning **soft mother** (because it is a delicate membrane). **Mater** was used because the Arabians believed that the meninges were the mother of all other body membranes.

Organs of the Peripheral Nervous System

Term	Definition
nerve	cordlike structure that carries impulses from one part of the body to another. There are 12 pairs of cranial nerves and 31 pairs of spinal nerves (see Figures 15-1 and 15-4).
ganglion (*pl.* ganglia)	group of nerve cell bodies located outside the central nervous system
glia	cells that form support and nourish nervous tissue. Some cells assist in the secretion of cerebrospinal fluid and others assist with phagocytosis. They do not conduct impulses. Three types of glia are **astroglia, oligodendroglia,** and **microglia.** (also called **neuroglia**)
neuron	conducts nerve impulses to carry out the function of the nervous system. Destroyed neurons cannot be replaced.

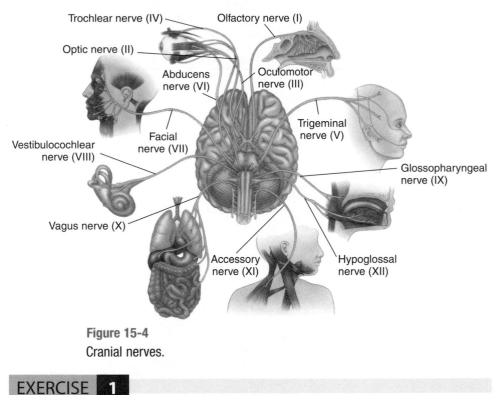

Figure 15-4
Cranial nerves.

EXERCISE 1

Fill in the blanks with the correct terms.

The layer of membrane that covers the brain and spinal cord is called the
(1) _____. Three layers that comprise this membrane are called
(2) _____ _____, (3) _____, and (4) _____
_____. Below the middle layer is a space called the (5) _____
_____ through which the (6) _____ _____ flows
around the brain and spinal cord.

EXERCISE 2

Match the definitions in the first column with the correct terms in the second column.

_____ 1. maintains balance

_____ 2. connects the cerebrum with the cerebellum and brainstem

_____ 3. spaces within the brain

_____ 4. contains the control center for respiration

_____ 5. carries impulses from one part of the body to another

_____ 6. conducts impulses to and from the brain and initiates reflex action to sensory information

_____ 7. group of nerve cell bodies outside the central nervous system

_____ 8. colorless fluid contained in the ventricles

_____ 9. supports and nourishes nervous tissue

a. nerve

b. ganglion

c. cerebrospinal fluid

d. cerebellum

e. medulla oblongata

f. pons

g. ventricles

h. spinal cord

i. pia mater

j. glia

WORD PARTS

Word parts you need to learn to complete this chapter are listed on the following pages. The exercises at the end of each list will help you learn their definitions and spellings.

Combining Forms of the Nervous System

Combining Form	Definition
cerebell/o	cerebellum
cerebr/o	cerebrum, brain
dur/o	hard, dura mater
encephal/o	brain
gangli/o, ganglion/o	ganglion
gli/o	glia (also called neuroglia), gluey substance
meningi/o, mening/o	meninges
myel/o	spinal cord

(NOTE: *myel/o* also means *bone marrow*; see Chapter 14.)

Combining Forms of the Nervous System—*cont'd*

Combining Form	Definition
neur/o.................. (NOTE: *neur/o* was intro- duced in Chapter 2.)	nerve
radic/o, radicul/o, rhiz/o.......	nerve root (proximal end of a peripheral nerve, closest to the spinal cord)

EXERCISE FIGURE A

Fill in the blanks with combining forms in this diagram of the brain and spinal cord.

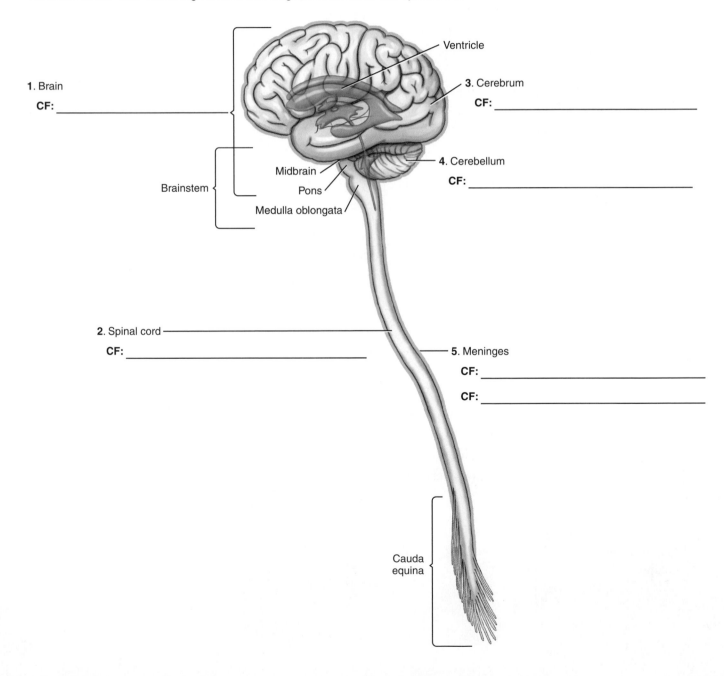

1. Brain

   CF: _____

2. Spinal cord

   CF: _____

Brainstem
 Midbrain
 Pons
 Medulla oblongata

Ventricle

3. Cerebrum

   CF: _____

4. Cerebellum

   CF: _____

5. Meninges

   CF: _____

   CF: _____

Cauda
equina

EXERCISE FIGURE B

Fill in the blanks with combining forms in this diagram of the spinal cord and layers of meninges.

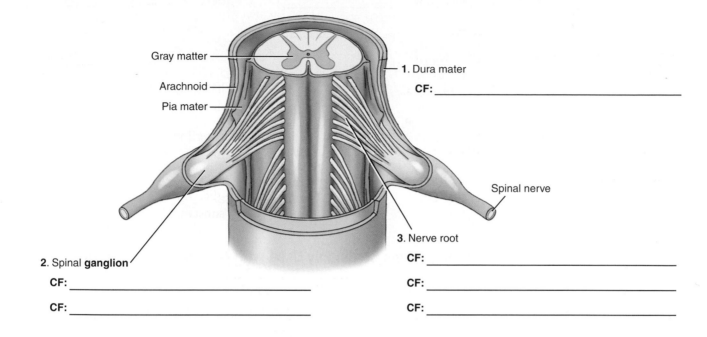

Gray matter

Arachnoid

Pia mater

1. Dura mater

CF: _____

Spinal nerve

3. Nerve root

CF: _____

CF: _____

2. Spinal **ganglion**

CF: _____

CF: _____

EXERCISE 3

Write the definitions of the following combining forms.

1. cerebell/o _____

2. neur/o _____

3. myel/o _____

4. meningi/o,
   mening/o _____

5. encephal/o _____

6. cerebr/o _____

7. radicul/o _____

8. gangli/o _____

9. radic/o _____

10. dur/o _____

11. ganglion/o _____

12. rhiz/o _____

13. gli/o _____

EXERCISE 4

Write the combining form for each of the following terms.

1. cerebellum   _____

2. nerve   _____

3. spinal cord   _____

4. meninges a. _____

            b. _____

5. brain   _____

6. cerebrum, brain   _____

7. nerve root a. _____

         b. _____

         c. _____

8. hard, dura mater   _____

9. ganglion a. _____

            b. _____

10. glia, gluey substance   _____

Combining Forms Commonly Used with Nervous System Terms

Combining Form	Definition
esthesi/o....................	sensation, sensitivity, feeling
ment/o, psych/o	mind
mon/o.....................	one, single
phas/o....................	speech
poli/o.....................	gray matter
quadr/i	four
(NOTE: an *i* is the combining vowel in *quadr/i*.)	

EXERCISE 5

Write the definitions of the following combining forms.

1. mon/o _____

2. psych/o _____

3. quadr/i _____

4. ment/o _____

5. phas/o _____

6. esthesi/o _____

7. poli/o_____

EXERCISE 6

Write the combining form for each of the following.

1. four _____   4. speech _____

2. one, single _____   5. gray matter _____

3. mind a. _____   6. sensation,
        b. _____   sensitivity,
                                   feeling _____

Suffixes

Suffix	Definition
-iatrist.....................	specialist, physician (-*logist* also means specialist)
-iatry.....................	treatment, specialty
-ictal.....................	seizure, attack
-paresis	slight paralysis (-*plegia*, meaning *paralysis*, was covered in Chapter 12)

EXERCISE 7

Write the definitions of the following suffixes.

1. –paresis _____

2. -iatry _____

3. -ictal_____

4. -iatrist _____

EXERCISE 8

Write the suffix for each of the following.

1. slight paralysis _____

2. treatment, specialty _____

3. seizure, attack _____

4. specialist, physician _____

MEDICAL TERMS

Disease and Disorder Terms

Built from Word Parts

The following terms are built from word parts you have already learned and can be translated literally to find their meanings. Further explanation of terms beyond the definition of their word parts, if needed, is included in parentheses.

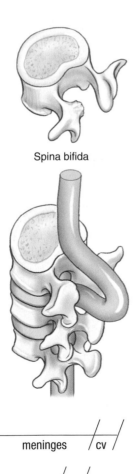

EXERCISE FIGURE C

Fill in the blanks to complete labeling of the diagram.

Spina bifida

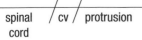

meninges	/ cv /		
spinal cord	/ cv /	protrusion	

Term	Definition
cerebellitis .... (ser-e-bel-Ī-tis)	inflammation of the cerebellum
cerebral thrombosis .... (se-RĒ-bral) (throm-BŌ-sis)	pertaining to the cerebrum, abnormal condition of a clot (blood clot in a blood vessel of the brain). Onset of symptoms may appear from minutes to days after an obstruction occurs (a type of **ischemic stroke**) (see Figure 15-11).
duritis .... (dū-RĪ-tis)	inflammation of the dura mater
encephalitis .... (*en*-sef-a-LĪ-tis)	inflammation of the brain
encephalomalacia .... (en-*sef*-a-lō-ma-LĀ-sha)	softening of the brain
encephalomyeloradiculitis ..... (en-*sef*-a-lō-*mī*-e-lō-ra-*dik*-ū-LĪ-tis)	inflammation of the brain, spinal cord, and nerve roots
gangliitis .... (*gang*-glē-Ī-tis)	inflammation of a ganglion
glioblastoma .... (*glī*-ō-blas-TŌ-ma)	tumor composed of developing glial tissue (the most malignant and most common primary tumor of the brain)
glioma .... (glī-Ō-ma)	tumor composed of the glial tissue (glioma is the term now used to describe all primary neoplasms of the brain and spinal cord)
meningitis .... (*men*-in-JĪ-tis)	inflammation of the meninges
meningioma .... (me-*nin*-jē-Ō-ma)	tumor of the meninges (benign and slow growing)
meningocele .... (me-NING-gō-sēl)	protrusion of the meninges (through a defect in the skull or vertebral column)
meningomyelocele .... (me-*ning*-gō-MĪ-e-lō-*sēl*)	protrusion of the meninges and spinal cord (through the vertebral column) (also called **myelomeningocele**) (Exercise Figure C)
mononeuropathy .... (mon-ō-nū-ROP-a-thē)	disease affecting a single nerve (such as carpal tunnel syndrome)
neuralgia .... (nū-RAL-ja)	pain in a nerve
neurasthenia .... (*nū*-ras-THĒ-nē-a)	nerve weakness

Term	Definition
neuritis (nū-RĪ-tis)	inflammation of a nerve
neuroarthropathy (nū-rō-ar-THROP-a-thē)	disease of nerves and joints
neuroma (nū-RŌ-ma)	tumor made up of nerve (cells)
neuropathy (nū-ROP-a-thē)	disease of the nerves (peripheral) (Figure 15-5)
poliomyelitis (pō-lē-ō-mī-e-LĪ-tis)	inflammation of the gray matter of the spinal cord. (This infectious disease, commonly referred to as *polio*, is caused by one of three polio viruses.)
polyneuritis (pol-ē-nū-RĪ-tis)	inflammation of many nerves
polyneuropathy (pol-ē-nū-ROP-a-thē)	disease of many nerves (most often occurs as a side effect of diabetes mellitus, but may also occur as a result of drug therapy, critical illness such as sepsis, or carcinoma; exhibiting symptoms of weakness, distal sensory loss, and burning)
radiculitis (ra-*dik*-ū-LĪ-tis)	inflammation of the nerve roots
radiculopathy (ra-*dik*-ū-LOP-a-thē)	disease of the nerve roots
rhizomeningomyelitis (*rī*-zō-me-*ning*-gō-*mī*-ē-LĪ-tis)	inflammation of the nerve root, meninges, and spinal cord
subdural hematoma (sub-DŪ-ral) (hē-ma-TŌ-ma)	pertaining to below the dura mater, tumor of blood (*hematoma*, translated literally, means *blood tumor*; however, a hematoma is a collection of blood resulting from a broken blood vessel) (Figure 15-6)

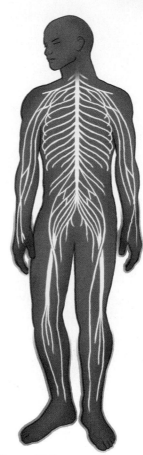

Figure 15-5
Peripheral neuropathy.

PERIPHERAL NEUROPATHY
refers to disorders of the peripheral nervous system, including **radiculopathy, neuropathy,** and **mononeuropathy.** The term is often used synonymously with **polyneuropathy.** Signs and symptoms vary and usually begin gradually, starting with tingling and numbness in the toes and spreading to the feet and upwards. Symptoms may be felt only at night, be constant, or be barely noticed by the patient. Other symptoms include numbness, loss of balance, tingling, burning or freezing sensation, and muscle weakness.

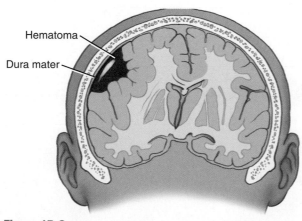

Hematoma

Dura mater

Figure 15-6
Subdural hematoma.

EXERCISE 9

Practice saying aloud each of the disease and disorder terms built from word parts on pp. 688-689.

 To hear the terms select Chapter 15, Chapter Exercises, Pronunciation.

☐ Place a check mark in the box when you have completed this exercise.

EXERCISE 10

Analyze and define the following terms.

1. neuritis _____

2. neuroma _____

3. neuralgia _____

4. neuroarthropathy _____

5. meningioma _____

6. neurasthenia _____

7. encephalomalacia _____

8. encephalitis _____

9. encephalomyeloradiculitis _____

10. meningitis _____

11. meningocele _____

12. meningomyelocele _____

13. radiculitis_____

14. cerebellitis _____

15. gangliitis _____

16. duritis _____

17. polyneuritis_____

18. poliomyelitis_____

19. cerebral thrombosis _____

20. subdural hematoma _____

21. rhizomeningomyelitis _____

22. mononeuropathy _____

23. neuropathy _____

24. radiculopathy _____

25. glioma _____

26. glioblastoma _____

27. polyneuropathy_____

EXERCISE 11

Build disease and disorder terms for the following definitions with the word parts you have learned.

1. inflammation of the nerve

   _____/_____
       WR   S

2. tumor made up of nerve (cells)

   _____/_____
       WR   S

3. pain in a nerve

   _____/_____
       WR   S

4. disease of nerves and joints

   _____/____/_____/____/_____
   WR CV WR CV S

5. disease of the nerve roots

   _____/____/_____
    WR   CV   WR

6. nerve weakness

   _____/_____
       WR   S

7. softening of the brain

   _____/____/_____
    WR   CV   S

8. inflammation of the brain

   _____/_____
       WR   S

9. inflammation of the brain, spinal cord, and nerve roots

   ____/____/_____/____/_____/____
   WR CV WR CV WR S

10. inflammation of the meninges

    _____/_____
        WR   S

11. protrusion of the meninges (through a defect in the skull or vertebral column)

    _____/____/_____
     WR   CV   S

12. protrusion of the meninges and spinal cord (through the vertebral column)

    _____/____/_____/____/_____
    WR CV WR CV S

13. inflammation of the (spinal) nerve roots

_____ / _____
      WR   /   S

14. inflammation of the cerebellum

_____ / _____
      WR   /   S

15. inflammation of the ganglion

_____ / _____
      WR   /   S

16. inflammation of the dura mater

_____ / _____
      WR   /   S

17. inflammation of many nerves

_____ / _____ / _____
   P   /   WR   /   S

18. inflammation of the gray matter of the spinal cord

_____ / ___ / _____ / _____
   WR   / CV /   WR   /   S

19. pertaining to the cerebrum; abnormal condition of a clot

_____ / _____   _____ / _____
  WR   /   S   WR   /   S

20. pertaining to below the dura mater; tumor of blood

____ / ____ / ____   _____ / _____
  P / WR / S   WR   /   S

21. inflammation of the nerve root, meninges, and spinal cord

_____ / ___ / _____ / ___ / _____ / _____
  WR   / CV /   WR   / CV /   WR   /   S

22. tumor of the meninges

_____ / _____
      WR   /   S

23. disease affecting a single nerve

_____ / ___ / _____ / _____
  WR   / CV /   WR   /   S

24. disease of the nerves

_____ / ___ / _____
      WR   / CV /   S

25. tumor composed of glial tissue

_____ / _____
      WR   /   S

26. tumor composed of developing glial tissue

_____ / ___ / _____ / _____
  WR   / CV /   WR   /   S

27. disease of many nerves

_____ / _____ / ___ / _____
   P   /   WR   / CV /   S

EXERCISE 12

Spell each of the disease and disorder terms built from word parts on pp. 688-689 by having someone dictate them to you.

 To hear and spell the terms select Chapter 15, Chapter Exercises, Spelling. You may type the terms on the screen or write them below in the spaces provided.

☐ Place a check mark in the box if you have completed this exercise using your CD-ROM.

1._____   15._____

2._____   16._____

3._____   17._____

4._____   18._____

5._____   19._____

6._____   20._____

7._____   21._____

8._____   22._____

9._____   23._____

10._____   24._____

11._____   25._____

12._____   26._____

13._____   27._____

14._____

Disease and Disorder Terms

Not Built from Word Parts

In some of the following terms, you may recognize word parts you have already learned; however, the full meaning of the terms cannot be discerned by the definition of their word parts.

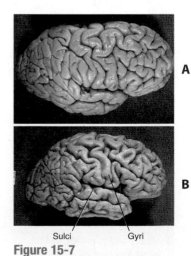

Sulci   Gyri

Figure 15-7

Alzheimer disease. **A,** Normal brain, age matched. **B,** Brain showing changes of Alzheimer disease. Note the brain is smaller, the gyri are narrower, and the sulci are wider than the normal brain.

Term	Definition
Alzheimer disease (AD) . . . . (AWLZ-hī-mer) (di-ZĒZ)	disease characterized by early senility, confusion, loss of recognition of persons or familiar surroundings, restlessness, and impaired memory (Figure 15-7)
amyotrophic lateral sclerosis (ALS) . . . . (a-mī-ō-TRŌ-fik) (LAT-er-al) (skle-RŌ-sis)	progressive muscle atrophy caused by hardening of nerve tissue on the lateral columns of the spinal cord (also called **Lou Gehrig disease**)

Disease and Disorder Terms—*cont'd*

Not Built from Word Parts

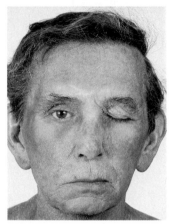

Figure 15-8
Bell palsy.

Term	Definition
Bell palsy (bel) (PAWL-zē)	paralysis of muscles on one side of the face, usually a temporary condition. Symptoms include a sagging mouth on the affected side and nonclosure of the eyelid (Figure 15-8).
cerebral aneurysm (se-RĒ-bral) (AN-ū-rizm)	aneurysm in the cerebrum (see Figure 15-11)
cerebral embolism (se-RĒ-bral) (EM-bō-lizm)	an embolus (usually a blood clot or a piece of atherosclerotic plaque arising from a distant site) lodges in a cerebral artery, causing sudden blockage of blood supply to the brain tissue. A common cause of cerebral embolism, a type of **ischemic stroke,** is atrial fibrillation (Figure 15-11).
cerebral palsy (CP) (se-RĒ-bral) (PAWL-zē)	condition characterized by lack of muscle control and partial paralysis, caused by a brain defect or lesion present at birth or shortly after
dementia (de-MEN-sha)	cognitive impairment characterized by a loss of intellectual brain function. Patients have difficulty in various ways, including difficulty in performing complex tasks, reasoning, learning, and retaining new information, orientation, word finding, and behavior. Dementia has several causes and is not considered part of normal aging.
epilepsy (EP-i-lep-sē)	disorder in which the main symptom is recurring seizures
hydrocephalus (*hī-dr*ō-SEF-a-lus)	increased amount of cerebrospinal fluid in the ventricles of the brain, which can cause enlargement of the cranium in infants
intracerebral hemorrhage (in-tra-SER-e-bral) (HEM-o-rij)	bleeding into the brain as a result of a ruptured blood vessel within the brain. Symptoms vary depending on the location of the hemorrhage; acute symptoms include dyspnea, dysphagia, aphasia, diminished level of consciousness, and hemiparesis. The symptoms often develop suddenly. Intracerebral hemorrhage, a type of **ischemic stroke,** is frequently associated with high blood pressure (see Figure 15-11).

Term	Definition
multiple sclerosis (MS)........ (MUL-ti-pl) (skle-RŌ-sis)	degenerative disease characterized by sclerotic patches along the brain and spinal cord
Parkinson disease (PD)........ (PAR-kin-sun) (di-ZĒZ)	chronic degenerative disease of the central nervous system. Symptoms include resting tremors of the hands and feet, rigidity, expressionless face, and shuffling gait. It usually occurs after the age of 50 years.
sciatica.................... (sī-AT-i-ka)	inflammation of the sciatic nerve, causing pain that travels from the thigh through the leg to the foot and toes; can be caused by injury, infection, athritis, herniated disk, or from prolonged pressure on the nerve from sitting for long periods (Figure 15-9)
shingles.................... (SHING-gelz)	viral disease that affects the peripheral nerves and causes blisters on the skin that follow the course of the affected nerves (also called **herpes zoster** [Figure 15-10])
stroke.................... (strōk)	occurs when there is an interruption of blood supply to a region of the brain, depriving nerve cells in the affected area of oxygen and nutrients. The cells cannot perform and may be damaged or die within minutes. The parts of the body controlled by the involved cells will experience dysfunction. Speech, movement, memory, and other CNS functions may be affected in varying degrees. **Ischemic stroke** is a result of a blocked blood vessel. **Hemorrhagic stroke** is a result of bleeding (also called **cerebrovascular accident [CVA]**, or **brain attack** [Figure 15-11])

Types of Dementia

Alzheimer disease is the most common type of dementia, making up 60% to 80% of all cases. The disease, the cause of which is unknown, is a progressive neurodegenerative disorder characterized by diffuse brain atrophy and the presence of senile plaques and neurofibrillary tangles within the brain cortex. Women are affected more than men, and the disease usually occurs after the age of 60. The disease is slowly progressive and usually results in profound dementia in 5 to 10 years.

Vascular or multiple infarct dementia affects approximately 10% to 20% of patients with dementia. It is secondary to cerebrovascular disease and usually occurs in older patients.

Central nervous system infection dementia may be caused by herpes simplex encephalitis or AIDS.

Lewy body dementia is usually a rapidly progressive form of dementia with Parkinson syndrome.

Parkinson disease dementia may develop in patients with advanced disease.

Wernicke-Korsakoff syndrome is a form of dementia found in chronic alcoholism.

Normal pressure hydrocephalus may cause dementia in elderly individuals and can be treated with a ventricular peritoneal shunt.

POSTHERPETIC NEURALGIA

is a complication of **shingles** (herpes zoster) and is caused by damage to the nerve fibers. Severe pain and hyperesthesia persist after the skin lesions disappear and may last months or even years.

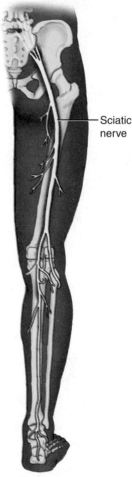

Sciatic nerve

Figure 15-9

The sciatic nerve, the longest in the body, travels through the hip from the spine to the thigh and continues with branches throughout the lower leg and foot. Sciatica is the inflammation of the nerve along its course.

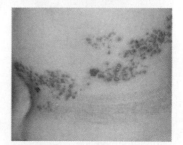

Figure 15-10

Shingles.

Term	Definition
subarachnoid hemorrhage . . . . . (sub-e-RAK-noid) (HEM-o-rij)	bleeding caused by a ruptured blood vessel just outside the brain (usually a ruptured cerebral aneurysm) that rapidly fills the space between the brain and skull (subarachnoid space) with blood. The patient may experience an intense, sudden headache accompanied by nausea, vomiting, and neck pain (a type of **hemorrhagic stroke**) (Figure 15-11).
transient ischemic attack (TIA) . . . . (TRAN-sē-ent) (is-KĒ-mik) (a-TAK)	sudden deficient supply of blood to the brain lasting a short time. The symptoms may be similar to those of stroke, but with TIA the symptoms are temporary and the usual outcome is complete recovery. TIAs are often warning signs for eventual occurrence of a stroke (Figure 15-12).

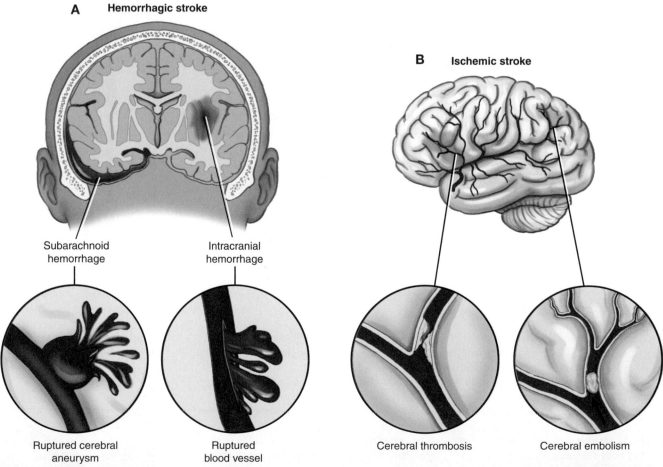

Figure 15-11

Causes of stroke. **A,** Hemorrhagic stroke is the result of bleeding caused by an **intracerebral hemorrhage** or a **subarachnoid hemorrhage,** usually a result of a ruptured cerebral aneurysm. **B,** Ischemic stroke is the result of a blocked blood vessel caused by a **cerebral thrombosis** or **cerebral embolism.**

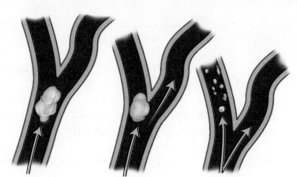

Embolus   Temporary   Embolus dislodged;
           blockage   return of blood flow

Figure 15-12
Transient ischemic attack (TIA).

EXERCISE 13

Practice saying aloud each of the disease and disorder terms not built from word parts on pp. 693-696.

 To hear the terms select Chapter 15, Chapter Exercises, Pronunciation.

☐ Place a check mark in the box when you have completed this exercise.

EXERCISE 14

Fill in the blanks with correct terms.

1. A stroke occurs when there is a disruption of blood supply to a region of the brain. Four causes of stroke are a) _____ _____, b) _____ _____, c)_____ _____, d) _____ _____.

2. A ruptured _____ _____ is often the cause of a subarachnoid hemorrhage.

3. _____ _____ is the paralysis of muscles on one side of the face.

4. The term to describe an increased amount of cerebrospinal fluid in the ventricles of the brain is _____.

5. Inflammation of the nerve that travels from the thigh to the toes is called _____.

6. A viral disease that affects peripheral nerves is _____.

7. The symptoms of a _____ _____ _____ are similar to a stroke but temporary and the patient usually experiences complete recovery.

8. A degenerative disease of the nervous system usually occurring after the age of 50 years is called _____ _____.

9. A disorder with the main symptoms being recurring seizures is _____.

> **PARKINSON DISEASE**
> is also called **parkinsonism, paralysis agitans,** and **shaking palsy.** Since James Parkinson, an English professor, described the disease in 1817 in his **Essay on the Shaking Palsy,** it has often been referred to as **Parkinson disease.**

10. _____ _____ _____ is caused by hardening of the nerve tissue along the lateral columns of the spinal cord.

11. _____ _____ is characterized by early senility, confusion, impaired memory, and loss of recognition.

12. _____ _____ is characterized by lack of muscle coordination and partial paralysis and is present at birth or shortly after.

13. A disease characterized by sclerotic patches along the brain and spinal cord is called _____ _____ .

14. A type of cognitive impairment that is not considered part of normal aging is called _____ .

EXERCISE 15

Match the diseases in the first column with the corresponding phrases in the second column.

_____ 1. cerebral embolism

_____ 2. sciatica

_____ 3. transient ischemic attack

_____ 4. Parkinson disease

_____ 5. cerebral palsy

_____ 6. hydrocephalus

_____ 7. dementia

_____ 8. stroke

_____ 9. Alzheimer disease

_____ 10. intracerebral hemorrhage

_____ 11. epilepsy

_____ 12. multiple sclerosis

_____ 13. shingles

_____ 14. amyotrophic lateral sclerosis

_____ 15. Bell palsy

_____ 16. cerebral aneurysm

_____ 17. subarachnoid hemorrhage

a. causes pain from the thigh to the toes

b. blocking of a cerebral artery by a blood clot or plaque

c. paralysis of muscles on one side of the face

d. hardened patches scattered along the brain and spinal cord

e. cognitive impairment

f. aneurysm in the cerebrum

g. occurs when there is an interruption of blood supply to the brain

h. blisters on the skin

i. early senility

j. resting tremors of the hands and feet and rigidity

k. inflammation of the spinal cord

l. lack of muscle control

m. bleeding within the brain tissue

n. deficient supply of blood to the brain

o. also called Lou Gehrig disease

p. increased amount of cerebrospinal fluid in the ventricles of the brain

q. recurring seizures

r. bleeding that fills space between the brain and skull

EXERCISE 16

Spell each of the disease and disorder terms not built from word parts on pp. 693-696 by having someone dictate them to you.

 To hear and spell the terms select Chapter 15, Chapter Exercises, Spelling. You may type the terms on the screen or write them below in the spaces provided.

☐ Place a check mark in the box if you have completed this exercise using your CD-ROM.

1. _____   10. _____
2. _____   11 _____
3. _____   12. _____
4. _____   13. _____
5. _____   14. _____
6. _____   15. _____
7. _____   16. _____
8. _____   17. _____
9. _____

Surgical Terms

Built from Word Parts

The following terms are built from word parts you have already learned and can be translated literally to find their meanings. Further explanation of terms beyond the definition of their word parts, if needed, is included in parentheses.

Term	Definition
ganglionectomy . . . . (*gang*-glē-o-NEK-to-mē)	excision of a ganglion (also called **gangliectomy**)
neurectomy . . . . (nū-REK-to-mē)	excision of a nerve
neurolysis . . . . (nū-ROL-i-sis)	separating a nerve (from adhesions)
neuroplasty . . . . (NŪR-ō-*plas*-tē)	surgical repair of a nerve
neurorrhaphy . . . . (nū-ROR-a-fē)	suture of a nerve
neurotomy . . . . (nū-ROT-o-mē)	incision into a nerve
radicotomy, rhizotomy . . . . (*rad*-i-KOT-o-mē) (rī-ZOT-o-mē)	incision into a nerve root (Exercise Figure D)

EXERCISE FIGURE D

Fill in the blanks to complete labeling of this diagram.

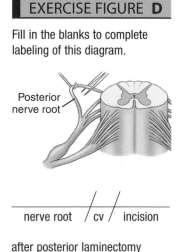

Posterior nerve root

_____ / cv / _____
nerve root   incision

after posterior laminectomy

Stereotactic radiosurgery is used to treat patients with **brain tumors or arteriovenous malformations (AVMs).** A special frame is mounted on the patient's head. Images of the brain are produced by MRI. A high-powered computer uses the images to design a plan for high-intensity radiation that matches the exact size and shape of the tumor. Radiation is then delivered directly to the tumor only, sparing surrounding tissue.

EXERCISE 17

Practice saying aloud each of the surgical terms built from word parts on p. 699.

 To hear the terms select Chapter 15, Chapter Exercises, Pronunciation.

☐ Place a check mark in the box when you have completed this exercise.

EXERCISE 18

Analyze and define the following surgical terms.

1. radicotomy _____

2. neurectomy _____

3. neurorrhaphy _____

4. ganglionectomy _____

5. neurotomy _____

6. neurolysis _____

7. neuroplasty _____

8. rhizotomy _____

EXERCISE 19

Build surgical terms for the following definitions by using the word parts you have learned.

1. incision into a nerve root   a. _____ / _____ / _____
                               WR   CV   S

                                 b. _____ / _____ / _____
                                 WR   CV   S

2. excision of a nerve _____ / _____
                                 WR   S

3. suture of a nerve _____ / _____ / _____
                                 WR   CV   S

4. excision of a ganglion _____ / _____
                                 WR   S

5. incision into a nerve _____ / _____ / _____
                                 WR   CV   S

6. separating a nerve (from adhesions) _____ / _____ / _____
                                 WR   CV   S

7. surgical repair of a nerve _____ / _____ / _____
                                 WR   CV   S

EXERCISE 20

Spell each of the surgical terms built from word parts on p. 699 by having someone dictate them to you.

 To hear and spell the terms select Chapter 15, Chapter Exercises, Spelling. You may type the terms on the screen or write them below in the spaces provided.

☐ Place a check mark in the box if you have completed this exercise using your CD-ROM.

1. _____   5. _____

2. _____   6. _____

3. _____   7. _____

4. _____   8. _____

Diagnostic Terms

Built from Word Parts

The following terms are built from word parts you have already learned and can be translated literally to find their meanings. Further explanation of terms beyond the definition of their word parts, if needed, is included in parentheses.

Term	Definition
DIAGNOSTIC IMAGING	
cerebral angiography . . . . (se-RĒ-bral) (*an*-jē-OG-ra-fē)	radiographic imaging of the blood vessels in the brain (after an injection of contrast medium)
CT myelography . . . . (*mī*-e-LOG-ra-fē)	process of recording (scan) the spinal cord (after an injection of a contrast agent into the subarachnoid space by lumbar puncture. Size, shape, and position of the spinal cord and nerve roots are demonstrated.) (Exercise Figure E)
NEURODIAGNOSTIC PROCEDURES	
electroencephalogram (EEG) . . . (ē-*lek*-trō-en-SEF-a-lō-gram)	record of the electrical impulses of the brain
electroencephalograph . . . . (ē-*lek*-trō-en-SEF-a-lō-graf)	instrument used to record the electrical impulses of the brain
electroencephalography . . . . (ē-*lek*-trō-en-sef-a-LOG-ra-fē)	process of recording the electrical impulses of the brain

EXERCISE FIGURE E

Fill in the blanks to complete labeling of the diagram.

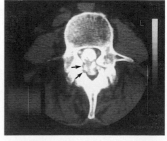

CT _____ / cv / _____
     spinal cord   process of recording

EXERCISE 21

Practice saying aloud each of the diagnostic terms built from word parts on p. 701.

 To hear the terms select Chapter 15, Chapter Exercises, Pronunciation.

☐ Place a check mark in the box when you have completed this exercise.

EXERCISE 22

Analyze and define the following diagnostic terms.

1. electroencephalogram _____

2. electroencephalograph _____

3. electroencephalography _____

4. CT myelography _____

5. cerebral angiography _____

EXERCISE 23

Build diagnostic terms that correspond to the following definitions by using the word parts you have learned.

1. record of the electrical impulses of the brain

　　　_____ / ____ / _____ / ____ / ____
　　　　WR 　 CV 　 WR 　 CV 　 S

2. instrument used for recording the electrical impulses of the brain

　　　_____ / ____ / _____ / ____ / ____
　　　　WR 　 CV 　 WR 　 CV 　 S

3. process of recording the electrical impulses of the brain

　　　_____ / ____ / _____ / ____ / ____
　　　　WR 　 CV 　 WR 　 CV 　 S

4. process of recording (scan) the spinal cord   CT _____ / ____ / ____
　　　　　　　　　　　　　　　　　　　　　　WR 　 CV 　 S

5. radiographic imaging of the blood vessels in the brain

　　　_____ / ____ 　 _____ / ____ / ____
　　　　WR 　 S 　　　　 WR 　 CV 　 S

EXERCISE 24

Spell each of the diagnostic terms built from word parts on p. 701 by having someone dictate them to you.

To hear and spell the terms select Chapter 15, Chapter Exercises, Spelling. You may type the terms on the screen or write them below in the spaces provided.

☐ Place a check mark in the box if you have completed this exercise using your CD-ROM.

1. _____   4. _____

2. _____   5. _____

3. _____

Diagnostic Terms

Not Built from Word Parts

Term	Definition
DIAGNOSTIC IMAGING	
computed tomography of the brain (CT scan) . . . . (com-PŪ-td) (tō-MOG-ra-fē)	process that includes the use of a computer to produce a series of brain tissue images at any desired depth. The procedure is noninvasive, painless, and particularly useful in diagnosing brain tumors (Figure 15-13).

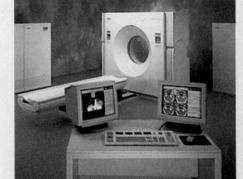 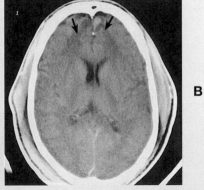

Figure 15-13
A, CT scanner. **B,** CT scan of the brain demonstrating bilateral and right temporal lobe brain contusions *(arrows)* caused by trauma.

magnetic resonance imaging of the brain or spine (MRI scan) . . . . (mag-NET-ik) (REZ-ō-nans) (IM-a-jing)	a noninvasive technique that produces sectional images of soft tissues of the brain or spine through a strong magnetic field. Unlike a CT scan, MRI produces images without use of radiation. It is used to visualize tumors, edema, multiple sclerosis, and herniated disks (Figure 15-14).

 The **first full-scale CT unit** for head scanning was installed in a hospital in **Wimbledon,** United Kingdom in **1971.** Its ability to provide neurological diagnostic information gained rapid recognition. The first units in the **United States** were used in **1973.** The first scanner for visualizing sections of the body other than the brain was developed in **1974** by Dr. Robert Ledly at Georgetown University Medical Center.

A **magnetic resonance imaging scanner** was first used in the **United States** in **1981.** The scanner was developed in England and installed there in 1975.

Diagnostic Terms—*cont'd*
Not Built from Word Parts

Term	Definition
positron emission tomography of the brain (PET scan) . . . . (POZ-i-tron) (ē-MISH-un) (tō-MOG-ra-fē)	an imaging technique with a radioactive substance that produces sectional imaging of the brain to examine blood flow and metabolic activity. Images are projected on a viewing screen (Figure 15-15).

NEURODIAGNOSTIC PROCEDURES

Term	Definition
evoked potential studies (EP studies) . . . . (i-VŌKD) (pō-TEN-shal)	a group of diagnostic tests that measure changes and responses in brain waves elicited by visual, auditory, or somatosensory stimuli. Visual evoked response (VER) is a response to visual stimuli. Auditory evoked response (AER) is a response to auditory stimuli.

OTHER

Term	Definition
lumbar puncture (LP) . . . . (LUM-bar) (PUNK-chur)	insertion of a needle into the subarachnoid space usually between the third and fourth lumbar vertebrae. It is performed for many reasons, including the removal of cerebrospinal fluid for diagnostic purposes (also called **spinal tap**) (Figure 15-16).

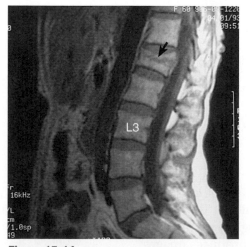

Figure 15-14

Sagittal MRI section of the lumbar spine demonstrating a compression fracture of L1 caused by trauma. (arrow)

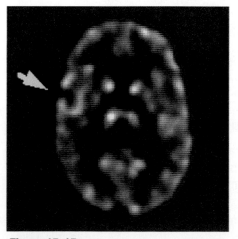

Figure 15-15

Positron emission tomography (PET) scan.

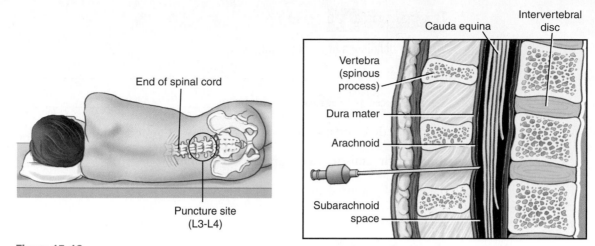

Figure 15-16
Lumbar puncture (spinal tap).

EXERCISE 25

Practice saying aloud each of the diagnostic terms not built from word parts on pp. 703-704.

To hear the terms select Chapter 15, Chapter Exercises, Pronunciation.

☐ Place a check mark in the box when you have completed this exercise.

EXERCISE 26

Fill in the blanks with the correct terms.

1. A computer is used to produce images during _____ _____ of the brain.

2. A needle is inserted into the subarachnoid space during a(n) _____ _____.

3. _____ _____ _____ produces images to examine blood flow and metabolic activity of the brain.

4. Uses a strong magnetic field to produce images of the brain or spine: _____ _____ _____.

5. Measures responses in brain waves from stimuli: _____ _____ _____.

EXERCISE 27

Write the definitions of the following terms.

1. lumbar puncture _____

2. computed tomography of the brain_____

3. magnetic resonance imaging of the brain or spine_____

4. positron emission tomography of the brain _____

5. evoked potential studies _____

EXERCISE 28

Spell each of the diagnostic terms not built from word parts on pp. 703-704 by having someone dictate them to you.

 To hear and spell the terms select Chapter 15, Chapter Exercises, Spelling. You may type the terms on the screen or write them below in the spaces provided.

☐ Place a check mark in the box if you have completed this exercise using your CD-ROM.

1. _____   4. _____

2. _____   5. _____

3. _____

Complementary Terms
Built from Word Parts

The following terms are built from word parts you have already learned and can be translated literally to find their meanings. Further explanation of terms beyond the definition of their word parts, if needed, is included in parentheses.

Term	Definition
anesthesia . . . . (*an*-es-THĒ-zha)	without (loss of) feeling or sensation
aphasia . . . . (a-FĀ-zha)	condition of without speaking (loss or impairment of the ability to speak)
cephalalgia . . . . (*sef*-el-AL-ja)	pain in the head (headache) (also called **cephalgia**)
cerebral . . . . (se-RĒ-bral)	pertaining to the cerebrum
craniocerebral . . . . (krā-nē-ō-su-RĒ-bral)	pertaining to the cranium and cerebrum
dysphasia . . . . (dis-FĀ-zha)	condition of difficulty speaking

HEADACHES
Migraine, tension headache, and cluster headaches account for nearly 90% of all headaches. Other types of headaches include posttraumatic headaches, giant cell (temporal) arteritis, sinus headaches, brain tumor, and chronic daily headache.

Term	Definition
encephalosclerosis.......... (en-*sef*-a-lō-skle-RŌ-sis)	hardening of the brain
gliocyte................... (GLI-ō-sīt)	glial cell
hemiparesis .... (*hem*-ē-pa-RĒ-sis)	slight paralysis of half (right or left side of the body)
hemiplegia .... (*hem*-ē-PLĒ-ja)	paralysis of half (right or left side of the body); stroke is the most common cause of hemiplegia (Exercise Figure F)
hyperesthesia............. (*hī*-per-es-THĒ-zha)	excessive sensitivity (to stimuli)
interictal .... (*in*-ter-IK-tal)	(occurring) between seizures or attacks
intracerebral.............. (*in*-tra-SER-e-bral)	pertaining to within the cerebrum
monoparesis.............. (*mon*-ō-pa-RĒ-sis)	slight paralysis of one (limb)
monoplegia .... (*mon*-ō-PLĒ-ja)	paralysis of one (limb)
myelomalacia............. (*mī*-e-lō-ma-LĀ-sha)	softening of the spinal cord
neuroid.................. (NŪ-royd)	resembling a nerve
neurologist .... (nū-ROL-o-jist)	physician who studies and treats diseases of the nerves (nervous system)
neurology .... (nū-ROL-o-jē)	study of nerves (branch of medicine dealing with diseases of the nervous system)
panplegia .... (pan-PLĒ-ja)	total paralysis (also spelled **pamplegia**)
paresthesia............... (*par*-es-THĒ-zha) (Note: the *a* is dropped from the prefix *para*)	abnormal sensation (such as burning, prickling, or tingling sensation, often in the extremities; may be caused by nerve damage or peripheral neuropathy)
postictal .... (pōst-IK-tal)	(occurring) after a seizure or attack
preictal .... (prē-IK-tal)	(occurring) before a seizure or attack
quadriplegia .... (kwod-ri-PLĒ-ja)	paralysis of four (limbs) (see Exercise Figure F)
subdural .... (sub-DŪ-ral)	pertaining to below the dura mater

EXERCISE FIGURE F

Fill in the blanks to complete labeling of this diagrams of types of paralysis.

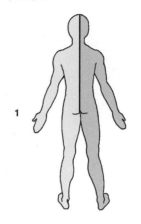

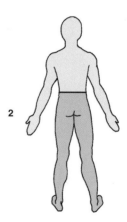

1. _____/_____
   half   paralysis

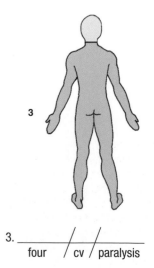

2. Paraplegia

3. _____/_____/_____
   four   cv   paralysis

EXERCISE 29

Practice saying aloud each of the complementary terms built from word parts on pp. 706-707.

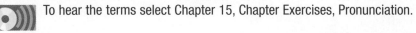 To hear the terms select Chapter 15, Chapter Exercises, Pronunciation.

☐ Place a check mark in the box when you have completed this exercise.

EXERCISE 30

Analyze and define the following complementary terms.

1. hemiplegia_____

2. paresthesia_____

3. neurologist _____

4. neurology _____

5. neuroid _____

6. quadriplegia _____

7. cerebral _____

8. monoplegia _____

9. aphasia_____

10. dysphasia _____

11. hemiparesis _____

12. anesthesia _____

13. hyperesthesia _____

14. subdural_____

15. cephalalgia_____

16. craniocerebral_____

17. myelomalacia _____

18. encephalosclerosis _____

19. postictal_____

20. panplegia_____

21. interictal _____

22. monoparesis _____

23. preictal_____

24. intracerebral _____

25. gliocyte _____

EXERCISE 31

Build the complementary terms for the following definitions by using the word parts you have learned.

1. slight paralysis of half (right or left side of the body)

    _____ / _____
    P   S(WR)

2. without (loss of) feeling or sensation

    _____ / _____ / _____
    P   WR   S

3. excessive sensitivity (to stimuli)

    _____ / _____ / _____
    P   WR   S

4. pertaining to below the dura mater

    _____ / _____ / _____
    P   WR   S

5. pain in the head (headache)

    _____ / _____
    WR   S

6. pertaining to the cranium and cerebrum

    _____ / CV / _____ / _____
    WR   WR   S

7. softening of the spinal cord

    _____ / CV / _____
    WR   S

8. hardening of the brain

    _____ / CV / _____
    WR   S

9. paralysis of half (left or right side) of the body

    _____ / _____
    P   S(WR)

10. physician who studies and treats diseases of the nervous system

    _____ / CV / _____
    WR   S

11. study of nerves (branch of medicine dealing with diseases of the nervous system)

    _____ / CV / _____
    WR   S

12. resembling a nerve

      WR   /   S

13. paralysis of four (limbs)

      WR   /   CV   /   S

14. pertaining to the cerebrum

      WR   /   S

15. paralysis of one (limb)

      WR   /   CV   /   S

16. condition of without speaking (loss or impairment of the ability to speak)

      P   /   WR   /   S

17. condition of difficulty speaking

      P   /   WR   /   S

18. (occurring) before a seizure or attack

      P   /   S(WR)

19. slight paralysis of one (limb)

      WR   /   CV   /   S

20. (occurring) after a seizure

      P   /   S(WR)

21. total paralysis

      P   /   S(WR)

22. (occurring) between seizures or attacks

      P   /   S(WR)

23. pertaining to within the cerebrum

      P   /   WR   /   S

24. glial cell

      WR   /   CV   /   S

25. abnormal sensation

      P   /   WR   /   S

EXERCISE 32

Spell each of the complementary terms built from word parts on pp. 706-707 by having someone dictate them to you.

 To hear and spell the terms select Chapter 15, Chapter Exercises, Spelling. You may type the terms on the screen or write them below in the spaces provided.

☐ Place a check mark in the box if you have completed this exercise using your CD-ROM.

1. _____
2. _____
3. _____
4. _____
5. _____
6. _____
7. _____
8. _____
9. _____
10. _____
11. _____
12. _____
13. _____

14. _____
15. _____
16. _____
17. _____
18. _____
19. _____
20. _____
21. _____
22. _____
23. _____
24. _____
25. _____

Complementary Terms

Not Built from Word Parts

In some of the following terms you may recognize word parts you have already learned; however, the full meaning of the terms cannot be discerned by the definition of their word parts.

Term	Definition
afferent . . . . (AF-er-ent)	conveying toward a center (for example, afferent nerves carry impulses to the central nervous system)
ataxia . . . . (a-TAK-sē-a)	lack of muscle coordination
cognitive . . . . (COG-ni-tiv)	pertaining to the mental processes of comprehension, judgment, memory, and reason
coma . . . . (KŌ-ma)	state of profound unconsciousness

TYPES OF COGNITIVE IMPAIRMENT

Mild cognitive impairment (MCI) is the presence of significant memory difficulty when adjusted for age-related norms. The patient usually has little difficulty performing activities of daily living. This condition may be an early manifestation of Alzheimer disease.

Age-associated memory impairment is when memory function tends to decline with aging when compared with young adults. This is not necessarily a forerunner of dementia.

Delirium is potentially reversible acute disturbance of consciousness with impairment of cognition. A number of conditions can cause delirium by interfering with brain metabolism. Drugs, alcohol, systemic infections, head trauma, hypoglycemia, and electrolyte disturbances are common examples.

Pseudodementia is a disorder resembling dementia but is not caused by a brain disease. This can be found in mental illness, such as major depression, and can be reversible with treatment.

Complementary Terms—*cont'd*
Not Built from Word Parts

Term	Definition
concussion . . . . (kon-KUSH-un)	jarring or shaking that results in an injury. Brain concussions are caused by slight or severe head injury; symptoms include vertigo, headache, and loss of consciousness.
conscious . . . . (KON-shus)	awake, alert, aware of one's surroundings
convulsion . . . . (kun-VUL-zhun)	sudden, involuntary contraction of a group of muscles (synonymous with **seizure**)
disorientation . . . . (dis-*or*-ē-en-TĀ-shun)	a state of mental confusion as to time, place, or identity
dysarthria . . . . (dis-AR-thrē-a)	the inability to use speech that is distinct and connected because of a loss of muscle control after damage to the peripheral or central nervous system
efferent . . . . (EF-er-ent)	conveying away from the center (for example, efferent nerves carry information away from the central nervous system)
gait . . . . (gāt)	a manner or style of walking
incoherent . . . . (*in*-kō-HĒR-ent)	unable to express one's thoughts or ideas in an orderly, intelligible manner
paraplegia . . . . (*par*-a-PLĒ-ja)	paralysis from the waist down caused by damage to the lower level of the spinal cord (see Exercise Figure F)
seizure . . . . (SĒ-zher)	sudden attack with an involuntary series of contractions (synonymous with **convulsion**)
shunt . . . . (shunt)	tube implanted in the body to redirect the flow of a fluid
syncope . . . . (SINC-o-pē)	fainting or sudden loss of consciousness caused by lack of blood supply to the cerebrum
unconsciousness . . . . (un-KON-shus-nes)	state of being unaware of surroundings and incapable of responding to stimuli as a result of injury, shock, or illness

PARAPLEGIA
is composed of the Greek **para**, meaning **beside**, and **plegia**, meaning **paralysis**. It has been used since Hippocrates' time and at first meant paralysis of any limb or side of the body. Since the nineteenth century, it has been used to mean paralysis from the waist down.

EXERCISE 33

Practice saying aloud each of the complementary terms not built from word parts on pp. 711-712.

 To hear the terms select Chapter 15, Chapter Exercises, Pronunciation.

☐ Place a check mark in the box when you have completed this exercise.

EXERCISE 34

Write the term for each of the following definitions.

1. jarring or shaking that results in an injury

   _____

2. state of being unaware of surroundings and incapable of responding to stimuli as a result of injury, shock, or illness

   _____

3. awake, alert, aware of one's surroundings

   _____

4. sudden attack with involuntary contractions

   _____

5. sudden, involuntary contraction of a group of muscles

   _____

6. tube implanted in the body to redirect the flow of a fluid

   _____

7. paralysis from the waist down caused by damage to the lower level of the spinal cord

   _____

8. state of profound unconsciousness

   _____

9. fainting

   _____

10. lack of muscle coordination _____

11. a manner or style of walking _____

12. inability to use speech that is distinctive and connected _____

13. unable to express one's thoughts or ideas in an orderly, intelligible manner _____

14. a state of mental confusion as to time, place, or identity _____

15. pertaining to the mental processes of comprehension, judgment, memory, and reason _____

16. conveying toward the center _____

17. conveying away from the center _____

EXERCISE 35

Write the definitions for the following terms.

1. shunt _____

2. paraplegia _____

3. coma _____

4. concussion _____

5. unconsciousness _____

6. conscious _____

7. seizure _____

8. convulsion _____

9. syncope _____

10. ataxia _____

11. dysarthria _____

12. gait _____

13. cognitive _____

14. disorientation _____

15. incoherent _____

16. efferent _____

17. afferent _____

EXERCISE 36

Spell each of the complementary terms not built from word parts on pp. 711-712 by having someone dictate them to you.

 To hear and spell the terms select Chapter 15, Chapter Exercises, Spelling. You may type the terms on the screen or write them below in the spaces provided.

☐ Place a check mark in the box if you have completed this exercise using your CD-ROM.

1._____   10._____

2._____   11._____

3._____   12._____

4._____   13._____

5._____   14._____

6._____   15._____

7._____   16._____

8._____   17._____

9._____

Behavioral Health

Although the terms below are listed as behavioral health terms, medications, physical changes, substance abuse, and illness may contribute to these conditions.

Built from Word Parts

The following terms are built from word parts you have already learned and can be translated literally to find their meanings. Further explanation of terms beyond the definition of their word parts, if needed, is included in parentheses.

Term	Definition
psychiatrist................ (sī-KĪ-a-trist)	a physician who studies and treats disorders of the mind
psychiatry................. (sī-KĪ-a-trē)	specialty of the mind (branch of medicine that deals with the treatment of mental disorders)
psychogenic............... (sī-kō-JEN-ik)	originating in the mind
psychologist............... (sī-KOL-o-jist)	specialist of the mind
psychology................ (sī-KOL-o-jē)	study of the mind (a profession that involves dealing with the mind and mental processes in relation to human behavior)

PSYCHIATRIST
a **physician** who has had **additional training** and experience in prevention, diagnosis, and treatment of mental disorders.

CLINICAL PSYCHOLOGIST
is one who has had **graduate study** in **psychology** and training in clinical psychology and who provides testing and counseling for mental and emotional disorders. A psychologist cannot prescribe medication or medical tests and treatments.

Behavioral Health—*cont'd*
Built from Word Parts

Term	Definition
psychopathy . . . . (sī-KOP-a-thē)	(any) disease of the mind

psychosis (*pl.* psychoses). . . . . .
  (sī-KO-sis)
  (sī-KO-sēz)
	abnormal condition of the mind (major mental disorder characterized by extreme derangement, often with delusions and hallucinations)

psychosomatic . . . . (*sī*-kō-sō-MAT-ik)	pertaining to the mind and body (interrelations of)

EXERCISE 37

Practice saying aloud each of the behavioral health terms built from word parts on pp. 715-716.

To hear the terms select Chapter 15, Chapter Exercises, Pronunciation.

☐ Place a check mark in the box when you have completed this exercise.

EXERCISE 38

Build the behavioral health terms for the following definitions by using the word parts you have learned.

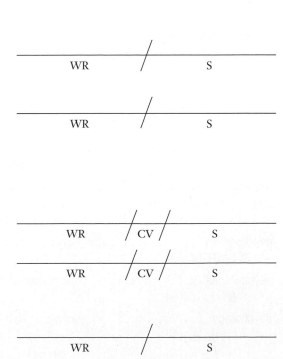

1. specialty of the mind (branch of medicine that deals with the treatment of mental disorders)

   WR   /   S

2. abnormal condition of the mind

   WR   /   S

3. study of the mind (a profession that involves dealing with the mind and mental processes in relation to human behavior)

   WR / CV / S

4. originating in the mind

   WR / CV / S

5. a physician who studies and treats disorders of the mind

   WR   /   S

6. specialist of the mind

———————— / ———— / ————
     WR   CV   S

7. pertaining to the mind
   and body

———————— / ———— / ———— / ————
     WR   CV   WR   S

8. disease of the mind

———————— / ———— / ————
     WR   CV   S

EXERCISE 39

Analyze and define the following terms.

1. psychosomatic _____

2. psychopathy _____

3. psychology _____

4. psychiatry _____

5. psychologist _____

6. psychogenic _____

7. psychiatrist _____

8. psychosis _____

EXERCISE 40

Spell each of the behavioral health terms built from word parts on pp. 715-716 by having someone dictate them to you.

 To hear and spell the terms select Chapter 15, Chapter Exercises, Spelling. You may type the terms on the screen or write them below in the spaces provided.

☐ Place a check mark in the box if you have completed this exercise using your CD-ROM.

1. _____
2. _____
3. _____
4. _____

5. _____
6. _____
7. _____
8. _____

Behavioral Health
Not Built from Word Parts

In some of the following terms, you may recognize word parts you have already learned; however, the full meaning of the terms cannot be discerned by the definition of their word parts.

> **CAM TERM**
> **Biofeedback** is a learned self-control of physiologic responses using electronic devices to provide monitoring information. Current research suggests that biofeedback is a viable alternative treatment for attention deficit–hyperactivity disorder (ADHD).

Term	Definition
anorexia nervosa . . . . (an-ō-REK-sē-a) (ner-VŌ-sa)	an eating disorder characterized by a disturbed perception of body image resulting in failure to maintain body weight, intensive fear of gaining weight, pronounced desire for thinness, and, in females, amenorrhea (introduced in Chapter 11)
anxiety disorder . . . . (ang-ZĪ-e-tē) (dis-OR-der)	an emotional disorder characterized by feelings of apprehension, tension, or uneasiness arising typically from the anticipation of unreal or imagined danger
attention deficit hyperactivity disorder (ADHD) . . . . (a-TEN-shun) (DEF-i-sit) (*hī*-per-ak-TIV-i-tē)	a disorder of learning and behavioral problems characterized by marked inattention, distractability, impulsiveness, and hyperactivity
autism. (AW-tizm)	a mental disorder, the features of which include onset during infancy or childhood, preoccupation with subjective mental activity, inability to interact socially, impaired communication, and repetitive body movements
bipolar disorder . . . . (bī-PŌ-lar) (dis-OR-der)	a major psychological disorder typified by a disturbance in mood. The disorder is manifested by manic and depressive episodes that may alternate or elements of both may occur simultaneously.
bulimia nervosa . . . . (bū-LĒ-mē-a) (ner-VŌ-sa)	an eating disorder characterized by uncontrolled binge eating followed by purging (induced vomiting) (introduced in Chapter 11)
major depression . . . . (MĀ-jor) (dē-PRESH-un)	a mood disturbance characterized by feelings of sadness, despair, discouragement, hopelessness, lack of joy, altered sleep patterns, and difficulty with decision making and daily function. Depression ranges from normal feelings of sadness (resulting from and proportional to personal loss or tragedy), through dysthymia (chronic depressive neurosis), to major depression (also referred to as **clinical depression, mood disorder**).

Term	Definition
obsessive-compulsive disorder (OCD)...................... (ob-SES-iv-kom-PUL-siv) (dis-OR-der)	a disorder characterized by intrusive, unwanted thoughts that result in the tendency to perform repetitive acts or rituals (compulsions), usually as a means of releasing tension or anxiety
panic attack................. (PAN-ik) (a-tak)	an episode of sudden onset of acute anxiety, occurring unpredictably, with feelings of acute apprehension, dyspnea, dizziness, sweating, and/or chest pain, depersonalization, paresthesia and fear of dying, loss of mind or control
phobia..................... (FŌ-bē-a)	a marked and persistent fear that is excessive or unreasonable cued by the presence or anticipation of a specific situation or object
pica....................... (PĪ-ka)	compulsive eating of nonnutritive substances such as clay or ice. This condition is often a result of an iron deficiency. When iron deficiency is the cause of pica the condition will disappear in 1 or 2 weeks when treated with iron therapy.
posttraumatic stress disorder (PTSD)...................... (pōst-tra-MAT-ik) (stress) (dis-OR-der)	a disorder characterized by an acute emotional response to a traumatic event perceived as life threatening or severe emotional stress such as an airplane crash, repeated physical or emotional trauma, or military combat. Symptoms include anxiety, sleep disturbance, nightmares, difficulty concentrating, and depression.
schizophrenia.............. (skit-sō-FRĒ-nē-a)	any one of a large group of psychotic disorders characterized by gross distortions of reality, disturbance of language and communication, withdrawal from social interaction, and the disorganization and fragmentation of thought, perception, and emotional reaction
somatoform disorders........ (sō-MAT-ō-form)	disorders characterized by physical symptoms for which no known physical cause exists

EXERCISE 41

Practice saying aloud each of the behavioral health terms not built from word parts on pp. 718-719.

 To hear the terms select Chapter 15, Chapter Exercises, Pronunciation.

☐ Place a check mark in the box when you have completed the exercise.

EXERCISE 42

Match the definitions in the first column with the correct terms in the second column.

_____ 1. manifested by manic and depressive episodes

_____ 2. an episode of acute anxiety

_____ 3. characterized by feelings of apprehension and tension

_____ 4. a disorder of learning and behavioral problems

_____ 5. a mood disturbance characterized by feelings of sadness, despair, and discouragement

_____ 6. a marked and persistent fear that is excessive or unreasonable

_____ 7. binge eating followed by purging

_____ 8. physical symptoms for which no known physical cause exists

_____ 9. eating of nonnutritive substances, such as ice

_____ 10. failure to maintain body weight

_____ 11. characterized by gross distortions of reality and disturbance of language and communication

_____ 12. preoccupation with subjective mental activity, inability to interact socially, and repetitive body movements

_____ 13. acute emotional response to a traumatic event

_____ 14. intrusive unwanted thoughts that result in rituals and/or repetitive acts

a. phobia

b. anxiety disorder

c. attention deficit hyperactivity disorder

d. somatoform disorders

e. schizophrenia

f. anorexia nervosa

g. bulimia nervosa

h. pica

i. bipolar disorder

j. major depression

k. obsessive-compulsive disorder

l. posttraumatic stress disorder

m. panic attack

n. autism

EXERCISE 43

Spell each of the behavioral health terms not built from word parts on pp. 718-719 by having someone dictate them to you.

 To hear and spell the term select Chapter 15, Chapter Exercises, Spelling. You may type the terms on the screen or write them below in the spaces provided.

☐ Place a check mark in the box if you have completed this exercise using your CD-ROM.

1. _____   8. _____

2. _____   9. _____

3. _____   10. _____

4. _____   11. _____

5. _____   12. _____

6. _____   13. _____

7. _____   14. _____

Refer to Appendix E for pharmacology terms related to the nervous system and behavioral health.

Abbreviations

AD	Alzheimer disease
ADHD	attention deficit hyperactivity disorder
ALS	amyotrophic lateral sclerosis
CNS	central nervous system
CP	cerebral palsy
CSF	cerebrospinal fluid
CVA	cerebrovascular accident
EEG	electroencephalogram
EP studies	evoked potential studies
LP	lumbar puncture
MRI scan	magnetic resonance imaging scan
MS	multiple sclerosis
OCD	obsessive-compulsive disorder
PD	Parkinson disease
PET scan	positron emission tomography scan
PNS	peripheral nervous system
PTSD	posttraumatic stress disorder
TIA	transient ischemic attack

Refer to Appendix D for a complete list of abbreviations.

EXERCISE 44

Write the meaning of the abbreviations in the following sentences.

1. Diagnostic tests used to diagnose patients with diseases of the nervous system include **EEG** _____, **MRI scan** _____ _____ _____ _____, **PET scan** _____ _____ _____ _____, **EP studies** _____ _____ _____, and **LP** _____ _____ _____.

2. Diseases that affect the nervous system are **AD**_____ _____, **ALS** _____ _____ _____, **CP** _____ _____, **MS** _____ _____, and **PD** _____ _____.

3. Stroke is the disruption of normal blood supply to the brain. It often occurs suddenly. Because of this, Hippocrates used the term *apoplexy*, which literally means *struck down*, to describe the condition. The term *stroke* grew out of the term *apoplexy*, meaning *struck down* or *stroke*. The term *brain attack* is a fairly new term used to signify that a stroke is in progress and an emergency situation exists. **CVA** _____ _____ is also used to describe a stroke. An ischemic stroke, which is caused by a thrombosis or embolus, is frequently preceded by a **TIA** _____ _____ _____.

4. The examination of **CSF** _____ _____ may assist in the diagnosis of cerebral hemorrhage, meningitis, encephalitis, and other diseases.

5. Three common psychiatric disorders are **PTSD,** _____ _____ _____, **OCD**_____ _____ _____, and **ADHD** _____ _____ _____ _____.

6. The nervous system may be divided into the **CNS** _____ _____ _____, and the **PNS** _____ _____ _____.

PRACTICAL APPLICATION

EXERCISE 45   *Interact with Medical Documents*

A. Complete the progress note by writing the medical terms in the blanks. Use the list of definitions with the corresponding numbers.

University Hospital and Medical Center
4700 North Main Street • Wellness, Arizona 54321 • (987) 555-3210

PATIENT NAME: Eldon Drake **CASE NUMBER:** 71086-NUR
DATE OF BIRTH: 08/12/19XX **DATE OF ADMISSION:** 01/02/20XX

PROGRESS NOTE

HISTORY: Eldon Drake is an 85-year-old Caucasian male who was admitted to the hospital on 01/02/20XX for fever and confusion. Mr. Drake was in his usual state of good health until 3 days before admission, when he began to show signs of confusion and 1. _____ accompanied by a fever of 38.5° C. His fever continued, and he showed a steady decline in 2. _____ function. He developed expressive 3. _____.

OBJECTIVE FINDINGS: On physical examination the patient was 4. _____ and alert but disoriented to time and place. Blood pressure was 160/80. Pulse, 96. Respirations, 20. Temperature 38.8° C. There were no focal neurologic deficits. Chest radiograph, urinalysis, and blood cultures were negative. A 5. _____ consultation was obtained. 6. _____ _____ _____ of the brain was performed, which disclosed 7. _____. An 8. _____ was markedly abnormal for his age.

TREATMENT SUMMARY: The patient was given acyclovir intravenous infusion. On the second hospital day, the patient developed a generalized 9. _____. He was placed on intravenous Dilantin and lorazepam. He later lapsed into a semicomatose state. He responded to tactile and verbal stimuli but was completely 10. _____. A nasogastric tube was placed, and enteral feedings were begun. After 14 days of IV acyclovir, the patient slowly began to improve and by the third week of his illness, he was talking normally and taking nourishment.

_____
Rashid Magolot, MD

RM/mcm

---

1. a state of mental confusion as to time, place, or identity
2. pertaining to the mental processes of comprehension, judgment, memory, and reason
3. loss of the ability to speak
4. awake, alert, and aware of one's surroundings
5. study of nerves (branch of medicine dealing with diseases of the nervous system)
6. noninvasive technique that produces cross-sectional and sagittal images of the brain by magnetic waves
7. inflammation of the brain
8. record of electrical impulses of the brain
9. sudden attack with involuntary series of contractions
10. unable to express one's thoughts or ideas in an orderly, intelligible manner

EXERCISE **45**   *Interact with Medical Documents—cont'd*

B. Read the consultation report and answer the questions following it.

32463 COOPER, STAN   _ □ X

File Patient Navigate Custom Fields Help

| Patient Chart | Lab | Rad | Notes | Documents | Rx | Scheduling | Images | Billing |

Name: **COOPER, STAN**   MR#: **32463**   Sex: **M**
                          DOB: **04/11/19XX**

NEUROLOGY CONSULTATION

ENCOUNTER DATE: 06/04/20XX

HISTORY: The patient is a 74-year-old Caucasian male referred to Neurology because of persistent low back and right leg pain and paresthesias of 6 months duration. The pain is described as dull and aching and is rated 6/10. The discomfort is worse when standing and intensifies after walking about a block. The pain improves when the patient is sitting or when bending over. His general health is good and there has been no weight loss.

NEUROLOGIC EXAM: The gait is somewhat wide based. Balance is normal. No muscle atrophy is present. Muscle strength is normal for age. The right Achilles reflex is absent. Sensation to pin prick is diminished over the right S1 dermatome.

LAB AND IMAGING: CBC and sed rate are normal. Fasting blood sugar is 106 mg%. A lumbosacral spine radiograph shows spondylosis and spondylolisthesis of L5 over S1. A CT scan shows a moderate degree of facet joint arthropathy and bulging discs at L2-3 and L4-5 levels along with narrowing of the spinal canal at these levels.

IMPRESSION: Lumbar spinal stenosis with radiculopathy of the S1 nerve root.

RECOMMENDATION: Referral to neuroanesthesia for a series of epidural steroid injections. Physical therapy is also advised. Surgical referral is not necessary at this time.

Electronically signed by: Susan Rand, MD 06/04/20XX 6:15 PM

SR/dlb

| Start | Log On/Off | Print | Edit |

---

1. Spinal stenosis causes compression of nerve roots demonstrated by which of the following symptoms for the patient?
   a. total paralysis
   b. abnormal sensation of prickling and tingling
   c. paralysis of one limb
   d slight paralysis

2. The patient's diagnosis is spinal stenosis with:
   a. disease of the nerve roots
   b. disease of peripheral nerves
   c. disease affecting a single nerve
   d. disease of many nerves

EXERCISE 46   *Interpret Medical Terms*

To test your understanding of the terms introduced in this chapter, circle the words that correctly complete the sentences. The italicized words refer to the correct answer.

1. *Paralysis of all four limbs* is (**paraplegia, monoplegia, hemiplegia, quadriplegia**).

2. The *inability to speak* or (**dysarthria, aphasia, dysphasia, dysphagia**) may be an after-effect of cerebrovascular accident.

3. A symptom of brain concussion that may cause a patient to be *unaware of his or her surroundings* and *unable to respond to stimuli* is (**subconscious, unconscious, convulsive**).

4. The newborn had *meninges protruding through a defect in his skull*, or a (**meningocele, myelomeningocele, myelomalacia**).

5. *The branch of medicine that deals with the treatment of mental disorders* is (**neurology, psychology, psychiatry**).

6. *Multiple sclerosis* is a disease of the nervous system and generally occurs in young adults. It is characterized by (**seizures, hardened patches along the brain and spinal cord, muscular tremors**).

7. *The process of recording of electrical impulses of the brain*, or (**electroencephalogram, electroencephalograph, electroencephalography**), is used to study brain function and is valuable for diagnosing epilepsy, tumors, and other brain diseases.

8. Cerebral *thrombosis*, or abnormal condition of a(n) (**blood clot, infection, hardened patches**), may cause a stroke.

9. The patient was admitted to the neurology unit of the hospital with a diagnosis of stroke. The physician ordered *a diagnostic procedure to examine blood flow and metabolic activity* or (**computed tomography, positron emission tomography, magnetic resonance imaging**).

10. The patient was diagnosed with (**ganglion, ganglia**) on both wrists.

EXERCISE **47** *Read Medical Terms in Use*

Practice pronunciation of terms by reading the following document. Use the pronunciation key following the medical term to assist you in saying the word.

 To hear these terms select Chapter 15, Chapter Exercises, Read Medical Terms in Use.

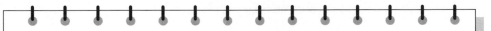

A 78-year-old right-handed male presented to the Emergency Department with a right **hemiparesis** (hem-ē-pa-RĒ-sis), expressive **aphasia** (a-FĀ-zha), and no apparent **cognitive** (COG-ni-tiv) decline. He has a history of hypertension and 2 years ago had a **transient ischemic** (is-KĒ-mik) **attack.** A **computed tomography** (tō-MOG-ra-fē) **scan of the brain** was negative for an **intracerebral** (in-tra-SER-e-bral) hemorrhage. A **neurologist** (nū-ROL-o-jist) was consulted. She confirmed the diagnosis of an **ischemic stroke** (strōk) after **magnetic resonance imaging** (mag-NET-ik) (REZ-ō-nans) (IM-a-jing) **of the brain** demonstrated an ischemic area of the left **cerebral** (se-RĒ-bral) cortex caused by a cerebral embolism (se-RĒ-bral) (EM-bo-lizm).

EXERCISE **48** *Comprehend Medical Terms in Use*

Test your comprehension of terms in the previous medical document by circling the correct answer.

1. While in the emergency department, the patient had:
   a. inability to swallow and paralysis from the waist down
   b. inability to speak and slight paralysis of the right side of the body
   c. inability to swallow and slight paralysis of the right side of the body
   d. inability to speak and paralysis from the waist down

2. T F A diagnosis of stroke was made after an MRI of the brain was performed.

3. The patient had a history of:
   a. sudden deficient supply of blood to the brain
   b. sudden loss of consciousness
   c. slight paralysis of one side
   d. a clot in the cerebrum

CHAPTER REVIEW

CHAPTER REVIEW ON CD-ROM

Use the CD-ROM that accompanies this textbook to play and practice what you have learned in this chapter. The Chapter Exercises, Practice Activities, Animations, and Games allow you to hear, see, and interact with the chapter content.

Chapter Exercises

Exercises in this section of your CD-ROM correlate to exercises in your textbook. You may have completed them as you worked through the chapter.

☐ Pronunciation
☐ Spelling
☐ Read Medical Terms in Use

Practice Activities

Practice in study mode, and then test your learning in assessment mode. Keep track of your scores from assessment mode if you wish.

SCORE

☐ Picture It   _____
☐ Define Word Parts   _____
☐ Build Medical Terms   _____
☐ Word Shop   _____
☐ Define Medical Terms   _____
☐ Use It   _____
☐ Hear It and Type It: _____
  Clinical Vignettes

Animations

☐ Brain Blood Clot Leading to Stroke
☐ Subdural Hematoma

Games

☐ Name that Word Part
☐ Term Storm
☐ Term Explorer
☐ Termbusters
☐ Medical Millionaire

REVIEW OF WORD PARTS

Can you define and spell the following word parts?

Combining Forms

cerebell/o	myel/o
cerebr/o	neur/o
dur/o	phas/o
encephal/o	poli/o
esthesi/o	psych/o
gangli/o	quadr/i
ganglion/o	radic/o
gli/o	radicul/o
mening/o	rhiz/o
meningi/o	
ment/o	
mon/o	

Suffixes

-iatrist
-iatry
-ictal
-paresis

REVIEW OF TERMS

Can you build, analyze, define, pronounce, and spell the following terms *built from word parts?*

Diseases and Disorders	Surgical	Diagnostic	Complementary	Behavioral Health
cerebellitis	ganglionectomy	cerebral angiography	anesthesia	psychiatrist
cerebral thrombosis	neurectomy	CT myelography	aphasia	psychiatry
duritis	neurolysis	electroencephalogram	cephalalgia	psychogenic
encephalitis	neuroplasty	(EEG)	cerebral	psychologist
encephalomalacia	neurorrhaphy	electroencephalograph	craniocerebral	psychology
encephalomyeloradiculitis	neurotomy	electroencephalography	dysphasia	psychopathy
gangliitis	radicotomy		encephalosclerosis	psychosis
glioblastoma	rhizotomy		gliocyte	psychosomatic
glioma			hemiparesis	
meningitis			hemiplegia	
meningioma			hyperesthesia	
meningocele			interictal	
meningomyelocele			intracerebral	
mononeuropathy			monoparesis	
neuralgia			monoplegia	
neurasthenia			myelomalacia	
neuritis			neuroid	
neuroarthropathy			neurologist	
neuroma			neurology	
neuropathy			panplegia	
poliomyelitis			paresthesia	
polyneuritis			postictal	
polyneuropathy			preictal	
radiculitis			quadriplegia	
radiculopathy			subdural	
rhizomeningomyelitis				
subdural hematoma				

Can you define, pronounce, and spell the following terms *not built from word parts?*

Diseases and Disorders	Diagnostic	Complementary	Behavioral Health
Alzheimer disease (AD)	computed tomography of the brain (CT scan)	afferent	anorexia nervosa
amyotrophic lateral sclerosis (ALS)	evoked potential studies (EP)	ataxia	anxiety disorder
Bell palsy	lumbar puncture (LP)	cognitive	attention deficit hyperactivity disorder (ADHD)
cerebral aneurysm	magnetic resonance imaging of the brain or spine (MRI scan)	coma	autism
cerebral embolism	positron emission tomography of the brain (PET scan)	concussion	bipolar disorder
cerebral palsy (CP)		conscious	bulimia nervosa
dementia		convulsion	major depression
epilepsy		disorientation	obsessive-compulsive disorder (OCD)
hydrocephalus		dysarthria	panic attack
intracerebral hemorrhage		efferent	phobia
multiple sclerosis (MS)		gait	pica
Parkinson disease (PD)		incoherent	posttraumatic stress disorder (PTSD)
sciatica		paraplegia	schizophrenia
shingles		seizure	somatoform disorders
stroke		shunt	
subarachnoid hemorrhage		syncope	
transient ischemic attack (TIA)		unconsciousness	

ANSWERS

Exercise Figures

Exercise Figure

A. 1. brain: encephal/o
2. spinal cord: myel/o
3. cerebrum: cerebr/o
4. cerebellum: cerebell/o
5. meninges: meningi/o, mening/o

Exercise Figure

B. 1. dura mater: dur/o
2. ganglion: gangli/o, ganglion/o
3. nerve root: radic/o, radicul/o, rhiz/o

Exercise Figure

C. mening/o/myel/o/cele

Exercise Figure

D. rhiz/o/tomy or radic/o/tomy

Exercise Figure

E. myel/o/graphy

Exercise Figure

F. 1. hemi/plegia
3. quadr/i/plegia

Exercise 1
1. meninges
2. dura mater
3. arachnoid
4. pia mater
5. subarachnoid space
6. cerebrospinal fluid

Exercise 2
1. d
2. f
3. g
4. e
5. a
6. h
7. b
8. c
9. j

Exercise 3
1. cerebellum
2. nerve
3. spinal cord
4. meninges
5. brain
6. cerebrum, brain
7. nerve root
8. ganglion
9. nerve root
10. hard, dura mater
11. ganglion
12. nerve root
13. glia, gluey substance

Exercise 4
1. cerebell/o
2. neur/o
3. myel/o
4. a. mening/o
   b. meningi/o
5. encephal/o
6. cerebr/o
7. a. radicul/o
   b. radic/o
   c. rhiz/o
8. dur/o
9. a. gangli/o
   b. ganglion/o
10. gli/o

Exercise 5
1. one, single
2. mind
3. four
4. mind
5. speech
6. sensation, sensitivity, feeling
7. gray matter

Exercise 6
1. quadr/i
2. mon/o
3. a. psych/o
   b. ment/o
4. phas/o
5. poli/o
6. esthesi/o

Exercise 7
1. slight paralysis
2. treatment, specialty
3. seizure, attack
4. specialist, physician

Exercise 8
1. -paresis
2. -iatry
3. -ictal
4. -iatrist

Exercise 9
Pronunciation Exercise

Exercise 10
1. WR   S
    neur/itis
    inflammation of a nerve
2. WR   S
    neur/oma
    tumor made up of nerve (cells)
3. WR   S
    neur/algia
    pain in a nerve
4. WR CV WR CV S
    neur/o/arthr/o/pathy
        CF   CF
    disease of nerves and joints
5. WR   S
    meningi/oma
    tumor of the meninges

6. WR   S
    neur/asthenia
    nerve weakness
7. WR   CV   S
    encephal/o/malacia
          CF
    softening of the brain
8. WR   S
    encephal/itis
    inflammation of the brain
9. WR CV WR CV WR   S
    encephal/o/myel/o/radicul/itis
           CF   CF
    inflammation of the brain, spinal
       cord, and nerve roots
10. WR   S
    mening/itis
    inflammation of the meninges
11. WR   CV S
    mening/o/cele
          CF
    protrusion of the meninges
12. WR CV WR CV S
    mening/o/myel/o/cele
          CF   CF
    protrusion of the meninges
       and spinal cord
13. WR   S
    radicul/itis
    inflammation of the nerve roots
14. WR   S
    cerebell/itis
    inflammation of the cerebellum
15. WR   S
    gangli/itis
    inflammation of a ganglion
16. WR S
    dur/itis
    inflammation of the dura mater
17. P   WR   S
    poly/neur/itis
    inflammation of many nerves
18. WR CV WR S
    poli/o/myel/itis
         CF
    inflammation of the gray matter
       of the spinal cord
19. WR S   WR   S
    cerebr/al thromb/osis
    pertaining to the cerebrum, abnormal
       condition of a clot

20. P WR S WR   S
sub/dur/al hemat/oma
pertaining to below the dura mater;
tumor of blood
21. WR CV WR CV WR S
rhiz/o/mening/o/myel/itis
CF   CF
inflammation of the nerve root,
meninges, and spinal cord
22. WR CV WR CV S
mon/o/neur/o/pathy
CF   CF
disease affecting a single nerve
23. WR CV S
neur/o/pathy
CF
disease of the nerves (peripheral)
24. WR   CV S
radicul/o/pathy
CF
disease of the nerve roots
25. WR   S
gli/oma
tumor composed of glial tissue
26. WR CV WR S
gli/o/blast/oma
CF
tumor composed of developing
glial tissue
27. P   WR CV S
poly/neur/o/pathy
CF
disease of many nerves

Exercise 11
1. neur/itis
2. neur/oma
3. neur/algia
4. neur/o/arthr/o/pathy
5. radicul/o/pathy
6. neur/asthenia
7. encephal/o/malacia
8. encephal/itis
9. encephal/o/myel/o/radicul/itis
10. mening/itis
11. mening/o/cele
12. mening/o/myel/o/cele
13. radicul/itis
14. cerebell/itis
15. gangli/itis
16. dur/itis
17. poly/neur/itis
18. poli/o/myel/itis
19. cerebr/al thromb/osis
20. sub/dur/al hemat/oma
21. rhiz/o/mening/o/myel/itis
22. meningi/oma
23. mon/o/neur/o/pathy

24. neur/o/pathy
25. gli/oma
26. gli/o/blast/oma
27. poly/neur/o/pathy

Exercise 12
Spelling Exercise; see text p. 693.

Exercise 13
Pronunciation Exercise

Exercise 14
1. a. intracerebral hemorrhage
b. cerebral embolism
c. subarachnoid hemorrhage
d. cerebral thrombosis
2. cerebral aneurysm
3. Bell palsy
4. hydrocephalus
5. sciatica
6. shingles
7. transient ischemic attack
8. Parkinson disease
9. epilepsy
10. amyotrophic lateral sclerosis
11. Alzheimer disease
12. cerebral palsy
13. multiple sclerosis
14. dementia

Exercise 15
1. b   10. m
2. a   11. q
3. n   12. d
4. j   13. h
5. l   14. o
6. p   15. c
7. e   16. f
8. g   17. r
9. i

Exercise 16
Spelling Exercise; see text p. 699.

Exercise 17
Pronunciation Exercise

Exercise 18
1. WR CV S
radic/o/tomy
CF
incision into a nerve root
2. WR   S
neur/ectomy
excision of a nerve
3. WR CV   S
neur/o/rrhaphy
CF
suture of a nerve

4. WR   S
ganglion/ectomy
excision of a ganglion
5. WR CV S
neur/o/tomy
CF
incision into a nerve
6. WR CV S
neur/o/lysis
CF
separating a nerve (from adhesions)
7. WR CV S
neur/o/plasty
CF
surgical repair of a nerve
8. WR CV S
rhiz/o/tomy
CF
incision into a nerve root

Exercise 19
1. a. radic/o/tomy
b. rhiz/o/tomy
2. neur/ectomy
3. neur/o/rrhaphy
4. ganglion/ectomy
5. neur/o/tomy
6. neur/o/lysis
7. neur/o/plasty

Exercise 20
Spelling Exercise; see text p. 701.

Exercise 21
Pronunciation Exercise

Exercise 22
1. WR CV   WR   CV S
electr/o/encephal/o/gram
CF   CF
record of the electrical impulses
of the brain
2. WR CV   WR   CV S
electr/o/encephal/o/graph
CF   CF
instrument used to record the
electrical impulses of the brain
3. WR CV   WR   CV S
electr/o/encephal/o/graphy
CF   CF
process of recording the electrical
impulses of the brain
4.   WR CV S
CT myel/o/graphy
CF
process of recording (scan)
the spinal cord

5. WR S WR CV S
   cerebr/al angi/o/graphy
                     CF
   radiographic imaging of the blood
      vessels in the brain

Exercise 23
1. electr/o/encephal/o/gram
2. electr/o/encephal/o/graph
3. electr/o/encephal/o/graphy
4. myel/o/graphy
5. cerebr/al angi/o/graphy

Exercise 24
Spelling Exercise; see text p. 703.

Exercise 25
Pronunciation Exercise

Exercise 26
1. computed tomography
2. lumbar puncture
3. positron emission tomography
4. magnetic resonance imaging
5. evoked potential studies

Exercise 27
1. insertion of a needle into the subarachnoid space
2. process that includes the use of a computer to produce a series of images of
   the brain tissues at any desired depth
3. produces sectional images of the brain
   or spine by a strong magnetic field
4. a technique that produces sectional
   imaging of the brain to examine blood
   flow and metabolic activity
5. a group of diagnostic tests that measure changes and responses in brain
   waves from stimuli

Exercise 28
Spelling Exercise; see text p. 706.

Exercise 29
Pronunciation Exercise

Exercise 30
1.   P   S(WR)
   hemi/plegia
   paralysis of half (left or right side
      of the body)
2.   P   WR S
   par/esthesi/a
   abnormal sensation

3. WR CV S
   neur/o/logist
           CF
   physician who studies and treats
      diseases of the nerves (nervous
      system)
4. WR CV S
   neur/o/logy
           CF
   study of nerves (branch of medicine
      dealing with diseases of the
      nervous system)
5. WR S
   neur/oid
   resembling a nerve
6. WR CV S
   quadr/i/plegia
           CF
   paralysis of four (limbs)
7. WR S
   cerebr/al
   pertaining to the cerebrum
8. WR CV S
   mon/o/plegia
           CF
   paralysis of one (limb)
9. P WR S
   a/phas/ia
   condition of without speaking
10. P   WR S
   dys/phas/ia
   condition of difficulty speaking
11. P   S(WR)
   hemi/paresis
   slight paralysis of half (right or left
      side of the body)
12. P   WR S
   an/esthesi/a
   without (loss of) feeling or sensation
13. P   WR S
   hyper/esthesi/a
   excessive sensitivity (to stimuli)
14. P WR S
   sub/dur/al
   pertaining to below the dura mater
15. WR S
   cephal/algia
   pain in the head (headache)
16. WR CV WR S
   crani/o/cerebr/al
           CF
   pertaining to the cranium
      and cerebrum
17. WR CV S
   myel/o/malacia
           CF
   softening of the spinal cord

18. WR   CV S
   encephal/o/sclerosis
               CF
   hardening of the brain
19.   P   S(WR)
   post/ictal
   (occurring) after a seizure or attack
20.   P   S(WR)
   pan/plegia
   total paralysis
21.   P   S(WR)
   inter/ictal
   (occurring) between seizures
      or attacks
22. WR CV S
   mon/o/paresis
           CF
   slight paralysis of one (limb)
23.   P S(WR)
   pre/ictal
   (occurring) before a seizure or attack
24.   P   WR S
   intra/cerebr/al
   pertaining to within the cerebrum
25. WRCV S
   gli/o/cyte
           CF
   glial cell

Exercise 31
1. hemi/paresis
2. an/esthesi/a
3. hyper/esthesi/a
4. sub/dur/al
5. cephal/algia
6. crani/o/cerebr/al
7. myel/o/malacia
8. encephal/o/sclerosis
9. hemi/plegia
10. neur/o/logist
11. neur/o/logy
12. neur/oid
13. quadr/i/plegia
14. cerebr/al
15. mon/o/plegia
16. a/phas/ia
17. dys/phas/ia
18. pre/ictal
19. mon/o/paresis
20. post/ictal
21. pan/plegia
22. inter/ictal
23. intra/cerebr/al
24. gli/o/cyte
25. par/esthesi/a

Exercise 32
Spelling Exercise; see text p. 711.

Exercise 33
Pronunciation Exercise

Exercise 34
1. concussion
2. unconsciousness
3. conscious
4. seizure
5. convulsion
6. shunt
7. paraplegia
8. coma
9. syncope
10. ataxia
11. gait
12. dysarthria
13. incoherent
14. disorientation
15. cognitive
16. afferent
17. efferent

Exercise 35
1. tube implanted in the body to redirect the flow of a fluid
2. paralysis from the waist down caused by damage to the lower level of the spinal cord
3. state of profound unconsciousness
4. jarring or shaking that results in injury
5. state of being unaware of surroundings and incapable of responding to stimuli as a result of injury, shock, or illness
6. awake, alert, aware of one's surroundings
7. sudden attack
8. sudden involuntary contraction of a group of muscles
9. fainting, or sudden loss of consciousness
10. lack of muscle coordination
11. the inability to use speech that is distinct and connected
12. a manner or style of walking
13. pertaining to the mental processes of comprehension, judgment, memory, and reasoning
14. a state of mental confusion regarding time, place, and identity
15. unable to express one's thoughts or ideas in an orderly, intelligible manner
16. conveying away from the center
17. conveying toward the center

Exercise 36
Spelling Exercise; see text p. 715.

Exercise 37
Pronunciation Exercise

Exercise 38
1. psych/iatry
2. psych/osis
3. psych/o/logy
4. psych/o/genic
5. psych/iatrist
6. psych/o/logist
7. psych/o/somat/ic
8. psych/o/pathy

Exercise 39
1. WR CV WR S
    psych/o/somat/ic
        ‿
        CF
    pertaining to the mind and body
2. WR CV S
    psych/o/pathy
        ‿
        CF
    (any) disease of the mind
3. WR CV S
    psych/o/logy
        ‿
        CF
    study of the mind
4. WR   S
    psych/iatry
    specialty of the mind (branch of medicine that deals with the treatment of mental disorders)
5. WR CV S
    psych/o/logist
        ‿
        CF
    specialist of the mind
6. WR CV S
    psych/o/genic
        ‿
        CF
    originating in the mind
7. WR   S
    psych/iatrist
    a physician who studies and treats disorders of the mind
8. WR   S
    psych/osis
    abnormal condition of the mind

Exercise 40
Spelling Exercise; see text p. 717.

Exercise 41
Pronunciation Exercise

Exercise 42
1. i
2. m
3. b
4. c
5. j
6. a
7. g
8. d
9. h
10. f
11. e
12. n
13. l
14. k

Exercise 43
Spelling Exercise; see text p. 721.

Exercise 44
1. electroencephalogram, magnetic resonance imaging scan, positron emission tomography scan, evoked potential studies, lumbar puncture
2. Alzheimer disease, amyotrophic lateral sclerosis, cerebral palsy, multiple sclerosis, Parkinson disease
3. cerebrovascular accident, transient ischemic attack
4. cerebrospinal fluid
5. posttraumatic stress disorder, obsessive-compulsive disorder, attention deficit hyperactivity disorder
6. central nervous system, peripheral nervous system

Exercise 45
A. 1. disorientation
    2. cognitive
    3. aphasia
    4. conscious
    5. neurology
    6. magnetic resonance imaging
    7. encephalitis
    8. electroencephalogram
    9. seizure
    10. incoherent

B. 1. b
    2. a

Exercise 46
1. quadriplegia
2. aphasia
3. unconscious
4. meningocele
5. psychiatry
6. hardened patches along brain and spinal cord
7. electroencephalography
8. blood clot
9. positron emission tomography
10. ganglia

Exercise 47
Reading Exercise

Exercise 48
1. b
2. *T*
3. a

CHAPTER 16
Endocrine System

OUTLINE

ANATOMY, 736

WORD PARTS, 741
Combining Forms, 741
Suffix, 743

MEDICAL TERMS, 744
Disease and Disorder Terms, 744
   Built from Word Parts, 744
   Not Built from Word Parts, 748
Surgical Terms, 753
   Built from Word Parts, 753
Diagnostic Terms, 754
   Not Built from Word Parts, 754
Complementary Terms, 757
   Built from Word Parts, 757
   Not Built from Word Parts, 760
Abbreviations, 761

PRACTICAL APPLICATION, 762
Interact with Medical Documents, 762
Interpret Medical Terms, 764
Read Medical Terms in Use, 765
Comprehend Medical Terms in Use, 765

CHAPTER REVIEW, 766

OBJECTIVES

Upon completion of this chapter you will be able to:

1. Identify organs and structures of the endocrine system.

2. Define and spell word parts related to the endocrine system.

3. Define, pronounce, and spell disease and disorder terms related to the endocrine system.

4. Define, pronounce, and spell surgical terms related to the endocrine system.

5. Define, pronounce, and spell diagnostic terms related to the endocrine system.

6. Define, pronounce, and spell complementary terms related to the endocrine system.

7. Interpret the meaning of abbreviations related to the endocrine system.

8. Interpret, read, and comprehend medical language in simulated medical statements and documents.

ANATOMY

Function

The endocrine system regulates body activities through the use of chemical messengers called *hormones*, which when released into the bloodstream influence metabolic activities, growth, and development (Figure 16-1). The nervous system also regulates body activities but does so through electrical impulses and activation of glandular secretions. *Hormones* secreted by the *endocrine glands* that make up the endocrine system go directly into the bloodstream and are transported throughout the body. They are referred to as *ductless glands* because they do not have ducts to carry their secretions. In contrast, the *exocrine* or *duct glands* have ducts that carry their secretions from the producing gland to other parts of the body. An example is the parotid gland, which produces saliva that flows through the parotid duct into the mouth. Only those terms related to the major endocrine glands—pituitary, thyroid, parathyroids, adrenals, and the islets of Langerhans in the pancreas—are presented in this chapter. The thymus and the male and female sex glands were discussed in previous chapters.

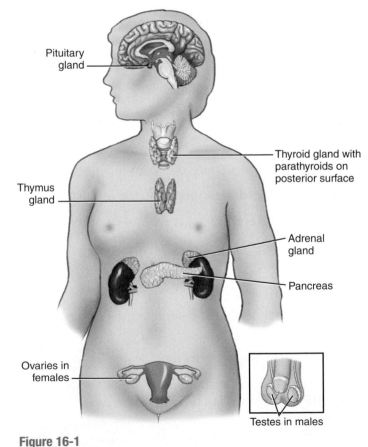

Figure 16-1

The endocrine system.

Endocrine Glands

Term	Definition
pituitary gland or hypophysis cerebri	approximately the size of a pea and located at the base of the brain. The pituitary is divided into two lobes. It is often referred to as the master gland because it produces hormones that stimulate the function of other endocrine glands (Figure 16-2).
anterior lobe or adenohypophysis	produces and secretes the following hormones:
growth hormone (GH)	regulates the growth of the body
adrenocorticotropic hormone (ACTH)	stimulates the adrenal cortex
thyroid-stimulating hormone (TSH)	stimulates the thyroid gland
gonadotropic hormones	affect the male and female reproductive systems
follicle-stimulating hormone (FSH), luteinizing hormone (LH)	regulate development, growth, and function of the ovaries and testes
prolactin or lactogenic hormone (PRL)	promotes development of glandular tissue during pregnancy and produces milk after birth of an infant
posterior lobe or neurohypophysis	stores and releases antidiuretic hormone and oxytocin
antidiuretic hormone (ADH)	stimulates the kidney to reabsorb water
oxytocin	stimulates uterine contractions during labor and postpartum
hypothalamus	located near the pituitary gland in the brain. The hypothalamus secretes "releasing" hormone that functions to stimulate or inhibit the release of pituitary gland hormones.
thyroid gland	largest endocrine gland. It is located in the neck below the larynx and comprises bilateral lobes connected by an isthmus (see Figure 16-3). The thyroid gland secretes the hormones triiodothyronine (T3) and thyroxine (T4), which require iodine for their production. Thyroxine is necessary for body cell metabolism.

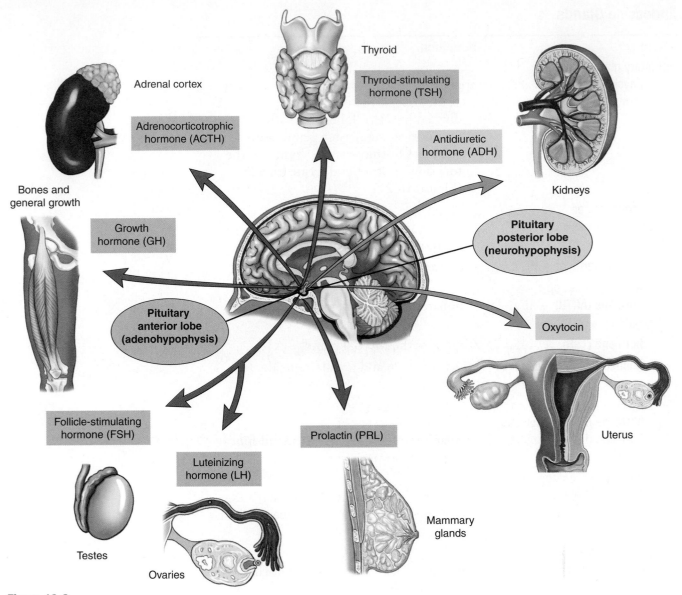

Figure 16-2
Pituitary gland, hormones secreted, and target organs.

Endocrine Glands—*cont'd*

Term	Definition
parathyroid glands	four small bodies lying directly behind the thyroid (Figure 16-3). Parathormone (PTH), the hormone produced by the glands, helps maintain the level of calcium in the blood.
islets of Langerhans	clusters of endocrine tissue found throughout the pancreas, made up of different cell types that secrete various hormones, including insulin and glucagon. Non-endocrine cells found throughout the pancreas produce enzymes that facilitate digestion (Figure 16-4).

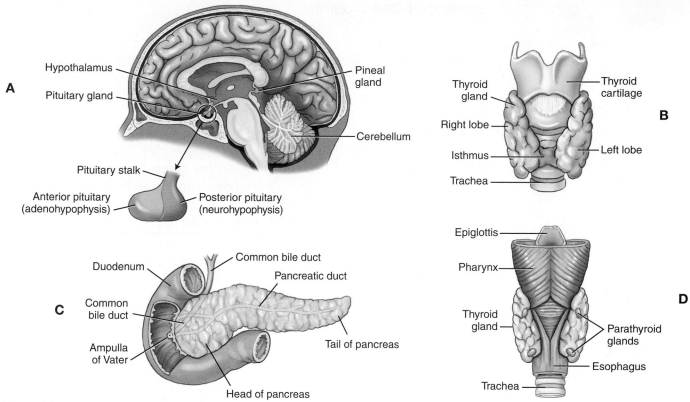

Figure 16-3
A, Pituitary and pineal glands. **B,** Thyroid gland. **C,** Pancreas. **D,** Parathyroid glands, posterior view.

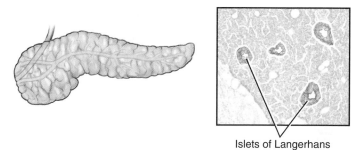

Islets of Langerhans

Figure 16-4
Pancreas, with islets of Langerhans.

Term	Definition
adrenal glands or suprarenals . . .	paired glands, one of which is located above each kidney. The outer portion is called the **adrenal cortex,** and the inner portion is called the **adrenal medulla.** The following hormones are secreted by the adrenal glands:
cortisol	secreted by the adrenal cortex. It aids the body during stress by increasing glucose levels to provide energy (also called **hydrocortisone).**

Endocrine Glands—*cont'd*

Term	Definition
aldosterone.	secreted by the adrenal cortex. Electrolytes (mineral salts) that are necessary for normal body function are regulated by this hormone.
epinephrine (adrenaline), norepinephrine (noradrenaline).	secreted by the adrenal medulla. These hormones help the body to deal with stress by increasing the blood pressure, heartbeat, and respirations.

EXERCISE 1

Match the terms in the first column with the correct definitions in the second column.

_____ 1. adrenal cortex

_____ 2. adrenal glands

_____ 3. adrenaline

_____ 4. adrenal medulla

_____ 5. adrenocorticotropic hormone

_____ 6. adenohypophysis

_____ 7. aldosterone

a. hormone that stimulates the adrenal cortex

b. tissue that secretes cortisol and aldosterone

c. anterior lobe of pituitary that secretes growth hormone and thyroid-stimulating hormone

d. another name for epinephrine

e. assists in regulating body electrolytes

f. another name for norepinephrine

g. located above each kidney

h. secretes epinephrine and norepinephrine

EXERCISE 2

Match the terms in the first column with the correct phrases in the second column.

_____ 1. antidiuretic hormone

_____ 2. islets of Langerhans

_____ 3. neurohypophysis

_____ 4. parathyroid glands

_____ 5. pituitary gland

_____ 6. thyroid gland

a. portions of the pancreas that secrete insulin

b. glands that maintain the blood calcium level

c. gland located in the neck that secretes thyroxine

d. hormone secreted by posterior lobe of the pituitary

e. gland that stores and releases antidiuretic hormone and oxytocin

f. another name for the anterior lobe of the pituitary

g. gland located at the base of the brain

WORD PARTS

Word parts you need to learn to complete this chapter are listed on the following pages. The exercises at the end of each list will help you learn their definitions and spellings.

Combining Forms of the Endocrine System

Combining Form	Definition
aden/o...................	gland
(NOTE: *aden/o* was introduced in Chapter 2.)	
adren/o, adrenal/o	adrenal glands
cortic/o..................	cortex (the outer layer of a body organ)
endocrin/o	endocrine
parathyroid/o	parathyroid glands
pituitar/o.................	pituitary gland
thyroid/o, thyr/o	thyroid gland

EXERCISE FIGURE A

Fill in the blanks with combining forms in this diagram of the endocrine glands.

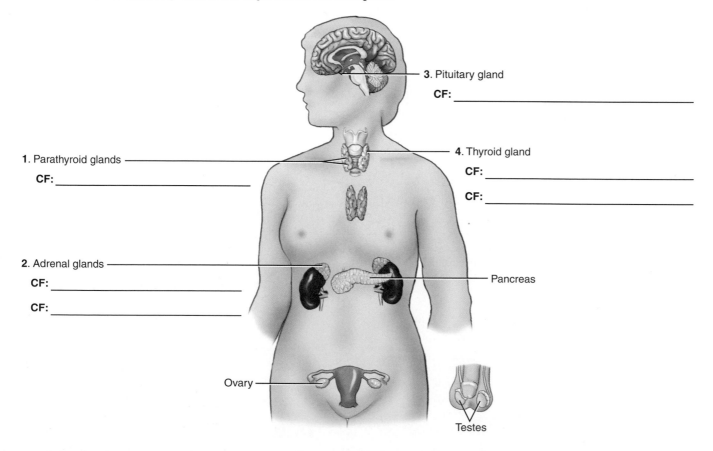

3. Pituitary gland

  CF: _____

1. Parathyroid glands

  CF: _____

4. Thyroid gland

  CF: _____

  CF: _____

2. Adrenal glands

  CF: _____

  CF: _____

Pancreas

Ovary

Testes

EXERCISE FIGURE B

Fill in the blank with the combining form in this diagram of adrenal glands (with transverse cross-sectional view).

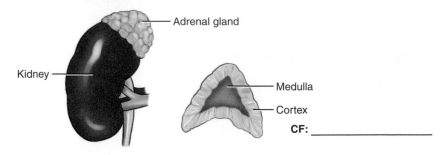

Adrenal gland

Kidney

Medulla

Cortex

CF: _____

EXERCISE 3

Write the definitions of the following combining forms.

1. cortic/o _____   6. thyr/o_____

2. adren/o _____   7. endocrin/o_____

3. parathyroid/o _____   8. aden/o _____

4. thyroid/o _____   9. pituitar/o _____

5. adrenal/o _____

EXERCISE 4

Write the combining form for each of the following terms.

1. adrenal gland a. _____   4. cortex   _____

                  b. _____   5. parathyroid
                                            gland   _____
2. thyroid gland a. _____
                                         6. gland   _____
                  b. _____
                                         7. pituitary gland   _____
3. endocrine   _____

Combining Forms Commonly Used with Endocrine System Terms

Combining Form	Definition
acr/o	extremities, height
calc/i . . . . (NOTE: The combining vowel is *i*.)	calcium
dips/o	thirst
kal/i . . . . (NOTE: the combining vowel is *i*.)	potassium
natr/o	sodium

EXERCISE 5

Write the definitions of the following combining forms.

1. dips/o _____   4. acr/o _____

2. kal/i _____   5. natr/o _____

3. calc/i _____

EXERCISE 6

Write the combining form for each of the following.

1. extremities, height   _____   4. potassium   _____

2. calcium   _____   5. sodium   _____

3. thirst   _____

Suffix

Suffix	Definition
-drome	run, running

Refer to Appendix A and Appendix B for a complete list of word parts.

EXERCISE 7

Write the definition of the following word part.

1. -drome _____

EXERCISE 8

Write the suffix for the following.

1. run, running _____

MEDICAL TERMS

The terms you need to learn to complete this chapter are listed below. The exercises following each list will help you learn the definition and spelling of each word.

Disease and Disorder Terms
Built from Word Parts

The following terms are built from word parts you have already learned and can be translated literally to find their meanings. Further explanation of terms beyond the definition of their word parts, if needed, is included in parentheses.

Term	Definition
acromegaly (*ak*-rō-MEG-a-lē)	enlargement of the extremities (and bones of the face, hands, and feet caused by excessive production of the growth hormone by the pituitary gland after puberty) (Exercise Figure C)
adenitis (ad-e-NĪ-tis)	inflammation of a gland
adenomegaly (*ad*-e-nō-MEG-a-lē)	enlargement of a gland
adenosis (ad-e-NŌ-sis)	abnormal condition of a gland
adrenalitis (a-*drē*-nal-Ī-tis)	inflammation of the adrenal glands
adrenomegaly (a-*drē*-nō-MEG-a-lē)	enlargement (of one or both) of the adrenal glands
hypercalcemia (*hī*-per-kal-SĒ-mē-a)	excessive calcium in the blood
hyperglycemia (*hī*-per-glī-SĒ-mē-a)	excessive sugar in the blood
hyperkalemia (*hī*-per-ka-LĒ-mē-a)	excessive potassium in the blood
hyperpituitarism (*hī*-per-pi-TOO-i-ta-*rizm*)	state of excessive pituitary gland activity (characterized by excessive secretion of pituitary hormones)
hyperthyroidism (*hī*-per-THĪ-royd-izm)	state of excessive thyroid gland activity (characterized by excessive secretion of thyroid hormones)
hypocalcemia (*hī*-pō-kal-SĒ-mē-a)	deficient calcium in the blood
hypoglycemia (*hī*-pō-glī-SĒ-mē-a)	deficient sugar in the blood
hypokalemia (*hī*-pō-ka-LĒ-mē-a)	deficient potassium in the blood

EXERCISE FIGURE C

Fill in the blanks to complete labeling of this photograph.

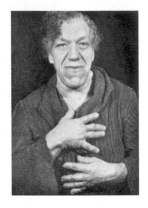

_____ / cv / _____,
extremities   enlargement

a metabolic disorder characterized by marked enlargement of the bones of the face, jaw, and extremities.

HYPOTHYROIDISM
is the state of deficient thyroid gland activity, resulting in the decreased production of the thyroid hormone called thyroxine. A severe form of hypothyroidism in adults is called **myxedema** and in children is called **cretinism.**

Term	Definition
hyponatremia . . . . (hī-pō-na-TRĒ-mē-a)	deficient sodium in the blood
hypopituitarism . . . . (hī-pō-pi-TŪ-i-ta-*rizm*)	state of deficient pituitary gland activity (characterized by decreased secretion of one or more of the pituitary hormones, which can affect the function of the target endocrine gland; for example, hypothyroidism results from decreased secretion of thyroid-stimulating hormone by the pituitary gland)
hypothyroidism . . . . (hī-pō-THĪ-royd-izm)	state of deficient thyroid gland activity (characterized by decreased secretion of thyroid hormones)
panhypopituitarism . . . . (pan-hī-po-pi-TŪ- i-ta-*rizm*) (NOTE: two prefixes contained in this term)	state of total deficient pituitary gland activity (characterized by decreased secretion of all the pituitary hormones; this is a more serious condition than hypopituitarism in that it affects the function of all the other endocrine glands)
parathyroidoma . . . . (*par*-a-*thī*-royd-Ō-ma)	tumor of a parathyroid gland
thyroiditis . . . . (thī-royd-Ī-tis)	inflammation of the thyroid gland

EXERCISE 9

Practice saying aloud each of the disease and disorder terms built from word parts on pp. 744-745.

 To hear the terms select Chapter 16, Chapter Exercises, Pronunciation.

☐ Place a check mark in the box when you have completed this exercise.

EXERCISE 10

Analyze and define the following terms.

1. adrenalitis _____

2. hypocalcemia _____

3. hyperthyroidism _____

4. hyperkalemia_____

5. hyperglycemia_____

6. adrenomegaly _____

7. adenomegaly _____

8. hypothyroidism _____

9. hypokalemia _____

10. adenitis _____

11. parathyroidoma _____

12. acromegaly _____

13. panhypopituitarism _____

14. hypoglycemia _____

15. hypercalcemia _____

16. hyperpituitarism _____

17. hyponatremia _____

18. adenosis _____

19. thyroiditis _____

20. hypopituitarism _____

EXERCISE 11

Build disease and disorder terms for the following definitions with the word parts you have learned.

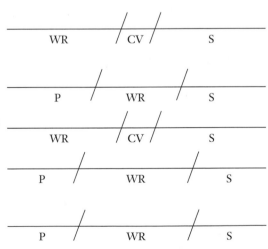

1. enlargement of (one or both) the adrenal glands

    _____ / ___ / _____
    WR   CV   S

2. state of deficient thyroid gland activity

    _____ / ___ / _____
    P   WR   S

3. enlargement of the extremities

    _____ / ___ / _____
    WR   CV   S

4. deficient sugar in the blood

    _____ / ___ / _____
    P   WR   S

5. excessive potassium in the blood

    _____ / ___ / _____
    P   WR   S

6. deficient calcium in the blood _____ / _____ / _____
   P   WR   S

7. state of excessive thyroid gland activity _____ / _____ / _____
   P   WR   S

8. state of deficient pituitary gland activity _____ / _____ / _____
   P   WR   S

9. excessive calcium in the blood _____ / _____ / _____
   P   WR   S

10. state of excessive pituitary gland activity _____ / _____ / _____
    P   WR   S

11. tumor of a parathyroid gland _____ / _____
    WR   S

12. excessive sugar in the blood _____ / _____ / _____
    P   WR   S

13. abnormal condition of a gland _____ / _____
    WR   S

14. deficient potassium in the blood _____ / _____ / _____
    P   WR   S

15. inflammation of the adrenal glands _____ / _____
    WR   S

16. enlargement of a gland _____ / _____ / _____
    WR   CV   S

17. deficient sodium in the blood _____ / _____ / _____
    P   WR   S

18. inflammation of a gland _____ / _____
    WR   S

19. inflammation of the thyroid gland _____ / _____
    WR   S

20. state of total deficient pituitary gland activity _____ / _____ / _____ / _____
    P   P   WR   S

EXERCISE 12

Spell each of the disease and disorder terms built form word parts on pp. 744-745 by having someone dictate them to you.

 To hear and spell the terms select Chapter 16, Chapter Exercises, Spelling. You may type the terms on the screen or write them below in the spaces provided.

☐ Place a check mark in the box if you have completed this exercise using your CD-ROM.

1._____	11._____
2._____	12._____
3._____	13._____
4._____	14._____
5._____	15._____
6._____	16._____
7._____	17._____
8._____	18._____
9._____	19._____
10._____	20._____

Disease and Disorder Terms
Not Built from Word Parts

In some of the following terms, you may recognize word parts you have already learned; however, the full meaning of the terms cannot be discerned by the definition of their word parts.

Term	Definition
acidosis . . . . (*as*-i-DŌ-sis)	condition brought about by an abnormal accumulation of acid products of metabolism seen in uncontrolled diabetes mellitus (see discussion of diabetes mellitus that follows)
Addison disease . . . . (AD-i-sun) (di-ZĒZ)	chronic syndrome resulting from a deficiency in the hormonal secretion of the adrenal cortex. Symptoms may include weakness, darkening of skin, loss of appetite, depression, and other emotional problems.
cretinism . . . . (KRĒ-tin-izm)	condition caused by congenital absence or atrophy (wasting away) of the thyroid gland, resulting in hypothyroidism. The disease is characterized by puffy features, mental deficiency, large tongue, and dwarfism.

 ADDISON DISEASE was named in **1855** for **Thomas Addison,** an English physician and pathologist. He described the disease as a "morbid state with feeble heart action, anemia, irritability of the stomach, and a peculiar change in the color of the skin."

Term	Definition
Cushing syndrome . . . . (KŪSH-ing) (SIN-drŏm)	group of symptoms attributed to the excessive production of cortisol by the adrenal cortices (*pl.* of cortex). This syndrome may be the result of a pituitary tumor or a primary adrenal gland dysfunction. Symptoms include abnormally pigmented skin, "moon face," pads of fat on the chest and abdomen, "buffalo hump" (fat on the upper back), and wasting away of muscle (Figure 16-5).
diabetes insipidus (DI) . . . . (dī-a-BĒ-tēz) (in-SIP-i-dus)	result of decreased secretion of antidiuretic hormone by the posterior lobe of the pituitary gland. Symptoms include excessive thirst (*polydipsia*) and large amounts of urine (*polyuria*) and sodium being excreted from the body.
diabetes mellitus (DM) . . . . (dī-a-BĒ-tēz) (MEL-li-tus)	chronic disease involving a disorder of carbohydrate metabolism caused by underactivity of the islets of Langerhans and characterized by elevated blood sugar (hyperglycemia). DM can cause chronic renal disease, retinopathy, and neuropathy. In extreme cases the patient may develop ketosis, acidosis, and finally coma.
gigantism . . . . (jī-GAN-tizm)	condition brought about by overproduction of growth hormone by the pituitary gland before puberty
goiter . . . . (GOY-ter)	enlargement of the thyroid gland (Figure 16-6)
Graves disease . . . . (grāvz) (di-ZĒZ)	a disorder of the thyroid gland characterized by the presence of hyperthyroidism, goiter, and exophthalmos
ketosis . . . . (kē-TŌ-sis)	condition resulting from uncontrolled diabetes mellitus, in which the body has an abnormal concentration of ketone bodies resulting from excessive fat metabolism
myxedema . . . . (*mik*-se-DĒ-ma)	condition resulting from a deficiency of the thyroid hormone thyroxine; a severe form of hypothyroidism in an adult. Symptoms include puffiness of the face and hands, coarse and thickened skin, enlarged tongue, slow speech, and anemia (Figure 16-7).

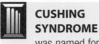

CUSHING SYNDROME was named for an American neurosurgeon, **Harvey Williams Cushing** (1869–1939), after he described adrenocortical hyperfunction.

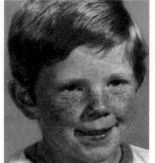
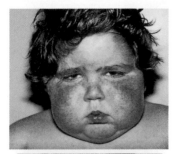

A

B

Figure 16-5

Cushing syndrome. **A,** At diagnosis. **B,** Four months after treatment.

GIGANTISM AND ACROMEGALY are both caused by overproduction of growth hormone. **Gigantism** occurs before puberty and before the growing ends of the bones have closed. If untreated, an individual may reach 8 feet tall in adulthood.

Acromegaly occurs after puberty. The bones most affected are those in the hands, feet, and jaw.

Insufficient production of growth hormone in children is one cause of **dwarfism,** or underdevelopment of the body. In adulthood, a dwarf may be as short as 2.5 feet tall.

Disease and Disorder Terms—*cont'd*
Not Built from Word Parts

GOITER
may be caused by Graves disease, thyroiditis, or a thyroid nodule, which is a lump on the thyroid gland. Goiter is a general term for the enlargement of the thyroid gland.

Because of early medical intervention and because iodine is in table salt and many foods, goiter is rare in the United States today.

Term	Definition
pheochromocytoma . . . . (*fe-ō-krō-*mō-sī-TŌ-ma)	tumor of the adrenal medulla, which is usually benign and characterized by hypertension, headaches, palpitations, diaphoresis, chest pain, and abdominal pain. Surgical removal of the tumor is the most common treatment. Though usually curable with early detection, it can be fatal if untreated.
tetany . . . . (TET-a-nē)	condition affecting nerves causing muscle spasms as a result of low amounts of calcium in the blood caused by a deficiency of the parathyroid hormone
thyrotoxicosis . . . . (*thī-*rō-*tok*-si-KŌ-sis)	a condition caused by excessive thyroid hormones

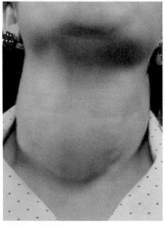

Figure 16-6
Goiter.

EXERCISE 13

Practice saying aloud each of the disease and disorder terms not built from word parts on pp. 748-750.

 To hear the terms select Chapter 16, Chapter Exercises, Pronunciation.

☐ Place a check mark in the box when you have completed this exercise.

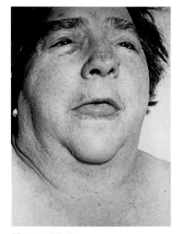

Figure 16-7
Myxedema.

Diabetes Mellitus
Two major forms of diabetes mellitus are **type 1,** previously called *insulin-dependent diabetes mellitus (IDDM)* or *juvenile-onset diabetes,* and **type 2,** previously called *noninsulin-dependent diabetes mellitus (NIDDM)* or *adult-onset diabetes (AODM).* Long-term complications of both types of diabetes mellitus include neuropathy, which can lead to amputation, chronic renal disease, retinopathy, atherosclerosis, coronary artery disease, stroke, and peripheral artery disease.

Type 1 diabetes mellitus

Cause	the beta cells of the pancreas that produce insulin are destroyed and eventually no insulin is produced
Characteristics	abrupt onset, occurs primarily in childhood or adolescence. Patients often are thin.
Symptoms	polyuria, polydipsia, weight loss, hyperglycemia, acidosis, and ketosis
Treatment	insulin injections and diet

Type 2 diabetes mellitus

Cause	resistance of body cells to the action of insulin, which may eventually lead to a decrease in insulin secretion
Characteristics	slow onset, usually occurs in middle-aged or elderly adults. Most patients are obese.
Symptoms	fatigue, blurred vision, thirst, and hyperglycemia; may have neural or vascular complications.
Treatment	diet, exercise, oral medication, and perhaps insulin

EXERCISE 14

Match the terms in the first column with the correct definitions in the second column.

_____ 1. acidosis

_____ 2. Addison disease

_____ 3. cretinism

_____ 4. Cushing syndrome

_____ 5. diabetes insipidus

_____ 6. diabetes mellitus

_____ 7. gigantism

_____ 8. goiter

_____ 9. ketosis

_____ 10. myxedema

_____ 11. tetany

_____ 12. thyrotoxicosis

_____ 13. Graves disease

_____ 14. pheochromocytoma

a. results from a deficiency in the hormonal secretion of the adrenal cortex

b. attributed to the excessive production of cortisol

c. chronic disease involving a disorder of carbohydrate metabolism

d. abnormal accumulation of acid products of metabolism

e. enlargement of the thyroid gland

f. results from low blood calcium

g. caused by excessive thyroid hormones

h. result of a decreased amount of antidiuretic hormone

i. caused by deficiency of the thyroid hormone thyroxine

j. caused by a wasting away of the thyroid gland

k. abnormal concentration of compounds resulting from excessive fat metabolism

l. caused by overproduction of the pituitary growth hormone

m. caused by an excessive amount of parahormone

n. characterized by hyperthyroidism, goiter, and exophthalmos

o. tumor of the adrenal medulla

EXERCISE 15

Write the name of the endocrine gland responsible for each of the following conditions.

1. myxedema _____

2. tetany _____

3. ketosis _____

4. gigantism _____

5. goiter _____

6. Addison disease _____

7. diabetes mellitus _____

8. cretinism _____

9. acidosis _____

10. Cushing syndrome _____

11. diabetes insipidus _____

12. Graves disease _____

13. thyrotoxicosis _____

14. pheochromocytoma _____

EXERCISE 16

Spell each of the disease and disorder terms not built from word parts on pp. 748-750 by having someone dictate them to you.

 To hear and spell the terms select Chapter 16, Chapter Exercises, Spelling. You may type the terms on the screen or write them below in the spaces provided.

☐ Place a check mark in the box if you have completed this exercise using your CD-ROM.

1. _____   8. _____

2. _____   9. _____

3. _____   10. _____

4. _____   11. _____

5. _____   12. _____

6. _____   13. _____

7. _____   14. _____

Surgical Terms
Built from Word Parts

The following terms are built from word parts you have already learned and can be translated literally to find their meanings. Further explanation of terms beyond the definition of their word parts, if needed, is included in parentheses.

Term	Definition
adenectomy . . . . (*ad*-en-EK-to-mē)	excision of a gland
adrenalectomy . . . . (ad-*rē*-nal-EK-to-mē)	excision of (one or both) adrenal glands
parathyroidectomy . . . . (*par*-a-*thī*-royd-EK-to-mē)	excision of (one or more) parathyroid glands
thyroidectomy. . . . . (*thī*-royd-EK-to-mē)	excision of the thyroid gland
thyroidotomy. . . . . (*thī*-royd-OT-o-mē)	incision of the thyroid gland
thyroparathyroidectomy . . . . (*thī*-rō-par-a-*thī*-royd- EK-to-mē)	excision of the thyroid and parathyroid glands

EXERCISE 17

Practice saying aloud each of the surgical terms built from word parts above.

 To hear the terms select Chapter 16, Chapter Exercises, Pronunciation.

☐ Place a check mark in the box when you have completed this exercise.

EXERCISE 18

Analyze and define the following surgical terms.

1. thyroidotomy _____

2. adrenalectomy _____

3. thyroparathyroidectomy _____

4. thyroidectomy _____

5. parathyroidectomy _____

6. adenectomy _____

EXERCISE 19

Build surgical terms for the following definitions by using the word parts you have learned.

1. excision of the thyroid gland

   _____ / _____
   WR   S

2. excision of the thyroid and parathyroid glands

   _____ / _____ / _____ / _____
   WR   CV   WR   S

3. excision of (one or both) adrenal glands

   _____ / _____
   WR   S

4. excision of (one or more) parathyroid glands

   _____ / _____
   WR   S

5. incision of the thyroid gland

   _____ / _____ / _____
   WR   CV   S

6. excision of a gland

   _____ / _____
   WR   S

EXERCISE 20

Spell each of the surgical terms built from word parts on p. 753 by having someone dictate them to you.

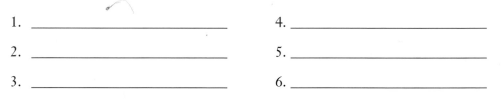 To hear and spell the terms select Chapter 16, Chapter Exercises, Spelling. You may type the terms on the screen or write them below in the spaces provided.

☐ Place a check mark in the box if you have completed this exercise using your CD-ROM.

1. _____   4. _____

2. _____   5. _____

3. _____   6. _____

Diagnostic Terms
Not Built from Word Parts

In some of the following terms, you may recognize word parts you have already learned; however, the full meaning of the terms cannot be discerned by the definition of their word parts.

Ultrasound and **computed tomography (CT scanning)** are also used to diagnose various other conditions of the endocrine system. Examples are CT of the adrenal glands and thyroid ultra-sonography.

Term	Definition
DIAGNOSTIC IMAGING radioactive iodine uptake **(RAIU)** .... (rā-dē-ō-AK-tiv) (Ī-ō-dīn)	a nuclear medicine scan that measures thyroid function. Radioactive iodine is given to the patient orally, after which its uptake into the thyroid gland is measured.

Term	Definition
thyroid scan .... (THĪ-royd)	a nuclear medicine test that shows the size, shape, and function of the thyroid gland. The patient is given a radioactive substance to visualize the thyroid gland. An image is recorded as the scanner is passed over the neck area; used to detect tumors and nodules.

LABORATORY

fasting blood sugar (FBS)......	a blood test performed after the patient has fasted for 8 to 10 hours to determine the amount of glucose (sugar) in the blood at the time of the test. Elevation may indicate diabetes mellitus.
glycosylated hemoglobin (HbA1C)................... (glī-KŌ-sa-*lāt*-ad) (HĒ-mō-*glō*-bin)	a blood test that measures the average blood sugar concentration over the life span of the red blood cell. Results indicate the patient's average blood sugar level for the 6 to 8 weeks before the test, making it a useful tool in monitoring diabetes treatment. (also called **hemoglobin A1C**)
thyroid-stimulating hormone level .... (THĪ-royd)	a blood test that measures the amount of thyroid-stimulating hormone in the blood; used to diagnose hyperthyroidism and to monitor patients on thyroid replacement therapy.
thyroxine level (T4)........... (thī-ROK-sin)	a blood study that gives the direct measurement of the amount of thyroxine in the patient's blood. A greater-than-normal amount indicates hyperthyroidism; a less-than-normal amount indicates hypothyroidism.

EXERCISE 21

Practice saying aloud each of the diagnostic terms not built from word parts on pp. 754-755.

 To hear the terms select Chapter 16, Chapter Exercises, Pronunciation.

☐ Place a check mark in the box when you have completed this exercise.

EXERCISE 22

Match the terms in the first column with their correct definitions in the second column.

_____ 1. fasting blood sugar

_____ 2. thyroid scan

_____ 3. thyroxine level

_____ 4. radioactive iodine uptake

_____ 5. thyroid-stimulating hormone level

_____ 6. glycosylated hemoglobin

a. a nuclear medicine test used to determine the size, shape, and function of the thyroid gland

b. determines the amount of glucose in the blood at the time of the test

c. used to determine hypernatremia

d. uses radioactive iodine to measure thyroid function

e. used to diagnose hyperthyroidism and to monitor thyroid replacement therapy

f. measures the amount of thyroxine in the blood

g. measures the average blood sugar concentration over a period of time

EXERCISE 23

Write the name of the procedure that measures each of the following.

1. thyroid function _____

2. amount of glucose in the blood at the time of the test _____

3. amount of thyroid-stimulating hormone in the blood _____

4. amount of thyroxine in the blood _____

5. size, shape, and function of the thyroid gland _____

6. average blood sugar concentration over a period of time _____

EXERCISE 24

Spell each of the diagnostic terms not built from word parts on pp. 754-755 by having someone dictate them to you.

 To hear and spell the terms select Chapter 16, Chapter Exercises, Spelling. You may type the terms on the screen or write them below in the spaces provided.

☐ Place a check mark in the box if you have completed this exercise using your CD-ROM.

1. _____   4. _____

2. _____   5. _____

3. _____   6. _____

Complementary Terms

Built from Word Parts

The following terms are built from word parts you have already learned and can be translated literally to find their meanings. Further explanation of terms beyond the definition of their word parts, if needed, is included in parentheses.

Term	Definition
adrenocorticohyperplasia (a-*drē*-nō-*kōr*-ti-kō-*hī*-per-PLĀ-zha) (NOTE: *hyper*, a prefix, appears within this word.)	excessive development of the adrenal cortex
adrenopathy (*ad*-ren-OP-a-thē)	disease of the adrenal gland
cortical (KŌR-ti-kal)	pertaining to the cortex
corticoid (KŌR-ti-koyd)	resembling the cortex
endocrinologist (en-dō-kri-NOL-o-jist)	a physician who studies and treats diseases of the endocrine (system)
endocrinology (en-dō-kri-NOL-o-jē)	the study of the endocrine (system) (a branch of medicine dealing with diseases of the endocrine system)
endocrinopathy (en-dō-kri-NOP-a-thē)	(any) disease of the endocrine (system)
euglycemia (*u*-glī-SĒ-mē-a)	normal (level of) sugar in the blood (within normal range)
euthyroid (ū-THĪ-royd)	resembling a normal thyroid gland (normal thyroid function)
polydipsia (*pol*-ē-DIP-sē-a)	abnormal state of much thirst
syndrome (SIN-drōm)	(set of symptoms that) run (occur) together

METABOLIC SYNDROME is a group of related health problems including insulin resistance, obesity characterized by excessive fat around the waist and abdomen, hypertension, hyperglycemia, elevated triglycerides, and low levels of the "good" cholesterol HDL. Risks include development of type 2 diabetes, coronary heart disease, or stroke. Lifestyle changes such as weight loss, regular exercise, healthy eating, and cessation of smoking are central in treatment and prevention; also called **syndrome X** and **insulin resistance syndrome.**

EXERCISE 25

Practice saying aloud each of the complementary terms built from word parts on p. 757.

 To hear the terms select Chapter 16, Chapter Exercises, Pronunciation.

☐ Place a check mark in the box when you have completed this exercise.

EXERCISE 26

Analyze and define the following complementary terms.

1. corticoid _____

2. syndrome_____

3. adrenopathy _____

4. endocrinologist_____

5. polydipsia _____

6. euglycemia _____

7. endocrinopathy_____

8. adrenocorticohyperplasia_____

9. euthyroid_____

10. cortical_____

11. endocrinology_____

EXERCISE 27

Build the complementary terms for the following definitions by using the word parts you have learned.

1. (any) disease of the endocrine (system)

2. resembling the cortex

3. (set of symptoms that) run (occur) together

4. excessive development of the adrenal cortex

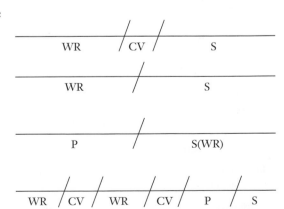

5. the study of the endocrine
   (system)

   _____/_____/_____
   WR   CV   S

6. abnormal state of much thirst

   _____/_____/_____
   P   WR   S

7. disease of the adrenal gland

   _____/_____/_____
   WR   CV   S

8. normal (level of) sugar
   in the blood

   _____/_____/_____
   P   WR   S

9. resembling a normal thyroid
   gland

   _____/_____/_____
   P   WR   S

10. pertaining to the cortex

    _____/_____
    WR   S

11. a physician who studies
    and treats diseases of the
    endocrine (system)

    _____/_____/_____
    WR   CV   S

EXERCISE 28

Spell each of the complementary terms built from word parts on p. 757 by having someone dictate them to you.

 To hear and spell the terms select Chapter 16, Chapter Exercises, Spelling. You may type the terms on the screen or write them below in the spaces provided.

☐ Place a check mark in the box if you have completed this exercise using your CD-ROM.

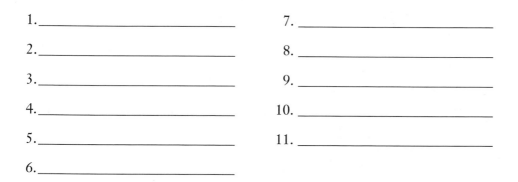

1. _____   7. _____

2. _____   8. _____

3. _____   9. _____

4. _____   10. _____

5. _____   11. _____

6. _____

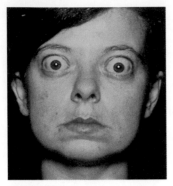

Figure 16-8
Abnormal protrusion of eyeballs, exophthalmos, a characteristic of thyroid disease.

 EXOPHTHALMOS
is derived from the Greek *ex*, meaning **outward**, and **ophthalmos**, meaning **eye**. Protrusion of the eyeball is sometimes a symptom of Graves disease, first described by Dr. Robert Graves, an Irish physician, in 1835.

Complementary Terms
Not Built from Word Parts

In some of the following terms, you may recognize word parts you have already learned; however, the full meaning of the terms cannot be discerned by the definition of their word parts.

Term	Definition
exophthalmos.............. (ek-sof-THAL-mos)	abnormal protrusion of the eyeball (Figure 16-8)
hormone................. (HOR-mōn)	a chemical substance secreted by an endocrine gland that is carried in the blood to a target tissue
isthmus.................. (IS-mus)	narrow strip of tissue connecting two large parts in the body, such as the isthmus that connects the two lobes of the thyroid gland (see Figure 16-3, *B*)
metabolism............... (me-TAB-ō-lizm)	sum total of all the chemical processes that take place in a living organism

EXERCISE 29

Practice saying aloud each of the complementary terms not built from word parts above.

To hear the terms select Chapter 16, Chapter Exercises, Pronunciation.

☐ Place a check mark in the box when you have completed this exercise.

EXERCISE 30

Fill in the blanks with the correct terms.

1. The total of all the chemical processes that take place in a living organism is called its _____.

2. A chemical substance secreted by an endocrine gland is called a(n) _____.

3. A narrow strip of tissue connecting larger parts in the body is called a(n) _____.

4. Abnormal protrusion of the eyeball is called _____.

EXERCISE 31

Write the definitions of the following terms.

1. isthmus _____

2. metabolism _____

3. hormone _____

4. exophthalmos _____

EXERCISE 32

Spell each of the complementary terms not built from word parts on p. 760 by having someone dictate them to you.

 To hear and spell the terms select Chapter 16, Chapter Exercises, Spelling. You may type the terms on the screen or write them below in the spaces provided.

☐ Place a check mark in the box if you have completed this exercise using your CD-ROM.

1. _____   3. _____

2. _____   4. _____

Refer to Appendix E for pharmacology terms related to the endocrine system.

Abbreviations

DI	diabetes insipidus
DM	diabetes mellitus
FBS	fasting blood sugar
HbA1C	glycosylated hemoglobin
RAIU	radioactive iodine uptake
T4	thyroxine level

EXERCISE 33

Write the meaning of the following abbreviations.

1. RAIU _____ _____ _____

2. FBS _____ _____ _____

3. DM _____ _____

4. DI _____ _____

5. T4 _____ _____

6. HbA1C _____ _____

Refer to Appendix D for a complete list of abbreviations.

PRACTICAL APPLICATION

EXERCISE 34 *Interact with Medical Documents*

A. Complete the history and physical by writing the medical terms in the blanks. Use the list of definitions with the corresponding numbers.

University Hospital and Medical Center
4700 North Main Street • Wellness, Arizona 54321 • (987) 555-3210

PATIENT NAME: Jane Nelson   **CASE NUMBER:** 021286-END
DATE OF BIRTH: 05/21/19XX   **DATE:** 06/20/20XX

HISTORY AND PHYSICAL

CHIEF COMPLAINT: Jane Nelson is a 33-year-old Caucasian female presenting with an episode of syncope at work, complaining of excessive urination and thirst and fatigue for approximately 1 month.

HISTORY OF PRESENT ILLNESS: For the past 4 weeks she has been having 1. _____ and 2. _____, drinking 3 to 4 quarts of water daily for the past 10 days. This has also resulted in nocturia, getting up 2 to 3 times a night to void. She denies anorexia, nausea, vomiting, 3. _____, or any abdominal pain.

MEDICAL HISTORY: No known allergies. No previous hospitalizations. She does not smoke or drink. She has had no recent illness.

FAMILY HISTORY: Mother died of a 4. _____ at age 78. Father is still living at the age of 85, but has had 5. _____ _____ for 20 years. She has two brothers, both in good health, and no sisters.

SOCIAL HISTORY: Unmarried without children. She does not smoke and uses alcohol rarely.

REVIEW OF SYSTEMS: She denies fever, chills, headache, palpitations, chest pain, or edema.

PHYSICAL EXAM: Temperature, 98.9. Pulse, 80. Respirations, 24. Her blood pressure is 125/80. Her weight is 143 pounds, down 10 pounds since her last routine visit 3 months ago. **HEENT:** Normal. **CHEST:** Clear to auscultation and percussion. **HEART:** Regular rhythm. No murmurs or extra heart sounds. **ABDOMEN:** Soft, nontender, bowel sounds normal, without evidence of organomegaly. **RECTAL:** Unremarkable. **EXTREMITIES:** No 6. _____ , clubbing, or edema. Pedal pulses are intact. **NEUROLOGIC:** Alert and oriented to time, person, and place. Cranial nerves II through XII are grossly intact.

LABORATORY FINDINGS: Random blood sugar was discovered to be greater than 600 mg/dl. Urinalysis showed moderate ketonuria. Guaiac was negative.

ASSESSMENT: Diabetic 7. _____, most likely caused by type 1 diabetes mellitus.

PLAN: Administer IV fluids and insulin. Schedule 8. _____ consult for this afternoon for complete diagnosis and treatment.

Christina Kraemer, MD

CK/mcm

1. excessive urine
2. excessive thirst
3. vomiting of blood
4. interruption of blood supply to a region of the brain
5. chronic disease involving a disorder of carbohydrate metabolism caused by underactivity of islets of Langerhans and characterized by hyperglycemia

6. abnormal condition of blue (bluish discoloration of skin) caused by inadequate supply of oxygen in the blood
7. abnormal concentration of ketone bodies
8. study of the endocrine system

B. Read the operative report and answer the questions on p. 764.

029210 GOMEZ, RUTH   _ □ X

File Patient Navigate Custom Fields Help

| ‹ | › | 👤 | 👥 | ▯ | ▤ | ▤ | ⌂ | 🕐 | 🔓 | ✂ | ▭ | ✉ | ▦ | ✔ | ? |

| Patient Chart | Lab | Rad | Notes | Documents | Rx | Scheduling | Images | Billing |

Name: **GOMEZ, RUTH**   MR#: **029210**   Sex: **Female**
DOB: **5/11/19XX**

DATE OF OPERATION: April 10, 20XX

SURGERY PERFORMED: Right laparoscopic adrenalectomy

PREOPERATIVE DIAGNOSIS: Primary hyperaldosteronism (Conn syndrome), adrenal adenoma.

INDICATIONS: The patient is a 39-year-old woman who has a history of hypertension and hypokalemia seen on referral from her endocrinologist. The patient complained of headache and muscle weakness. She underwent a 24-hour urine collection, a general metastatic workup, and evaluation for Cushing syndrome. Laboratory studies indicated elevated plasma and urinary aldosterone levels. CT scan revealed the presence of a 3.5-cm right adrenal mass, and adrenal sampling confirmed that it was an aldosterone-producing adenoma.

PROCEDURE: The procedure was performed with the patient under general endotracheal anesthesia and with an arterial line, a Foley catheter, and a central venous pressure line in place. A Veress needle was inserted into the abdominal cavity between the midclavicular and anterior axillary lines. The abdominal cavity was then insufflated with CO_2. A 10- to 11-mm trocar was placed at the site of the Veress needle, and a 30-degree videotelescope was inserted. A third 10- to 11-mm port was placed 3 to 4 cm behind the posterior axillary line, and a fourth port inserted after mobilization of the right lobe of the liver. The superior pole and lateral border of the adrenal gland were mobilized first, with the dissection proceeding carefully along the lateral edge of the inferior vena cava. The right adrenal vein was ligated with endoscopic clips and divided, freeing the adrenal gland from its surrounding attachments. The gland was placed in an impermeable entrapment sac and removed from the most anterior port site. After evacuation of CO_2, all ports were removed, and the incisions were closed with absorbable sutures.

POSTOPERATIVE DIAGNOSIS: Aldosteronoma

Electronically signed by: Merriam Fitch, MD 4/11/20XX 11:24 AM

MF/abr

| Start | Log On/Off | Print | Edit |

1. Which procedure was performed during surgery:
   a. excision of a parathyroid gland
   b. surgical repair of the thyroid gland
   c. excision of an adrenal gland
   d. surgical repair of the thymus

2. The patient had a history of:
   a. excessive sugar in the blood
   b. deficient potassium in the blood
   c. excessive sodium in the blood
   d. deficient calcium in the blood

3. The patient was evaluated for a:
   a. group of symptoms from the excessive production of cortisol
   b. condition caused by congenital absence of the thyroid gland
   c. syndrome caused by deficient secretion from the adrenal cortex
   d. condition causing muscle spasms resulting from low amounts of calcium

EXERCISE 35 *Interpret Medical Terms*

To test your understanding of the terms introduced in this chapter, circle the words that correctly complete the sentences. The italicized words refer to the correct answer.

1. A patient who has an *enlargement of the thyroid gland* has (**myxedema, tetany, goiter**).

2. A condition that results from *uncontrolled diabetes mellitus* is (**calcipenia, ketosis, tetany**).

3. *Addison disease* is caused by an *underfunctioning* of the (**adrenal, pituitary, thyroid**) gland.

4. *Decreased secretion* of (**ACTH, antidiuretic hormone, TSH**) may cause diabetes insipidus.

5. *Cushing syndrome* is caused by (**overactivity, underactivity**) of the *adrenal cortices*.

6. A *wasting away of the thyroid gland* may result in (**cretinism, myxedema, tetany**).

7. The primary treatment for *tumor of the adrenal medulla* (**pheochromocytoma, adenomegaly, thyrotoxicosis**) is surgical removal of the tumor by laparoscopic *excision of an adrenal gland* (**adenectomy, adrenalectomy, thyroidectomy**).

8. Unlike *the blood test measuring the amount of glucose in the blood at the time of the test* (**fasting blood sugar, glycosylated hemoglobin, radioactive iodine uptake test**), *the test measuring average blood sugar level for the previous 6 to 8 weeks* (**fasting blood sugar, glycosylated hemoglobin, radioactive iodine uptake test**) test results are not altered by eating habits the day before the test.

EXERCISE **36**   *Read Medical Terms in Use*

Practice pronunciation of the terms by reading the following medical document. Use the pronunciation key following the medical terms to assist you.

 To hear these terms select Chapter 16, Chapter Exercises, Read Medical Terms in Use.

A 55-year-old female patient presented to her doctor because of a 10-pound weight gain, fatigue, hair loss, dry skin, and cold intolerance. She was referred to an **endocrinologist** (en-dō-kri-NOL-o-jist), who established a diagnosis of **hypothyroidism** (hī-pō-THĪ-royd-izm) after test results indicated an elevated **thyroid** (THĪ-royd)-**stimulating hormone level** and a low **thyroxine** (thī-ROX-sin) **level.** Thyroid hormone therapy was prescribed. Approximately 20 years ago she was diagnosed with Graves disease characterized by hyperthyroidism, **exophthalmos** (ek-sof-THAL-mos), fatigue, irritability, weight loss, and **goiter** (GOY-ter). At this time she had an increased **radioactive iodine** (ra-dē-ō-AK-tiv) (Ī-ō-dīn) **uptake** (RAIU). Treatment included a **thyroidectomy** (thī‾-royd-EK-to-mē) with subsequent thyroid hormone therapy. She remained in a **euthyroid** (ū-THĪ‾-royd) state until she stopped taking the medication 6 months ago. Consequently she became hypothyroid and could easily have developed **myxedema** (mik-se-DĒ-ma) if she had not sought treatment.

EXERCISE **37**   *Comprehend Medical Terms in Use*

Test your comprehension of terms in the previous medical document by circling the correct answer.

1. On a recent visit to the endocrinologist the patient was diagnosed with:
   a. a state of deficient thyroid gland activity
   b. an enlargement of the thyroid gland
   c. a state of excessive thyroid gland activity
   d. Graves disease

2. After a thyroidectomy the patient remained in a state resembling a:
   a. stressed thyroid gland
   b. normal thyroid gland
   c. hyperactive thyroid gland
   d. hypoactive thyroid gland

3. The patient's earlier diagnosis of Graves disease was characterized by:
   a. thirst, excessive thyroid activity, protruding eyes
   b. protruding eyes, spasms, excessive thyroid activity
   c. excessive thyroid activity, enlargement of the thyroid gland, protruding eyes
   d. enlargement of the extremities, excessive thyroid activities, protruding eyes

4. What type of diagnostic procedure was used to assist in diagnosing hypothyroidism?
   a. computed tomography
   b. nuclear medicine
   c. ultrasound
   d. blood test

CHAPTER REVIEW

CHAPTER REVIEW ON CD-ROM

Use the CD-ROM that accompanies this textbook to play and practice what you have learned in this chapter. The Chapter Exercises, Practice Activities, Animations, and Games allow you to hear, see, and interact with the chapter content.

Chapter Exercises

Exercises in this section of your CD-ROM correlate to exercises in your textbook. You may have completed them as you worked through the chapter.
☐ Pronunciation
☐ Spelling
☐ Read Medical Terms in Use

Practice Activities

Practice in study mode, and then test your learning in assessment mode. Keep track of your scores from assessment mode if you wish.

SCORE
☐ Picture It _____
☐ Define Word Parts _____
☐ Build Medical Terms _____
☐ Word Shop _____
☐ Define Medical Terms _____
☐ Use It _____
☐ Hear It and Type It: _____
Clinical Vignettes

Animations
☐ Adrenal Function

Games
☐ Name that Word Part
☐ Term Storm
☐ Term Explorer
☐ Termbusters
☐ Medical Millionaire

REVIEW OF WORD PARTS

Can you define and spell the following word parts?

Combining Forms

acr/o	endocrin/o
aden/o	kal/i
adren/o	natr/o
adrenal/o	parathyroid/o
calc/i	pituitar/o
cortic/o	thyr/o
dips/o	thyroid/o

Suffix

-drome

REVIEW OF TERMS

Can you build, analyze, define, pronounce, and spell the following terms *built from word parts?*

Diseases and Disorders	**Surgical**	**Complementary**
acromegaly	adenectomy	adrenocorticohyperplasia
adenitis	adrenalectomy	adrenopathy
adenomegaly	parathyroidectomy	cortical
adenosis	thyroidectomy	corticoid
adrenalitis	thyroidotomy	endocrinologist
adrenomegaly	thyroparathyroidectomy	endocrinology
hypercalcemia		endocrinopathy
hyperglycemia		euglycemia
hyperkalemia		euthyroid
hyperpituitarism		polydipsia
hyperthyroidism		syndrome
hypocalcemia		
hypoglycemia		
hypokalemia		
hyponatremia		
hypopituitarism		
hypothyroidism		
panhypopituitarism		
parathyroidoma		
thyroiditis		

Can you define, pronounce, and spell the following terms *not built from word parts?*

Diseases and Disorders	**Diagnostic**	**Complementary**
acidosis	fasting blood sugar (FBS)	exophthalmos
Addison disease	glycosylated hemoglobin (HbA1C)	hormone
cretinism	radioactive iodine uptake (RAIU)	isthmus
Cushing syndrome	thyroid scan	metabolism
diabetes insipidus (DI)	thyroid-stimulating hormone level	
diabetes mellitus (DM)	thyroxine level (T4)	
gigantism		
goiter		
Graves disease		
ketosis		
myxedema		
pheochromocytoma		
tetany		
thyrotoxicosis		

ANSWERS

Exercise Figures

Exercise Figure
A. 1. parathyroid glands: parathyroid/o
2. adrenal glands: adren/o, adrenal/o
3. pituitary gland: pituitar/o
4. thyroid gland: thyroid/o, thyr/o

Exercise Figure
B. cortex: cortic/o

Exercise Figure
C. acr/o/megaly

Exercise 1
1. b
2. g
3. d
4. h
5. a
6. c
7. e

Exercise 2
1. d
2. a
3. e
4. b
5. g
6. c

Exercise 3
1. cortex
2. adrenal glands
3. parathyroid glands
4. thyroid gland
5. adrenal glands
6. thyroid gland
7. endocrine
8. gland
9. pituitary gland

Exercise 4
1. a. adren/o
   b. adrenal/o
2. a. thyroid/o
   b. thyr/o
3. endocrin/o
4. cortic/o
5. parathyroid/o
6. aden/o
7. pituitar/o

Exercise 5
1. thirst
2. potassium
3. calcium
4. extremities, height
5. sodium

Exercise 6
1. acr/o
2. calc/i
3. dips/o
4. kal/i
5. natr/o

Exercise 7
1. run, running

Exercise 8
1. -drome

Exercise 9
Pronunciation Exercise

Exercise 10
1. WR   S
   adrenal/itis
   inflammation of the adrenal glands
2. P   WR   S
   hypo/calc/emia
   deficient calcium in the blood
3. P   WR   S
   hyper/thyroid/ism
   state of excessive thyroid gland activity
4. P   WR   S
   hyper/kal/emia
   excessive potassium in the blood
5. P   WR   S
   hyper/glyc/emia
   excessive sugar in the blood
6. WR CV S
   adren/o/megaly
   CF
   enlargement of the adrenal glands
7. WR CV S
   aden/o/megaly
   CF
   enlargement of a gland
8. P   WR   S
   hypo/thyroid/ism
   state of deficient thyroid gland activity
9. P   WR S
   hypo/kal/emia
   deficient potassium in the blood
10. WR   S
    aden/itis
    inflammation of a gland
11. WR   S
    parathyroid/oma
    tumor of a parathyroid gland
12. WR CV S
    acr/o/megaly
    CF
    enlargement of the extremities
13. P   P   WR   S
    pan/hypo/pituitar/ism
    a state of total deficient pituitary gland activity
14. P   WR   S
    hypo/glyc/emia
    deficient sugar in the blood

15. P   WR   S
    hyper/calc/emia
    excessive calcium in the blood
16. P   WR   S
    hyper/pituitar/ism
    state of excessive pituitary gland activity
17. P   WR   S
    hypo/natr/emia
    deficient sodium in the blood
18. WR   S
    aden/osis
    abnormal condition of a gland
19. WR   S
    thyroid/itis
    inflammation of the thyroid gland
20. P   WR   S
    hypo/pituitar/ism
    a state of deficient pituitary gland activity

Exercise 11
1. adren/o/megaly
2. hypo/thyroid/ism
3. acr/o/megaly
4. hypo/glyc/emia
5. hyper/kal/emia
6. hypo/calc/emia
7. hyper/thyroid/ism
8. hypo/pituitar/ism
9. hyper/calc/emia
10. hyper/pituitar/ism
11. parathyroid/oma
12. hyper/glyc/emia
13. aden/osis
14. hypo/kal/emia
15. adrenal/itis
16. aden/o/megaly
17. hypo/natr/emia
18. aden/itis
19. thyroid/itis
20. pan/hypo/pituitar/ism

Exercise 12
Spelling Exercise; see text p. 748.

Exercise 13
Pronunciation Exercise

Exercise 14

1. d	8. e
2. a	9. k
3. j	10. i
4. b	11. f
5. h	12. g
6. c	13. n
7. l	14. o

Exercise 15

1. thyroid
2. parathyroid
3. islets of Langerhans (pancreas)
4. pituitary
5. thyroid
6. adrenal
7. islets of Langerhans (pancreas)
8. thyroid
9. islets of Langerhans (pancreas)
10. adrenal
11. pituitary
12. thyroid
13. thyroid
14. adrenal

Exercise 16
Spelling Exercise; see text p. 752.

Exercise 17
Pronunciation Exercise

Exercise 18

1. WR CV S
    thyroid/o/tomy
         CF
    incision of the thyroid gland
2. WR   S
    adrenal/ectomy
    excision of (one or both) adrenal glands
3. WR CV WR   S
    thyr/o/parathyroid/ectomy
        CF
    excision of the thyroid and parathyroid
       glands
4. WR   S
    thyroid/ectomy
    excision of the thyroid gland
5. WR   S
    parathyroid/ectomy
    excision of (one or more) parathyroid
       glands
6. WR   S
    aden/ectomy
    excision of a gland

Exercise 19

1. thyroid/ectomy
2. thyr/o/parathyroid/ectomy
3. adrenal/ectomy
4. parathyroid/ectomy
5. thyroid/o/tomy
6. aden/ectomy

Exercise 20
Spelling Exercise; see text p. 754.

Exercise 21
Pronunciation Exercise

Exercise 22

1. b	4. d
2. a	5. e
3. f	6. g

Exercise 23

1. radioactive iodine uptake
2. fasting blood sugar
3. thyroid-stimulating hormone level
4. thyroxine level
5. thyroid scan
6. glycosated hemoglobin

Exercise 24
Spelling Exercise; see text p. 757.

Exercise 25
Pronunciation Exercise

Exercise 26

1. WR   S
    cortic/oid
    resembling the cortex
2. P   S(WR)
    syn/drome
    (set of symptoms that) run (occur)
       together
3. WR CV S
    adren/o/pathy
         CF
    disease of the adrenal glands
4. WR   CV S
    endocrin/o/logist
            CF
    a physician who studies and treats
       diseases of the endocrine (system)
5. P   WR S
    poly/dips/ia
    abnormal state of much thirst
6. P WR   S
    eu/glyc/emia
    normal (level of) sugar in the blood
7. WR   CV S
    endocrin/o/pathy
            CF
    (any) disease of the endocrine (system)
8. WR CV WR CV P   S
    adren/o/cortic/o/hyper/plasia
         CF   CF
    excessive development of the adrenal
       cortex

9. P WR   S
    eu/thyr/oid
    resembling normal thyroid
       gland
10. WR   S
    cortic/al
    pertaining to the cortex
11.   WR   CV S
    endocrin/o/logy
            CF
    study of the endocrine (system)

Exercise 27

1. endocrin/o/pathy
2. cortic/oid
3. syn/drome
4. adren/o/cortic/o/hyper/plasia
5. endocrin/o/logy
6. poly/dips/ia
7. adren/o/pathy
8. eu/glyc/emia
9. eu/thyr/oid
10. cortic/al
11. endocrin/o/logist

Exercise 28
Spelling Exercise; see text p. 759.

Exercise 29
Pronunciation Exercise

Exercise 30

1. metabolism	3. isthmus
2. hormone	4. exophthalmos

Exercise 31

1. narrow strip of tissue connecting large
   parts in the body
2. total of all chemical processes that take
   place in living organisms
3. a chemical substance secreted by an
   endocrine gland
4. abnormal protrusion of the eyeball

Exercise 32
Spelling Exercise; see text p. 761.

Exercise 33

1. radioactive iodine uptake
2. fasting blood sugar
3. diabetes mellitus
4. diabetes insipidus
5. thyroxine level
6. glycosylated hemoglobin

Exercise 34

A.
1. polyuria
2. polydipsia
3. hematemesis
4. stroke
5. diabetes mellitus
6. cyanosis
7. ketosis
8. endocrinology

B.
1. c
2. b
3. a

Exercise 35
1. goiter
2. ketosis
3. adrenal
4. antidiuretic hormone
5. overactivity
6. cretinism
7. pheochromocytomas, adrenalectomy
8. fasting blood sugar, glycosylated hemoglobin

Exercise 36
Reading Exercise

Exercise 37
1. a
2. b
3. c
4. d

NOTES

APPENDIX A

Combining Forms, Prefixes, and Suffixes Alphabetized According to Word Part

Combining Forms	Definition	Chapter
A		
abdomin/o	abdomen, abdominal cavity	11
acr/o	extremities, height	16
aden/o	gland	2, 16
adenoid/o	adenoids	5
adren/o	adrenal gland	16
adrenal/o	adrenal gland	16
albumin/o	albumin	6
alveol/o	alveolus	5
amni/o	amnion	9
amnion/o	amnion	9
andr/o	male	7
angi/o	vessel	10
ankyl/o	crooked, stiff, bent	14
an/o	anus	11
anter/o	front	3
antr/o	antrum	11
aort/o	aorta	10
aponeur/o	aponeurosis	14
appendic/o	appendix	11
arche/o	first, beginning	8
arteri/o	artery	10
arthr/o	joint	14
atel/o	imperfect, incomplete	5
ather/o	yellowish, fatty plaque	10
atri/o	atrium	10
aur/i	ear	13
aur/o	ear	13
aut/o	self	4
azot/o	urea, nitrogen	6
B		
balan/o	glans penis	7
bi/o	life	4

Combining Forms	Definition	Chapter
blast/o	developing cell	6
blephar/o	eyelid	12
bronch/i	bronchus	5
bronchi/o	bronchus	5
burs/o	bursa (cavity)	14

C

Combining Forms	Definition	Chapter
calc/i	calcium	16
cancer/o	cancer	2
capn/o	carbon dioxide	5
carcin/o	cancer	2
cardi/o	heart	10
carp/o	carpals (wrist bones)	14
caud/o	tail (downward)	3
cec/o	cecum	11
celi/o	abdomen (abdominal cavity)	11
cephal/o	head	3, 9
cerebell/o	cerebellum	15
cerebr/o	cerebrum, brain	15
cervic/o	cervix	8
cheil/o	lip	11
chlor/o	green	2
cholangi/o	bile duct	11
chol/e	gall, bile	11
choledoch/o	common bile duct	11
chondr/o	cartilage	14
chori/o	chorion	9
chrom/o	color	2
clavic/o	clavicle (collarbone)	14
clavicul/o	clavicle (collarbone)	14
cochle/o	cochlea	13
col/o	colon	11
cocle/o	cochlea	13
colon/o	colon	11
colp/o	vagina	8
coni/o	dust	4
conjunctiv/o	conjunctiva	12
cor/o	pupil	12
core/o	cornea	12
corne/o	pupil	12
cortic/o	cortex (outer layer of body organ)	16
cost/o	rib	14

Combining Forms	Definition	Chapter
crani/o	cranium (skull)	14
cry/o	cold	12
crypt/o	hidden	4
culd/o	cul-de-sac	8
cutane/o	skin	4
cyan/o	blue	2
cyst/o	bladder, sac	6
cyt/o	cell	2

D

Combining Forms	Definition	Chapter
dacry/o	tear, tear duct	12
dermat/o	skin	4
derm/o	skin	4
diaphragmat/o	diaphragm	5
dipl/o	two, double	12
dips/o	thirst	16
disk/o	intervertebral disk	14
dist/o	away (from the point of attachment of a body part)	3
diverticul/o	diverticulum	11
dors/o	back	3
duoden/o	duodenum	11
dur/o	hard, dura mater	15

E

Combining Forms	Definition	Chapter
ech/o	sound	10
electr/o	electricity, electrical activity	10
embry/o	embryo, to be full	9
encephal/o	brain	15
endocrin/o	endocrine	16
enter/o	intestine	11
epididym/o	epididymis	7
epiglott/o	epiglottis	5
episi/o	vulva	8
epitheli/o	epithelium	2
erythr/o	red	2
esophag/o	esophagus	9, 11
esthesi/o	sensation, sensitivity, feeling	15
eti/o	cause (of disease)	2

F

Combining Forms	Definition	Chapter
femor/o	femur (upper leg bone)	14
fet/i	fetus, unborn child	9
fet/o	fetus, unborn child	9

Combining Forms	Definition	Chapter
fibr/o	fiber	2
fibul/o	fibula (lower leg bone)	14

G

gangli/o	ganglion	15
ganglion/o	ganglion	15
gastr/o	stomach	11
gingiv/o	gum	11
gli/o	glia	15
glomerul/o	glomerulus	6
gloss/o	tongue	11
glyc/o	sugar	6
glycos/o	sugar	6
gno/o	knowledge	2
gravid/o	pregnancy	9
gynec/o	woman	8
gyn/o	woman	8

H

hemat/o	blood	5
hem/o	blood	5
hepat/o	liver	11
herni/o	hernia	11
heter/o	other	4
hidr/o	sweat	4
hist/o	tissue	2
humer/o	humerus (upper arm bone)	14
hydr/o	water	6
hymen/o	hymen	8
hyster/o	uterus	8

I

iatr/o	medicine, physician, treatment	2
ile/o	ileum	11
ili/o	ilium	14
infer/o	below	3
irid/o	iris	12
ir/o	iris	12
ischi/o	ischium	14
isch/o	deficiency, blockage	10

J

jejun/o	jejunum	11

Combining Forms	Definition	Chapter
K		
kal/i	potassium	16
kary/o	nucleus	2
kerat/o	cornea	12
kerat/o	horny tissue, hard	4
kinesi/o	movement, motion	14
kyph/o	hump	14
L		
labyrinth/o	labyrinth, inner ear	13
lacrim/o	tear duct, tear	12
lact/o	milk	9
lamin/o	lamina (thin, flat plate or layer)	14
lapar/o	abdomen, abdominal cavity	11
laryng/o	larynx (voice box)	5
later/o	side	3
lei/o	smooth	2
leuk/o	white	2
lingu/o	tongue	11
lip/o	fat	2
lith/o	stone, calculus	6
lob/o	lobe	5
lord/o	bent forward	14
lumb/o	loin (or lumbar region of the spine)	14
lymphaden/o	lymph node	10
lymph/o	lymph, lymph tissue	10
M		
mamm/o	breast	8
mandibul/o	mandible (lower jawbone)	14
mast/o	breast	8
mastoid/o	mastoid	13
maxill/o	maxilla (upper jawbone)	14
meat/o	meatus (opening)	6
melan/o	black	2
meningi/o	meninges	15
mening/o	meninges	15
menisc/o	meniscus (crescent)	14
men/o	menstruation	8
ment/o	mind	15
metr/i	uterus	8
metr/o	uterus	8

Combining Forms	Definition	Chapter
mon/o	one, single	15
muc/o	mucus	5
myc/o	fungus	4
myel/o	bone marrow	10
myel/o	spinal cord	15
my/o	muscle	2, 14
myos/o	muscle	14
myring/o	eardrum	13

N

nas/o	nose	5
nat/o	birth	9
necr/o	death (cells, body)	4
nephr/o	kidney	6
neur/o	nerve	2, 15
noct/i	night	6

O

ocul/o	eye	12
olig/o	scanty, few	6
omphal/o	umbilicus, navel	9
onc/o	tumor, mass	2
onych/o	nail	4
oophor/o	ovary	8
ophthalm/o	eye	12
opt/o	vision	12
orchid/o	testis, testicle	7
orchi/o	testis, testicle	7
orch/o	testis, testicle	7
organ/o	organ	2
or/o	mouth	11
orth/o	straight	5
oste/o	bone	14
ot/o	ear	13
ox/i	oxygen	5
ox/o	oxygen	5

P

pachy/o	thick	4
palat/o	palate	11
pancreat/o	pancreas	11
parathyroid/o	parathyroid gland	16
par/o	bear, give birth to, labor	9

Combining Forms	Definition	Chapter
part/o	bear, give birth to, labor	9
patell/o	patella (kneecap)	14
path/o	disease	2
pelv/i	pelvis, pelvic bone	9, 14
pelv/o	pelvis, pelvic bone	9, 14
perine/o	perineum	8
peritone/o	peritoneum	11
petr/o	stone	14
phalang/o	phalanx (finger or toe bone)	14
pharyng/o	pharynx (throat)	5
phas/o	speech	15
phleb/o	vein	10
phon/o	sound	5
phot/o	light	12
phren/o	diaphragm	5
pituitar/o	pituitary	16
plasm/o	plasma	10
pleur/o	pleura	5
pne	breathing	5
pneumat/o	lung, air	5
pneum/o	lung, air	5
pneumon/o	lung, air	5
poli/o	gray matter	15
polyp/o	polyp, small growth	11
poster/o	back, behind	3
prim/i	first	9
proct/o	rectum	11
prostat/o	prostate gland	7
proxim/o	near (the point of attachment of a body part)	3
pseud/o	false	9
psych/o	mind	15
pub/o	pubis	14
puerper/o	childbirth	9
pulmon/o	lung	5
pupill/o	pupil	12
pyel/o	renal pelvis	6
pylor/o	pylorus (pyloric sphincter)	9, 11
py/o	pus	5

Q

quadr/i	four	15

Combining Forms	Definition	Chapter
R		
rachi/o	spinal or vertebral column	14
radic/o	nerve root	15
radicul/o	nerve root	15
radi/o	radius (lower arm bone)	14
rect/o	rectum	11
ren/o	kidney	6
retin/o	retina	12
rhabd/o	rod-shaped, striated	2
rhin/o	nose	5
rhiz/o	nerve root	15
rhytid/o	wrinkles	4
S		
sacr/o	sacrum	14
salping/o	uterine (fallopian) tube	8
sarc/o	flesh, connective tissue	2
scapul/o	scapula (shoulder bone)	14
scler/o	sclera	12
scoli/o	crooked, curved	14
seb/o	sebum (oil)	4
sept/o	septum	5
sial/o	saliva	11
sigmoid/o	sigmoid	11
sinus/o	sinus	5
somat/o	body	2
somn/o	sleep	5
son/o	sound	6
sperm/o	spermatozoan, sperm	7
spermat/o	spermatozoan, sperm	7
spir/o	breathe, breathing	5
splen/o	spleen	10
spondyl/o	vertebra	14
staped/o	stapes (middle ear bone)	13
staphyl/o	grapelike clusters	4
stern/o	sternum (breastbone)	14
stomat/o	mouth	11
steat/o	fat	11
strept/o	twisted chains	4
super/o	above	3
synovi/o	synovia, synovial membrane	14
system/o	system	2

Combining Forms	Definition	Chapter
T		
tars/o	tarsals (ankle bones)	14
tendin/o	tendon	14
tend/o	tendon	14
ten/o	tendon	14
terat/o	malformation (monster)	9
test/o	testis, testicle	7
therm/o	heat	10
thorac/o	thorax (chest)	5
thromb/o	clot	10
thym/o	thymus gland	10
thyroid/o	thyroid gland	16
thyr/o	thyroid gland	16
tibi/o	tibia (lower leg bone)	14
tom/o	cut, section	6
ton/o	tension, pressure	12
tonsill/o	tonsil	5
trache/o	trachea (windpipe)	5
trachel/o	cervix	8
trich/o	hair	4
tympan/o	eardrum, middle ear	13
U		
uln/o	ulna (lower arm bone)	14
ungu/o	nail	4
ureter/o	ureter	6
urethr/o	urethra	6
ur/o	urine, urinary tract	6
urin/o	urine, urinary tract	6
uter/o	uterus	8
uvul/o	uvula	11
V		
vagin/o	vagina	8
valv/o	valve	10
valvul/o	valve	10
vas/o	vessel, duct	7
ven/o	vein	10
ventricul/o	ventricle	10
ventr/o	belly, front	3
vertebr/o	vertebra	14
vesic/o	bladder, sac	6

Combining Forms	Definition	Chapter
vesicul/o	seminal vesicles	7
vestibul/o	vestibule	13
viscer/o	internal organs	2
vulv/o	vulva	8

X

xanth/o	yellow	2
xer/o	dry	4

Prefix	Definition	Chapter
a-	without, absence of	5
an-	without, absence of	5
ante-	before	9
bi-	two	3, 12
bin-	two	12
brady-	slow	10
dia-	through, complete	2
dys-	painful, abnormal, difficult, labored	2
endo-	within	5
epi-	on, upon, over	4
eu-	normal, good	5
hemi-	half	11
hyper-	above, excessive	2
hypo-	below, incomplete, deficient	2
inter-	between	14
intra-	within	4
meta-	after, beyond, change	2
micro-	small	9
multi-	many	9
neo-	new	2
nulli-	none	9
pan-	all, total	5
para-	beside, beyond, around, abnormal	4
per-	through	4
peri-	surrounding (outer)	8
poly-	many, much	5
post-	after	9
pre-	before	9
pro-	before	2
sub-	under, below	4
supra-	above	14

Prefix	Definition	Chapter
sym-	together, joined	14
syn-	together, joined	14
tachy-	fast, rapid	5
trans-	through, across, beyond	4
uni-	one	3

Suffix	Definition	Chapter
-a	no meaning	4
-ac	pertaining to	10
-ad	toward	3
-al	pertaining to	2
-algia	pain	5
-amnios	amniotic fluid, amnion	9
-apheresis	removal	10
-ar	pertaining to	5
-ary	pertaining to	5
-asthenia	weakness	14
-atresia	absence of a normal body opening, occlusion, closure	8
-cele	hernia, protrusion	5
-centesis	surgical puncture to aspirate fluid	5
-clasia	break	14
-clasis	break	14
-clast	break	14
-coccus (*pl.* cocci)	berry-shaped (a form of bacterium)	4
-cyesis	pregnancy	9
-cyte	cell	2
-desis	surgical fixation, fusion	14
-drome	run, running	16
-eal	pertaining to	5
-ectasis	stretching out, dilatation, expansion	5
-ectomy	excision, surgical removal	4
-emia	blood condition	5
-esis	condition	6
-gen	substance or agent that produces or causes	2
-genesis	origin, cause	2
-genic	producing, originating, causing	2
-gram	record, radiographic image	6
-graph	instrument used to record; record	10
-graphy	process of recording, radiographic imaging	5

Suffix	Definition	Chapter
-ia	diseased or abnormal state, condition of	4
-ial	pertaining to	8
-iasis	condition	6
-iatrist	specialist, physician	15
-iatry	treatment, specialty	15
-ic	pertaining to	2
-ictal	seizure, attack	15
-ior	pertaining to	3
-is	no meaning	9
-ism	state of	7
-itis	inflammation	4
-logist	one who studies and treats, specialist, physician	2
-logy	study of	2
-lysis	loosening, dissolution, separating	6
-malacia	softening	4
-megaly	enlargement	6
-meter	instrument used to measure	5
-metry	measurement	5
-odynia	pain	10
-oid	resembling	2
-oma	tumor, swelling	2
-opia	vision (condition)	12
-opsy	view of, viewing	4
-osis	abnormal condition (means *increase* when used with blood cell word roots)	2
-ous	pertaining to	2
-paresis	slight paralysis	15
-partum	childbirth, labor	9
-pathy	disease	2
-penia	abnormal reduction (in number)	10
-pepsia	digestion	11
-pexy	surgical fixation, suspension	5
-phagia	eating, swallowing	4
-phobia	abnormal fear of or aversion to specific things	12
-physis	growth	14
-plasia	condition of formation, development, growth	2
-plasm	growth, substance, formation	2
-plasty	surgical repair	4
-plegia	paralysis	12
-poiesis	formation	10
-ptosis	drooping, sagging, prolapse	6

Suffix	Definition	Chapter
-rrhagia	rapid flow of blood	5
-rrhaphy	suturing, repairing	6
-rrhea	flow, discharge	4
-rrhexis	rupture	9
-salpinx	uterine (fallopian) tube	8
-sarcoma	malignant tumor	2
-schisis	split, fissure	14
-sclerosis	hardening	10
-scope	instrument used for visual examination	5
-scopic	pertaining to visual examination	5
-scopy	visual examination	5
-sis	state of	2
-spasm	sudden, involuntary muscle contraction	5
-stasis	control, stop, standing	2
-stenosis	constriction or narrowing	5
-stomy	creation of an artificial opening	5
-thorax	chest	5
-tocia	birth, labor	9
-tome	instrument used to cut	4
-tomy	cut into or incision	5
-tripsy	surgical crushing	6
-trophy	nourishment, development	6
-um	no meaning	9
-uria	urine, urination	6
-us	no meaning	10

Combining Forms, Prefixes, and Suffixes Alphabetized According to Definition

Definition	Combining Form	Chapter
A		
abdomen	abdomin/o	11
abdomen	lapar/o	11
abdomen (abdominal cavity)	celi/o	11
above	super/o	3
adenoids	adenoid/o	5
adrenal gland	adren/o	16
adrenal gland	adrenal/o	16
albumin	albumin/o	6
alveolus	alveol/o	5
amnion	amni/o	9
amnion	amnion/o	9
antrum	antr/o	11
anus	an/o	11
aorta	aort/o	10
aponeurosis	aponeur/o	14
appendix	appendic/o	11
artery	arteri/o	10
atrium	atri/o	10
away (from the point of attachment of a body part)	dist/o	3
B		
back	dors/o	3
back, behind	poster/o	3
bear, give birth to, labor, childbirth	part/o	9
bear, give birth to, labor, childbirth	par/o	9
belly, front	ventr/o	3
below	infer/o	3
bent forward	lord/o	14
bile duct	cholangi/o	11
birth	nat/o	9
black	melan/o	2
bladder, sac	cyst/o	6

Definition	Combining Form	Chapter
bladder, sac	vesic/o	6
blood	hemat/o	5
blood	hem/o	5
blue	cyan/o	2
body	somat/o	2
bone	oste/o	14
bone marrow	myel/o	10
brain	encephal/o	15
breast	mamm/o	8
breast	mast/o	8
breathe, breathing	spir/o	5
bronchus	bronch/o	5
bursa (cavity)	burs/o	14

C

Definition	Combining Form	Chapter
calcium	calc/i	16
cancer	cancer/o	2
cancer	carcin/o	2
carbon dioxide	capn/o	5
carpus (wrist bone)	carp/o	14
cartilage	chondr/o	14
cause (of disease)	eti/o	2
cecum	cec/o	11
cell	cyt/o	2
cerebellum	cerebell/o	15
cerebrum, brain	cerebr/o	15
cervix	cervic/o, trachel/o	8
childbirth	puerper/o	9
chorion	chori/o	9
clavicle (collarbone)	clavic/o	14
clavicle (collarbone)	clavicul/o	14
clot	thromb/o	10
cochlea	cochle/o	13
cold	cry/o	12
colon	col/o, colon/o	11
color	chrom/o	2
common bile duct	choledoch/o	11
conjunctiva	conjunctiv/o	12
cornea	corne/o	12
cornea	kerat/o	12
cortex	cortic/o	16
cranium, skull	crani/o	14

Definition	Combining Form	Chapter
crooked, curved	scoli/o	14
crooked, stiff, bent	ankyl/o	14
cul-de-sac	culd/o	8
cut, section	tom/o	6

D

death (cells, body)	necr/o	4
deficiency, blockage	isch/o	10
developing cell	blast/o	6
diaphragm	diaphragmat/o	5
disease	path/o	2
diverticulum	diverticul/o	11
dry	xer/o	4
duodenum	duoden/o	11
dust	coni/o	4

E

ear	ot/o	13
ear	aur/i, aur/o	13
eardrum	myring/o	13
eardrum, middle ear	tympan/o	13
electricity, electrical activity	electr/o	10
embryo, to be full	embry/o	9
endocrine	endocrin/o	16
epididymis	epididym/o	7
epiglottis	epiglott/o	5
epithelium	epitheli/o	2
esophagus	esophag/o	9, 11
extremities, height	acr/o	16
eye	ophthalm/o	12
eye	ocul/o	12
eyelid	blephar/o	12

F

fallopian tube	salping/o	8
false	pseud/o	9
fat	lip/o	2
fat	steat/o	11
femur (upper leg bone)	femor/o	14
fetus, unborn child	fet/o, fet/i	9
fiber	fibr/o	2
fibula (lower leg bone)	fibul/o	14
first	prim/i	9

Definition	Combining Form	Chapter
first, beginning	arche/o	8
flesh, connective tissue	sarc/o	2
four	quadr/i	15
fungus	myc/o	3

G

gall, bile	chol/e	11
ganglion	gangli/o	15
ganglion	ganglion/o	15
gland	aden/o	2, 16
glans penis	balan/o	7
glia	gli/o	15
glomerulus	glomerul/o	6
grapelike clusters	staphyl/o	4
gray matter	poli/o	15
green	chlor/o	2
gum	gingiv/o	11

H

hair	trich/o	4
hard, dura mater	dur/o	15
head	cephal/o	3, 9
hearing	audi/o	13
heart	cardi/o	10
heat	therm/o	10
hernia	herni/o	11
hidden	crypt/o	4
horny tissue, hard	kerat/o	4
humerus (upper arm bone)	humer/o	14
hump	kyph/o	14
hymen	hymen/o	8

I

ileum	ile/o	11
ilium	ili/o	14
imperfect, incomplete	atel/o	5
inner ear	labyrinth/o	13
internal organs	viscer/o	2
intervertebral disk	disk/o	14
intestine	enter/o	11
iris	irid/o	12

Definition	Combining Form	Chapter
iris	ir/o	12
ischium	ischi/o	14

J

jejunum	jejun/o	11
joint	arthr/o	14

K

kidney	nephr/o	6
kidney	ren/o	6
knowledge	gno/o	2

L

labyrinth	labyrinth/o	13
lamina (thin flat plate or layer)	lamin/o	14
larynx	laryng/o	5
life	bi/o	4
light	phot/o	12
lip	cheil/o	11
liver	hepat/o	11
lobe	lob/o	5
lung	pulmon/o	5
lung, air	pneumat/o	5
lung, air	pneum/o	5
lung, air	pneumon/o	5
lymph node	lymphaden/o	10
lymph, lymph tissue	lymph/o	10

M

male	andr/o	7
malformation (monster)	terat/o	9
mandible (lower jaw bone)	mandibul/o	14
mastoid	mastoid/o	13
maxilla (upper jaw bone)	maxill/o	14
meatus (opening)	meat/o	6
medicine (treatment)	iatr/o	2
meninges	mening/o, meningi/o	15
meniscus (crescent)	menisc/o	14
menstruation	men/o	8
middle	medi/o	3
mind	ment/o	15
mind	psych/o	15
mouth	or/o	11
mouth	stomat/o	11

Definition	Combining Form	Chapter
movement, motion	kinesi/o	14
mucus	muc/o	5
muscle	my/o	2, 14
muscle	myos/o	14
N		
nail	ungu/o	4
nail	onych/o	4
near (the point of attachment of a body part)	proxim/o	3
nerve	neur/o	2, 15
nerve root	radicul/o	15
nerve root	radic/o	15
nerve root	rhiz/o	15
night	noct/i	6
nose	rhin/o	5
nose	nas/o	5
nucleus	kary/o	2
O		
one, single	mon/o	15
organ	organ/o	2
other	heter/o	4
ovary	oophor/o	8
oxygen	ox/o, ox/i	5
P		
palate	palat/o	11
pancreas	pancreat/o	11
parathyroid gland	parathyroid/o	16
patella (kneecap)	patell/o	14
pelvis, pelvic bone	pelv/i, pelv/o	14
perineum	perine/o	8
peritoneum	peritone/o	11
phalanx (finger or toe)	phalang/o	14
pharynx	pharyng/o	5
physician (treatment)	iatr/o	2
plasma	plasm/o	10
pleura	pleur/o	5
potassium	kal/i	16
pregnancy	gravid/o	9
prostate gland	prostat/o	7
pubis	pub/o	14

Definition	Combining Form	Chapter
pupil	core/o, cor/o	12
pupil	pupill/o	12
pus	py/o	5
pylorus, pyloric sphincter	pylor/o	9, 11
R		
radius (lower arm bone)	radi/o	14
rectum	proct/o	11
rectum	rect/o	11
red	erythr/o	2
renal pelvis	pyel/o	6
retina	retin/o	12
rib	cost/o	14
rod-shaped, striated	rhabd/o	2
S		
sacrum	sacr/o	14
saliva	sial/o	11
scanty, few	olig/o	6
scapula (shoulder blade)	scapul/o	14
sclera	scler/o	12
sebum (oil)	seb/o	4
self	aut/o	4
seminal vesicles	vesicul/o	7
sensation, sensitivity, feeling	esthesi/o	14
septum	sept/o	5
side	later/o	3
sigmoid	sigmoid/o	11
sinus	sinus/o	5
skin	cutane/o	4
skin	dermat/o	4
skin	derm/o	4
sleep	somn/o	5
small growth	polyp/o	11
smooth	lei/o	2
sound	son/o	6
sound	ech/o	10
speech	phas/o	15
spermatozoa, sperm	sperm/o	7
spermatozoa, sperm	spermat/o	7
spinal cord	myel/o	15
spleen	splen/o	10

Definition	Combining Form	Chapter
stapes	staped/o	13
sternum (breast bone)	stern/o	14
stomach	gastr/o	11
stone	petr/o	14
stone, calculus	lith/o	6
straight	orth/o	5
sugar	glycos/o	6
sugar	glyc/o	6
sweat	hidr/o	4
synovia, synovial membrane	synovi/o	14
system	system/o	2

T

Definition	Combining Form	Chapter
tail (downward)	caud/o	3
tarsus (ankle bone)	tars/o	14
tear duct, tear	lacrim/o	12
tear, tear duct	dacry/o	12
tendon	ten/o	14
tendon	tendin/o	14
tendon	tend/o	14
tension, pressure	ton/o	12
testis, testicle	orch/o	7
testis, testicle	test/o	7
testis, testicle	orchi/o	7
testis, testicle	orchid/o	7
thick	pachy/o	4
thirst	dips/o	16
thorax (chest)	thorac/o	5
thymus gland	thym/o	10
thyroid gland	thyroid/o	16
thyroid gland	thyr/o	16
tibia (lower leg bone)	tibi/o	14
tissue	hist/o	2
tongue	lingu/o	11
tongue	gloss/o	11
tonsils	tonsill/o	5
trachea	trache/o	5
tumor	onc/o	2
twisted chains	strept/o	4
two, double	dipl/o	12

Definition	Combining Form	Chapter
U		
ulna (lower arm bone)	uln/o	14
umbilicus, navel	omphal/o	9
urea, nitrogen	azot/o	6
ureter	ureter/o	6
urethra	urethr/o	6
urinary bladder	vesic/o, cyst/o	6
urine, urinary tract	urin/o	6
urine, urinary tract	ur/o	6
uterus	uter/o	8
uterus	metr/o, metr/i	8
uterus	hyster/o	8
uvula	uvul/o	11
V		
vagina	vagin/o	8
vagina	colp/o	8
valve	valv/o	10
valve	valvul/o	10
vein	phleb/o	10
vein	ven/o	10
ventricle	ventricul/o	10
vertebra	vertebr/o	14
vertebral or spinal column	rachi/o	14
vessel	angi/o	10
vessel, duct	vas/o	7
vestibule	vestibul/o	13
vision	opt/o	12
vulva	vulv/o	8
vulva	episi/o	8
W		
water	hydr/o	6
white	leuk/o	2
woman	gyn/o	8
woman	gynec/o	8
wrinkles	rhytid/o	4
Y		
yellow	xanth/o	2
yellowish, fatty plaque	ather/o	10

Definition	Prefix	Chapter
above	supra-	14
above, excessive	hyper-	2
after	post-	9
after, beyond, change	meta-	2
all, total	pan-	5
before	ante-, pre-	9
before	pro-	2
below, incomplete, deficient	hypo-	2
beside, beyond, around, abnormal	para-	4
between	inter-	14
difficult, labored, painful, abnormal	dys-	2
fast, rapid	tachy-	10
four	quadri-	14
half	hemi-	11
many	multi-	9
many, much	poly-	5
new	neo-	2
none	nulli-	9
normal	eu-	5
on, upon, over	epi-	4
one	uni-	3
outside, outward	ex-, exo-	16
slow	brady-	10
small	micro-	9
surrounding (outer)	peri-	8
through, complete	per-	4
through	dia-	2
through, across, beyond	trans-	4
together, joined	sym-	14
together, joined	syn-	14
two	bin-	14
two	bi-	2, 14
under, below	sub-	4
within	intra-	4
within	endo-	5
without, absence of	a-, an-	5

Definition	Suffix	Chapter
abnormal condition (means *increase* when used with blood cell word roots)	-osis	2
abnormal fear of or aversion to specific things	-phobia	12
abnormal reduction (in number)	-penia	10
absence of a normal opening, occlusion, closure	-atresia	8
amnion, amniotic fluid	-amnios	9
berry-shaped (a form of bacterium)	-coccus (*pl.* -cocci)	4
birth, labor	-tocia	9
blood condition	-emia	5
break	-clasis	14
break	-clasia	14
break	-clast	14
breathing	-pnea	5
cell	-cyte	2
chest	-thorax	5
childbirth	-partum	9
condition	-iasis	6
condition	-esis	6
condition of formation, development, growth	-plasia	2
constriction, narrowing	-stenosis	5
control, stop, standing	-stasis	2
creation of an artificial opening	-stomy	5
cut into or incision	-tomy	5
digestion	-pepsia	11
disease	-pathy	2
diseased or abnormal state	-ia	4
drooping, sagging, prolapse	-ptosis	6
eating, swallowing	-phagia	4
enlargement	-megaly	6
excision, surgical removal	-ectomy	4
fallopian tube	-salpinx	7
flow, discharge	-rrhea	4
formation	-poiesis	10
growth	-physis	14
growth, substance, formation	-plasm	2
hardening	-sclerosis	10
hernia, protrusion	-cele	5
inflammation	-itis	4

Definition	Suffix	Chapter
instrument used for visual examination	-scope	5
instrument used to measure	-meter	5
instrument used to cut	-tome	4
instrument used to record; record	-graph	10
labor	-partum	9
loosening, dissolution, separating	-lysis	6
malignant tumor	-sarcoma	2
measurement	-metry	5
nourishment, development	-trophy	6
one who studies and treats (specialist, physician)	-logist	2
origin, cause	-genesis	2
oxygen	-oxia	5
pain	-dynia	10
pain	-algia	5
paralysis	-plegia	12
pertaining to	-ac	10
pertaining to	-ous	2, 6
pertaining to	-ar	5
pertaining to	-ic	2
pertaining to	-ial	8
pertaining to	-ior	3
pertaining to	-eal	5
pertaining to	-ary	5
pertaining to	-al	2
pertaining to sound or voice	-phonia	5
pertaining to visual examination	-scopic	5
physician, specialist	-iatrist	15
pregnancy	-cyesis	9
process of recording, radiographic imaging	-graphy	5
producing, originating, causing	-genic	2
rapid flow of blood	-rrhagia	5
record, radiographic image	-gram	5
removal	-apheresis	10
resembling	-oid	2
run, running	-drome	16
rupture	-rrhexis	9
seizure, attack	-ictal	15
slight paralysis	-paresis	15

Definition	Suffix	Chapter
softening	-malacia	4
split, fissure	-schisis	14
state of	-ism	7
state of	-sis	2
stretching out, dilation, expansion	-ectasis	5
study of	-logy	2
substance or agent that produces or causes	-gen	2
sudden, involuntary muscle contraction	-spasm	5
surgical crushing	-tripsy	6
surgical fixation, fusion	-desis	14
surgical fixation, suspension	-pexy	5
surgical puncture to aspirate fluid	-centesis	5
surgical repair	-plasty	4
suturing, repairing	-rrhaphy	6
toward	-ad	3
treatment, specialty	-iatry	15
tumor, swelling	-oma	2
urine, urination	-uria	6
view of, viewing	-opsy	4
vision (condition)	-opia	12
visual examination	-scopy	5
weakness	-asthenia	14

Additional Combining Forms, Prefixes, and Suffixes

The following word parts were not included in the text. They are listed here for your easy reference. *As you discover word parts not included in this list, add them to the space provided at the end of Appendix C.*

Combining Form	Definition
acanth/o	thorny, spiny
acetabul/o	acetabulum (hip socket)
actin/o	ray, radius
aer/o	air, gas
algesi/o	pain
ambly/o	dull, dim
amyl/o	starch
anis/o	unequal, dissimilar
arteriol/o	arteriole (small artery)
articul/o	joint
axill/o	armpit
bacteri/o	bacteria
bil/i	bile
brachi/o	arm
bucc/o	cheek
cerumin/o	cerumen (earwax)
chir/o	hand
cry/o	cold
dactyl/o	fingers or toes
dent/i	tooth
dextr/o	right
diaphor/o	sweat
dynam/o	power, strength
ectop/o	located away from usual place
emmetr/o	a normal measure
faci/o	face
ger/o	old age, aged
geront/o	old age, aged
gluc/o	sweetness, sugar

Combining Form	Definition
gnath/o	jaw
gon/o	seed
home/o	sameness, unchanging
hom/o	same
hypn/o	sleep
ichthy/o	fish
immun/o	immune
is/o	equal, same
kin/e	movement
labi/o	lips
macr/o	abnormal largeness
morph/o	form, shape
myelon/o	spinal cord
narc/o	stupor
nyct/o	night
nyctal/o	night
oo/o	egg, ovum
ov/i	egg
ov/o	egg
papill/o	nipple
pector/o	chest
ped/o	child, foot
phac/o	lens of the eye
phak/o	lens of the eye
physi/o	nature
pil/o	hair
pod/o	foot
poikil/o	varied, irregular

Combining Form	Definition
pyr/o	fever, heat
scirrh/o	hard, relationship to hard cancer
stear/o	fat
tars/o	edge of the eyelid, tarsal (instep of foot)
top/o	place
toxic/o	poison

Prefix	Definition
ab-	from, away from
ana-	up, again, backward
anti-	against
apo-	upon
cata-	down
con-	together
contra-	against
de-	from, down from, lack of
di-	two
dis-	to undo, free from
ecto-	outside, outer
eso-	inward
ex-	outside, outward
exo-	outside, outward
extra-	outside of, beyond
in-	in, into, not
infra-	under, below
mal-	bad
meso-	middle
re-	back
retro-	back, behind
semi-	half

Prefix	Definition
tetra-	four
toc-	childbirth, labor
tri-	three
ultra-	beyond, excess

Suffix	Definition
-agra	excessive pain
-ase	enzyme
-cidal	killing
-clysis	irrigating, washing
-crine	separate, secrete
-crit	to separate
-ectopia	displacement
-emesis	vomiting
-er	one who
-ician	one who
-lepsy	seizure
-lytic	destroy, reduce
-mania	madness, insane desire
-morph	form, shape
-odia	smell
-opia	vision
-philia	love
-phily	love
-phoria	feeling
-porosis	passage
-prandial	meal
-praxia	in front of, before
-ptysis	spitting
-sepsis	infection
-stalsis	contraction
-ule	little

Record additional word parts below that you have discovered:

Abbreviations

These abbreviations are written as they appear most commonly in the medical and health care environment. Some may also appear in both capital and small letters and with or without periods.

Common Medical Abbreviations	Definitions
ab	abortion
abd	abdomen
ABE	acute bacterial endocarditis
ABGs	arterial blood gases
a.c.	before meals
ACS	acute cardiac syndrome
ACTH	adrenocorticotropic hormone
AD	Alzheimer disease
ADH	antidiuretic hormone
ADL	activities of daily living
ad lib	as desired
Adm	admission
AFB	acid-fast bacillus
AFib	atrial fibrillation
AHD	arteriosclerotic heart disease
AI	aortic insufficiency
AICD	automatic implantable cardioverter defibrillator
AIDS	acquired immune deficiency syndrome
AKA	above-knee amputation
ALB	albumin
alk phos	alkaline phosphatase
ALL	acute lymphocytic leukemia
ALS	amyotrophic lateral sclerosis
AM	between midnight and noon

Common Medical Abbreviations	Definitions
AMA	against medical advice; American Medical Association
amb.	ambulate, ambulatory
AMI	acute myocardial infarction
AML	acute myelocytic leukemia
amp.	ampule
amt	amount
ant	anterior
AODM	adult-onset diabetes mellitus
AOM	acute otitis media
AP	anteroposterior; angina pectoris
A&P	auscultation and percussion; anterior and posterior colporrhaphy
ARDS	adult respiratory distress syndrome
ARM	artificial rupture of membranes
ARMD	age-related macular degeneration
ART	assisted reproductive technology
ASA	aspirin
ASCVD	arteriosclerotic cardiovascular disease
ASD	atrial septal defect
ASHD	arteriosclerotic heart disease

Common Medical Abbreviations	Definitions
Ast	astigmatism
as tol	as tolerated
AUL	acute undifferentiated leukemia
AV	arteriovenous
AVR	aortic valve replacement
ax	axillary
BA	bronchial asthma
BBB	bundle branch block
BCC	basal cell carcinoma
BE	barium enema
b.i.d.	twice a day
BK	below knee
BKA	below-knee amputation
BM	bowel movement
BOM	bilateral otitis media
BP	blood pressure
BPH	benign prostatic hyperplasia
BR	bedrest
BRP	bathroom privileges
BS	blood sugar; bowel sounds; breath sounds
BSO	bilateral salpingo-oophorectomy
BUN	blood urea nitrogen
Bx	biopsy
$\bar{c}$	with
C	Celsius
C_1-C_7	cervical vertebrae
Ca	calcium
CA	cancer; carcinoma
CABG	coronary artery bypass graft
CAD	coronary artery disease
CAL	calorie
CAP	capsule
CAPD	continuous ambulatory peritoneal dialysis
cath	catheterization
CBC	complete blood count

Common Medical Abbreviations	Definitions
CBR	complete bed rest
CBS	chronic brain syndrome
CC	chief complaint or colony count
CCU	coronary care unit
CDH	congenital dislocation of the hip
CEA	carcinoembryonic antigen
CF	cystic fibrosis
CHB	complete heart block
CHD	coronary heart disease
CHF	congestive heart failure
CHO	carbohydrate
chemo	chemotherapy
chol	cholesterol
CI	coronary insufficiency
circ	circumcision
CIS	carcinoma in situ
Cl	chloride
CLD	chronic liver disease
CLL	chronic lymphocytic leukemia
cl liq	clear liquid
cm	centimeter
CML	chronic myelogenous leukemia
CNS	central nervous system
c/o	complains of
CO	carbon monoxide
CO_2	carbon dioxide
COB	coordination of benefits
COLD	chronic obstructive lung disease
comp	compound
cond	condition
COPD	chronic obstructive pulmonary disease
CP	cerebral palsy
CPAP	continuous positive airway pressure
CPD	cephalopelvic disproportion

Common Medical Abbreviations | Definitions

Common Medical Abbreviations	Definitions
CPK	creatine phosphokinase
CPN	chronic pyelonephritis
CPR	cardiopulmonary resuscitation
CRD	chronic respiratory disease
creat	creatinine
CRF	chronic renal failure
CRP	C-reactive protein
C&S	culture and sensitivity
C/S, CS, C-section	cesarean section
CSF	cerebrospinal fluid
CT	computed tomography
CTS	carpal tunnel syndrome
Cu	copper
CVA	cerebrovascular accident
CVP	central venous pressure
Cx	cervix
CXR	chest x-ray
DAT	diet as tolerated
D&C	dilation and curettage
del	delivery
derm	dermatology
DI	diabetes insipidus
DIC	diffuse intravascular coagulation
diff	differential (part of complete blood count)
disch	discharge
DLE	discoid lupus erythematosus
DM	diabetes mellitus
DNA	deoxyribonucleic acid
DOA	dead on arrival
DOB	date of birth
Dr	dram
DRG	diagnosis-related group
DSA	digital subtraction angiography
DVT	deep vein thrombosis
DW	distilled water

Common Medical Abbreviations	Definitions
D/W	dextrose in water
Dx	diagnosis
E	enema
EBL	estimated blood loss
ECG	electrocardiogram
echo	echocardiogram
ECT	electroconvulsive herapy
ED	emergency department
EDD	estimated date of delivery
EEG	electroencephalogram
EENT	eyes, ears, nose, and throat
EGD	esophagogastroduodenoscopy
EKG	electrocardiogram
Elix	elixir
EM	emmetropia
EMG	electromyogram
ENG	electronystagmography
ENT	ears, nose, and throat
EP	ectopic pregnancy
EP studies	evoked potential studies
ERCP	endoscopic retrograde cholangiopancreatography
ERT	estrogen replacement therapy
ESR	erythrocyte sedimentation rate
ESRD	end-stage renal disease
ESWL	extracorporeal shock-wave lithotripsy
etio	etiology
exam	examination
ext	extract; external
F	Fahrenheit
FAS	fetal alcohol syndrome
FBD	fibrocystic breast disease
FBS	fasting blood sugar
Fe	iron

Common Medical Abbreviations	Definitions
FHT	fetal heart tones
flu	influenza
FOBT	fecal occult blood test
Fr	French (catheter size)
FS	frozen section
FSH	follicle-stimulating hormone
FTT	failure to thrive
FUO	fever of undetermined origin
Fx	fracture
g	gram
GC	gonorrhea culture
GERD	gastroesophageal reflux disease
GI	gastrointestinal
GSW	gunshot wound
gtt	drops
GTT	glucose tolerance test
GU	genitourinary
Gyn	gynecology
h	hour
H	hypodermic
HAART	highly active antiretroviral therapy
HB	heart block
HCVD	hypertensive cardiovascular disease
HD	hemodialysis
HHD	hypertensive heart disease
H&H	hemoglobin and hematocrit
HCl	hydrochloric acid
HCO_3	bicarbonate
Hct	hematocrit
Hg	mercury
hgb	hemoglobin
HIV	human immunodeficiency virus
HMD	hyaline membrane disease
HNP	herniated nucleus pulposus

Common Medical Abbreviations	Definitions
H_2O	water
H_2O_2	hydrogen peroxide (hydrogen dioxide)
HOB	head of bed
H&P	history and physical examination
H. pylori	*Helicobacter pylori*
HRT	hormone replacement therapy
ht	height
HTN	hypertension
Hx	history
hypo	hypodermic
IBS	irritable bowel syndrome
ICD	implantable cardiac defibrillator
ICU	intensive care unit
ID	intradermal
IDDM	insulin-dependent diabetes mellitus
I&D	incision and drainage
IHD	ischemic heart disease
IM	intramuscular
inf	inferior
INR	international normalized ratio
I&O	intake and output
IOP	intraocular pressure
IPG	impedance plethysmography
IPPB	intermittent positive pressure breathing
irrig	irrigation
isol	isolation
IUD	intrauterine device
IV	intravenous
IVC	intravenous cholangiogram
IVF	in vitro fertilization
IVP	intravenous pyelogram
K	potassium

Common Medical Abbreviations	Definitions
KCl	potassium chloride
kg	kilogram
KO	keep open
KUB	kidney, ureter, bladder (x-ray)
KVO	keep vein open
L	liter
L_1-L_5	lumbar vertebrae
lab	laboratory
lac	laceration
LAP	laparotomy
lat	lateral
L&D	labor and delivery
LDH	lactic dehydrogenase
LE	lupus erythematosus
lg	large
LLL	left lower lobe
LLQ	left lower quadrant
LMP	last menstrual period
LNMP	last normal menstrual period
LOC	loss of consciousness, level of consciousness
LP	lumbar puncture
LPN	licensed practical nurse
LR	lactated Ringer (IV solution)
lt	left
LTB	laryngotracheobronchitis
LUL	left upper lobe
LUQ	left upper quadrant
mcg	microgram
MCH	mean corpuscular hemoglobin
MCV	mean corpuscular volume
MD	muscular dystrophy
mEq	milliequivalent
mets	metastasis
mg	milligram
MG	myasthenia gravis
MI	myocardial infarction

Common Medical Abbreviations	Definitions
ml	milliliter
mm	millimeter
MM	multiple myeloma
MOM	milk of magnesia
MR	may repeat
MRCP	magnetic resonance cholangiopancreatography
MRSA	methicillin-resistant *Staphylococcus aureus*
MS	multiple sclerosis
MVP	mitral valve prolapse
Na	sodium
NaCl	sodium chloride (salt)
NAS	no added salt
NB	newborn
neg	negative
neuro	neurology
NG	nasogastric
NICU	neurological intensive care unit; neonatal intensive care unit
NIDDM	non-insulin-dependent diabetes mellitus
NIVA	noninvasive vascular assessment
noc	night
noct	night
NPO	nothing by mouth
NS	normal saline
NSR	normal sinus rhythm
N&V	nausea and vomiting
NVS	neurovital signs
O_2	oxygen
OB	obstetrics
OD	overdose
oint	ointment
OM	otitis media
OOB	out of bed
OP	outpatient
Ophth	ophthalmic
OR	operating room

Common Medical Abbreviations	Definitions
Ortho	orthopedics
OSA	obstructive sleep apnea
OT	occupational therapy
OTC	over-the-counter drugs
oto	otology
oz	ounce
p̄	after
P	phosphorus
P	pulse
PA	physician's assistant or posteroanterior
PAC	premature atrial contractions
PAD	peripheral arterial disease
PAT	paroxysmal atrial tachycardia
pc	after meals
PCP	*Pneumocystis carinii*
PCU	progressive care unit
PCV	packed cell volume
PD	Parkinson disease
PDA	patent ductus arteriosus
PDR	*Physicians' Desk Reference*
PE	pulmonary embolism
Peds	pediatrics
PEEP	positive end expiratory pressure
PEG	percutaneous endoscopic gastrostomy
per	by
PERRLA	pupils equal, round, reactive to light and accommodation
PET scan	positron emission tomography scan
PFTs	pulmonary function tests
PICC	peripherally inserted central catheter
PICU	pediatric intensive care unit

Common Medical Abbreviations	Definitions
PID	pelvic inflammatory disease
PKU	phenylketonuria
PM	between noon and midnight
PMS	premenstrual syndrome
PNS	peripheral nervous system
PO	orally; postoperative; phone order
post-op	postoperatively
PP	postpartum or post-prandial (after meals)
PPD	purified protein derivative
pr	per rectum
PRBC	packed red blood cells
pre-op	preoperatively
primip.	primipara
PRN	as needed
PSA	prostate specific antigen
pt	patient; pint
PT	physical therapy
PT	prothrombin time
PTCA	percutaneous transluminal coronary angioplasty
PT/INR	prothrombin time/ international normalized ratio
PTT	partial thromboplastin time
PUL	percutaneous ultrasound lithotripsy
PVC	premature ventricular contractions
PVD	peripheral vascular disease
Px	prognosis
q	every
q_h	every (number) hour (e.g., q2h)
qt	quart
R	rectal
RA	rheumatoid arthritis

Common Medical Abbreviations / Definitions

Common Medical Abbreviations	Definitions
RAD	reactive airway disease
RAIU	radioactive iodine uptake
RBC	red blood cell count
RDS	respiratory distress syndrome
reg	regular
REM	rapid eye movement
resp.	respirations
RHD	rheumatic heart disease
RLL	right lower lobe
RLQ	right lower quadrant
RN	registered nurse
R/O	rule out
ROM	range of motion
ROM	rupture of membranes
RP	radical prostatectomy
RR	recovery room
rt	right; routine
RT	respiratory therapy
RUL	right upper lobe
Rx	prescription
$\bar{s}$	without
SAB	spontaneous abortion
SARS	severe acute respiratory syndrome
SBE	subacute bacterial endocarditis; self breast examination
SHG	sonohystogram
SICU	surgical intensive care unit
SIDS	sudden infant death syndrome
SLE	systemic lupus erythematosus
SMAC	sequential multiple analysis computer
SMR	submucous resection
SO	salpingo-oophorectomy
SPECT	single-photon emission computed tomography

Common Medical Abbreviations	Definitions
ss.	one-half
SSE.	soapsuds enema
STAPH or staph	staphylococcus
stat	immediately
STD	sexually transmitted disease
STREP or strep.	streptococcus
subling	sublingual
sup	superior
supp	suppository
surg.	surgical
SVD	spontaneous vaginal delivery
SVN	small-volume nebulizer
SWL	shock wave lithotripsy
T_1-T_{12}	thoracic vertebrae
T4	thyroxine
tab	tablet
TAB	therapeutic abortion
T&A	tonsillectomy and adenoidectomy
TAH	total abdominal hysterectomy
TAH-BSO	total abdominal hysterectomy-bilateral salpingo-oophorectomy
TAT	tetanus antitoxin
TB	tuberculosis
TCDB	turn, cough, deep breathe
TCT	thrombin clotting time
TD	transdermal
TEE	transesophageal echocardiogram
temp	temperature
TENS	transcutaneous electrical nerve stimulation
THA	total hip arthroplasty
THR	total hip replacement
TIA	transient ischemic attack
tid	three times per day
tinct	tincture

Common Medical Abbreviations — Definitions

Common Medical Abbreviations	Definitions
TKA	total knee arthroplasty
TPN	total parenteral nutrition
tr	tincture
trach	tracheostomy
TSH	thyroid-stimulating hormone
TSS	toxic shock syndrome
TUIP	transurethral incision of the prostate
TULIP	transurethral laser incision of the prostate
TUMP	transurethral microwave thermotherapy
TURP	transurethral resection of the prostate
TVH	total vaginal hysterectomy
TVS	transvaginal sonography
TWE	tap water enema
Tx	treatment
UA	urinalysis
UAE	uterine artery embolization
UGI	upper gastrointestinal
UGISBFT	upper gastrointestinal, small bowel follow through
UNG	ointment

Common Medical Abbreviations	Definitions
UPPP	uvulopalatopharyngoplasty
URI	upper respiratory infection
US	ultrasound
UTI	urinary tract infection
UV	ultraviolet
UVR	ultraviolet radiation
vag	vaginal
VATS	video-assisted thoracic surgery
VBAC	vaginal birth after cesarean section
VCUG	voiding cystourethrogram
VD	venereal disease
VDRL	Venereal Disease Research Laboratory
VLAP	visual ablation of the prostate
VPS	ventilation/perfusion scanning
VS	vital signs
WA	while awake
WBC	white blood cell count
W/C	wheelchair
wt	weight
XRT	radiotherapy; radiation therapy

Institute for Safe Medication Practices' List of *Error-Prone Abbreviations, Symbols,* and *Dose Designations*

The abbreviations, symbols, and dose designations found in this table have been reported to ISMP through the USP=ISMP Medication Error Reporting Program as being frequently misinterpreted and involved in harmful medication errors. They should NEVER be used when communicating medical information. This includes internal communications, telephone/verbal prescriptions, computer-generated labels, labels for drug storage bins, medication administration records, as well as pharmacy and prescriber computer order entry screens.

The Joint Commission (TJC; formerly the Joint Commission on Accreditation of Healthcare Organizations [JCAHO]) has established a National Patient Safety Goal that specifies that certain abbreviations must appear on an accredited organization's do-not-use-list; we have highlighted these items with a double asterisk (**). However, we hope that you will consider others beyond the minimum TJC requirements. By using and promoting safe practices and by educating one another about hazards, we can better protect our patients.

Abbreviations	Intended Meaning	Misinterpretation	Correction
μg	Microgram	Mistaken as "mg"	Use "mcg"
AD, AS, AU	Right ear, left ear, each ear	Mistaken as OD, OS, OU (right eye, left eye, each eye)	Use "right ear," "left ear," or "each ear"
OD, OS, OU	Right eye, left eye, each eye	Mistaken as AD, AS, AU (right ear, left ear, each ear)	Use "right eye," "left eye," or "each eye"
BT	Bedtime	Mistaken as "BID" (twice daily)	Use "bedtime"
cc	Cubic centimeters	Mistaken as "u" (units)	Use "mL"
D/C	Discharge or discontinue	Premature discontinuation of medications if D/C (intended to mean "discharge") has been misinterpreted as "discontinued" when followed by a list of discharge medications	Use "discharge" and "discontinue"
IJ	Injection	Mistaken as "IV" or "intrajugular"	Use "injection"
IN	Intranasal	Mistaken as "IM" or "IV"	Use "intranasal" or "NAS"

**These abbreviations are included on the TJC's "minimum list" of dangerous abbreviations, acronyms, and symbols that must be included on an organization's "Do Not Use" list, effective January 1, 2004. Visit www.jointcommission.org for more information about this TJC requirement.

Abbreviations	Intended Meaning	Misinterpretation	Correction
HS	Half-strength	Mistaken as bedtime	Use "half-strength" or "bedtime"
hs	At bedtime, hours of sleep	Mistaken as half-strength	
IU**	International unit	Mistaken as IV (intravenous) or 10 (ten)	Use "units"
o.d. or OD	Once daily	Mistaken as "right eye" (OD-oculus dexter), leading to oral liquid medications administered in the eye	Use "daily"
OJ	Orange juice	Mistaken as OD or OS (right or left eye); drugs meant to be diluted in orange juice may be given in the eye	Use "orange juice"
Per os	By mouth, orally	The "os" can be mistaken as "left eye" (OS-oculus sinister)	Use "PO," "by mouth," or "orally"
q.d. or QD**	Every day	Mistaken as q.i.d., especially if the period after the "q" or the tail of the "q" is misunderstood as an "i"	Use "daily"
qhs	Nightly at bedtime	Mistaken as "qhr" or every hour	Use "nightly"
qn	Nightly or at bedtime	Mistaken as "qh" (every hour)	Use "nightly" or "at bedtime"
q.o.d. or QOD**	Every other day	Mistaken as "q.d." (daily) or "q.i.d." (four times daily) if the "o" is poorly written	Use "every other day"
q1d	Daily	Mistaken as q.i.d. (four times daily)	Use "daily"
q6PM, etc.	Every evening at 6 PM	Mistaken as every 6 hours	Use "6 PM nightly" or "6 PM daily"
SC, SQ, sub q	Subcutaneous	SC mistaken as SL (sublingual); SQ mistaken as "5 every;" the "q" in "sub q" has been mistaken as "every" (e.g., a heparin dose ordered "sub q 2 hours before surgery" misunderstood as every 2 hours before surgery)	Use "subcut" or "subcutaneously"
ss	Sliding scale (insulin) or ½ (apothecary)	Mistaken as "55"	Spell out "sliding scale;" use "one-half" or "½"

Abbreviations	Intended Meaning	Misinterpretation	Correction
SSRI	Sliding scale regular insulin	Mistaken as selective-serotonin reuptake inhibitor	Spell out "sliding scale (insulin)"
SSI	Sliding scale insulin	Mistaken as Strong Solution of Iodine (Lugol's)	
i/d	Once daily	Mistaken a "tid"	Use "1 daily"
TIW or tiw	3 times a week	Mistaken as "3 times as day" or "twice in a week"	Use "3 times weekly"
U or u**	Unit	Mistaken as the number 0 or 4, causing a 10-fold overdose or greater (e.g., 4U seen as "40" or 4u seen as "44"); mistaken as "cc" so dose given in volume instead of units (e.g., 4u seen as 4cc)	Use "unit"

Dose Designations and Other Information	Intended Meaning	Misinterpretation	Correction
Trailing zero after decimal point (e.g., 1.0 mg)**	1 mg	Mistaken as 10 mg if the decimal point is not seen	Do not use trailing zeros for doses expressed in whole numbers
"Naked" decimal point (e.g., .5 mg)**	0.5 mg	Mistaken as 5 mg if the decimal point is not seen	Use zero before a decimal point when the dose is less than a whole unit
Drug name and dose run together (especially problematic for drug names that end in "l" such as Inderal40mg; Tegretol300 mg)	Inderal 40 mg Tegretol 300 mg	Mistaken as Inderal 140 mg Mistaken as Tegretol 1300 mg	Place adequate space between the drug name, dose, and unit of measure
Numerical dose and unit of measure run together (e.g., 10mg, 100mL)	10 mg 100 mL	The "m" is sometimes mistaken as a zero or two zeros, risking a 10- to 100-fold overdose	Place adequate space between the dose and unit of measure

---

**These abbreviations are included on the TJC's "minimum list" of dangerous abbreviations, acronyms, and symbols that must be included on an organization's "Do Not Use" list, effective January 1, 2004. Visit www.jointcommission.org for more information about this TJC requirement.

Dose Designations and Other Information

Dose Designations and Other Information	Intended Meaning	Misinterpretation	Correction
Abbreviations such as mg. or mL. with a period following the abbreviation	mg mL	The period is unnecessary and could be mistaken as the number 1 if written poorly	Use mg, mL, etc. without a terminal period
Large doses without properly placed commas (e.g., 100000 units; 1000000 units)	100,000 units 1,000,000 units	100000 has been mistaken as 10,000 or 1,000,000; 1000000 has been mistaken as 100,000	Use commas for dosing units at or above 1,000, or use words such as 100 "thousand" or 1 "million" to improve readability

Drug Name Abbreviations

Drug Name Abbreviations	Intended Meaning	Misinterpretation	Correction
ARA A	vidarabine	Mistaken as cytarabine (ARA C)	Use complete drug name
AZT	Zidovudine (Retrovir)	Mistaken as azathioprine or aztreonam	Use complete drug name
CPZ	Compazine (prochlorperazine)	Mistaken as chlorpromazine	Use complete drug name
DPT	Demerol-Phenergan-Thorazine	Mistaken as diphtheria-pertussis-tetanus (vaccine)	Use complete drug name
DTO	Diluted tincture of opium, or deodorized tincture of opium (Paregoric)	Mistaken as tincture of opium	Use complete drug name
HCl	hydrochloric acid or hydrochloride	Mistaken as potassium chloride (the "H" is misinterpreted as "K")	Use complete drug name unless expressed as a salt of a drug
HCT	hydrocortisone	Mistaken as hydrochlorothiazide	Use complete drug name
HCTZ	hydrochlorothiazide	Mistaken as hydrocortisone (seen as HCT250 mg)	Use complete drug name
MgSO4**	magnesium sulfate	Mistaken as morphine sulfate	Use complete drug name
MS, MSO4**	morphine sulfate	Mistaken as magnesium sulfate	Use complete drug name
MTX	methotrexate	Mistaken as mitoxantrone	Use complete drug name
PCA	procainamide	Mistaken as patient controlled analgesia	Use complete drug name
PTU	propylthiouracil	Mistaken as mercaptopurine	Use complete drug name

Drug Name Abbreviations	Intended Meaning	Misinterpretation	Correction
T3	Tylenol with codeine No. 3	Mistaken as lithothyronine	Use complete drug name
TAC	triamcinolone	Mistaken as tetracaine, Adrenalin, cocaine	Use complete drug name
TNK	TN Kase	Mistaken as "TPA"	Use complete drug name
ZnS04	zinc sulfate	Mistaken as morphine sulfate	Use complete drug name

Stemmed Drug Names	Intended Meaning	Misinterpretation	Correction
"Nitro" drip	nitroglycerin infusion	Mistaken as sodium nitroprusside infusion	Use complete drug name
"Norflox"	norfloxacin	Mistaken as Norflex	Use complete drug name
"IV Vanc"	intravenous vancomycin	Mistaken as Invanz	Use complete drug name

Symbols	Intended Meaning	Misinterpretation	Correction
ʒ	Dram	Symbol for dram mistaken as "3"	Use metric system
♍	Minim	Symbol for minim mistaken as "mL"	
X3D	For three days	Mistaken as "3 doses"	Use "for three days"
> and <	Greater than and less than	Mistaken as opposite of intended; mistakenly use incorrect symbol; "< 10" mistaken as "40"	Use "greater than" or "less than"
/ (slash mark)	Separates two doses or indicates "per"	Mistaken as the number 1 (e.g., "25 units/10 units" misread as "25 units and 110" units)	Use "per" rather than a slash mark to separate doses
@	At	Mistaken as "2"	Use "at"
&	And	Mistaken as "2"	Use "and"
+	Plus or and	Mistaken as "4"	Use "and"
°	Hour	Mistaken as a zero (e.g., q2° seen as q 20)	Use "hr," "h," or "hour"

**These abbreviations are included on the TJC's "minimum list" of dangerous abbreviations, acronyms, and symbols that must be included on an organization's "Do Not Use" list, effective January 1, 2004. Visit www.jointcommission.org for more information about this TJC requirement.

Permission is granted to reproduce material for internal newsletters or communications with proper attribution. Other reproduction is prohibited without written permission. Unless noted, reports were received through the USP-ISMP Medication errors Reporting Program (MERP). Report actual and potential medication errors to the MERP via the web at www.ismp.org or by calling 1-800-FAIL-SAF(E). ISMP guarantees confidentiality of information received and respects reporters' wishes as to the level of detail included in publications.

Pharmacology Terms

Chapter 2: Oncology

antineoplastic agent.............	a drug used to destroy or halt the rapid replication of cancer cells
chemotherapy (also called **chemo**)	the treatment of cancer with chemical agents
cytotoxic.....................	an agent that causes cell death

Chapter 4: Integumentary

antipsoriatic..................	a drug that treats psoriasis
astringent....................	an agent that reduces inflammation and irritation and provides a protective barrier on mucosa and skin by contracting the surface tissue
keratolytic	an agent that augments the shedding of the top layer of dead skin
pediculicide	an agent that kills lice
retinoid......................	a derivative of vitamin A that regulates the growth of epithelial cells; often used to treat acne
scabicide.....................	an agent that kills scabies

Chapter 5: Respiratory

antitussive	a drug that suppresses coughing
bronchodilator................	a drug that expands the airways by relaxing smooth muscle in the lungs
decongestant	a drug that breaks up nasal and head congestion
expectorant	a drug that breaks up mucus in the lungs so that it can be expelled
mucolytic	a drug that breaks up mucus in the lungs so that it can be expelled

Chapter 6: Kidney (Renal) and Electrolytes

aldosterone receptor antagonist (ARA).......................	a drug that prevents reabsorption of water and sodium; used in chronic heart failure to minimize edema
angiotensin-converting enzyme inhibitor (ACEI or ACE inhibitor)	a drug that prevents the formation of angiotensin, which is a major contributor to high blood pressure
angiotensin receptor blocker (ARB) (also called **angiotensin II antagonist**)	a drug that blocks the angiotensin molecule from binding to its receptors throughout the body to reduce high blood pressure
diuretic......................	a drug that promotes the formation and excretion of urine to reduce the volume of extracellular fluid; commonly referred to as a water pill

Chapter 6: Kidney (Renal) and Electrolytes—cont'd

urinary alkalinizer . . . . an agent that increases the urine pH to make it more basic to treat acidosis

vasopressin (also called **antidiuretic hormone** or **ADH**). . . . . a drug that contracts blood vessels to retain water and increase blood pressure

Chapter 7: Male Reproductive System

androgen . . . . natural and synthetic hormones involved in male reproduction and secondary gender attributes

antiandrogen . . . . a drug that blocks the effects of androgen hormones in the body

phosphodiesterase inhibitor . . . . a drug that blocks the inactivation of cyclic adenosine monophosphate either to increase cardiac output or to increase vasodilation in the penis

spermicide . . . . an agent that kills sperm

Chapter 8: Female Reproductive System

antiestrogen. . . . . a drug used to block the action of estrogen hormones in the body

birth control (BC) . . . . exogenous hormones to prevent pregnancy

contraceptive . . . . an agent (drug or barrier) used to prevent conception or pregnancy

estrogens . . . . natural and synthetic hormones involved in female reproduction and secondary gender characteristics

hormone replacement therapy . . . . . a regimen that mimics the body's normal levels of female hormones when they are no longer produced; typically used during menopause

intrauterine device (IUD) . . . . a hormone-containing device that is inserted directly in the vagina or uterus to prevent pregnancy

oral contraceptive . . . . exogenous hormones taken by mouth to prevent pregnancy

ovulation stimulant . . . . a drug that enhances the release of an egg from the ovary to promote pregnancy

progestin . . . . synthetic or natural hormones involved in female reproduction and secondary sex characteristics

vaginal ring . . . . a device containing estrogens and progestins that is inserted in the vagina to prevent pregnancy

Chapter 9: Obstetrics

abortifacient. . . . . a drug that causes uterine muscles to contract with subsequent abortion of the fetus

oxytocic . . . . a hormone that stimulates the uterine muscles to contract, thereby inducing labor in a pregnant woman

pregnancy category . . . . a level of risk the Food and Drug Administration assigns a drug based on documented problems with the use of that drug during pregnancy; risk categories from safest to most harmful are A, B, C, D, and X

tocolytic . . . . an agent that suppresses labor contractions

Chapter 10: Cardiovascular System and Blood

aggregation inhibitor. . . . .   a drug that stops platelets from bonding together

antianginal . . . .   a drug that relieves the chest pain paroxysms caused by lack of oxygen delivery to the heart; typically involves vasodilation

antiarrhythmic. . . . .   a drug that treats abnormal heart rhythm

anticoagulant . . . .   a drug that prevents blood clotting and coagulation

antihypertensive. . . . .   a drug that lowers blood pressure

antiplatelet . . . .   a drug that prevents platelet formation or causes platelet destruction

antithrombin . . . .   a drug that prevents fibrin production, thereby reducing blood coagulation

beta-blocker (BB) . . . .   a drug that inhibits beta-adrenergic receptors; mostly used to lower blood pressure

bile acid sequestrant . . . .   a type of antihyperlipidemic drug used to lower high cholesterol levels by increasing the excretion of bile acid

calcium channel blocker (CCB) . . . .   a drug that regulates the entry of calcium into muscle cells of the heart and blood vessels to lower blood pressure

hemostatic . . . .   a drug that stops bleeding or hemorrhaging

nitrate. . . . .   a drug that dilates the blood vessels

thrombolytic . . . .   a drug that dissolves blood clots

vasodilator . . . .   a drug that expands blood vessels to lower blood pressure

vasopressor (also called
vasoconstrictor) . . . .   a drug that contracts blood vessels to raise blood pressure

Chapter 11: Digestive System and Lipids

antacid . . . .   a drug that neutralizes acid in the stomach

antidiarrheal. . . . .   a drug that treats diarrhea by increasing water absorption, decreasing muscle contraction of the intestines, altering electrolyte exchange, or absorbing toxins or microorganisms

antiemetic . . . .   a drug that reduces or prevents nausea and vomiting

antihyperlipidemic. . . . .   a drug used to treat high cholesterol by affecting low-density lipoprotein, high-density lipoprotein, total cholesterol, and/or triglyceride levels, which are collectively called lipids

enema. . . . .   a liquid agent administered rectally to clear the contents of the bowel

fibrate. . . . .   a type of antihyperlipidemic drug that raises high-density lipoprotein levels and lowers total cholesterol, low-density lipoprotein, and triglyceride levels

histamine H$_2$ receptor antagonist
(H2RA) (also called **H$_2$ blocker**) . . .   a drug that reduces stomach acid

laxative . . . .   a drug that aids the evacuation of the bowels

proton pump inhibitor (PPI) . . . . . .   a drug that blocks acid production in the stomach

statin. . . . .   a drug used to treat dyslipidemia by inhibiting 3-hydroxy-3-methylglutaryl coenzyme A reductase

Chapter 12: Eye

antiglaucoma . . . .   a drug that treats glaucoma of the eye

miotic. . . . .   an agent that contracts the pupil

mydriatic . . . .   an agent that dilates the pupil

ophthalmic. . . . .   an agent that is intended to be used in the eye

Chapter 13: Ear

ceruminolytic. . . . .   an agent that breaks down ear wax

otic . . . .   an agent intended to be used in the ear

Chapter 14: Musculoskeletal System

antiarthritic . . . .   a drug used in the treatment of arthritis

antispasmodic. . . . .   a drug that prevents or relieves muscle spasms

bisphosphonates. . . . .   drugs that bind to bone matrix to treat osteoporosis

colony-stimulating factor (CSF). . . .   aids in the replication of blood cells in the bone marrow

muscle relaxant . . . .   a drug that reduces muscle contractility to relieve tension- or spasm-induced pain

neuromuscular blocking agent
(NMBA). . . . .   a drug that blocks all nerve stimulation of the skeletal muscles to cause paralysis

Chapter 15: Nervous System and Behavioral Health

adrenergic agonist . . . .   a drug that stimulates aspects of the sympathetic nervous system

amphetamine . . . .   a drug that stimulates the central nervous system

anticonvulsant . . . .   a drug that reduces the incidence and severity of seizures and convulsions (may also be referred to as an antiepileptic drug)

analgesic. . . . .   a drug that relieves pain; a *narcotic analgesic* is used for severe pain but can result in dependence and tolerance; a *nonnarcotic analgesic* is used for mild to moderate pain and is less likely to cause dependence and tolerance

anesthetic.   a drug that causes numbness or a loss of feeling that can be used locally or systemically; often used systemically to put a patient "to sleep" during extensive procedures

anticholinergic. . . . .   a drug that blocks the action of acetylcholine and therefore opposes the parasympathetic nervous system

anticholinesterase . . . .   a drug that prevents the breakdown of acetylcholine to yield a cholinergic or parasympathetic effect

antidepressant . . . .   a drug used to treat depression

antiparkinsonian agent . . . .   a drug that treats Parkinson disease and parkinsonism by elevating the levels of dopamine in the brain

antipsychotic (also called
neuroleptic) . . . .   a drug that treats psychosis disorders by inducing a calming or tranquilizing effect and/or by adjusting neurotransmitter levels in the brain

antipyretic . . . .   a drug that reduces fever

anxiolytic . . . .   a drug that relieves anxiety

Chapter 15: Nervous System and Behavioral Health—cont'd

barbiturate . . . . a drug used to produce relaxation and sleep

benzodiazepine (BZD) . . . . a drug that binds to receptors in the brain to calm and sedate the central nervous system

central nervous system stimulant . . . a drug that excites the central nervous system; can be used for many brain disorders

cholinergic . . . . an agent that acts like acetylcholine to activate the parasympathetic nervous system

dopaminergic . . . . a drug that acts like dopamine; mostly used to treat Parkinson disease by increasing dopamine-dependent activity in the brain

hypnotic . . . . a drug used to induce sleep; may also be used as a sedative

mood stabilizer . . . . a drug that balances neurotransmitters in the brain to prevent periods of either mania or depression in bipolar patients

neuroleptic (also called
antipsychotic) . . . . a drug that reduces abnormal psychomotor activities in psychotic patients

nonsteroidal anti-inflammatory
drug (NSAID) . . . . a drug that reduces pain, inflammation, and fever

sedative . . . . a drug that depresses the central nervous system to calm a patient

tranquilizer . . . . a drug that reduces anxiety or agitation

tricyclic antidepressant (TCA) . . . . . a type of drug used to treat depression

Chapter 16: Endocrine System

antihistamine . . . . a drug that treats allergic and hypersensitivity reactions by blocking histamine

anti-inflammatory . . . . a drug that reduces inflammation

antirheumatic . . . . a drug that prevents or relieves rheumatism by affecting the immune system

antithyroid agent . . . . a drug that counters hyperthyroidism by reducing the production of thyroid hormones

antiretroviral . . . . a drug that suppresses the replication of HIV; highly active antiretroviral therapy (HAART) is the combination of three or more of these drugs to treat HIV infection

corticosteroid . . . . a drug that mimics hormones produced by the adrenal glands and has antiinflammatory and immunosuppressive effects

disease-modifying antirheumatic
drug (DMARD) . . . . a drug that slows the progression of rheumatoid arthritis

hypoglycemic . . . . a drug that lowers blood sugar levels

immunosuppressant (also called
immunomodulator) . . . . a drug that reduces the response of the immune system; used in autoimmune diseases and to prepare a patient for an organ transplant

leukotriene receptor antagonist . . . . a drug that blocks late-stage regulators of allergic and hypersensitivity reactions

thyroid hormone . . . . a replacement hormone to regulate metabolism and endocrine functions

Chapter 16: Endocrine System—cont'd

vaccine (also called
immunization) . . . . A preparation of microbial antigen that will confer a degree of immunity to the disease caused by that microbial

General Drug Categories

antibacterial . . . . a drug that targets bacteria to kill or halt growth or replication

antibiotic . . . . a drug that targets microorganisms to kill or halt growth or replication

antifungal . . . . a drug that targets fungus to kill or halt growth or replication

antigout . . . . a drug that opposes the buildup of uric acid crystals in the joints to prevent and treat gout attacks

antimicrobial . . . . a drug that targets microorganisms to kill or halt growth or replication

antiviral . . . . a drug that targets viruses to kill or halt growth or replication

antiadrenergic agent . . . . a drug that blocks adrenergic receptors to reduce sympathetic nervous system activity in the body

antiseptic . . . . a chemical agent that can safely be applied to external tissues to halt the growth of microorganisms

bactericidal . . . . the designation for an antimicrobial agent that kills or destroys bacteria

bacteriostatic . . . . the designation for an antimicrobial agent that halts the growth or replication of bacteria but does not destroy them

disinfectant . . . . a chemical agent that can be applied to inanimate objects to destroy microorganisms

emollient . . . . an external agent that softens or soothes the skin

herbal supplement . . . . a naturally derived dietary product that may have some therapeutic effect; rigorous proof of safety and effectiveness is not required because it is not regulated as a drug

narcotics . . . . a class of drugs that have opiumlike effects to cause drowsiness, pain relief, and sedation; can be habit forming and are considered controlled substances.

parasympatholytic . . . . an agent that blocks the actions of the parasympathetic nervous system

parasympathomimetic . . . . an agent that enhances the actions of the parasympathetic nervous system

radiopharmaceutical . . . . a drug with a radioactive component; used for diagnosis or treatment

smoking cessation agent . . . . a drug that helps a patient quit smoking; may be a behavioral deterrent or a nicotine substitute

sympatholytic . . . . an agent that blocks the actions of the sympathetic nervous system

sympathomimetic . . . . an agent that enhances the actions of the sympathetic nervous system

vitamin . . . . an organic compound essential in small quantities for normal physiologic and metabolic functioning

General Pharmacy Terms

absorption . . . . the process in which a drug is taken up into the body, organ, tissue, or cell

adverse drug reaction (ADR) . . . . . . any harmful or unintended reaction to a drug administered at a normal dose

ampoule (or ampule) . . . . a small, sterile glass or plastic container that usually holds a single dose of a solution to be administered parenterally

aseptic technique . . . . the method used to minimize the microbial contamination of sterile drugs

bioavailability . . . . the percentage of administered drug available to affect the body and target site(s) after absorption, metabolism, and other factors

capsule (cap) . . . . a small, digestible container (usually made of gelatin) used to hold a dose of medication for oral administration

chemical name . . . . the exact designation of the chemical structure of a drug

compounding . . . . the act of combining drug ingredients to prepare a customized prescription or drug order for a patient

contraindications . . . . factors that prohibit administration of a drug

controlled substance . . . . a drug that has been identified as having the potential for abuse or addiction; designated as schedule I, II, III, IV, or V under the Controlled Substance Act

cream . . . . a water-based, semisolid preparation that usually contains a drug and is applied topically to external parts of the body

distribution . . . . the uptake pattern of drug molecules by various tissues throughout the body

dose . . . . the amount of a drug or other substance to be administered at one time

drug . . . . any substance taken by mouth; injected into a muscle, the skin, a blood vessel, or a cavity of the body; or applied topically to treat, cure, prevent, or diagnose a disease or condition

drug-drug interaction (DDI) . . . . . . a modification of the effect of a drug when administered with another drug; food can also interact with a drug to cause a modification of the drug's effect

elimination . . . . the removal of a substance from the body by any route, including the kidneys, liver, lungs, and sweat glands

elixir . . . . a liquid containing sweeteners, flavorings, water, and/or alcohol in which an oral medication may be dispersed

emulsion . . . . a stable mixture that contains one component suspended within another component that it cannot normally dissolve in or mix with

Food and Drug Administration (FDA) . . . . a federal agency responsible for the enforcement of federal regulations regarding the manufacturing and distribution of food, drugs, and cosmetics as protection against the sale of impure or dangerous substances

formulary . . . . a listing of drugs and drug information used by health practitioners within an institution to prescribe treatment that is medically appropriate

General Pharmacy Terms—cont'd

generic name	the official, established nonproprietary name assigned to a drug
mechanism of action (MOA)	the means by which a drug exerts a desired effect
metabolism	the chemical changes that a drug or other substance undergoes in the body
ointment	an oil-based, semisolid preparation that usually contains a drug and is applied topically to external parts of the body
over-the-counter (OTC) drug (also called **nonprescription drug**)	a drug that may be purchased without a prescription
pharmaceutical	a drug used for medicinal purposes
pharmacist	a person formally trained to formulate and dispense medications
pharmacodynamics	the study of the actions of a drug on the body
pharmacogenomics	the study of the correlation between genetics and response to a drug
pharmacokinetics	the study of the actions of the body on a drug
pharmacology	the study of the preparation, properties, uses, and actions of drugs
pharmacy	a place for preparing and dispensing drugs
placebo	an inactive substance, prescribed as if it were an effective dose of a needed medication
prescription	an order for medication, therapy, or a therapeutic device given by a properly authorized person to a person properly authorized to dispense or perform the order for the specified patient
preservative	a substance included in some parenteral and topical medications used to prevent the growth of microorganisms in the product
route of administration	any one of the ways in which a drug or agent may be given to a patient
side effect	any reaction or result from a medication other than what was intended
solution	a homogenous mixture of one or more substances dissolved into another substance
state board of pharmacy	the agency responsible for regulating the practice of pharmacy within the state
suppository	a topical form of drug that is inserted into the rectum, vagina, or penis
suspension	a liquid in which particles of a solid are dispersed, but not dissolved, and in which the dispersal is maintained by stirring or shaking the mixture
tablet	a small, solid dose form of a medication
toxicity	the level at which a drug's concentration within the body produces serious adverse effects
trade name (also called **brand name**)	a proprietary name assigned to a drug by its manufacturer that is registered as part of the drug's identity

General Pharmacy Terms—cont'd

United States Pharmacopeia
(USP)........................ a compendium, recognized officially by the federal Food, Drug, and Cosmetic Act, that contains descriptions, uses, strengths, and standards of purity for selected drugs and for all their dosage forms

Routes of Administration

enteral .... the use of oral ingestion as a mode of drug administration

epidural .... injection of a drug into the epidural space of the spine

infusion .... the prolonged administration of a fluid substance directly into a vein, artery, or under the skin in which the flow rate is driven by gravity or a mechanical pump

inhalation.................... a method of drug administration that involves the breathing in of a spray, vapor, or powder

injection..................... the introduction of a substance into the body by using a needle

intramuscular (IM) .... the administration of a medication into a muscle

intrathecal .... the administration of a drug into the subarachnoid space of the meninges in the spine

intravenous (IV)................ the administration of a medication directly into a vein

oral.......................... the administration of a medication by mouth

parenteral.................... a drug or agent that is administered into the body by an injection, thereby bypassing the digestive tract

subcutaneous .... the introduction of a medication into the tissue just beneath the skin

sublingual.................... a form of drug that dissolves under the tongue

topical....................... a dosage form of a medication that is applied directly to an external area of the body

transdermal .... a method of applying a drug to unbroken skin so that it is continuously absorbed through the skin to produce a systemic effect; a transdermal patch is a drug delivery system that controls the rate of absorption through the skin

ILLUSTRATION CREDITS

Chapter 1

Figure 1-2 reprinted by permission of Tribune Media Services.

Chapter 2

Figure 2-3 from Kamal A, Brockelhurst JC: *Color atlas of geriatric medicine*, ed 2, St. Louis, 1991, Mosby.

Figure 2-5 from Kumar VK: *Basic pathology*, ed 7, Philadelphia, 2003, Saunders.

Figure 2-7 from Damjanov I: *Pathology, A color atlas*, ed 2, St. Louis, 2000, Mosby.

Figure 2-8 from Ballinger PW, Frank ED: *Merrill's atlas of radiographic positions and radiologic procedures*, ed 10, St. Louis, 2003, Mosby.

Exercise Figure C from (1) Mace JD: *Radiography pathology*, ed 4, St. Louis, 2004, Elsevier Mosby; (2) Habif TP: *Clinical dermatology*, ed 4, St. Louis, 2004, Elsevier Mosby; (3) Stevens A: *Pathology*, ed 2, London, 2000, Mosby; (4) Damjanov I, Linder J: *Anderson's pathology*, ed 10, St. Louis, 1996, Mosby.

Chapter 3

Table 3-1 figures and Exercise Figure C from Bontrager KL: *Radiographic positioning and related anatomy*, ed 5, St. Louis, 2002, Mosby.

Chapter 4

Figure 4-2 from Zitelli BJ, David HW: *Atlas of pediatric physical diagnosis*, ed 4, St. Louis, 2002, Mosby.

Dermatology poem courtesy Julia Frank, MD.

Exercise Figure C (1), Figures 4-3 (A), 4-6, 4-11, 4-12, 4-13 and 4-15 and Unn Fig 4 from Bork K, Brauninger W: *Skin diseases in clinical practice*, ed 2, Philadelphia, 1998, WB Saunders.

Figure 4-3 (B), 4-4 from Callen JP: *Color atlas of dermatology*, ed 2, Philadelphia, 2000, Saunders.

Figure 4-3 (C) from Chabner DE: *The language of medicine*, ed 7, Philadelphia, 2004, Saunders.

Figure 4-5 from *Dorland's illustrated medical dictionary*, ed 31, Philadelphia, 2007, Saunders.

Table 4-1 figures from Frazier M: *Essentials of human disease and conditions*, ed 3, St. Louis, 2004, Elsevier Mosby.

Figure 4-14 and Exercise Figure D (1 and 2) from Shiland B: *Mastering healthcare teminology*, ed 2, St. Louis, 2006, Elsevier Mosby.

Figure 4-3 (D, E), 4-7, 4-8, 4-10, and Table 4-1 figures from Habif TP: *Clinical dermatology*, ed 4, St. Louis, 2004, Elsevier Mosby.

Chapter 5

Figure 5-3 from Eisenberg RL, Johson NM: *Comprehensive radiographic pathology*, ed 3, St. Louis, 2003, Mosby.

Figure 5-7 from Kumar V et al: *Robbins basic pathology*, ed 7, Philadelphia, 2003, Saunders.

Figure 5-11 from Potter PA, Perry AG: *Fundamentals of nursing: concepts, process, and practice*, ed 5, St. Louis, 2001, Mosby.

Figure 5-12 courtesy Nelcor Puritan Bennett.

Figure 5-13 (A) from Lewis SM et al: *Medical-surgical nursing*, ed 6, St. Louis, 2004, Elsevier Mosby.

Table 5-1 figures from Ruppel GL: *Manual pulmonary function testing*, ed 7, St. Louis, 1998, Mosby; Siemens Medical Systems, Inc., New Jersey; Ballinger PW, Frank ED: *Merrill's atlas of radiographic positions and radiologic procedures*, ed 10, St. Louis, 2003, Mosby; GE Medical Systems, Waukesha, Wis; Pagana KD, Pagana TJ: *Mosby's manual of diagnostic and laboratory test reference*, ed 7, St. Louis, 2004, Elsevier Mosby. Shiland B: *Mastering healthcare teminology*, ed 2, St. Louis, 2006, Elsevier Mosby.

Chapter 6

Figure 6-4 (A), 6-5 from Damjanov I: *Pathology, a color atlas*, ed 2, St. Louis, 2000, Mosby.

Figure 6-7 from Shiland B: *Mastering healthcare teminology*, ed 2, St. Louis, 2006, Elsevier Mosby.

Figures 6-10, 6-11, and Exercise Figure I from Ballinger PW, Frank ED: *Merrill's atlas of radiographic positions and radiologic procedures*, ed 10, St. Louis, 2003, Mosby.

Figures 6-12 and 6-13 from Bontrager KL: *Textbook of radiographic positioning and related anatomy*, ed 6, St. Louis, 2002, Mosby.

Figure 6-16 courtesy Baxter Healthcare Corp, Deerfield, Ill.

Exercise Figure E courtesy Dornier Medical Systems, Kennesaw, Ga.

Exercise Figure I courtesy Fisher Scientific, Pittsburgh, Pa.

Chapter 7

Figure 7-8 from Ignatiavicius DD, et al: *Medical-surgical nursing: a nursing process approach*, ed 4, 2002, Saunders.

Figure 7-10 courtesy EDAP Technomed, Inc., Vaulx-en-Velin, France.

Exercise Figure B from Bork K, Brauninger W: *Skin diseases in clinical practice*, ed 2, Philadelphia, 1998, WB Saunders.

Chapter 8

Figure 8-12 (A) courtesy Biopsys Medical, Inc, Irvine, Calif.

Figure 8-12 (B, C) from Pagana KD, Pagana TJ: *Mosby's manual of diagnostic and laboratory test reference*, ed 7, St. Louis, 2004, Elsevier Mosby.

Figures 8-13 (A), 8-14 (B), and Exercise Figure H from Ballinger PW, Frank ED: *Merrill's atlas of radiographic positions and radiologic procedures*, ed 10, St. Louis, 2003, Mosby.

Figure 8-13 (B) courtesy Martin K. Portnoff.

Figure 8-16 courtesy Richard Wolf Medical Instruments Corp., Vernon Hills, Ill.

Chapter 9

Figure 9-2 from Dickason EJ, Schultz MO, Silverman BL: *Maternal-infant nursing care*, ed 3, St. Louis, 1998, Mosby.

Figure 9-6, 9-7, 9-9, and 9-10 and Exercise Figure C from Zitelli BJ, David HW: *Atlas of pediatric physical diagnosis*, ed 4, St. Louis, 2002, Mosby.

Figure 9-12 from Ballinger PW, Frank ED: *Merrill's atlas of radiographic positions and radiologic procedures*, ed 10, St. Louis, 2003, Mosby.

Exercise Figure B from Lowdermilk DL: *Maternity and women's health care*, ed 8, St. Louis, 2004, Elsevier Mosby.

Chapter 10

Figure 10-11 (A) from Thibodeau GA, Patton KT: *Anatomy and physiology*, ed 4, St. Louis, 2001, Mosby.

Figure 10-11 (B) from Bork K, Brauninger W: *Skin diseases in clinical practice*, ed 2, Philadelphia, 1998, WB Saunders.

Figures 10-13 (B), 10-18 (B, C), 10-20, 10-21, 10-22, and 10-24 (B) from Ballinger PW, Frank ED: *Merrill's atlas of radiographic positions and radiologic procedures*, ed 10, St. Louis, 2003, Mosby.

Figure 10-24 (A) courtesy GE Medical Systems, Inc, Waukesha, Wis.

Figure 10-27 from Seidel H et al: *Mosby's guide to physical examination*, ed 5, St. Louis, 2003, Mosby.

Chapter 11

Figure 11-9 from Shiland B: *Mastering healthcare teminology*, ed 2, St. Louis, 2006, Elsevier Mosby.

Figure 11-10 from Anderson KN: *Mosby's medical, nursing and allied health dictionary*, St. Louis, 2003, Mosby.

Figure 11-10 from LaFleur Brooks M, LaFleur Brooks D: *Basic medical language*, ed 2, St. Louis, 2004, Elsevier Mosby.

Figure 11-14 from White RA, Klein SR: *Endoscopic surgery*, St. Louis, 1991, Mosby.

Figure 11-17, and Exercise G (2) from Ballinger PW, Frank ED: *Merrill's atlas of radiographic positions and radiologic procedures*, ed 10, St. Louis, 2003, Mosby.

Figure 11-19 from Chabner DE: *The language of medicine*, ed 7, Philadelphia, 2004, Saunders.

Exercise Figure G (1) from Hagen-Ansert S: *Textbook of diagnostic ultrasonography*, ed 5, St. Louis, 2001, Mosby.

Chapter 12

Figure 12-2 and Exercise Figures B and D from Zitelli BJ, David HW: *Atlas of pediatric physical diagnosis*, ed 4, St. Louis, 2002, Mosby.

Figure 12-4 (A, B) from Seidel H et al: *Mosby's guide to physical examination*, ed 5, St. Louis, 2003, Mosby.

Exercise Figure C from Stein HA, Slatt BJ, Stein RM: *The ophthalmic assistant: fundamentals and clinical practice*, ed 5, St. Louis, 1998, Mosby.

Figure 12-5 from Newell FW: *Ophthalmology*, ed 7, St. Louis, 1992, Mosby.

Figure 12-6 from Apple DJ, Robb MF: *Ocular pathology*, ed 5, St. Louis, 1998, Mosby.

Figure 12-7 copyright Mayo Foundation for Medical Education and Research. All rights reserved. Used with permission.

Figure 12-8 from Bedford MA: *Ophthalmological diagnosis*, London, 1986, Wolfe.

Figure 12-9 from Chabner DE: *The language of medicine*, ed 7, Philadelphia, 2004, Saunders.

2004 Conn's current therapy, Philadelphia, 2006, Saunders.

Age-related macular degeneration, *Women's Healthsource Mayo Clinic*, 4(3), 2000.

Alternative medicine, Payallup, Wash, 1994, Future Medicine Publishing.

American Journal of Nursing, 2006-2007, Lippincott Williams & Wilkins.

Applegate EJ: *The anatomy and physiology learning system*, ed 3, St. Louis, 2006, Saunders.

Awan, MA, Tarin, SA: Review of photodynamic therapy. *Surgeon*, 4(4), 231-6, (2006).

Ballinger PW, Frank ED: *Merrill's atlas of radiographic positions and radiologic procedures*, ed 10, St. Louis, 2003, Mosby.

Bontrager KL: *Textbook of radiographic positioning and related anatomy*, ed 6, St. Louis, 2005, Mosby.

Callen J et al: *Color atlas of dermatology*, ed 2, Philadelphia, 2000, WB Saunders.

Chabner D: *The language of medicine*, ed 8, Philadelphia, 2007, Saunders.

Chung UL et al: Effects of LI4 and BL67 acupressure on labor pain and uterine contractions in the first stage of labor. *Journal of Nursing Research, 11*, 251-260, (2003).

Diehl M: *Medical transcription guide: do's and don'ts*, ed 3, St. Louis, 2005, Saunders.

Diehl M: *Diehl and Fordney's medical transcription, techniques and procedures*, ed 5, 2002, Saunders.

Dorland's illustrated medical dictionary, 30th Edition. Philadelphia, 2003, Saunders.

Fitzpatrick JE, Aeling JL: *Dermatology secrets in color*, ed 2, Philadelphia, 2001, Hanley and Belfus.

Fox DJ et al: Neurofeedback: an alternative and efficacious treatment for attention deficit hyperactivity disorder, *Applied Psychophysiology and Biofeedback*, 30 (4), 365-73, (2005).

Frazier M, Drzymkowski JW: *Essentials of human diseases and conditions*, ed 3, Philadelphia, 2004, Elsevier.

Habif T: *A color guide to diagnosis and therapy, clincial dermatology*, ed 4, Philadelphia, 2004, Mosby.

Haubrich WS: *Medical meanings: a glossary of word origins*, Philadelphia, 1997, American College of Physicians.

Herlihy B, Maebius N: *The human body in health and illness*, ed 3, Philadelphia, 2007, Saunders.

Hernandez-Reif M et al: Natural killer cells and lymphocytes increase in woman with breast cancer following massage therapy. *International Journal of Neuroscience*, 115 (4), 495-510, (2005).

Ignatavicius DD et al: *Medical-surgical nursing: a nursing process approach*, ed 5, Philadelphia, 2006, Saunders.

Itamura R, Hosoya R: Homeopathic treatment of Japanese patients with intractable atopic dermatitis. *Homeopathy*, 92 (2), 108-14, (2003).

Kawakita K et al: How do acupuncture and moxibustion act? Focusing on the progress of Japanese acupuncture research. *Journal of Pharmacological Sciences*, 100 (5), 443-59, (2006).

Kohatsu W: *Complementary and alternative medicine secrets*, Philadelphia, 2002, Hanley and Belfus.

Kurtz ME et al: Primary care physicians' attitudes and practices regarding complementary and alternative medicine, *JAOA 103* (12), 2003.

LaFleur Brooks M, Gillingham EA: *Health unit coordinating*, ed 5, Philadelphia, 2004, Saunders.

LaFleur Brooks M, LaFleur Brooks D: *Basic medical language*, ed 2, St. Louis, 2004, Mosby.

Langford R, Thompson JM: *Mosby's handbook of diseases*, St. Louis, 1996, Mosby.

Lee MK et al: Effects of SP6 acupressure on labor pain and length of delivery time in women during labor. *Journal of Alternative and Complementary Medicine*, 10, 959-65, (2004).

Lewis SM et al: *Medical-surgical nursing*, ed 6, St. Louis, 2004, Mosby.

Littleton LY, Engebretson JC: *Maternal, neonatal, and women's health nursing*, Albany, 2002, Delmar.

Malhotra V et al: The beneficial effect of yoga in diabetes, *Nepal Medical College Journal*, 7 (2), 145-47, (2005).

Mayo Clinic Health Letter, Rochester, 2000-2007, Mayo Foundation for Medical Education and Research.

Mayo Clinic Women's Health Source, Rochester, 2005-2007, Mayo Foundation for Medical Education and Research.

Medline Plus, http://www.nlm.nih.gov/medlineplus, 2006-2007, National Library of Medicine and the National Institutes of Health.

Miller-Keane encyclopedia and dictionary of medicine, nursing, and allied health, ed 6, Philadelphia, 1997, WB Saunders.

Mosby's medical, nursing, and allied health dictionary, ed 6, St. Louis, 2002, Mosby.

Masters RM, Gylys BA: *Medical terminology simplified*, ed 3, Philadelphia, 2005, FA Davis.

Medicine in quotations, Philadelphia, 2000, American College of Physicians.

Mercier LM: *Practical orthopedics*, ed 4, St. Louis, 1995, Mosby.

National Institutes of Health: *Age-related eye disease study.* http://www.nei.nih.gov/neitrials/static/study44.html. Accessed April 10, 2004.

Nath JL: *Using medical terminology, a practical approach*, Baltimore, 2006, Lippincott Williams & Wilkins.

New England Journal of Medicine, 2006-2007, Massachusetts Medical Society.

Nickel AK et al: Outcome research in music therapy: a step on the long road to an evidence-based treatment. *Annals of the New York Academy of Sciences, 1060*, 283-93, (2005).

Novey D: *Clinicians' complete reference to complementary and alternative medicine*, St. Louis, 2000, Mosby.

Pagana KD, Pagana TJ: *Mosby's manual of diagnostic and laboratory test reference*, ed 3, St. Louis, 2006, Mosby.

Paul-Labrador M et al: Effects of a randomized controlled trial of transcendental meditation on components of the metabolic syndrome in subjects with coronary heart disease. *Archives of Internal Medicine*, 166: 1218-24, (2006).

Phillips N: *Berry & Kohn's operating room technique*, ed 11, St. Louis, 2007, Mosby.

Potter PA, Perry AG: *Fundamentals of nursing: concepts, process, and practice*, ed 5, St. Louis, 2001, Mosby.

Rakel D: *Integrative medicine*, Philadelphia, 2003, Saunders.

Safarinejad MR: Urtica dioica for treatment of benign prostatic hyperplasia: a prospective, randomized, double-blind, placebo-controlled crossover study. *Journal of Herbal Pharmacotherapy, 5* (4), 1-11, (2005).

Shiland B: *Mastering healthcare terminology*, ed 2, St Louis, 2006, Mosby.

Spencer JW, Jacobs JJ: *Complementary and alternative medicine: an evidence-based approach*, St Louis, 2003, Mosby.

Stedman's abbreviations, acronyms, and symbols, ed 3, Baltimore, 2003, Lippincott Williams & Wilkins.

Tan G et al: Hypnosis and irritable bowel syndrome: a review of efficacy and mechanism of action. *The American Journal of Clinical Hypnosis, 47* (3), 161-78, (2005).

Taylor-Piliae RE et al: Improvement in balance, strength, and flexibility after 12 weeks of Tai Chi exercise in ethnic Chinese adults with cardiovascular risk factors. *Alternative Therapies in Health and Medicine, 12(2)*, 50-8, (2006).

Thibodeau GA, Patton KT: *Anthony's textbook of anatomy and physiology*, ed 18, St. Louis, 2007, Mosby.

Torpy JM: The metabolic syndrome, *JAMA, 295* (7), 850, (2006).

UpToDate, http://www.uptodate.com, 2007.

Whiteside MM et al: Sensory impairment in older adults: part 2, vision loss, *Consultant, 106* (11), 52-62, (2006).

A

-a, 96
a-, 149
A&P (abdominoperineal) resection, 501, 520
A&P (anterior and posterior) repair, 319, 335
AAA (abdominal aortic aneurysm), 414f
Abbreviations/acronyms
  for cardiovascular, lymphatic systems, and blood, 455-456
  for digestive system, 523
  directional, 80
  for the ear, 597
  for endocrine system, 761
  for the eye, 568
  for female reproductive system, 337
  for integumentary system, 128-129
  for male reproductive system, 286
  for musculoskeletal system, 662
  for obstetrics and neonatology, 379
  for oncology, 51
  related to behavioral health, 721
  for respiratory system, 191-192
  for urinary system, 242
Abdomen/abdominal, 472f, 475, 515
Abdominal aortic aneurysm (AAA), 414f
Abdominal cavity, 21-23
abdomin/o, celi/o, lapar/o, 480
Abdominocentesis, 494
Abdominopelvic cavity, 21-23
Abdominopelvic quadrants, 78-80
Abdominopelvic regions, 75-77
Abdominoperineal (A&P) resection, 501, 520
Abdominoplasty, 494
Abducens nerve (VI), 682f
Abduction, 618-619
ABGs (arterial blood gases), 179, 191
Ablation, atrial fibrillation, 414f, 425
Ablation, endometrial, 319, 321f
Abortion, 361
Abrasion, 102
Abruptio placentae, 361, 362f
Abscess, 102
-ac, 406
Acapnia, 181
Accessory nerve (XI), 682f
Acetabulum, 610-612, 644t
Achilles tendon, 617f
Acid-fast bacilli (AFB) smear, 179, 191
Acidosis, 748
Acne, 102, 123t
Acoustic nerve (VIII), 580
Acoustic neuroma, 587
Acquired immunodeficiency syndrome (AIDS), 282, 286
acr/o, 743
Acromegaly, 744, 749
Acromium process, 609, 611f
Acronyms, 4-5. See also Abbreviations/acronyms.
ACS (acute coronary syndrome), 413, 455
ACTH (adrenocorticotropic hormone), 737, 738f
Actinic keratosis, 102, 103f
Active immunity, 453
Acupressure, 367b
Acupunture, 221
Acute coronary syndrome (ACS), 413, 455

Acute myocardial infarction (AMI), 413, 427b
Acute (or adult) respiratory distress syndrome (ARDS), 155, 160, 191
Acute otitis media (AOM), 597
Acute renal failure (ARF), 221
-ad, 29, 66
AD (Alzheimer disease), 693, 695, 721
Adam's apple (thyroid cartilage), 142, 739f
Addison disease, 748
Addison, Thomas, 748
Adduction, 618-619
Adenectomy, 753
Adenitis, 744
aden/o, 23, 741
Adenocarcinoma, 31
Adenohypophysis, 737
Adenoidectomy, 166
Adenoiditis, 153
adenoid/o, 145
Adenoids, 142
Adenoma, 31
Adenomegaly, 744
Adenosis, 744
Adenotome, 166
ADH (antidiuretic hormone), 737, 738f
ADHD (attention deficit hyperactivity disorder), 718, 721
Adhesions, 489
Adipose, 121
Adjuvant chemotherapy, 46
Adrenal cortex, 738f, 739
Adrenal glands, 736f, 738f, 739
Adrenal medulla, 739
Adrenalectomy, 753
Adrenaline (epinephrine), 740
Adrenalitis, 744
adren/o, adrenal/o, 741
Adrenocorticohyperplasia, 757
Adrenocorticotropic hormone (ACTH), 737, 738f
Adrenomegaly, 744
Adrenopathy, 757
Adult (or acute) respiratory distress syndrome (ARDS), 155, 160, 191
AFB (acid-fast bacilli) smear, 179, 191
Afferent, 711
AFib (atrial fibrillation), 455
Age-associated memory impairment, 711
Age-related macular degeneration (ARMD), 552, 568
AI (artificial insemination), 282, 286
AIDS (acquired immunodeficiency syndrome), 282, 286
Airway, 187
alb, 104f
Albinism, 102, 104f
albumin/o, 213
Albuminuria, 238
Aldosterone, 740
-algia, 150
Alimentary canal. See Digestive system.
Allergists, 453
Allergy/allergens, 121, 402f, 453
Alopecia, 121
ALS (amyotrophic lateral sclerosis), 693, 721
Alteplase (rtPA, recombinant tissue plasminogen activator), 427b
alveol/o, 145
Alveolus (pl.-alveoli), 143-144, 161f
Alzheimer disease (AD), 693, 695

Amblyopia (lazy eye), 551
Amenorrhea, 305
AMI (acute myocardial infarction), 413
amni/o, amnion/o, 354
Amniocentesis, 369, 370f
Amniochorial, 372
Amnion, 352, 353f
Amnionitis, 359
Amniorrhea, 372
Amniorrhexis, 372
-amnios, 358
Amnioscope/amnioscopy, 369
Amniotic/amnionic sac and fluid, 352, 353f, 370f
Ampulla of Vater, 739f
Amyotrophic lateral sclerosis (ALS), 693
an-, 149
Anal sphincter, 490f
Anaphylaxis/anaphylactic shock, 453
Anastomosis/ses, 502
Anatomic planes, 72-74
Anatomic position, 64-66
Anatomy and physiology
  of body cavities, 21-23
  for body organization, 20-23
  of cardiovascular system, 394-396, 414f
  of digestive system, 474-475
  of the ear, 427b
  of endocrine system, 736-740
  of the eye, 540-541
  of female reproductive system, 352-353
  of integumentary system, 90-91
  of male reproductive system, 260-261
  of musculoskeletal system, 608-612, 614-618
  of nervous system, 678-682
  of respiratory system, 142-144
  of urinary system, 208-211
andr/o, 264
Andropathy, 280
Anemia of chronic inflammation, 417b
Anemias, 417b
Anesthesia, 706
Aneurysmectomy, 425
Aneurysms
  cardiovascular, 413, 414f
  cerebral, 694, 696f, 697f
Angina pectoris, 413
angi/o, 403
Angiography
  coronary, 438
  defined, 431, 432f, 432t
  fluorescein, 561
Angioma, 408
Angioplasty, 422, 427, 428f
Angioscope/angioscopy, 431
Angiostenosis, 408
ankyl/o, 626
Ankylosing spondylitis, 636
Ankylosis, 629
Anmniotomy, 368
an/o, 477
Anoplasty, 494
Anorchism, 265
Anorexia nervosa, 489, 718
Anoxia, 181
ante-, pre-, 357
Antepartum, 372
Anterior (ant), 68f, 80
anter/o, 64

Page numbers followed by f indicate figures; t, tables; b, boxes.

829

Anteroposterior (AP), 68, 80
Antibiotic, 453
Antibodies, 453, 513
Antidiuretic hormone (ADH), 737, 738f
Antigens, 453
Antrectomy, 494
antr/o, 477
Antrum, 473-474
Anuria, 238
Anus/anal
    defined, 210f, 513
    structure and function of, 261f, 299, 472,
        474-475
Anxiety disorder, 718
AOM (acute otitis media), 597
Aorta, 395f
Aortic aneurysm, 414
Aortic stenosis, 408
Aortic valve, 395f
aort/o, 403
Aortogram, 431
Aphagia, 515
Aphasia, 706
-apheresis, 406
Aphonia, 181
Apical pulse, 82
Aplastic anemia, 417b
aponeur/o, 625
Aponeurorrhaphy, 643
Aponeurosis, 614
Appendectomy/appendicectomy, 494
Appendicitis, 483
appendic/o, 480
Appendix, 472f, 475
Aqueous humor, 540, 541f
-ar, 150
Arachnoid, 679f, 681, 705f
arche/o, 301
ARDS (adult (or acute) respiratory distress
    syndrome), 155, 160, 191
Areola, 299-300
ARF (acute renal failure), 221
Aristotle, 27
ARMD (age-related macular degeneration),
    552, 568
Arrhythmias, 415, 445
ART (assisted reproductive technology), 380f
Arterial blood gases (ABGs), 179, 191
Arterial pulses, 82
Arteries
    coronary, 431-432, 438f
    defined, 395
    pulmonary, 395f, 432f
    renal, 209f, 229f
    uterine, 320
    visualization of, 431-432, 438f
arteri/o, 403
Arteriogram
    coronary, 428f
    defined, 431, 432f
Arterioles, 209f
Arteriosclerosis, 408
Arteriovenous malformations (AVMs), 699
Arthralgia, 653
Arthritis
    in knee joint, 629f
    in spinal column, 631, 636
arthr/o, 625
Arthrocentesis, 643
Arthroclasia, 643
Arthrodesis, 643
Arthrography, 650
Arthroplasty, 643, 644t
Arthroscopes/arthroscopy, 328t, 651

Articular cartilage, 608f, 614, 629f
Articulations. *See* Joints.
Artificial immunity, 453
Artificial insemination (AI), 282, 286
-ary, 150
Ascending colon, 475f, 508f, 513f
Ascending limb, renal, 209f
Ascites, 519
Aspermia, 280
Asphyxia, 187
Aspirate, 187
Aspiration of bone marrow, 428b, 429f
Assisted reproductive technology (ART), 380f
Ast (astigmatism), 551, 568
-asthenia, 628
Asthma, 160
Astigmatism (Ast), 551, 568
Ataxia, 711
Atelectasis, 153
atel/o, 148
Atherectomy, 422
ather/o, 405
Atherosclerosis, 408
-atresia, 304
Atrial fibrillation (AFib), 414f, 415, 425, 455
atri/o, 403
Atrioventricular (AV), 445, 455
Atrium/atria, 395f
Atrophy, 629f, 653
Attention deficit hyperactivity disorder
    (ADHD), 718
audi/o, 582
Audiogram, 592, 593f
Audiology/audiologists, 595
Audiometer/audiometry, 592
Aural, 595
aur/i, aur/o, ot/o, 582
Auricle (pinna), 580f, 581
Auscultation, 438
Autism, 718
aut/o, 94
Autoimmune diseases, 453
AV (atrioventricular), 445, 455
AVMs (arteriovenous malformations), 699
Azoospermia, 280
Azotemia, 238
azot/o, 213

B

Bacteria/bacterium, 121
Bacterium/bacteria. *See also specific bacteria.*
Bag of water, 352
Balanitis, 265
balan/o, 262
Balanoplasty, 272
Balanorrhea, 265
Balloon angioplasty, 427, 428f
Balloon catheters, 427, 428f
Bariatric surgery, 502-503
Barium enema (BE), 512-513, 520, 523
Bartholin adenitis (Bartholinitis), 305
Bartholin, Casper, 299
Bartholin gland, 299
Basal cell carcinoma (BCC), 102, 103f, 123t,
    128
Basophils, 398
BE (barium enema), 512-513, 520, 523
Bed sores, 122, 128
Behavioral health
    abbreviations related to, 721
    disorders of, 718-719
    terms related to, 715-716
Bell palsy, 694
Bell, Sir Charles, 694

Benign, 46, 47
Benign prostatic hyperplasia (BPH), 265-266,
    275-277, 286
bi-, 66, 545
Biceps brachii muscle, 616f
Bilateral, 67
Bile ducts, 473, 475
Bilevel positive airway pressure (BiPAP), 192
Biliary tract, 472-473, 475
bin-, 545
Binocular, 563
bi/o, 94
Biofeedback, 718
Biomarkers, 439f
Biopsy/ies (bx)
    of bone marrow, 428b, 429f
    of breasts, 320, 323f
    endoscopic, 328t
    of skin, 111, 128
BiPAP (bilevel positive airway pressure), 192
Bipolar disorder, 718
Birmingham hip resurfacing, 644t
Biventricular pacing, 427b
Blanket continuous sutures, 114f
blast/o, 213
Blepharitis, 547
blephar/o, 543
Blepharoplasty, 555
blepharoptosis, 547
Blood
    combining forms for, 403, 405
    complementary terms for, 445-446, 450
    composition of, 398f
    defined, 398
    diseases and disorders of, 409, 417
    red blood cells, 37, 143f, 398, 436f, 456
    structure and function of, 398
    study of, 445
    suffixes for, 406
    surgical terms for, 428, 429f
    white blood cells, 37, 398, 436f, 456
    word parts for, 403-407
Blood clots. *See* Embolus/embolism
    (pl.-emboli); Thrombus/thrombosis
    (pl.-thrombi).
Blood pressure (BP), 438, 455
Blood urea nitrogen (BUN), 236, 245
Blood vessels, defined, 395. *See also specific
    vessels.*
Body cavities, 21-23
Body cells. *See* Cell/cells.
Body movement, 618-619
Body of stomach, 473-474
Body structure
    combining forms for, 23
    prefixes for, 28
    suffixes for, 29-31
    terms for, 37-41, 57
Bombeck, Erma, 305
Bone densitometry, 652t
Bone marrow
    aspiration of, 428b, 429f
    defined, 608f, 609
    transplantation of, 428
    tumor of, 630
Bone scan (nuclear medicine test), 652t
Bone spurs, 637
Bone tissue. *See also* Musculoskeletal system.
    compact vs. cancellous, 608
    cortical vs. spongy, 429f
    fractures of. *See* Fracture (Fx).
    osteoporosis in, 631, 639, 640f, 646t, 652t
    structure and function of, 608-612, 614-
        618

Borrelia burgdorferi bacteria, 638
BP (blood pressure), 438, 455
BPH (benign prostatic hyperplasia), 265-266
Brachial plexus, 678f
Brachial pulse, 82
Brachytherapy, 46
Bradycardia, 408
Bradykinesia, 653
Brain
   appearance with Alzheimer disease, 693f
   CT of, 703
   defined, 680
   MRI of, 703, 704f
   PET of, 704
   structure and function of, 678-682
   tumors of, 699
Brain attack. *See* Cerebrovascular accident
   (CVA).
Brainstem, 679f, 680
Breasts (mammary glands)
   biopsy of, 320, 323f
   cancer of, 310, 315t, 341
   fibrocysts in, 310
   online information on, 340
   prolactin and, 737, 738f
   structure and function of, 299-300, 738f
   surgeries on, 314, 315t
Breathing/respiration, 142
Breech presentation, 378
Bronchial tree, 142
Bronchiectasis, 153
bronchi/o, bronch/o, 145
Bronchioles, 142-143
Bronchitis, 153, 161f
Bronchoalveolar, 181
Bronchoconstrictor, 187
Bronchodilator, 187
Bronchoplasty, 166
Bronchopneumonia, 154, 155f
Bronchoscope/bronchoscopy, 169f, 171-172
Bronchospasm, 181
Bronchus (pl.-bronchi)
   endoscopy of, 169f
   primary, 162f
   structure and function of, 142-143
Broncogenic carcinoma, 153
Bulbourethral (Cowper's) gland and duct,
   261f
Bulimia nervosa, 489, 718
BUN (blood urea nitrogen), 236
Bunion/bunionectomy, 637
Burn keloid, 122
Bursa/bursae, 614
Bursectomy, 643
Bursitis, 630
burs/o, 625
bx (biopsy), 111, 128, 428b, 429f

C

C1-C7 (cervical vertebrae), 662
CABG (coronary artery bypass graft), 425,
   455
CAC (coronary artery calcification), 432t
CAD (coronary artery disease), 415, 455
Calcaneal tendon, 617f
Calcaneous, 611-612
calc/i, 743
Calculus/calculi
   of coronary artery, 432t
   in gallbladder, 484f
   prostatic, 266f
   renal, 216-217, 221, 228, 232
CAM. *See* Complementary and alternative
   medicine (CAM).

Camera/capsule endoscopy, 504
Cancellous bone, 429f, 608
Cancer. *See also* Carcinoma (Ca).
   of bone marrow, 630
   of breast, 310, 315t, 326f, 341
   of cervix, 310, 341
   of colon, 489f, 497f, 501, 506f
   of endometrium, 310, 341
   origination of term, 26
   of ovaries, 311, 341
   of prostate gland, 269, 270t
   of synovium, 631
   of testes, 269
   TNM staging system for, 31
   of uterus, 310
cancer/o, 26
Cancerous, 41
Candida/candidiasis, 104
Cannulae, uterine, 322f
Capillaries, 143f, 395
capn/o, 148
Capnometer, 173
Capsule
   of joints, 629f
   prostatic, 266f
   renal, 209f
Carbon dioxide (CO_2), 142, 191
Carbuncle, 104
carcin/o, 26
Carcinogen/carcinogenic, 41
Carcinoma (Ca), 31, 47f, 123, 341. *See also*
   Cancer.
Carcinoma in situ, 46
Cardia, 474
Cardiac arrest, 415
Cardiac catheterization, 432t, 438f
Cardiac muscle, 615, 618f
Cardiac resynchronization therapy (CRT),
   427b
Cardiac tamponade, 415
Cardiac/cardiogenic, 445
cardi/o, 403
Cardiodynia, 408
Cardiology/cardiologists, 445
Cardiomegaly, 408
Cardiomyopathy, 408
Cardiopulmonary resuscitation (CPR), 448,
   455
Cardiovalvulitis, 408
Cardiovascular system
   abbreviations for, 455-456
   combining forms for, 403, 405
   complementary terms for, 445-446,
     448-450
   diagnostic imaging for, 431-433, 436-437
   diagnostic terms for, 431-440
   diseases and disorders of, 408-409, 413-416
   structure and function of, 394-396, 414f
   suffixes for, 406
   surgical terms for, 422-423, 425, 427
   word parts for, 403-407
Carotid pulse, 82
Carpal, 653
Carpal bones, 610, 612
Carpal tunnel syndrome (CTS), 637, 662
Carpectomy, 643
carp/o, 620
Cartilage
   articular, 614
   costal, 610f
   structure and function of, 608f, 629f
Case studies, 194, 570
Castration, 272
Cataracts, 551

Catheters (caths)
   balloon type, 321f, 427, 428f
   coronary, 431-432, 438f
   for urinary system, 241-242, 245
Cauda equina, 678f, 679f, 705f
Caudad/caudal, 67, 68f
caud/o, 64
Cauterization, 113
Cavernous urethra, 261f
CBC (complete blood count), 439, 455
CCS (coronary calcium score), 432t
CCTA (coronary computed tomography
   angiography), 432t
CCU (coronary care unit), 455
cec/o, 477
Cecum, 472, 474-475, 508f, 513f
-cele, 150
Celiotomy, 494
Cell membrane, 20
Cell/cells. *See also specific cells.*
   defined, 20
   as formed elements of blood, 398
Cellulitis, 104
-centesis, 150
Central nervous system (CNS)
   defined, 678-682
   dementia-related infection in, 695
Central nervous system infection dementia,
   695
Cephalad, 67
Cephalgia/cephalalgia, 706
Cephalic, 67, 68f
Cephalic presentation, 378
cephal/o, 64, 356
Cerebellitis, 688
cerebell/o, 683
Cerebellum (hindbrain), 678-680, 739f
Cerebral, 706
Cerebral aneurysms, 694, 696f, 697f
Cerebral embolism, 694, 696f, 697f
Cerebral palsy (CP), 694, 721
Cerebral thrombosis, 688
cerebr/o, 683
Cerebrospinal fluid (CSF), 680, 681, 721
Cerebrovascular accident (CVA), 688, 695,
   696f
Cerebrum, 678-680
Ceruminoma, 587
Cervical vertebrae, 609, 610f, 611f
Cervicectomy, 314
Cervicitis, 305, 311f
cervic/o, 301
Cervix (Cx)
   abbreviations for, 337
   cancer of, 310
   structure and function of, 298-299, 353f
Cesarean section (C-section, CS), 379
CF (cystic fibrosis), 160, 191
Chalazion (meibomian cyst), 540, 551
Chart notes, 339, 665
cheil/o, 480
Cheilorraphy, 494
Chemical barriers, 402f
Chemical stress tests, 436
Chemotherapy (chemo), 46
Chest cavity, 21-23, 173
Chest computed tomography (CT) scans, 179
Chest physiotherapy (CPT), 192
Chest radiograph (CXR, chest x-ray), 179,
   191, 426f
CHF (congestive heart failure), 415, 455
Chiropodist, 660
Chiropractic/chiropractors, 660
Chlamydia, 282

Chloasma, 352
chlor/o, 27
Chloroma, 31
cholangi/o, 480
Cholangiogram/cholangiography, 504
Cholangioma, 483
chol/e, choledoch/o, 480
Cholecystectomy, 494
Cholecystitis, 484
Cholecystogram, 504
Choledocholithotomy, 494
Cholelithiasis, choledocholithiasis, 484, 505f
Cholesteatoma, 587
Cholesterol, 440t
Chondrectomy, 643
chondr/o, 625
Chondromalacia, 630
Chondroplasty, 645
chori/o, 354
Chorioanmionitis, 359
Choriocarcinoma, 359
Chorion, 352, 353f
Choroid, 540, 541f, 552f
chrom/o, 27
Chromosomes, 20
Chronic obstructive pulmonary disease
    (COPD), 160, 191
Chronic renal failure (CRF), 221
Cicatrix, 121
Ciliary body, 541f
Circumcision, 275
Cirrhosis, 489
-clasia, -clasis, -clast, 628
Clavicle, 609, 610f, 611f
clavic/o, clavicul/o, 620
Cleft lip and palate, 366
Clinical depression, 718
Clinical notes, 133, 290, 461, 599
Clitoris, 300
CMV (cytomegalovirus), 121, 128
CNS. See Central nervous system (CNS).
CO₂ (carbon dioxide), 142, 191
Coagulation time, 439
Coarctation of the aorta, 415
Coccidioidomycosis (valley fever), 160
-coccus (pl.-cocci), 96
Coccyx, 609, 610f, 611f
Cochlea, 580f, 581
Cochlear, 595
Cochlear implants, 590
cochle/o, 582
Coenzyme Q10, 160
Cognition/cognitive, 711
Cognitive impairment, 711
Coitus, 282
Colectomy, 494
Collecting duct, renal, 209f
Colles, Abraham, 642
Colles fractures, 637, 642, 652f
col/o, colon/o, 477
Colon
    cancer of, 506f
    diseases and disorders of, 489-491
    polyps of, 506f
    structure and function of, 472, 474-475
    visualization of, 508f
Colonoscopes/colonoscopy, 328t, 497f, 506f,
    508f
Colorectal, 515
Colors, 27
Colostomy, 501
Colostrum, 379
Colpitis, 305
colp/o, 301

Colpoplasty, 314
Colporrhaphy/colpoperineorraphy, 314, 319
Colposcope/colposcopy, 325
Coma, 711
Combining forms
    for body structure, 23
    for cardiovascular, lymphatic systems,
        and blood, 403, 405
    for color, 27
    defined, 9-10, 14
    for digestive system, 477, 480
    for directional terms, 64-65
    for the ear, 582
    for endocrine system, 741, 743
    for the eye, 543, 545
    for female reproductive system, 301-302
    for integumentary system, 92, 94
    lists of, 23, 26, 27
    for male reproductive system, 262, 264
    for musculoskeletal system, 620-621,
        625-626
    for nervous system, 683-684, 686
    for obstetrics and neonatology, 354, 356
    for respiratory system, 148
    for urinary system, 211, 213
Combining vowels, 7-9, 10t, 14
Comminuted fractures, 637
Common bile duct, 473f, 475, 484f, 739f
Compact bone, 429f, 608
Complementary and alternative medicine
    (CAM)
    acupressure, 367b
    acupuncture, 221
    biofeedback, 718
    defined, 38
    herbal therapy, 266
    homeopathy, 98
    hypnotherapy, 491b
    light therapy, 552
    massage therapy, 311
    meditation, 409
    music therapy, 588
    vitamin therapy, 160
    yoga, 751
Complementary terms
    for cardiovascular, lymphatic systems, and
        blood, 445-446, 448-450
    for digestive system, 515-516, 519-520
    for the ear, 595
    for endocrine system, 757, 760
    for the eye, 563-564, 566
    for female reproductive system, 333, 335
    for immune system, 453-454
    for integumentary system, 116-128
    for male reproductive system, 280, 282-283
    for musculoskeletal system, 653-655, 660
    for neonatology, 371-373, 378-379
    for nervous system, 706-707, 711-712
    for obstetrics, 371-373, 378-379
    for oncology, 41-48, 57
    for respiratory system, 181-190
    for urinary system, 238-239, 241-242
Complete blood count (CBC), 439, 455, 652
Compound fractures, 637
Compression fractures, 637
Computed tomography angiography (CTA),
    432t
Computed tomography (CT) scans
    abbreviation for, 191
    in behavioral health, 718
    of blood vessels, 432t
    of brain, 703
    of chest, 179
    of colon, 504

Computed tomography (CT) scans
    (Continued)
    documentation of, 195
    for endocrine system, 754
    helical (spiral), 179
    machine for, 174t
    for musculoskeletal system, 652t
    for myelography, 701
    scanner for, 703f
    single-photon emission (SPECT), 436,
        437f, 456, 652
Conception/fertilization, 352, 353f
Concussion, 712
Congenital anomaly, 379
Congenital heart diaease, 415
Congestive heart failure (CHF), 415, 455
coni/o, 94
Conization/cone biopsy, 319
Conjunctiva, 540, 541f
Conjunctivitis, 547
conjunctiv/o, 543
Connective tissue, 21
Consciousness, 712
Consultation reports, 723
Contact dermatitis, 99t, 123t
Continuous positive airway pressure (CPAP),
    160, 188f, 192
Continuous sutures, 114f
Contusion, 104
Convulsions, 712
Cooled ThermoTherapy, 276-277
COPD (chronic obstructive pulmonary
    disease), 160, 191
Copulation, 282
Cor pulmonale, 160
Cornea, 540, 541f, 551f
Corneal, 563
corne/o, 543
Cornified layer, 90
cor/o, core/o, pupill/o, 543
Coronal, 72-74
Coronary arteries, 431-432, 438f
Coronary artery bypass graft (CABG), 425,
    455
Coronary artery calcification (CAC), 432t
Coronary artery disease (CAD), 415, 455
Coronary calcium score (CCS), 432t
Coronary care unit (CCU), 455
Coronary computed tomography angiogra-
    phy (CCTA), 432t
Coronary occlusion, 415
Coronary stent, 426f
Corpus (body) of uterus, 298-299
Corpuscle, renal, 209f
Cortex, renal, 209f
Cortical bone, 429f
Cortical/corticoid, 757
cortic/o, 741
Cortisol, 739
Costal cartilage, 610f
Costectomy, 645
cost/o, 620
Cough, 187
Cowper's (bulbourethral) gland and duct,
    261f
CP (cerebral palsy), 694, 721
CPAP (continuous positive airway pressure),
    160, 188f, 192
CPK (creatine phosphokinase), 439, 455
CPR (cardiopulmonary resuscitation), 448,
    455
CPT (chest physiotherapy), 192
Cranial, 653
Cranial cavity, 21-23

Cranial nerves, 678, 682f
crani/o, 620
Craniocerebral, 706
Cranioplasty, 645
Cranioschisis, 630
Craniotomy, 645
Cranium, 610-611
C-reactive protein (CRP), 439, 455
Creatine phosphokinase (CPK), 439, 455
Creatinine, 236
Crepitus/crepitation, 660
Cretinism, 744
CRF (chronic renal failure), 221
Crohn disease, 490
Croup (laryngotracheobronchitis), 154, 160, 191
CRP (C-reactive protein), 439, 455
CRT (cardiac resynchronization therapy), 427b
cry/o, 545
Cryoretinopexy, 555
Cryosurgery, 113
crypt/o, 94
Cryptorchidism, 266
C-section (cesarean section), 379
CSF (cerebrospinal fluid), 680, 681, 721
CT colonography, 504
CT scan. See Computed tomography (CT) scans.
CTA (computed tomography angiography), 432t
CTS (carpal tunnel syndrome), 637, 662
culd/o, 301
Culdocentesis, 325
Culdoscope/culdoscopy, 325
Curettes, 319, 321f
Cushing, Harvey Williams, 749
Cushing syndrome, 749
cutane/o, 92
Cx. See Cervix (Cx).
CXR (chest radiograph or chest x-ray), 179, 191, 426f
cyan/o, 27
Cyanosis, 41, 43f
-cyesis, 358
Cyst, 121, 123t
Cystectomy, 223
Cystic duct, 473f, 475, 484f
Cystic fibrosis (CF), 160, 191
Cystitis, 216, 217f
cyst/o, 211
Cystocele, 216
Cystogram/cystography, 230, 231f
Cystolith, 216
Cystolithotomy, 223
Cystorrhaphy, 223
Cystoscope/cystoscopy, 232
Cystostomy, 223
Cystotomy/vesicotomy, 223
Cystourethroscopes, 228f
Cysts, 221f
-cyte, 29
cyt/o, 23
Cytogenic, 37
Cytoid, 37
Cytology, 37
Cytomegalovirus (CMV), 121, 128
Cytoplasm, 20, 37

D

D&C (dilation and curettage), 319, 321f, 337
dacry/o, 543
Dacryocystitis, 547
Dacryocystorhinostomy, 555

Dacryocystotomy, 555
Date of birth (DOB), 379
De Graaf, Reinier, 298
Debridement, 113
Decub (pressure ulcer), 122, 128
Decubitus ulcer, 122, 128
Deep vein thrombosis (DVT), 415, 455
Defibrillation, 449
Delirium, 711
Deltoid muscle, 616f, 617f
Dementia
    of Alzheimer disease, 693
    defined, 694
    types of, 695
Deoxyribonucleic acid (DNA), 20
Depression, 718
Derm (dermatology), 92, 128
Dermabrasion, 113
Dermatitis, 98-99
dermat/o, 92
Dermatoautoplasty, 111
Dermatoconiosis, 98
Dermatofibroma, 98
Dermatoheteroplasty, 111
Dermatologist, 116
Dermatology, 116, 124
Dermatome, 111
Dermatoplasty, 111
Dermis, 90-91
derm/o, 92, 128
Descending colon, 475f, 508f, 513f
Descending limb, renal, 209f
-desis, 628
Detached retina, 551, 552f, 558f
Deviated septum, 160
DEXA (dual-energy X-ray absorptiometry) scan, 652t
DI (diabetes insipidus), 749, 761
Diabetes insipidus (DI), 749, 761
Diabetes mellitus (DM), 749-750, 761
Diagnosis (Dx), 42
Diagnostic imaging
    for cardiovascular, lymphatic system, and blood, 431-433, 436-437
    for digestive system, 504-508, 512-513
    for endocrine system, 754-755
    for the eye, 561
    for female reproductive system, 325, 330
    for male reproductive system, 279
    for musculoskeletal system, 650, 652t
    for nervous system, 701, 703-704
    in obstetrics, 369
    for respiratory system, 174, 179
    for urinary system, 230-232, 236
Diagnostic terms
    for cardiovascular, lymphatic system, and blood, 431-440
    for digestive system, 504-508, 512-513
    for the ear, 592-593
    for endocrine system, 754-755
    for the eye, 561
    for female reproductive system, 325, 330, 331f
    for male reproductive system, 279
    for musculoskeletal system, 650-652
    for nervous system, 701, 703-705
    in obstetrics, 369
    for respiratory system, 171-181
    for urinary system, 230-232, 236-237
Diaphoresis, 121
Diaphragm, 143-144
Diaphragmatic (phrenic), 181
diaphragmat/o, 145
Diaphragmatocele, 154

Diaphysis, 608f, 609
Diarrhea, 519
Diastole, 449
Differential count (diff.), 439, 455
Digestive system
    abbreviations for, 523
    complementary terms for, 515-516, 519-520
    diagnostic terms for, 504-508, 512-513
    diseases and disorders of, 483-485, 489-491
    prefixes and suffixes for, 483
    structure and function of, 474-475
    surgical terms for, 494-496, 501-504
    word parts and combining forms for, 477, 480
Digital rectal examination (DRE), 279, 286
Digital subtraction angiography (DSA), 432t, 436, 455
Dilatation. See Dilation and curettage (D&C).
Dilation and curettage (D&C), 319, 321f, 337
Dilators, uterine, 321f
dipl/o, 545
Diplopia, 547
dips/o, 743
Directional terms, 64-65, 67-68
Discharge summaries, 247
Diseases and disorders. See also under specific body systems.
    oncologic, 31-32
Diskectomy, 638f, 645
Diskitis, 630
disk/o, 625
Disks/discs. See Intervertebral disks.
Disorientation, 712
Distal, 67, 68f
Distal tubules, renal, 209f
Distended/distension, 241
dist/o, 64
Diuretic/diuresis, 238, 241
Diurnal enuresis, 241
Diverticulectomy, 494
Diverticulitis/diverticulosis, 484, 506f
diverticul/o, 480
DM (diabetes mellitus), 749-750, 761
DNA (deoxyribonucleic acid), 20
DOB (date of birth), 379
Documentation, medical
    case studies, 194, 570
    chart notes, 339, 665
    clinical notes, 133, 290, 461, 599
    consultation reports, 723
    CT scan reports, 195
    discharge summaries, 247
    emergency department notes, 197, 288
    endoscopy reports, 524b
    history and physical forms, 762
    medical consult report, 193
    operative reports, 130, 247, 664, 763
    pathology reports, 131
    progress notes, 81, 83, 289, 338, 384, 385, 458-459, 569, 598, 723
    radiology reports, 385, 525-526
Donor organs, 228, 229f
Doppler ultrasound, 436
Dorsal, 68
Dorsalis pedis pulse, 82
dors/o, 64
Douglas cul-de-sac
    procedures on, 325
    structure and function of, 298-299
Down syndrome, 366
DPI (dry powder inhaler), 192

DRE (digital rectal examination), 279, 286
Drugs. *See specific drugs.*
Dry powder inhaler (DPI), 192
DSA (digital subtraction angiography), 432t, 436, 455
Dual-energy X-ray absorptiometry (DEXA) scan, 652t
Ductus deferens, 260, 273
Duodenal ulcers, 490, 491f
duoden/o, 477
Duodenum, 473-474, 484f, 495f, 503, 739f
Dura mater, 679f, 681, 689f, 705f
Duritis, 688
dur/o, 683
DVT (deep vein thrombosis), 415, 455
Dwarfism, 749
Dx (diagnosis), 42
Dysarthria, 712
Dyscrasia, 450
Dysentery, 519
Dyskinesia, 653
Dysmenorrhea, 305
Dyspareunia, 335
Dyspepsia, 515
Dysphagia, 515
Dysphasia, 706
Dysphonia, 181
Dysplasia, 37, 47f
Dyspnea, 181
Dystocia, 359
Dystrophy, 653
Dysuria, 238

E

-e, 358
-eal, 150
Ear
    abbreviations for, 597
    combining forms for, 582
    complementary terms for, 595
    diagnostic terms for, 592-593
    diseases and disorders of, 584-585, 587-588
    structure and function of, 580-581
    surgical terms for, 590
    word parts and combining forms for, 582
Ear wax, 402f
Eardrum (tympanic membrane), 580f, 581, 585f
Ears, nose, and throat (ENT), 597
EBCT (electronic beam CT) scanner, 432t
Ecchymosis, 121
ECG. *See* Electrocardiogram/graph/graphy (EKG, ECG).
ech/o, 405
Echocardiogram (ECHO), 433, 436-437, 455
Eclampsia, 361
-ectasis, 150
-ectomy, 96
Ectopic pregnancy, 361
Eczema, 104
EDD (expected/estimated date of delivery), 379
Edema, 121
EEG (electroencephalogram/graph/graphy), 701, 721
EENT (eyes, ears, nose, and throat), 597
Efferent, 712
EGD (esophagogastroduodenoscopy), 505, 523
EKG. *See* Electrocardiogram/graph/graphy (EKG, ECG).
Elective abortion, 361
electr/o, 405
Electrocardiogram/graph/graphy (EKG, ECG), 433, 455, 662

Electroencephalogram/graph/graphy (EEG), 701, 721
Electrolytes, 740
Electromyelogram/graphy (EMG), 651, 662
Electronic beam CT (EBCT) scanner, 432t
Electrophysiologists, 445
Em (emmetropia), 551, 568
Embolecyomy, 425
Embolus/embolism (pl.-emboli)
    cerebral, 694, 696f, 697f
    defined, 417
    pulmonary, 162f, 163
Embryo, 260, 352
embry/o, 354
Embryogenic/embryoid, 372
Emergency department notes/reports, 197, 288
Emesis, 520
EMG (electromyelogram/graphy), 651, 662
-emia, 151
Emmetropia (Em), 551, 568
Emollient, 122
Emphysema, 160, 161f
Encapsulated, 46, 47f
Encephalitis, 688
encephal/o, 683
Encephalomalacia, 688
Encephalomyeloradiculitis, 688
Encephalosclerosis, 707
Endarterectomy, 422
endo-, 150
Endocarditis, 408
Endocardium, 395
Endocervicitis, 305
Endocrine glands. *See also* Endocrine system.
    defined, 736
Endocrine system. *See also specific glands.*
    abbreviations for, 761
    complementary terms for, 757, 760
    diagnostic terms for, 754-755
    diseases and disorders of, 744-745, 748-750
    structure and function of, 736-740
    surgical terms for, 753
    word parts and combining forms for, 741, 743
endocrin/o, 741
Endocrinology/endocrinologist, 757
Endocrinopathy, 757
Endometrial ablation, 319, 321f
Endometriosis, 310
Endometritis, 305, 311f
Endometrium
    ablation of, 321f
    cancer of, 310
    inflammation of, 305, 311f
    structure and function of, 298-299
Endophthalmitis, 547
Endoscope/endoscopic, 171-172, 175t, 504
Endoscopic retrograde cholangiopancreatography (ERCP), 512, 523
Endoscopic ultrasound (EUS), 512, 523
Endoscopy reports, 524b
Endoscopy/endoscopic surgery
    with camera, 504
    defined, 504
    for digestive system, 494f
    documentation of, 524b
    for female reproductive system, 325
    for musculoskeletal system, 651
    for respiratory system, 171-172, 175t
    types of, 328t, 504-508
    for urinary system, 232
Endosteum, 608f, 609
Endotracheal, 181

Endotracheal tube, 176f
Endovenous laser ablation, 417
End-stage renal disease (ESRD), 221
End-to-end anastomosis, 502f
End-to-side anastomosis, 502f
Enema, barium, 512-513
ENT (ears, nose, and throat), 597
Enteritis, 490
enter/o, 477
Enterorrhaphy, 495
Enucleation, 558
Enuresis, 241
Eosinophils, 398
EP (evoked potential) studies, 721
epi-, 95
Epicardium, 395
Epidermal, 116
Epidermis, 90-91
Epididymectomy, 272
Epididymitis, 266
epididym/o, 262
Epididymus, 260, 261f
Epigastric region, 75-77
Epiglottis, 142-143, 161f, 739f
Epiglottitis, 154
epiglott/o, 145
Epilepsy, 694
Epinephrine (adrenaline), 740
Epiphyseal plates, 608f
Epiphysis/epiphyses, 608f
episi/o, 301
Episioperineoplasty, 314
Episiorrhaphy, 314
Episiotomy, 368
Epispadias, 220
Epistaxis (rhinorrhagia), 155, 160
Epithelial, 37
Epithelial tissue, 21
epitheli/o, 23
Epithelioma, 31
Epithelium, 23
Eponyms, defined, 4-5
Epstein-Barr virus, 417
ERCP (endoscopic retrograde cholangiopancreatography), 512, 523
Erectile dysfunction (ED), 269
Erector pilli muscle, 90
Erythema, 122
erythr/o, 27
Erythroblastosis fetalis, 366
Erythrocytes (RBCs), 37, 143f, 398, 436f, 456
Erythrocytosis, 37
Erythroderma, 116
-esis, 214
Esophageal atresia, 366
Esophagitis, 484
esophag/o, 356, 477
Esophagogastroduodenoscopy (EGD), 505, 523
Esophagogastroplasty, 495
Esophagogram/barium swallow, 504
Esophagoscope/esophagoscopy, 505
Esophagus, 472f, 473, 495f, 503, 739f
ESRD (end-stage renal disease), 221
esthesi/o, 686
ESWL (extracorporeal shock wave lithotripsy), 223, 224f, 228, 245
eti/o, 26
Etiology, 42
eu-, 150
Euglycemia, 757
Eupnea, 181
EUS (endoscopic ultrasound), 512, 523
Eustachian tubes, 580f, 581

Euthyroid, 757
Eversion, 618-619
Evoked potential (EP) studies, 721
Exacerbation, 46
Excimer lasers, 558f
Excision, 113
Excisional biopsy, 111
Exercise stress tests, 436
Exfoliative erythroderma, 116f
Exocrine glands, 736
Exopthalmos, 760
Exostosis/bone spurs, 637
Expected (estimated) date of delivery (EDD), 379
Extension, 618-619
Extensor digitorum longus muscle, 616f
External abdominal oblique muscle, 616f, 617f
External auditory meatus, 580f, 581
External ear, 580f, 581
Extracorporeal, 449
Extracorporeal shock wave lithotripsy (ESWL), 223, 224f, 228, 245
Extravasation, 449
Eye
    abbreviations for, 568
    complementary terms for, 563-564, 566
    diseases and disorders of, 547-548, 551-553
    prefixes and suffixes for, 546
    structure and function of, 540-541
    surgical terms for, 555-556, 558-559
    word parts and combining forms for, 543, 545
Eyebrows/eyelids, 541f, 547f
Eyes, ears, nose, and throat (EENT), 597

F
Facets, spinal, 640f
Facial muscles, 616f
Facial nerve (VII), 682f
Fallopian tubes
    ligation of, 320
    removal of, 315
    structure and function of, 298-299
Fallopius, Gabrielle, 298
FAS (fetal alcohol syndrome), 367, 379
Fasting blood sugar (FBS), 755, 761
Fatty tissue, 90, 116, 128, 261f
FBD (fibrocystic breast disease), 310, 319, 337
FBS (fasting blood sugar), 755, 761
Fecal occult blood test (FOBT), 512, 523
Feces, 520
Femoral, 653
Femoral head, 644t
Femoral nerve, 678f
Femoral pulse, 82
Femoral vein, 432f
    bypass of, 426f, 427
    structure and function of, 432f
femor/o, 620
Femoropopliteal bypass graft, 426f, 427
Femur, 610-612, 640f, 644t
Fertilization/conception
    assisted reproductive technology (ART) for, 380f
    defined, 352, 353f
    in vitro, 379, 380f
Fetal, 372
Fetal alcohol syndrome (FAS), 367, 379
fet/o, fet/i, 354
Fetus, 352, 353f
Fever, 402f
Fiberoptic light cords, 228f

Fibrillation, 449
fibr/o, 23
Fibrocystic breast disease (FBD), 310, 319, 337
Fibroid tumors, 311
Fibroma, 31
Fibromyalgia, 630
Fibrosarcoma, 32
Fibula, 610-612
fibul/o, 620
Fimbria (pl. fimbriae), 298-299, 353f
Fissure, 105
Fistula, 335, 364
Flatus, 520
Flexion, 618-619
Flu (influenza), 160, 191
Fluorescein angiography, 561
FOBT (fecal occult blood test), 512, 523
Follicle-stimulating hormone (FSH), 737, 738f
Foreign agents, 402f
Formed elements, 398
Fracture (Fx), 637, 640f, 642, 646t, 652f, 662. *See also specific fractures.*
Freckle, 123t
Frontal, 72-74
FSH (follicle-stimulating hormone), 737, 738f
Fulguration, 228
Fundus, stomach, 473-474
Fundus, uterine, 298-299, 353f
Fungus, 122
Furuncle, 104f, 105
Fx (fracture), 637, 640f, 642, 646t, 652f, 662. *See also specific fractures.*

G
Gait/gaits, 712
Gallbladder
    diagnostic terms for, 504-505
    diseases and disorders of, 483-484
    structure and function of, 473-475, 483-484
    surgery on, 494-496
Gallstones, 484f
Gamete, 352, 353f
Gangliectomy, ganglionectomy, 699
Gangliitis, 688
gangli/o, ganglion/o, 683
Ganglion/ganglia, 679f, 682
Gangrene, 105
Gastrectomy, 495
Gastric bypass surgery, 503
Gastric lavage, 520
Gastric ulcers, 490
Gastritis, gastroenteritis, 484
gastr/o, 477
Gastrocnemius muscle, 616f
Gastrodynia, 515
Gastroenterocolitis, 485
Gastroenterology/gastroenterologists, 515
Gastroesophageal reflux disease (GERD), 490, 512, 523
Gastrointestinal (GI) tract. *See Digestive system.*
Gastrojejunostomy, 495
Gastromalacia, 515
Gastroplasty, 495
Gastroschisis, 367
Gastroscope/gastroscopy, 505, 507f
Gastrostomy, 496
Gavage, 520
-gen, 29
Gene therapy, 20

Genes, 20
-genesis, 29
-genic, 29
Genital herpes, 282
Genitals/genitalia, 261
Genome, 20
Genomics, 20
GERD (gastroesophageal reflux disease), 490, 512, 523
Gestation/gestation period, 352
GH (growth hormone), 737, 738f
GI (gastrointestinal), 523
Gigantism, 749
Gingivectomy, 496
Gingivitis, 485
gingiv/o, 480
Glands
    adrenal glands, 736f, 738f, 739
    bulbourethral (Cowper's) gland and duct, 261f
    of female reproductive system, 299, 736f, 738f
    hypothalamus gland, 737, 739f
    lacrimal glands, 540, 541f
    of male reproductive system, 260-261, 269-270, 736f, 738f
    mammary glands, 299-300, 738f
    meibomian glands, 551, 5540
    pancreas/islets of Langerhans, 736f, 738, 739f
    pineal gland, 739f
    pituitary gland, 736, 737-739
    prostate. *See Prostate gland.*
    salivary glands, 474
    sebaceous glands, 90-91
    sudoriferous glands, 90-91
    thymus gland, 399f, 400, 736f
    thyroid/parathyroid glands, 736f, 737
Glans penis, 261
Glaucoma, 552
Glia/neuroglia, 679f, 682
gli/o, 683
Gliocytes, 707
Glioma/glioblastoma, 688
glomerul/o, 211
Glomerulonephritis, 216
Glomerulus (pl. glomeruli), 208, 209f, 211
gloss/o/, lingu/o, 480
Glossopathy, 515
Glossopharyngeal nerve (IX), 682f
Glossorrhaphy, 496
Glucagon, 738
Gluteus maximus muscle, 617f
glyc/o, 213
glycos/o, 213
Glycosuria, 238
Glycosylated hemoglobin (HbA1C), 755, 761
gno/o, 26
Goiter, 749, 750
Gonadotropic hormones, 737. *See also Repro-ductive systems.*
Gonads, 282
Gonorrhea, 282
Gout, 638
Graafian follicles, 298-299
Gracilis muscle, 617f
-gram, 214
-graph/-graphy, 151, 406
Graves disease, 749
gravid/o, 354, 372
Gravidopuerpural, 372
Gray matter, 679f
Greater duodenal papilla, 484f
Greater trochanter, 610f

Greek language, 4-5
Greenstick fractures, 637
Growth hormone (GH), 737, 738f
GYN (gynecology), 337
gynec/o, 301
Gynecology/gynecologists, 333, 337
gyn/o, 301
Gynopathic, 333
Gyri, 693f

H

H. pylori (*Helicobacter pylori*), 513, 523
Hair, 91
Hair follicle, 90
Hair shaft, 90
Hallux valgus, 637
Hard palate, 473
HbA1C (glycosylated hemoglobin, hemoglobin A1C), 755, 761
HCT (hematocrit), 439, 440, 455
HDL (high-density lipoprotein), 440t
Headaches, 706
Heart. *See also* Cardiovascular system.
    anatomy of, 395f, 396f, 414f
    defined, 394
    rhythm patterns of, 414f
Heart attack (myocardial infarction), 416
Heart failure (HF), 415
Heart murmurs, 449
Helical computed tomography (CT) scan, 179
Helicobacter pylori antibodies test, 513, 523
Hematemesis, 520
Hematochezia, 520
Hematocrit (HCT), 439, 440, 455
Hematology/hematologists, 445
Hematoma, 409, 689f
Hematopoiesis, 445
Hematosalpinx, 305
Hematuria, 238
hemi-, 483
Hemicolectomy, 496
Hemiparesis, 707
Hemiplegia, 707
hem/o, hemat/o, 148
Hemochromatosis, 490
Hemodialysis (HD), 241, 242f, 245
Hemoglobin A1C (HbA1C), 755
Hemoglobin (Hgb), 439, 440, 455
Hemolysis, 445
Hemolytic anemia, 417b
Hemophilia, 417
Hemorrhage, 450, 694, 696
Hemorrhagic stroke. *See* Cerebrovascular accident (CVA).
Hemorrhoids, 490
Hemostasis, 445
Hemothorax, 154
Hepatic duct, 473f, 475, 484f
Hepatic flexure, 475f, 513f
Hepatitis, 485
hepat/o, 480
Hepatoma, 485
Herbal therapy, 266
Hernias/herniation
    hiatal, 480f
    inguinal, 480f, 489f
    of intervertebral disks, 638, 640, 646t
    types of, 480f
    umbilical, 364, 365f, 480f, 489f
Herniated nucleus pulposus (HNP), 638, 640, 646t, 662
herni/o, 480
Herniorrhaphy, 496
Herpes, 99t, 105

Herpes simplex, 123t
Herpes simplex virus, 282
Herpes zoster (shingles), 99t, 105, 106, 123t, 695
heter/o, 94
Heterosexuality, 282
HF (heart failure), 415
Hgb (hemoglobin), 439, 440, 455
HHD (hypertensive heart disease), 416, 456
Hiatal hernias, 480f
Hiccup/hiccough, 187
Hidradenitis, 98
hidr/o, 92
High-density lipoprotein (HDL), 440t
Hilum of kidney, 208
Hip joint, 610-612, 640f
Hippocrates, 31
hist/o, 23
Histology, 37
History and physical forms, 762
HIV (human immunodeficiency virus), 283, 286, 453
HNP (herniated nucleus pulposus), 638, 640, 646t, 662
Hodgkin disease, 417
Homeopathy, 98
Homocysteine, 439
Homosexuality, 282
Hordeolum, 553
Hormone replacement therapy (HRT), 335, 337
Hormones. *See also specific hormones.*
    defined, 736, 760
    secreted by pituitary gland, 738f
HPV (human papillomavirus), 283, 286
HRT (hormone replacement therapy), 335, 337
Human immunodeficiency virus (HIV), 283, 286, 453
Human papillomavirus (HPV), 283, 286
Humeral, 653
humer/o, 620
Humerus, 609, 610f, 611f
Hunchback/humpback, 630
Hyaline membrane disease, 160
Hydramnios, 359
hydr/o, 213
Hydrocele, 269
Hydrocelectomy, 275
Hydrocephalus, 694, 695
Hydrocortisone, 739
Hydronephrosis, 216
Hydrosalpinx, 305
Hymen, 298-299
Hymenectomy/hymenotomy, 314
hymen/o, 301
Hypercalcemia/hypocalcemia, 744
Hypercapnia, 181
Hypercholesterolemia, 449
Hyperesthesia, 707
Hyperglycemia/hypoglycemia, 744
Hyperkalemia/hypokalemia, 744
Hyperkinesia, 653
Hyperlipidemia, 449
Hyperopia (farsightedness), 551f, 552
Hyperpituitarism/hypopituitarism/ panhypopituitarism, 744-745
Hyperplasia
    benign prostatic (BPH), 275-277, 286
    defined, 37, 47f
Hyperpnea, 181, 197
Hypertension, 221, 449
Hypertensive heart disease (HHD), 416, 456
Hyperthyroidism/hypothyroidism, 744

Hypertriglyceridemia, 449
Hypertrophy, 653
Hyperventilation, 187
Hypnotherapy, 491b
Hypocapnia, 181
Hypochondriac, 75
Hypochondriac regions, 75-77
Hypodermic, 116
Hypogastric region, 75-77
Hypoglossal nerve (XII), 682f
Hyponatremia, 745
Hypophysis cerebri, 737
Hypoplasia, 37
Hypopnea, 182
Hypospadias, 220
Hypotension, 450
Hypothalamus gland, 737, 738f, 739f
Hypothermia, 445
Hypoventilation, 187
Hypoxemia, 182
Hypoxia, 182
Hysteratresia, 305
Hysterectomy
    defined, 314
    total (TAH), 337
    types of, 315t
hyster/o, 301
Hysteropexy, 314
Hysteroptosis, 311
Hysterorrhexis, 359
Hysterosalpingo-oophorectomy (TAH, BS&O), 314, 337
Hysteroscope/hysteroscopy, 325, 328t

I

I and D (incision and drainage), 113, 128
-ia, 96
-ial, 304
-iasis, 214
iatr/o, 26
Iatrogenic, 42
Iatrology, 42
-iatry/-iatrist, 687
IBS (irritable bowel syndrome), 491, 523
-ic, 29
ICD (implantable cardiac defibrillator), 427, 456
-ictal, 687
ID (intradermal), 116, 128
Idiopathic, 46
Ileitis, 490
ile/o, 477
Ileocecal, 515
Ileostomy, 496
Ileum, 472, 474, 513f
Ileus, 491
Iliac regions, 75-77
Iliac vein, 432f
ili/o, 620
Iliofemoral, 653
Iliotibial tract, 617f
Ilium, 610-612
Immune system
    complementary terms for, 453-454
    lymphatic system's role in, 394
    structure and function of, 401-402
    three lines of defense in, 401, 402f
Immune/immunity
    specific, 401, 402f
    types of, 453
Immunity, 541f
Immunodeficiency, 453
Immunoglobulins, 453
Immunology/immunologists, 453

Impacted fractures, 637
Impedance plethysmography (IPG), 438, 456
Impetigo, 99t, 105
Impetigo acne, 123t
Implantable cardiac defibrillator (ICD), 427, 456
Implantation, 352, 353f
In situ, 46, 47
In vitro, 46
In vitro fertilization (IVF), 367, 379, 380f
In vivo, 46
Incidentaloma, 29
Incision and drainage (I and D), 113, 128
Incisions
    anterior (ant), 175t
    defined, 113
    posterior, 175t
Incoherent, 712
Incontinence, urinary, 242
Incus (anvil), 580f, 581, 585f, 590f
Induced abortion, 361
Induration, 122
Infant respiratory distress syndrome of
    newborns (IRDS), 160
Infection/s
    defined, 104f, 453
    of male reproductive system, 266
    nosocomial, 187
    of respiratory tract, 162f, 191
    of urinary tract, 217f, 221
Infectious mononucleosis, 417
Inferior (inf), 67, 68f, 80
infer/o, 64
Inflammation
    C-reactive protein (CRP) and, 439
    defined, 46
    as line of defense, 402f
Influenza (flu), 160, 191
Infraspinatus muscle, 617f
Inguinal hernias, 480f, 489f
Insulin, 738
Integrative medicine, 38
Integumentary system. See also Skin.
    abbreviations for, 128-129
    combining forms for, 92, 94
    complementary terms for, 116-128
    diseases and disorders of, 98-111
    online information on, 132
    prefixes for, 95-96
    structure and function of, 90, 90-91
    suffixes for, 96-97
    surgical terms for, 111-115
    word parts for, 92-93
inter-, 627
Intercostal, 654
Intercostal nerves, 678f
Interferons, 401
Interictal, 707
Intermittent claudication, 416, 436
Intermittent sutures, 114f
Intervertebral, 654
Intervertebral disks
    defined, 614, 625
    herniation of, 638, 640, 646t, 662
Intestinal obstructions, 489f
Intestines. See Colon; Small intestine/bowel.
intra-, 95
Intracerebral, 707
Intracerebral hemorrhage, 694
Intracranial, 654
Intradermal, 116, 128
Intraocular, 563
Intrapartum, 372
Intrapleural, 182

Intravenous (IV), 445, 456
Intravenous urogram or pyelogram (IVU/
    IVP), 230, 245
Intussusception, 489f, 491
Invasive procedures, 432
Inversion, 618-619
-ior, 66
IPG (impedance plethysmography), 438, 456
Iridectomy, 555
irid/o, ir/o, 543
Iridoplegia, 547
Iridotomy, 555
Iris, 540, 541f
Iritis, 547
Iron deficiency anemia, 417b
Irritable bowel syndrome (IBS), 491, 523
-is, 358
Ischemia, 408
Ischemic stroke. See Cerebrovascular accident
    (CVA).
ischi/o, 620
Ischiofibular, 654
Ischiopubic, 654
Ischium, 610-612
isch/o, 405
-ism, 264
Isthmus, 760
-itis, 96
IV (intravenous), 445, 456
IVF (in vitro fertilization), 367, 379, 380f
IVU/IVP (intravenous urogram or
    pyelogram), 230, 245

J
Jaundice, 117, 122
jejun/o, 477
Jejunum, 472, 474
Joints
    combining forms for, 625-626
    defined, 614
    replacement of, 644t
    structure and function of, 614, 629f

K
kal/i, 743
Kaposi sarcoma, 103f, 105
kary/o, 23
Karyocyte, 37
Karyoplasm, 37
Keloid, 122
Keratin, 91
Keratitis, 547
kerat/o, 92, 543
Keratogenic, 116
Keratomalacia, 547
Keratoplasty, 556
Ketatometer, 561
Ketosis, 749
Kidneys
    antidiuretic hormone and, 738f, 739f
    cysts in, 221
    as donor organs, 228, 229f
    infection of, 216, 217f
    radiation of, 236
    stones in, 216-217, 221, 228, 232
    structure and function of, 208-211, 414f
    transplantation of, 228, 229f
kinesi/o, 626
Knee joints
    arthritis in, 629f
    arthroscopy of, 328t, 651
    replacement of, 664t
    structure and function of, 622f, 629f
KUB (kidneys, ureters, and bladder), 236

kyph/o, 626
Kyphoplasty, 646t
Kyphosis, 630

L
L1-L5 (lumbar vertebrae), 662
Laboratory evaluations
    for cardiovascular, lymphatic system, and
        blood, 439
    for digestive system, 512-513
    for endocrine system, 755
    for female reproductive system, 331
    for male reproductive system, 279
    for musculoskeletal system, 650-652
    for nervous system, 701, 703-705
    for prostate gland, 279
    for respiratory system, 171-181
    specimen collection for, 175t
    for urinary system, 236-237
Labyrinth (inner ear), 580f, 581
Labyrinthectomy, 590
Labyrinthitis, 584
labyrinth/o, 582
Laceration, 105
Lacrimal, 563
Lacrimal glands and ducts, 540, 541f
lacrim/o, 543
Lactation, 379
Lactic/lactogenic, 372
lact/o, 354
Lactorrhea, 372
Lamaze, 384
Lamina/laminae, 609, 610f, 611f
Laminectomy, 645
lamin/o, 626
Laparoscopes/laparoscopy, 319, 322f, 328t, 506
Laparoscopic adjustable gastric banding
    (LAGB), 503
Laparoscopic cholecystectomy, 494
Laparoscopic-assisted vaginal hysterectomy,
    315t
Laparotomy, 496
Large intestine. See Colon.
Laryngeal, 182
Laryngectomy, 166
Laryngitis, 154
laryng/o, 145
Laryngoplasty, 166
Laryngoscope/laryngoscopy, 172, 176f
Laryngospasm, 182
Laryngostomy, 166
Laryngotracheobronchitis (LTB or croup),
    154, 160, 191
Laryngotracheotomy, 166
Larynx, 162f
Laser surgery, 113, 277, 417
Laser-assisted in situ keratomileusis (LASIK),
    558
LASIK (laser-assisted in situ keratomileusis),
    558
Last menstrual period (LMP), 383
Last normal menstrual period (LNMP), 383
Lateral (lat), 67, 68f, 80
later/o, 64
Latin language, 4-5
Lavage, gastric, 520
LDL (low-density lipoprotein), 440t
Left lower lobe (LLL), 191
Left lower quadrant (LLQ), 78-80
Left upper lobe (LUL), 191
Left upper quadrant (LUQ), 78-80
Legionnaire disease, 160
lei/o, 26

Leioderma, 98
Leiomyoma, 32, 311
Leiomyosarcoma, 32
Lens, 540, 541f, 551f
Lesion, 105
Lesser trochanter, 610f
Leukemia, 417
leuk/o, 27, 104f
Leukocoria, 547
Leukocytes (WBCs), 37, 398, 436f, 456
Leukocytosis, 37
Leukoderma, 116
Leukoplakia, 122
Leukorrhea, 333
Levator ani muscle, 490f
Lewy body dementia, 695
LH (luteinizing hormone), 737, 738f
Ligaments, 614
Ligamentum flavum, 640f
Light therapy, 552
Light waves, 551f
Linea alba, 616f
Linea nigra, 352
Lipid profile, 439, 440t
Lipids, 450
lip/o, 23
Lipoid, 37
Lipoma, 32, 123t
Liposarcoma, 32
lith/o, 213
Lithotripsy. *See* Extracorporeal shock wave lithotripsy (ESWL).
Liver
   cirrhosis of, 489
   structure and function of, 473f, 474
LLL (left lower lobe), 191
LLQ (left lower quadrant), 78-80
LMP (last menstrual period), 383
LNMP (last normal menstrual period), 383
Lobar pneumonia, 154
Lobectomy, 167
lob/o, 145
Lochia, 379
-logist, 29
-logy, 29
lord/o, 626
Lordosis, 630
Lou Gehrig disease, 693
Low-density lipoprotein (LDL), 440t
Lower GI series, 512-513
Lower respiratory tract infection, 162f
LP (lumbar puncture), 704-705, 721
LTB (laryngotracheobronchitis), 154, 160, 191
LUL (left upper lobe), 191
Lumbar, 654
Lumbar puncture (LP), 704-705, 721
Lumbar regions, 75-77
Lumbar vertebrae, 609, 610f, 611f, 652t
lumb/o, 620
Lumbocostal, 654
Lumbosacral, 654
Lumen, 450
Lumpectomy, 315t
Lung scan, 179
Lungs, 142-144, 161f, 162f, 168f
Lunula, 91
LUQ (left upper quadrant), 78-80
Luteinizing hormone (LH), 737, 738f
Lyme disease, 638, 639f
Lymph, 400
Lymph nodes
   biopsy of, 320, 322
   structure and function of, 322f
   types and locations of, 399f, 400

lymphaden/o, 403
Lymphadenopathy, 409
Lymphadenitis, 409
Lymphatic ducts and vessels, 399f, 400
Lymphatic system
   combining forms for, 403, 405
   diseases and disorders of, 409, 417
   and immunity, 394
   structure and function of, 399-400
   suffixes for, 406
   surgical terms for, 423
   word parts for, 403-407
lymph/o, 403
Lymphocytes, 398
Lymphoma, 409
-lysis, 214

M
Macula lutea, 552
Macular degeneration, 552
Macule, 122, 123t
Magnetic resonance angiography (MRA), 432t
Magnetic resonance imaging (MRI)
   of brain or spinal cord, 703, 704f
   defined, 174t
   for musculoskeletal system, 650, 652t
Major depression, 718
-malacia, 96
Malignancies. *See* Cancer.
Malignant, 46
Malleus (hammer), 580f, 581, 585f, 590f
Mammary glands, 299-300, 738f. *See also* Breasts (mammary glands).
Mammary papilla (nipple), 299-300
mamm/o, 301
Mammography/mammograms, 325, 326f, 341
Mammoplasty, 314
Mandible, 609
mandibul/o, 620
Marshall-Marchetti Krantz technique, 223
Massage therapy, 311
Mastalgia, 333
Mastectomy, 314
Mastitis, 305
mast/o, 301
Mastoid bone and cells, 580f, 581
Mastoidectomy, 590
Mastoiditis, 584
mastoid/o, 582
Mastoidotomy, 590
Mastoptosis, 333
Maxilla, 609, 610f, 611f
Maxillectomy, 645
Maxillitis, 630
maxill/o, 621
MCI (mild cognitive impairment), 711
MD (muscular dystrophy), 639, 662
MDI (metered-dose inhaler), 192
meat/o, 211
Meatoscope/meatoscopy, 232
Meatotomy, 223
Meatus/meatal, 238
Meconium, 379
Medial (med), 67, 68f, 80
Mediastinum, 143-144
Medical consult reports, 193
Medical genomics, 20
Medical language
   learning techniques for, 10-14
   origins of, 4-5
Medical records, 52

Medical terms
   analysis of, 10, 14
   for body structure, 57
   building of, 12-14
   for cardiovascular, lymphatic system, and blood, 408-417
   complementary, 57
   defining of, 11, 14
   for female reproductive system, 305-311
   for integumentary system, 92-93, 97-111
   for male reproductive system, 265-270
   for obstetrics, 359, 361-362
   for oncology, 31-36, 33f, 51, 54, 57
   for respiratory system, 153-160
   for urinary system, 216-221
medi/o, 64
Mediolateral, 67
Meditation, 409
Medulla oblongata, 679f, 680
Medulla, renal, 209f
Medullary cavity, 608f
-megaly, 214
Meibomian glands, 540, 551
Melanin, 91
melan/o, 27
Melanocarcinoma, 32
Melanoma, 32, 103f
Melena, 520
Menarche, 333
Ménière disease, 587
Meninges, 679f, 681
Meningioma, 688
Meningitis, 688
mening/o, meningi/o, 683
Meningocele/myelomeningocele/meningo-myelocele, 367f, 688
Meniscectomy, 645
Meniscitis, 630
menisc/o, 625
Meniscus, 614
men/o, 301
Menometrorrhagia, 305
Menopause, 335
Menorrhagia, 305
ment/o, psych/o, 686
Mesenteric vascular occlusion, 489f
Mesothelioma, 32
Metabolic syndrome, 757
Metabolism, 760
Metacarpal bones, 610, 612
Metacarpus, 620
Metastasis/metastases (mets), 42, 43f
Metastatic carcinoma, 123t
Metatarsal arthroplasty, 644t
-meter, 151
Metered-dose inhaler (MDI), 192
Methicillin-resistant *Staphylococcus aureus* (MRSA), 116
Metrorrhagia, 305
metr/o, metr/i, 301
-metry, 151
MG (myasthenia gravis), 639, 662
MI (myocardial infarction), 413, 416, 427b, 456
micro-, 357
Microcephalus, 364
Micturate/micturition, 242
Midbrain, 679f, 681
Middle ear, 580f, 581
Midsagittal view, 72-74
Midwife/midwifery, 379
Mild cognitive impairment (MCI), 711
Miotic, 566

Mirza (palmar uniportal endoscopic carpal tunnel release), 637
Mitral valve, 394, 395f
Mitral valve stenosis, 416
Modified radical mastectomy, 315t
Mohs, Frederick E., 113
Mohs surgery, 113
Mole, 122f
Mongolism, 368
mon/o, 686
Monocytes, 398
Mononeuropathy, 688
Monoparesis, 707
Monoplegia, 707
Mood disorder, 718
Motion sickness (vertigo), 588
Mouth, 472f, 473, 516
Movement, body, 618-619
MRA (magnetic resonance angiography), 432t
MRI. *See* Magnetic resonance imaging (MRI).
MRSA (methicillin-resistant *Staphylococcus aureus*), 116
MS (multiple sclerosis), 695, 721
MSCT (multislice spiral CT scanner), 432t
muc/o, 148
Mucoid, 182
Mucopurulent, 187
Mucous, 182-183
Mucus, 183, 187
Multigravida, 372
multi-, 357
Multipara (multip), 372, 383
Multiple myeloma, 409
Multiple sclerosis (MS), 695, 721
Multislice spiral CT (MSCT) scanner, 432t
Muscle tissue, 20, 615, 618f. *See also specific muscles.*
Muscular dystrophy (MD), 639, 662
Musculoskeletal system. *See also specific bones; specific muscles.*
    abbreviations for, 662
    complementary terms for, 653-655, 660
    diagnostic terms for, 650-652
    diseases and disorders of, 629-630, 636-640
    movements of, 618-619
    prefixes and suffixes for, 627-628
    structure and function of, 608-612, 614-618
    surgical terms for, 643-646
    word parts and combining forms for, 620-621, 625-626
Music therapy, 588
Myasthenia, 630
Myasthenia gravis (MG), 639, 662
myc/o, 94
Mydriatic, 566
myel/o, 403, 626, 683
Myelography, 701
Myeloma, 630
Myelomalacia, 707
Myelopoiesis, 445
my/o, 23
my/o, myos/o, 626
Myocardial infarction (MI), 413, 416, 427b, 456
Myocarditis, 408
Myocardium, 395, 618f
Myoma, 32
Myoma of the uterus, 311
Myometritis, 305
Myometrium, 298-299
Myopathy, 38
Myopia (nearsightedness), 551f, 552

Myorrhaphy, 645
Myringitis, 584
myring/o, 582
Myringoplasty, 590
Myringotomy (tympanocentesis), 590
Myxedema, 744, 749, 750f

N
N&V (nausea and vomiting), 520, 523
Nails, 91
Nasal bone, 610f
Nasal cavity, 162f
Nasal polyps, 485f
Nasal septum, 142-143
nas/o, 145
Nasogastric, 515
Nasopharyngeal, 182
Nasopharyngitis, 154
Natal, 372
nat/o, 354
natr/o, 743
Natural immunity, 453
Natural killer (NK) cells, 401, 402f
Nausea, 520, 523
NBs (newborns), 372, 383
Nebulizer, 187
necr/o, 94
Necrosis, 116, 439
Neoadjuvant therapy, 46
Neonate, 372
Neonatologists, 372
Neonatology
    abbreviations for, 379
    combining forms for, 354, 356
    defined, 373
    diseases and disorders in, 364, 366-367
    prefixes for, 357
    suffixes for, 358
    terms related to, 352-353
    word parts for, 354, 356
Neopathy, 42
Neoplasm, 32, 489f
Nephrectomy, 223
Nephritis, 216
nephr/o, 211
Nephroblastoma, 216
Nephrogram/nephrography, 230
Nephrohypertrophy, 216
Nephrolithiasis, 216, 232f
Nephrology/nephrologist, 238
Nephrolysis, 223
Nephroma, 216
Nephromegaly, 216
Nephron, 208-209
Nephropexy, 223
Nephroptosis, 216
Nephropyelolithotomy, 223
Nephroscope/nephroscopy, 232
Nephrosonography, 230, 231f
Nephrostomy, 223
Nephrotomogram, 230
Nerves/nervous tissue, 20, 678, 679f, 682
Nervous system
    complementary terms for, 706-707, 711-712
    diagnostic terms for, 701, 703-705
    diseases and disorders of, 688-690, 693-697
    of the skin, 90
    structure and function of, 678-682
    suffixes for, 687
    surgical terms for, 699
    word parts and combining forms for, 683-684, 686
Neuralgia, 688
Neurasthenia, 688

Neurectomy, 699
Neuritis, 689
neur/o, 23, 684
Neurodiagnostic procedures, 701, 704-705
Neurohypophysis, 737, 738f
Neuroid, 38, 707
Neurology/neurologists, 707
Neurolysis, 699
Neuroma, 32, 689
Neurons, 682
Neuropathy/neuroarthropathy, 689
Neuroplasty, 699
Neurorrhaphy, 699
Neurotomy, 699
Neutrophils, 398
Nevus (nevi), 122, 122f
Newborns (NBs), 372, 383
Nipples (mammary papillae), 299-300, 310f
noct/i, 213
Nocturia, 238, 241
Nodule, 122, 123t
Nonalcoholic steatohepatitis (NASH), 485
Noninvasive procedures, 432t
Noradrenaline (norepinephrine), 740
Norepinephrine (noradrenaline), 740
Normal pressure hydrocephalus dementia, 695
Nose, 142-143
Nosebleed, 155
Nosocomial infection, 187
Nuclear medicine
    defined, 174t
    SPECT procedure in, 436, 437f
    thyroid scans in, 755
Nucleus, 20
Nucleus pulposus, herniated (HNP), 638, 662
nulli-, 357
Nulligravida, 373
Nullipara, 373
Nyctalopia (night blindness), 552
Nystagmus, 552

O
O₂ (oxygen), 142, 148, 191
OA (osteoarthritis), 629f, 630, 639, 644t, 662
OB. *See* Obstetrics (OB).
Obesity, 491
Obsessive-compulsive disorder (OCD), 719
Obstetricians, 379
Obstetrics (OB)
    abbreviations for, 379
    combining forms for, 354, 356
    defined, 379, 383
    diagnostic terms in, 369
    diseases and disorders in, 359, 361-362
    prefixes for, 357
    pregnancy-related terms, 352-353
    suffixes for, 358
    surgical terms in, 368
    word parts for, 354, 356, 358
Obstruction, intestinal, 489f
Obstructive sleep apnea (OSA), 160-161, 191
Occlude/occlusions, 450, 489f
OCD (obsessive-compulsive disorder), 719, 721
ocul/o, ophthalm/o, 543
Oculomotor nerve (III), 682f
Oculomycosis, 547
-odynia, 406
Office visit reports, 53, 55
-oid, 29
Oil (sebum), 90
Olecranon process, 610-612

Olfactory nerve (I), 682f
olig/o, 213
Oligohydramnios, 359
Oligomenorrhea, 306
Oligospermia, 280
Oliguria, 239
OM (otitis media), 587, 597
-oma, 29
Omphalitis, 364
omphal/o, 354
Omphalocele, 364
onc/o, 26
Oncogenic, 42
Oncologist, 42
Oncology
    abbreviations for, 51
    complementary terms for, 41-48, 57
    defined, 42
    word parts for, 56
Online information
    on breast health, 340
    on heart disease, 461
    on integumentary system, 132
    on lung diseases, 197
Onychectomy, 111
onych/o, 92
Onychocryptosis, 98
Onychomalacia, 98
Onychomycosis, 98
Onychophagia, 98
Oophorectomy, 314
Oophoritis, 306
oophor/o, 301
Operative cholangiography, 504
Operative reports, 130, 247, 664, 763
Ophth, 561
Ophthalmalgia, 547
Ophthalmic, 563
Ophthalmic evaluations, 561
Ophthalmology/ophthalmologists, 564
Ophthalmoplegia, 547
Ophthalmoscope/ophthalmoscopy, 561
-opia, 545
-opsy, 96
Optic, 564
Optic nerve (II), 540, 541f, 682f
optician, 566
opt/o, 543
Optometry/optometrists, 561, 566
Oral, 515
Oral cavity, 472f, 473
Orbit (eye), 540, 610f
orchid/o, orchi/o orch/o, test/o, 262
Orchiectomy/orchidectomy, 272
Orchiepididymitis, 266
Orchiopexy/orchidopexy, 272
Orchioplasty, 272
Orchiotomy/orchidotomy, 272
Orchitis, orchiditis, testitis, 266
organ/o, 23
Organ/organs. *See also specific organs and systems.*
    defined, 21
    donor organs, 228, 229f
Orgasm, 283
or/o, stomat/o, 477
Oropharynx, 161f
orth/o, 148
Ortho, 662
Orthopedics/orthopedists, 660
Orthopnea, 182
Orthotics/orthotist, 660
OSA (obstructive sleep apnea), 160-161, 191
-osis, 29
Ossicles (ear), 580f, 581, 585f, 590f

Ostectomy, 645
Osteitis, 630
oste/o, 626
Osteoarthritis (OA), 629f, 630, 639, 644t, 662
Osteoblasts, 654
Osteochondritis, 630
Osteoclasis, 645
Osteocytes, 654
Osteofibroma, 630
Osteomalacia, 630
Osteomyelitis, 631
Osteonecrosis, 654
Osteopathy/osteopaths, 660
Osteopenia, 631
Osteoporosis, 631, 639, 640f, 646t, 652t
Osteosarcoma, 631
Otalgia, 584
Otitis externa, 587
Otitis media (OM), 587, 597
Otolaryngologists/otorhinolaryngologists, 595
Otology/otologists, 595
Otomastoiditis, 584
Otomycosis, 584
Otopyorrhea, 584
Otorrhea, 585
Otosclerosis, 585
Otoscopes/otoscopy, 592
Oval window, 580f, 581, 590f
Ovary/ies
    cancer of, 311
    defined, 353f
    removal of, 314
    structure and function of, 298-299, 736f, 738f
Ovulation, 352, 353f
Ovum/ova, 298-299, 353f
Oximeter, 173, 175t, 179
ox/o, ox/i, 148
Oxygen (O$_2$), 142, 148, 191
Oxytocin, 737, 738f

P
PA (posteroanterior), 68, 80
Pacemakers, cardiac, 425, 426f, 427b
Pachyderma, 98
pachy/o, 94
PAD (peripheral arterial disease), 416, 456
PAF (paroxysmal atrial fibrillation), 415
Palate, 473
Palatitis, 485
palat/o, 480
Palatoplasty, 496
Pallor, 122
Palmar uniportal endoscopic carpal tunnel
    release (Mirza), 637
pan-, 150
Pancreas
    islets of Langerhans in, 738
    structure and function of, 736f, 739f
Pancreatic, 473f, 475, 515
Pancreatitis, 485
pancreat/o, 480
Pancytopenia, 409
Panhysterectomy, 315t
Panic attacks, 719
Panplegia, 707
Pansinusitis, 153
Pap smears, 331, 332f
Papanicolaou, George, 331
Papillae, renal, 209f
Papule, 122, 123t
para-, 95, 373
Paralysis agitans, 697

Paranasal sinuses, 142-143
Paraplegia, 712
Parathormone (PTH), 738
Parathyroid glands, 736f, 738, 739f
Parathyroidectomy, 753
parathyroid/o, 741
Parathyroidoma, 745
-paresis, 687
Paresthesia, 707
Parietal pleura, 168f
Parkinson disease (PD)/Parkinsonism, 695, 697, 721
par/o, part/o, 354
Paronychia, 98
Paroxysm, 187
Paroxysmal atrial fibrillation (PAF), 415
-partum, 358
Parturition, 379
Patch, skin, 118f
Patella/patellae, 610, 612
Patellar tendon, 616f
Patellectomy, 645
patell/o, 621
Patent, 187
path/o, 26
Pathogenic, 42
Pathogens, 402f
Pathology reports, 131
Pathology/pathologists, 42
-pathy, 29
PCI (percutaneous coronary intervention), 422b
PD (Parkinson disease), 695, 697, 721
PE (pulmonary embolism) (pl.-emboli), 162f, 163, 191
Pectoralis major muscle, 299f, 616f
Pediculosis, 105
PEG (percutaneous endoscopic gastrostomy), 496f, 523
pelv/i, pelv/o, 356, 621
Pelvic, 654
Pelvic bone/pelvic girdle, 610-612
Pelvic cavity, 21-23
Pelvic inflammatory disease (PID), 311, 337
Pelvic sonography, 369
Pelvisacral, 654
-penia, 406
Penis, 210f, 261, 269
PEP (positive expiratory pressure), 192
-pepsia, 483
Peptic ulcers, 491
per-, 95
Percussion, 438-439
Percutaneous, 116
Percutaneous coronary intervention (PCI), 422b
Percutaneous diskectomy, 638f, 645
Percutaneous endoscopic gastrostomy (PEG), 496f, 523
Percutaneous transluminal coronary angio-plasty (PTCA), 427, 428f, 456
Percutaneous vertebroplasty (PV), 646t
peri-, 304
Pericardiocentesis, 423
Pericarditis, 409
Pericardium, 395
Perimetritis, 306
Perimetrium, 298-299
perine/o, 301
Perineorrhaphy, 315
Perineotomy, 368
Perineum (pelvic floor), 300
Periosteum, 608
Peripheral arterial disease (PAD), 416, 456

Peripheral nervous system (PNS), 678-682
Peripheral neuropathy, 689f
Peristalsis, 520
Peritoneal dialysis, 242
peritone/o, 480
Peritoneum/peritoneal, 475, 515
Peritonitis, 485
Pernicious anemia, 417b
Peroneus brevis muscle, 616f, 617f
Peroneus longus muscle, 616f, 617f
Pertussis (whooping cough), 161
PET (positron emission tomography) scan, 704, 721
Petechia (petechiae), 122
petr/o, 626
-pexy, 151
PFTs (pulmonary function tests), 173, 175t, 179, 191
Phacoemulsification, 558
-phagia, 96
Phagocytes/phagocytosis, 401, 402f, 453
Phalangectomy, 645
Phalanges, 610, 612
phalang/o, 621
Pharyngitis, 154
pharyng/o, 145
Pharynx (throat), 142-143, 162f, 176f, 472f, 473, 739f
phas/o, 686
Pheochromocytoma, 750
Phimosis, 269
Phlebectomy, 417, 423
Phlebitis, 409
phleb/o, ven/o, 403
Phlebology/phlebologists, 445
Phlebotomy, 423
-phobia, 545
Phobias, 719
phon/o, 148, 545
Photophobia, 547
Photorefractive keratectomy (PRK), 558
Phrenalgia, 182
Phrenic, 181
phren/o, 145
Phrenospasm, 182
-physis, 628
Pia mater, 679f, 681
Pica, 719
PID (pelvic inflammatory disease), 311, 337
Pigmentation, 27, 91, 352
Pimple, 122f
Pineal gland, 739f
Pinguecula, 552
pituitar/o, 741
Pituitary gland
    defined, 737
    hormones secreted by, 737-739
    structure and function of, 736f, 738f
Placenta previa, 361, 362f
Placenta/afterbirth, 352, 353f, 370f
Plaque, atherosclerotic, 408f
-plasia, 29
-plasm, 29
Plasma, 398
Plasmapheresis, 445
plasm/o, 403
-plasty, 96
Platelets, 398
-plegia, 545
Pleura, 143-144
Pleural effusion, 161, 168f
Pleuritis (pleurisy), 154, 155f
pleur/o, 145
Pleuropexy, 167

Plural endings, 49-51
PMMA (polymethylmethacrylate), 646t
PMS (premenstrual syndrome), 335, 337
-pnea, 151
Pneumatocele, 154
pneum/o, pneumat/o, pneumon/o, 145
Pneumobronchotomy, 167
Pneumoconiosis, 155
Pneumonectomy, 167
Pneumonia
    defined, 155
    Pneumocystis carinii–related (PCP), 155
Pneumonitis, 155
Pneumothorax, 155
PNS (peripheral nervous system), 678-682, 721
Podiatry/podiatrists, 660
-poiesis, 406
poli/o, 686
Poliomyelitis, 689
poly-, 150
Polyarteritis, 409
Polycystic kidney disease, 221
Polydipsia, 757
Polyhydramnios, 359
Polymethylmethacrylate (PMMA), 646t
Polymyositis, 631
Polyneuritis, 689
Polyneuropathy, 689
Polypectomy, 496, 497f
polyp/o, 480
Polyps/polyposis, 485, 489f, 491, 506f
Polysomnography (PSG), 160, 173, 191
Polyuria, 239
Pons, 679f, 680
Popliteal vein
    bypass of, 426f, 427
    structure and function of, 432f
Positive expiratory pressure (PEP), 192
Positron emission tomography (PET) scan, 704, 721
post-, 357
Posterior, 68
Posterior tibial pulse, 82
poster/o, 64
Posteroanterior (PA), 68, 80
Postherpetic neuralgia, 695
Postictal, 707
Postnatal, 373
Postpartum, 373
Posttraumatic stress disorder (PTSD), 719, 721
PPD (purified protein derivative) skin test, 179
Preeclampsia, 362
Prefixes
    for body structure, 28
    defined, 6, 10t, 14
    for digestive system, 483
    directional, 66
    for the eye, 546
    for integumentary system, 95-96
    for musculoskeletal system, 627-628
    for obstetrics and neonatology, 357
    for respiratory system, 149-150
Pregnancy
    ectopic, 361
    false pregnancy, 373
    terms related to, 352-353
Preictal, 707
Premature infant, 379
Premenstrual syndrome (PMS), 335, 337
Prenatal, 373
Prepuce (foreskin), 261

Presbycusis, 587
Pressure ulcer, 122, 128
Priapism, 269
Primagravida, 373
prim/i, 356
Primipara (primip), 373, 383
PRK (photorefractive keratectomy), 558
PRL (prolactin/lactogenic hormone), 737, 738f
Proctology/proctologists, 515
Proctoptosis, 485
Proctoscopes/proctoscopy, 506-507
Prognosis (Px), 42
Progress notes, 81, 83, 289, 338, 384, 458-459, 569, 598, 723
Prolactin/lactogenic hormone (PRL), 737, 738f
Pronation, 619
Pronunciation guide, 34
Prostate gland
    calculi of, 266f
    cancer of, 242, 269, 270t
    excision of, 272, 275, 276f
    infection of, 266
    structure and function of, 210f, 260, 261f, 266f
Prostatectomy, 272, 275
Prostate-specific antigen (PSA), 279, 286
Prostatitis, 266
prostat/o, 262
Prostatocystitis, 266
Prostatocystotomy, 272
Prostatolithotomy, 272
Prostatoliths, 266, 272
Prostatorrhea, 266
Prostatovesiculectomy, 273
Prostatovesiculitis, 266
Prosthesis/prostheses
    defined, 660
    for hip and knee joints, 644t
    penile, 283
    for stapes, 590f
Proteins, protective, 401, 402f
Prothrombin time (PT), 440, 456
provt/o, rect/o, 477
Proximal, 67, 68f
proxim/o, 64
Pruritis, 122
PSA (prostate-specific antigen), 279, 286
pseud/o, 356
Pseudocyesis, 373
Pseudodementia, 711
PSG (polysomnography), 160, 173, 191
Psoriasis, 105
Psychiatry/psychiatrists, 715
Psychogenic, 715
Psychology/psychologists, 715
Psychopathy, 716
Psychosis/psychoses, 716
Psychosomatic, 716
PT (prothrombin time), 440, 456
PTCA (percutaneous transluminal coronary angioplasty), 427, 428f, 456
Pterygium, 552, 553
PTH (parathormone), 738
-ptosis, 214
PTSD (posttraumatic stress disorder), 719, 721
Puberty, 283
Pubic, 654
Pubic symphysis, 610f, 614
Pubis, 610-612
pub/o, 621
Pubofemoral, 654

Puerpera/puerperal, 373
Puerperium, 379
puerper/o, 354
Pulmonary, 182
Pulmonary artery, 395f, 432f
Pulmonary edema, 161
Pulmonary embolism (pl.-emboli) (PE), 162f, 163, 191
Pulmonary function tests (PFTs), 173, 175t, 179, 191
Pulmonary neoplasm, 155
Pulmonary valve, 395f
Pulmonary veins, 395f
pulmon/o, 145
Pulmonologist, 182
Pulmonology, 182
Pulse oximetry, 173, 175t, 179
Pulses
    defined, 438
    palpation of, 82
Punch biopsy, 111f
Pupil, 540, 541f
Pupillary, 564
pupill/o, 543
Pupillometer, 561
Pupilloscope, 561
Purified protein derivative (PPD) skin test, 179
Purpura, 122
Pustule, 122, 123t
PV (percutaneous vertebroplasty), 646t
Pyelitis, 216
pyel/o, 211
Pyelolithotomy, 223
Pyelonephritis, 216, 217f
Pyeloplasty, 223
Pyloric sphincter, 474
Pyloric stenosis, 364
pylor/o, 356, 480
Pyloromyotomy, 496
Pyloroplasty, 496
Pylorus, 473-474
py/o, 148
Pyosalpinx, 306
Pyothorax (empyema), 155
Pyrami, 209f
Pyuria, 239

Q

quadr/i, 686
Quadriplegia, 707
Quickening, 379

R

RA (rheumatoid arthritis), 453, 639, 662
rachi/o, 621
Rachiotomy, 645
Rachischisis, 631
Radial pulse, 82
Radiation therapy (XRT), 46, 47f
Radical hysterectomy, 315t
Radical mastectomy, 315t
Radical prostatectomy (RP), 275, 276f, 286
radic/o, radicul/o, 684
Radicotomy, 699
Radiculitis, 689
Radiculopathy, 689
Radioactive iodine uptake (RAIU), 754, 761
Radiography, 151, 214. See also Diagnostic imaging.
Radiology reports, 385, 525-526
Radius, 610-612
RAIU (radioactive iodine uptake), 754, 761
Raynaud disease, 416b

RBCs (red blood cells, erythrocytes), 37, 143f, 398, 436f, 456
RDS (respiratory distress syndrome), 367, 383
Reactive airway disease, 163
Recombinant tissue plasminogen activator (rtPA), 427b
Rectocele, 485
Rectouterine pouch, 298-299
Rectum/rectal
    barium enema of, 513f
    defined, 515
    endoscopy of, 508f
    polyps of, 485f
    structure and function of, 210f, 261f, 299, 472, 474-475
    valves of, 490f
    visualization of, 506-507
Rectus abdominis muscle, 616f
Rectus femoris muscle, 616f
Red blood cells (RBCs), 37, 143f, 398, 436f, 456
Red marrow, 608f, 609
Reflux, 520
Refraction errors, 551f
Remission, 46
Renal anatomy and physiology, 208-211
Renal corpuscle, 209f
Renal failure, acute (ARF), 221
Renal hypertension, 221
Renal transplant, 228, 229f
ren/o, 211
Renogram, 230
Repetitive motion syndrome, 639
Reproductive system, female. See also Obstetrics.
    abbreviations for, 337
    cancers of, 341
    diagnostic terms for, 325-326, 330-332
    diseases and disorders of, 305-311
    prefixes for, 304
    structure and function of, 298-301
    suffixes for, 304
    surgical terms for, 314-315, 319-320
    word parts and combining forms for, 301-304
Reproductive system, male
    abbreviations for, 286
    complementary terms for, 280, 282-283
    diagnostic terms for, 279
    diseases and disorders of, 265-266, 269-270
    structure and function of, 260-261
    suffixes for, 264
    surgical terms for, 272-273, 275-277
    word parts and combining forms for, 262-264
Respiration/breathing, 142
Respiratory distress syndrome (RDS), 367, 383
Respiratory system
    abbreviations for, 191-192
    combining forms for, 148
    complementary terms for, 181-190
    diagnostic terms for, 171-181
    diseases and disorders of, 153-165
    endoscopic surgery for, 171-172, 175t
    prefixes for, 149-150
    structure and function of, 142-144
    suffixes for, 150-151
    surgical terms for, 166-172
    word parts for, 145
Retention sutures, 114f
Reteplase (rtPA, recombinant tissue plasminogen activator), 427b

Retina, 540, 541f, 543f, 551f
Retinaculum, 616f
Retinal, 564
Retinal photocoagulation, 558
Retinitis pigmentosa, 553
retin/o, 543
Retinoblastoma, 548
Retinopathy, 548
Retinoscopy, 561
Retrograde urogram, 230
rhabd/o, 26
Rhabdomyolysis, 631
Rhabdomyoma, 32
Rhabdomyosarcoma, 32
Rheumatic fever, 416b
Rheumatic heart disease, 416
Rheumatoid arthritis (RA), 453, 639, 662
Rheumatoid nodule, 123t
Rheumatoid spondylitis, 636
Rhinitis, 155
rhin/o, 145
Rhinomycosis, 155
Rhinoplasty, 167
Rhinorrhagia (epistaxis), 155, 160
Rhinorrhea, 182
rhiz/o, 684
Rhizomeningomyelitis, 689
Rhizotomy, 699
Rhytidectomy, 111
rhytid/o, 94
Rhytidoplasty, 111
Ribs, 168f
Right lower lobe (RLL), 191
Right middle lobe (RML), 191
Right upper lobe (RUL), 191
Right upper quadrant (RUQ), 78-80
RLL (right lower lobe), 191
RLQ (right lower quadrant), 78-80
RML (right middle lobe), 191
Rosacea, 105
Rotation, 619
Rotator cuff injuries and repair, 639
Routes of administration, 117
Roux-en-Y gastric bypass (RYGB), 503
RP (radical prostatectomy), 275, 276f, 286
-rrhagia, 151
-rrhaphy, 214
-rrhea, 96
-rrhexis, 358
rtPA (Alteplase, recombinant tissue plasminogen activator), 427b
RUL (right upper lobe), 191
Ruptured disks. See Herniated nucleus pulposus (HNP).
RUQ (right upper quadrant), 78-80

S

Sacral, 654
sacr/o, 621
Sacrum, 609, 610f, 611f
Sagittal view
    defined, 72-74
    of urinary system, 210f
Saliva, 402f
Salivary glands, 474
Salpingectomy, 315
Salpingitis, 306, 311f
salping/o, 301
Salpingocele, 306
Salpingo-oophorectomy (BS&O), 315
Salpingostomy, 315
Salpinx, 301, 304
sarc/o, 23
-sarcoma, 29
Sarcoma, 32

Sartorius muscle, 616f
Scabies, 106
Scapula/scapulae, 609, 610f, 611f
scapul/o, 621
-schisis, 628
Schizophrenia, 719
Sciatic nerve, 678f, 695
Sciatica, 695
Sclera, 540, 541f
Scleral buckling, 558f, 559
scler/o, 543
Scleroderma, 106
Sclerokeratitis, 548
Scleromalacia, 548
-sclerosis, 406
Sclerotherapy, 417
Sclerotomy, 556
scoli/o, 626
Scoliosis, 631
-scope/-scopic/-scopy, 151, 172
Scrotum, 261
Sebaceous (oil) glands, 90-91
seb/o, 92
Seborrhea, 98
Seborrheic dermatitis, 99t
Segmental resection (lung), 167f
Seizures, 712
Semen, 261
Semicircular canals and vestibule, 580f, 581
Semilunar valves, 395, 416f
Seminal duct, 260, 261f, 273
Seminal vesicles, 260, 261f
Seminiferous tubules, 260, 261f
Senile cataracts, 551f
Sentinel lymph node biopsy, 320, 322
Sepsis/septicemia, 221
sept/o, 145
Septoplasty, 167
Septotomy, 168
Septum (heart), 395f
Serratus anterior muscle, 616f
Sestamibi, 436
Sexually transmitted diseases (STDs), 282-283, 286
SG (specific gravity), 237, 245
Shave biopsy, 111
SHG (sonohysterography), 325, 335, 337
Shingles (herpes zoster), 99t, 105, 106, 123t, 695
Shock wave lithotripsy, 223, 224f, 228
Shunts, 712
sial/o, 480
Sialoliths, 485
Side-to-side anastomosis, 502f
Sigmoid colon, 475f, 490f, 508f, 513f
sigmoid/o, 477
Sigmoidoscope/sigmoidoscopy, 507
Silent STDs, 282
Silicosis, 155
Simple mastectomy, 315t
Single-photon emission computed tomography (SPECT), 436, 437f, 456, 652t
Sinus rhythm, 414f
sinus/o, 145
Sinusotomy, 168
-sis, 29
Situ, 46, 47
Skeletal muscles, 615, 616f, 618f
Skeleton, 609-611. See also Musculoskeletal system.
Skin. See also Integumentary system.
    accessory structures of, 91
    biopsy of, 111f
    dimpling of, 310f

Skin (Continued)
    lesions of, 122-124
    as mechanical barrier, 402f
    pregnancy-related changes in, 352
    structure and function of, 90-91
Skin dimpling, 310
Skin patch, 118f
Skin tag, 123t
SLE (systemic lupus erythematosus), 106, 128, 453
Sleep studies, 173
Slipped disks. See Herniated nucleus pulposus (HNP).
Small intestine/bowel, 474
Small-volume nebulizer (SVN), 192
Smooth muscles, 615, 618f
Snowflake cataracts, 551f
Soft palate, 161f, 473
Soleus muscle, 616f, 617f
Somatic, 38
somat/o, 26
Somatoform disorders, 719
Somatogenic, 38
Somatopathy, 38
Somatoplasm, 38
somn/o, 148
son/o, 213
Sonography/sonograms
    defined, 174t
    pelvic, 369
    transducers for, 370f
    transrectal, 279
    transvaginal (TVS), 331f, 337
    uterine, 325
Sonohysterography (SHG), 325, 335, 337
Sound waves, 580
-spasm, 151
Specific gravity (SG), 237, 245
Specific immunity, 401, 402f
SPECT (single-photon emission computed tomography), 436, 437f, 456, 652t
Speculum/a, 321f, 332f, 335, 335f, 541f
Spermatic cord, 260, 261f
Spermatolysis, 280
sperm/o, spermat/o, 264
Sperm/spermatozoa, 260, 264f
Sphygmomanometer, 438
Spina bifida, 367, 631, 688f
Spinal cavity, 21-23
Spinal column, 210f, 609f, 610f, 611f
Spinal cord
    compression of, 639-640
    defined, 681-682
    disk herniation into, 638
    MRI of, 703, 704f
    structure and function of, 678-682
Spinal nerves, 678-679, 682
Spinal stenosis, 639, 640f
Spinal tap, 704-705
Spiral CT scan, 179
spir/o, 148
Spirometer/spirometry, 173
Spleen, 399f, 400
Splenectomy, 423
Splenic flexure, 475f, 513f
Splenius capitis muscle, 617f
splen/o, 403
Splenomegaly, 409
Splenopexy, 423
Spondylarthritis, 631
spondyl/o, vertebr/o, 621
Spondylolisthesis, 639, 640f
Spondylolysis, 631
Spondylosyndesis, 645

Spongy bone, 429f
Spontaneous abortion, 361
Spurs, bone, 637
Sputum, 187
Squamous cell carcinoma (SqCCA), 103f, 106, 128
Staging, cancer, 31
Stapedectomy, 590
staped/o, 582
Stapes (stirrup), 580f, 581, 585f, 590f
Staph (Staphylococcus), 104f, 128
staphyl/o, 94
Staphylococcus aureus, 104f, 116, 311
-stasis, 29
STDs (sexually transmitted diseases), 282-283, 286
steat/o, 480
Steatohepatitis, 485
Steatorrhea, 516
Steatosis, 516
-stenosis, 151
Stenosis
    aortic, 408
    arterial, 408
    mitral, 416
    pyloric, 364
    tracheal, 155
    ureteral, 217
Stents, 425, 426f
Stereotactic breast biopsy, 320, 323f
Stereotactic radiosurgery, 699
Sterilization (fertility-related), 283, 322f
stern/o, 621
Sternoclavicular, 654
Sternocleidomastoid muscle, 616f, 617f
Sternoid, 654
Sternum, 609, 610f
Stethoscope, 438
Stinging nettles, 266
Stoma, 520
Stomach
    banding or bypass of, 503
    structure and function of, 472-474
    surgical removal of, 495f
    ulcers of, 490-491
    visualization of, 506-507
Stomatogastric, 516
-stomy, 151
Stones. See Calculus/calculi.
Strabismus, 553
Strangulated inguinal hernia, 489f
Strep (Streptococcus), 116, 128
strept/o, 94
Streptococcus pyogenes, 116
Streptokinase, 427b
Stress hormones, 739-740
Stress incontinence, 223
Stress tests, exercise or chemical, 436
Striae gravidarum, 352
Striated muscles, 615, 616f, 618f
Strictures, 242
Stroke. See Cerebrovascular accident (CVA).
Strümpell-Marie arthritis, 636
Sty, stye, 553
sub-, 95
Subarachnoid hemorrhage, 696
Subarachnoid space, 679f, 681, 705f
Subcostal, 654
Subcu (subcutaneous), 116, 128, 261f
Subcutaneous fatty tissue, 90
Subcutaneous mastectomy, 315t
Subcutaneous (subcu), 116, 128, 261f
Subdural, 707
Subdural hematoma, 689

Sublingual, 516
Submandibular, 654
Submaxillary, 654
Subscapular, 654
Substernal, 654
Subtotal hysterectomy, 315t
Sudoriferous (sweat) glands, 90-91
Suffixes
  for body structure, 29-31
  for cardiovascular, lymphatic system, and
    blood, 406
  defined, 6, 10t, 14
  for digestive system, 483
  directional, 66
  for the eye, 546
  for integumentary system, 96-97
  for male reproductive system, 264
  for musculoskeletal system, 627-628
  for nervous system, 687
  for obstetrics and neonatology, 358
  for respiratory system, 150-151, 172
  for urinary system, 214
Sulci, 693f
Superior extensor retinaculum, 616f
Superior (sup), 67, 68f
super/o, 64
Supination, 619
supra-, 627
Suprapatellar, 654
Suprapubic prostatectomy, 276f
Suprascapular, 654
Surgical terms
  blood-related, 428, 429f
  for cardiovascular, lymphatic system, and
    blood, 422-423, 425-428
  for digestive system, 494-496, 501-504
  for endocrine system, 753
  for the eye, 555-556, 558-559
  for female reproductive system, 314-315,
    319-320
  for integumentary system, 111-115
  for male reproductive system, 272-273,
    275-277
  for musculoskeletal system, 643-646
  for nervous system, 699
  in obstetrics, 368
  for respiratory system, 166-172
  for urinary system, 223, 228
Sutures, 114f
Suturing, 113, 114f
SVN (small-volume nebulizer), 192
Swayback, 630
sym-, 627
Symphysis, 654
Symphysis pubis, 261f
syn-, 627
Syncope, 712
Syndrome/syndromal, 757
Synovectomy, 646
Synovial membrane, 629f
synovi/o, 625
Synoviosarcoma, 631
Synovium/synovia, 614
Syphilis, 283
Systemic, 38
Systemic lupus erythematosus (SLE), 106,
  128, 453
system/o, 23
System/systems, 21. *See also specific systems.*
Systole, 450

T

T1-T12 (thoracic vertebrae), 639, 662
T3 (triiodothyronine), 737
T4 (thyroxine), 737, 761

tachy-, 150
Tachycardia, 409
Tachypnea, 182
Talus, 611f
Tamponade, cardiac, 415
Tarsal bones, 610, 612
Tarsectomy, 646
tars/o, 621
TB skin test, 179
TB (tuberculosis), 163, 191
TD (transdermal), 116, 128
TEE (transesophageal echocardiogram), 437,
  456
Telescopes, 228f
Temporal pulse, 82
Tendonitis/tendinitis, 631
Tendons, 614
ten/o, tend/o, tendin/o, 625
Tenomyoplasty, 646
Tenorrhaphy, 646
Tenosynovitis, 631
Tensor faciae latae muscle, 616f
terat/o, 356
Testes/testicles
  cancer of, 269
  defined, 260, 261f
  structure and function of, 736f, 738f
  tortion of, 270
Testicular tortion, 270
Testosterone, 260
Tetany, 750
Tetralogy, 373
Tetratogen/tetratogenic, 373
TGs (triglycerides), 440t
THA (total hip arthroplasty), 643, 644t, 662
Thallium testing, 436-437
Therapeutic abortion, 361
therm/o, 405
Thermotherapy, 276-277
Thoracalgia, 155
Thoracic, 182
Thoracic (chest) cavity, 21-23
Thoracic duct, 399f
Thoracic vertebrae, 609, 610f, 611f
thorac/o, 145
Thoracocentesis (thoracentesis), 168
Thoracoscope/thoracoscopy, 173, 328t
Thoracotomy, 168, 175t
-thorax, 151
Throat, 142
thromb/o, 405
Thrombolysis/thrombolytic therapy, 456
  defined, 445
  intracoronary, 427
Thrombophlebitis, 409
Thrombus/thrombosis (pl.-thrombi), 409
Thymectomy, 423
thym/o, 403
Thymoma, 409
Thymus gland, 399f, 400, 736f
thyr/o, thyroid/o, 741
Thyroid cartilage, 10t, 142, 739f
Thyroid gland, 736-739
Thyroid scans, 755
Thyroidectomy, 753
Thyroiditis, 745
Thyroidotomy, 753
Thyroid-stimulating hormone (TSH), 737,
  738f, 755
Thyroparathyroidectomy, 753
Thyrotoxicosis, 750
Thyroxine (T4), 737, 755
TIA (transient ischemic attack), 696, 697f,
  721

Tibia, 610-612
Tibialis anterior muscle, 616f
tibi/o, 621
Tinea, 99t, 106
Tinnitus, 588
Tissue/tissues. *See also specific tissues.*
  defined, 20
TKA (total knee arthroplasty), 622, 644t
TNM staging system, 31
-tocia, 358
-tome, 96
tom/o, 213
-tomy, 151
Tongue, 161f, 176f, 472f, 473
ton/o, 545
Tonometer/tonometry, 561
Tonsillectomy, 168
Tonsillitis, 155
tonsill/o, 145
Tonsils, 142
Tophi, 638
Total abdominal hysterectomy (TAH), 337
Total cholesterol, 440t
Total hip arthroplasty (THA), 643, 644t, 662
Total hysterectomy, 315t
Total knee arthroplasty (TKA), 622, 644t
Total vaginal hysterectomy (TVH), 337
Toxic shock syndrome (TSS), 311, 337
Trabeculectomy, 559
Trachea, 142-143, 161f, 162f, 169f, 176f, 739f
Tracheitis, 155
Trachelectomy, 315
trachel/o, 301
Trachelorraphy, 315
Tracheoesophageal fistula, 364
Tracheoplasty, 168
Tracheostenosis, 155
Tracheotomy/tracheostomy, 167f, 168
trans-, 95
Transdermal (TD), 116, 128
Transducer, ultrasound, 370f
Transesophageal echocardiogram (TEE),
  437, 456
Transient ischemic attack (TIA), 696, 697f
Transplantation
  of bone marrow, 428
  of kidney, 228, 229f
Transrectal ultrasound, 279
Transurethral incision of the prostate gland
  (TUIP), 276-277, 286
Transurethral microwave thermotherapy
  (TUMT), 276-277, 286
Transurethral resection of the prostate gland
  (TURP), 276-277, 286
Transvaginal sonography (TVS), 330, 331f,
  337
Transverse, 72-74
Transverse colon, 475f, 508f, 513f
Trapezius muscle, 616f, 617f
Treponema pallidum, 283
trich/o, 92
Trichomonas, 283
Trichomoniasis, 283
Trichomycosis, 98
Tricuspid valve, 395, 395f
Trigeminal nerve (V), 682f
Triglycerides (TGs), 440t
Trigone (bladder), 210f
Triiodothyronine (T3), 737
Trimesters, 352
-tripsy, 214
Trochanters, 610f
Trochlear nerve (IV), 682f
-trophy, 214

Troponin, 439
TSH (thyroid-stimulating hormone), 737, 738f
TSS (toxic shock syndrome), 311, 337
Tubal ligation/sterilization, 320
Tuberculosis (TB), 163, 191
TUIP (transurethral incision of the prostate gland), 276-277, 286
TUMT (transurethral microwave thermotherapy), 276-277, 286
TURP (transurethral resection of the prostate gland), 276-277, 286
TVH (total vaginal hysterectomy), 337
TVS (transvaginal sonograply), 330, 331f, 337
Tympanic membrane (eardrum), 580f, 581, 585f
Tympanitis, 585
tympan/o, 582
Tympanocentesis, 590
Tympanometers/tympanometry, 592
Tympanoplasty, 590

U

UA (urinalysis), 237, 245
UAE (uterine artery embolism), 320, 337
UGI (upper gastrointestinal), 523
Ulcerative colitis, 491
Ulcers, 122, 124, 490-491. See also specific ulcers.
Ulna, 610-612
uln/o, 621
Ultrasonography (ultrasound)
    abdominal, 505f, 512
    defined, 174t
    Doppler ultrasound, 436
    echocardiograms, 433, 436-437
    for endocrine system, 754
    endoscopic ultrasound, 512
    pelvic, 369
    transducers for, 370f
    transrectal, 279
    transvaginal (TVS), 331f, 337
    uterine, 325
-um, 358
Umbilical cord, 353f
Umbilical hernias, 364, 365f, 480f
Umbilical region, 75-77
Umbilicus, 75
Unconsciousness, 712
Ungual, 116
ungu/o, 92
uni-, 66
Unilateral, 67
Upper gastrointestinal (UGI), 523
Upper GI series, 512
Upper respiratory infection (URI), 162f, 163, 191
UPPP (uvulopalatopharyngoplasty), 160, 496, 523
Uremia, 216
Ureterectomy, 223
Ureteritis, 217
Ureterocele, 217
Ureterolithiasis, 217
Ureteroscopy, 232
Ureterostenosis, 217
Ureterostomy, 223
Ureters
    infection of, 217f
    structure and function of, 208-211
Urethra
    infection of, 216, 217f
    length of, 210f
    prostatic, 261f, 266f
    structure and function of, 208-211, 299
    surgery through, 276, 286

Urethritis, 217f
urethr/o, 211
Urethrocystitis, 217
Urethroplasty, 223
Urethroscopes, 232
URI (upper respiratory infection), 162f, 163, 191
-uria, 214
Urinal, 242
Urinalysis (UA), 237, 245
Urinary bladder
    catheterization of, 241-242, 245
    infection of, 216, 217f, 221
    structure and function of, 208-211, 261f, 266f, 299, 414f
Urinary meatus, 210f, 211
Urinary rertention, 221
Urinary suppression, 221
Urinary system
    abbreviations for, 245
    combining forms for, 211, 213
    complementary terms for, 238-239, 241-242
    diagnostic terms for, 230-232, 236-237
    diseases and disorders of, 216-217, 220-221
    endoscopic surgery for, 232
    female vs. male, 210f
    structure and function of, 208-211
    suffixes for, 214
    surgical terms for, 223, 228
    word parts for, 211-216
Urinary tract infection (UTI), 221
Urine/urinary, 239
urin/o, 213
Urinometers, 232
ur/o, 213
Urodynamics, 242
Urology/urologist, 239
Urtica dioica (stinging nettles), 266
Urticaria (hive), 106, 123t
-us, 358
Uterine artery embolization (UAE), 320, 337
Uterine sound, 321f
Uterine tubes, 298-299
uter/o, 301
Uterus
    amniocentesis through, 370f
    cancer of, 310
    catheterization of, 321f
    fixation of, 314
    oxytocin and, 737, 738f
    prolapsed, 311
    removal of, 314
    structure and function of, 210f, 298-299
uteter/o, 211
UTI (urinary tract infection), 221
Uvula, 473
Uvulectomy, 496
Uvulitis, 485
uvul/o, 480
Uvulopalatopharyngoplasty (UPPP), 160, 496, 523

V

VA (visual acuity), 566, 568
Vaccines/vaccinations, 453
Vagina, 210f, 298-299, 353f
Vaginal, 333
Vaginitis, 305, 311f
vagin/o, 301
Vagus nerve (X), 682f
Valley fever (coccidioidomycosis), 160
Valves, heart, 395f. See also specific heart valves.
valv/o, valvul/o, 403

Valvuloplasty, 423
VAP (ventilator-associated pneumonia), 192
Varicocele, 270
Varicose veins, 416
Vas deferens, 260, 261f, 273
Vascular or multiple infarct dementia, 695
Vasectomy, 273
vas/o, 262
Vasoconstrictors, 450
Vasodilators, 450
Vasovasectomy, 273
Vastus lateralis muscle, 616f
Vastus medialis muscle, 616f
VATS (video-assisted thoracic surgery), 168
Veins
    defined, 395
    femoral, 426f, 427, 432f
    iliac, 432f
    popliteal, 426f, 427, 432f
    pulmonary, 395f
    renal, 209f, 229f
    structure and function of, 416f
    study of, 445
    thrombosis of, 415
    varicose, 416
Vena cava, 395f
Venogram/venography, 431, 432f
Ventilation, 142
Ventilation-perfusion scanning (VPS), 179, 191
Ventilator, 187
Ventilator-associated pneumonia (VAP), 192
Ventral, 68
Ventricles, brain, 679f, 680
Ventricles, heart
    derivation of, 403
    left, 395f
    right, 395f
ventricul/o, 403
ventr/o, 64
Venules, 395
Verruca (wart), 124
Vertebral column. See Spinal column.
Vertebra/vertebrae
    anatomy of, 640f
    displacement of, 640f
    fractures of, 638f, 646t
    herniated disk in, 640, 646t
Vertebrocostal, 654
Vertebroplasty, 646
Vertical banded gastroplasty (VBG), 503
Vertigo (motion sickness), 588
Very-low-density lipoprotein (VLDL), 440t
Vesicle, 123t, 124
vesic/o, 211
Vesicourethral suspension, 223
Vesicovaginal fistula, 311
Vesiculectomy, 273
vesicul/o, 262
Vestibular, 595
vestibul/o, 582
Vestibulocochlear, 595
Vestibulocochlear nerve (VIII), 682f
Video cameras, 175t
Video-assisted thoracic surgery (VATS), 168
Virtual colonoscopy, 504
Virus/es
    Epstein-Barr virus, 417
    herpes simplex virus, 282
    human immunodeficiency virus (HIV), 283
    human papillomavirus (HPV), 283
Visceral, 38
Visceral pleura, 168f
viscer/o, 23

Visual acuity (VA), 566, 568
"Vital air," 403
Vitamin therapy, 160
Vitrectomy, 559
Vitreous fluid, 552f
Vitreous humor, 540, 541f
VLDL (very low-density lipoprotein), 440t
Voiding cystourethrography (VCUG), 231, 245
Void/voiding, 242
Voluntary/involuntary muscles, 615
Volvulus, 489f, 491
Vomiting, 520, 523
Vowels, combining of, 7-8, 10t, 14
VPS (ventilation-perfusion scanning), 179, 191
Vulva, 300
Vulvectomy, 315
vulv/o, 301
Vulvovaginal, 333
Vulvovaginitis, 306

W
Warts (verruca), 124
WBCs (white blood cells), 37, 398, 456

Wedge resection (lung), 167f
Wernicke-Korsakoff dementia, 695
Wheal, 123t, 124
White blood cells (WBCs), 37, 398, 456
Whooping cough (pertussis), 161
Windpipe, 142
Word parts
    for body structure, 23
    for cardiovascular, lymphatic system, and
        blood, 403-407
    for digestive system, 477, 480
    for the ear, 582
    for endocrine system, 741, 743
    for the eye, 543, 545
    for female reproductive system, 301-304
    four types of, 4-5, 10t, 14
    for integumentary system, 92-93
    for male reproductive system, 262-264
    for musculoskeletal system, 620-621,
        625-626
    for nervous system, 683-684, 686
    for obstetrics and neonatology, 354, 356,
        358
    for oncology, 56
    for respiratory system, 145
    for urinary system, 211-216

Word roots, 10t, 14
Wrist, 652t

X
xanth/o, 27
Xanthochromic, 42
Xanthoderma, 116, 122
Xanthosis, 42
xer/o, 94
Xeroderma, 98
Xerophthalmia, 548
X-ray film, 179
X-rays. See Diagnostic imaging; Radiography.
Xyphoid process, 609, 610f

Y
Yellow marrow, 608f, 609
Yoga, 751

Z
Zygote, 352, 353f